ANGIOLOGY IN PRACTICE

Developments in Cardiovascular Medicine

VOLUME 187

The titles published in this series are listed at the end of this volume.

Angiology in Practice

edited by

ABDUL-MAJEED SALMASI
*Department of Cardiology, Central Middlesex Hospital,
London, UK*

and

ANTONIO STRANO
*Department of Internal Medicine, University 'Tor Vergata' of Rome,
Rome, Italy*

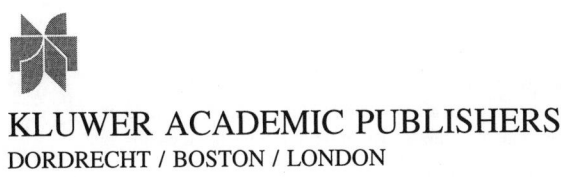

KLUWER ACADEMIC PUBLISHERS
DORDRECHT / BOSTON / LONDON

Library of Congress Cataloging-in-Publication Data

```
Angiology in practice / edited by A.M. Salmasi and A. Strano.
     p.   cm. -- (Developments in cardiovascular medicine ; v. 187)
   Includes index.
   ISBN 0-7923-4143-0 (HB)
   1. Arteries--Diseases.   I. Salmasi, Abdul-Majeed. II. Strano,
Antonio.  III. Series.
   [DNLM: 1. Vascular Diseases--diagnosis. 2. Vascular Diseases-
-therapy. 3. Blood Vessels--physiopathology. 4. Angiography-
-methods.   W1 DE997VME v.187 1996 / WG 500 A5883 1996]
 RC691.A546   1996
 616.1'3--dc20
 DNLM/DLC
 for Library of Congress                                     96-30909
                                                                  CIP
```

ISBN 0–7923–4143–0

Published by Kluwer Academic Publishers,
P.O. Box 17, 3300 AA Dordrecht, The Netherlands.

Kluwer Academic Publishers incorporates
the publishing programmes of
D. Reidel, Martinus Nijhoff, Dr W. Junk and MTP Press.

Sold and distributed in the U.S.A. and Canada
by Kluwer Academic Publishers
101 Philip Drive, Norwell, MA 02061, U.S.A.

In all other countries, sold and distributed
by Kluwer Academic Publishers Group,
P.O. Box 322, 3300 AH Dordrecht, The Netherlands.

Printed on acid-free paper

Printed and bound in Great Britain by
Hartnolls Limited, Bodmin, Cornwall

All Rights Reserved
© 1996 by Kluwer Academic Publishers
No part of the material protected by this copyright notice may be reproduced or utilized
in any form or by any means, electronic or mechanical, including photocopying, recording or
by any information storage and retrieval system, without written permission from the copyright
owners.

Table of contents

List of Contributors	ix
Foreword	
by Andrew Nicolaides	xiii
Preface	xiv

PART ONE: General pathophysiological considerations

1. Blood flow dynamics and mechanics of circulation
   by Susan B. Sherriff   1

2. Pathology of atherosclerosis
   by Simon Trotter and Mufeed Ali   21

3. Thrombosis and thromboembolism
   by Michael Schachter   31

4. Hemorheology and hemorheological mechanisms
   by Michael Rampling   41

5. The role of vascular endothelium in the modulation of coronary vasomotor tone
   by Juan Carlos Kaski   53

PART TWO: Diseases of the cerebrovascular system

6. Cerebrovascular flow dynamics and pathophysiology
   by Susan B. Sherriff   63

7. Stroke epidemiology and risk factors
   by Munther I. Aldoori, Peter A. Gaines and Jonathan D. Beard   73

8. The investigation of extracranial carotid disease
   by Peter A. Gaines, Timothy J. Hodgson, Munther I. Aldoori and Jonathan D. Beard   87

9. Management of extracranial carotid disease
   by Jonathan D. Beard, Munther I. Aldoori and Peter A. Gaines   97

PART THREE: Diseases of the coronary arteries

10. Hemodynamics of coronary flow in normal and abnormal states
    by Mario Mariani and Alberto Balbarini   109

vi   *Table of contents*

11. The pathology and pathophysiology of coronary artery disease
    by Ian Cox and Robert Crook — 121

12. Epidemiology and risk factors of coronary artery disease
    by Timothy J. Bowker, Mahmoud Barbir and Charles Ilsley — 139

13. Symptomatology and diagnosis of coronary artery diseases
    by Piers Clifford and Petros Nihoyannopoulos — 167

14. Angina pectoris in patients with normal coronary arteriograms: Syndrome X
    by Juan Carlos Kaski — 179

15. Management of coronary artery disease
    by John G.F. Cleland — 187

PART FOUR: Diseases of the aorta and arteries of the upper limb

16. Aortic aneurysm and dissection of the aorta
    by Jack Collin — 209

17. Diseases of the arteries of the upper limb
    by Michele Cospite, Filippo Ferrara and Valentina Cospite — 219

18. Raynaud's syndrome
    by Sherryl A. Wagstaff and Michael J. Grigg — 241

PART FIVE: Diseases of the arteries of the lower limb

19. Flow dynamics and pathophysiological mechanisms of diseases of lower limb arteries
    by Giuseppe Maria Andreozzi — 251

20. Epidemiology and risk factors of diseases of lower limb arteries
    by Gillian C. Leng and F. Gerry R. Fowkes — 271

21. Clinical assessment of diseases of lower limb arteries
    by Kenneth A. Myers and Winston Chong — 289

22. Management of peripheral obstructive arterial disease of the lower limbs
    by Salvatore Novo — 307

PART SIX: Diseases of the renal, celiac and mesenteric arteries

23. Pathophysiology and clinical manifestations of diseases of the renal, celiac and mesenteric arteries
    by Paolo Fiorani, Francesco Speziale, Marco Massucci, Enrico Sbarigia and Maurizio Taurino — 323

24. Management of diseases of the renal, celiac and mesenteric arteries
by Paolo Fiorani, Francesco Speziale, Marco Massucci, Luigi Rizzo
and Alvaro Zaccaria 333

PART SEVEN: Hypertension

25. Classification, epidemiology, risk factors, and clinical
manifestations of hypertension
by Luigi Corea and Maurizio Bentivoglio 343
26. Diagnosis, complications and management of hypertension
by Giuseppe Licata, Rosario Scaglione and Antonio Pinto 355

PART EIGHT: Diseases of the venous system

27. Varicose veins and varicose ulcers
by Claudio Allegra, Marisa Bonifacio, Antonio Frezzotti,
Anita Carlizza, Michele Bartolo, Bruna Carioti and
Daniela Cassiani 371
28. Deep vein thrombosis
by Sergio Coccheri 403

PART NINE: Associated general illnesses and related conditions

29. Cardiovascular manifestations and complications of diabetes
mellitus
by Jaffar Allawi 419
30. Autonomic dysfunction and hypotension
by Giuseppe Nuzzaci and I. Nuzzaci 431
31. Hemostatic defects and venous thromboembolism
by Catherine Ozanne and Hannah Cohen 443
32. Pulmonary embolism and venous thromboembolism
by Derek Bell 459
33. Vascular restenosis
by Philip Chan 473
34. Vascular emergencies
by Mauro Bartolo and Anna Rita Todini 485
35. Prevention of cardiovascular disease
by Mahmoud Barbir, Fawzi Lazem and Charles Ilsley 495

Index 519

List of Contributors

Munther I. Aldoori, PhD, FRCS, FRCS(G)
Consultant Vascular Surgeon, The Royal Infirmary, Lindley, Huddersfield, UK

Mufeed Ali, MB, ChB, FRCPath
Consultant Histopathologist, Wexham Park Hospital, Slough, UK

Jaffar Allawi, MD, MPH, FACE
Unit for Metabolic Medicine, Guy's Hospital, London, UK

Claudio Allegra, MD
Director Medical Angiology Department, S. Giovanni Hospital, Rome, Italy

Giuseppe M. Andreozzi, MD
Director Chair of Medical Angiology, University of Catania, Catania, Italy

Alberto Balbarini, MD
Director Chair of Medical Angiology, University of Pisa, Pisa, Italy

Mahmoud Barbir, MRCP
Consultant Cardiologist, Harefield Hospital, Harefield, Middlesex, UK

Mauro Bartolo, MD
Director Medical Angiology Department, San Camillo Hospital, Rome, Italy

Michele Bartolo, MD
Medical Angiology Department, S. Giovanni Hospital, Rome, Italy

Jonathan D. Beard, ChM, FRCS
Sheffield Vascular Institute, Northern General Hospital, Sheffield, UK

Derek Bell
Consultant Chest Physician, Central Middlesex Hospital, London, UK

Maurizio Bentivoglio, MD
Chair of Cardiology, University of Perugia, Perugia, Italy

Marisa Bonifacio, MD
Registrar, Medical Angiology Department, S. Giovanni Hospital, Rome, Italy

Timothy J. Bowker
Clinical Lecturer, National Heart & Lung Institute, London, UK

Bruna Carioti, MD
Medical Angiology Department, S. Giovanni Hospital, Rome, Italy

Anita Carlizza, MD
Medical Angiology Department, S. Giovanni Hospital, Rome, Italy

Daniela Cassiani, MD
Medical Angiology Department, S. Giovanni Hospital, Rome, Italy

Philip Chan, MChir, FRCS
Clinical Sciences Centre, Northern General Hospital, Sheffield, UK

List of contributors

Winston K.W. Chong, FRACAR
Department of Diagnostic Imaging, Monash Medical Center, Melbourne, Australia

John G.F. Cleland, MD, FRCP, FESC
Clinical Research Initiative in Heart Failure, University of Glasgow, Glasgow, UK

Piers Clifford, MRCP
Cardiology, Hammersmith Hospital, London, UK

Sergio Coccheri, MD
Director of Medical Angiology Institute, University of Bologna, Bologna, Italy

Hannah Cohen, MD, FRCP, FRCPath
Senior Lecturer in Haematology, Imperial College School of Medicine at St Mary's Hospital, London, UK

Jack Collin, MA, MD, FRCS
Consultant Surgeon, Nuffield Department of Surgery, John Radcliffe Hospital, Oxford, UK

Luigi Corea, MD
Chair of Cardiology, University of Perugia, Perugia, Italy

Michele Cospite, MD
Director Medical Institute of Angiology, University of Palermo, Palermo, Italy

Valentina Cospite, MD
Medical Angiology Institute, University of Palermo, Palermo, Italy

Ian Cox, MA, MRCP
Coronary Artery Disease Research Group, Department of Cardiological Sciences. St. George's Hospital Medical School, London, UK

Robert Crook, MB, BS, BSc, MRCP
Coronary Artery Disease Research Group, Department of Cardiological Sciences. St. George's Hospital Medical School, London, UK

Filippo Ferrara, MD
Medical Angiology Institute, University of Palermo, Palermo, Italy

Paolo Fiorani, MD
Director Vascular Surgery Institute, University of Rome, Italy

F. Gerry R. Fowkes, FRCPE
The Wolfson Unit for Prevention of Peripheral Vascular Diseases, Department of Public Health Sciences, University of Edinburgh, Edinburgh, UK

Antonio Frezzotti, MD
Medical Angiology Department, S. Giovanni Hospital, Rome, Italy

Peter A. Gaines, MRCP, FRCR
Sheffield Vascular Institute, Northern General Hospital, Sheffield, UK

Michael J. Grigg, MB, BS, FRACS
Consultant Vascular Surgeon, Albert Hospital, Melbourne, Australia

Timothy J. Hodgson, FRCS, FRCR
Consultant Neuroradiologist, Royal Hallamshire Hospital, Sheffield, UK

Charles Ilsley, FRCP
Consultant Cardiologist, Harefield Hospital, Harefield, UK

Juan Carlos Kaski, MD, FESC, FACC
Department of Cardiological Sciences, St. George's Hospital Medical School, London, UK

List of contributors xi

Fawzi Lazem, MD
Heart Sciences Centre, Harefield Hospital, Harefield, Middlesex, UK

Gillian C. Leng, MD
Wolfson Unit for Prevention of Peripheral Vascular Diseases, University of Edinburgh, Edinburgh, UK

Giuseppe Licata, MD
Director Institute of Internal Medicine, University of Palermo, Palermo, Italy

Mario Mariani, MD
Director Institute of Cardiology, University of Pisa, Pisa, Italy

Marco Massucci, MD
Vascular Surgery Institute, University of Rome, Rome, Italy

Kenneth A. Myers, MS, FACS, FRACS
Head of Department of Vascular Surgery, Monash Medical Centre, Melbourne, Australia

Petros Nihoyannopoulos, MD, FACC, FESC
Senior Lecturer in Cardiology, Hammersmith Hospital, London, UK

Salvatore Novo, MD, FESC
Head Chair of Clinical Pathophysiology, University of Palermo, Palermo, Italy

Giuseppe Nuzzaci, MD
Director Chair of Angiology, University of Firenze, Firenze, Italy

Ines Nuzzaci, MD
Chair of Angiology, University of Firenze, Firenze, Italy

Catherine Ozanne, BSc, MRCP, MRCPath
Senior Registrar in Haematology, St. Mary's Hospital, London, UK

Antonio Pinto, MD
Chair of Medical Pathophysiology, University of Catania, Catania, Italy

Michael Rampling, BSc, ARCS, PhD
Department of Physiology and Biophysics, Imperial College School of Medicine at St. Mary's Hospital, London, UK

Luigi Rizzo, MD
Vascular Surgery Institute, University of Rome, Rome, Italy

Abdul-Majeed Salmasi, MB, ChB, PhD, FACA
Cardiac Department, Central Middlesex Hospital, NHS Trust, London, UK

Enrico Sbarigia, MD
Vascular Surgery Institute, University of Rome, Rome, Italy

Rosario Scaglione, MD
Chair of Medical Therapy, University of Palermo, Palermo, Italy

Mike Schachter
Department of Clinical Pharmacology, Imperial College School of Medicine at St. Mary's Hospital, London, UK

Susan B. Sherriff, PhD, FIPSM
Department of Medical Physics and Clinical Engineering, Northern General Hospital, Sheffield, UK

Francesco Speziale, MD
Vascular Surgery Institute, University of Rome, Rome, Italy

Antonio Strano, MD, FESC
Director Department of Internal Medicine, University 'Tor Vergata' of Rome, Rome, Italy

Anna Rita Todini, MD
Medical Angiology Department, San Camillo Hospital, Rome, Italy

Simon Trotter, MRCPath
Department of Histopathology, Royal Brompton Hospital, London, UK

Sherryl A. Wagstaff, MB, BS
General Surgical Registrar, Alfred Hospital, Melbourne, Australia

Alvaro Zaccaria, MD
Vascular Surgery Institute, University of Rome, Rome, Italy

Foreword

Cardiovascular diseases are a major cause of death in the western world and are the result of atherosclerotic changes involving the arterial wall. Their clinical manifestations, depending on the vessels predominantly involved, range from stroke to angina pectoris and myocardial infarction, blindness, hypertension, and intermittent claudication.

The advent of new diagnostic techniques has given greater insight into the pathophysiology of vascular diseases. These techniques have also helped towards better and earlier diagnosis and a greater understanding of the nature of the arterial and venous processes involved, factors leading ultimately to a clearer understanding of their epidemiology. This, in turn, will help in the prevention of the major catastrophic events associated with these diseases.

Angiology in Practice deals in great depth with the mechanism, clinical manifestations, diagnosis and management of arterial and venous diseases. The international experts in various fields who have contributed chapters have made an immense effort in presenting this information in a clear and concise form, incorporating the most recent findings in the field as well as their own personal areas of expertise.

This book will be an invaluable aid to all those interested in the better understanding of the nature of vascular diseases and their clinical presentations, diagnosis and management. It will be of assistance not only to angiologists, cardiovascular physicians and surgeons, but also to diabetologists, epidemiologists and general physicians who wish to extend their knowledge of these diseases in a simple clinical text.

The editors are to be congratulated on their success in contriving to present such a tremendous amount of information in an understandable and readable format. I think this book is an admirable contribution to the literature of angiology and is destined to become a classic of its kind.

Andrew Nicolaides, MS, FRCS
Professor of Vascular Surgery
Director, Irvine Laboratory for Cardiovascular Investigation and Research
Imperial College School of Medicine at St Mary's
London

October 1996

Preface

Arterial diseases present a major ubiquitous threat to the life of mankind. Coronary artery disease *per se* is the commonest and the major cause of mortality in the developed countries, where one of the highest death rates dominates. Stroke resulting from atherosclerotic disorders of the carotid circulation is another single major ailment leading to morbidity and mortality. Additional to these remain complications resulting from atherosclerotic disorders of the aorta, the ilio-femoro-popliteal tree and the renal arteries. Hypertension with its major complications and threat to life is probably the focus in these conditions as it is a risk factor and sometimes a result of some of these arterial illnesses such as stenosis of the renal arteries.

A major contributory factor to the cardiovascular diseases is diabetes mellitus which is also directly related to hypertension. Other risk factors include disturbances in the coagulability of the blood and haemorrheological factors, as well as hyperlipidaemia and smoking. The majority of these factors also predispose to venous thrombosis, which by itself may present as a medical emergency and can be life-threatening.

We therefore thought that all these issues could be discussed in a practical and clinically applicable way in one book, since they are all intimately related. We invited a distinguished group of leading world authors in various fields to present their experience and the expertise of other leading groups, to be collected in a textbook. We emphasised the importance of the clinical aspects of various arterial and venous problems, paying special attention to basic haemodynamic principles. Special attention was paid to the management, epidemiology and prevention.

Finally we are grateful to Kluwer Academic Publishers for their interest, help and support.

Abdul-Majeed Salmasi *Antonio Strano*
London, UK *Rome, Italy*

1. Blood flow dynamics and mechanics of circulation
SUSAN B. SHERRIFF

When attempting to understand the mechanics of circulation it is necessary to consider the laws of physics which refer to the characteristics of fluids at rest and in motion, during steady and pulsatile flow, and in rigid and flexible pipes. As in many other areas of medicine as soon as one tries to apply these laws to the *in vivo* situation a number of complicating factors come into play. The heart which supplies the driving pressure is a complex intermittent pump. The blood vessels are multi-branched elastic walled conduits of varying diameter and length, the diameter of the vessel varying with the pressure of the blood within the vessel and the smooth muscle tone of the vessel wall. In addition the blood is not a simple homogeneous fluid but a suspension of red and other blood cells dispersed in a colloidal solution of proteins.

The systemic circulatory system consists of: a pump, the heart; a system of branching elastic pipes, the arteries and arterioles; the tissue beds supplied by the capillaries; and finally a system of converging pipes, the venules and veins. The heart pumps in an intermittent but regular fashion forcing the entire stroke volume of blood into the arterial system during systole. Not all of the stroke volume is dispatched to the capillary beds during systole, much is retained by the distensable arteries. This allows a proportion of the energy of the cardiac contraction to be dissipated during diastole when, as the elastic recoil of the artery walls takes place, the stored potential energy is converted into blood flow. The pulsations generated by the pumping action of the heart radiate out along the arteries and at discontinuities such as vessel bifurcations, the pulsations are partially reflected, back toward the heart, and partially transmitted along the vessel, becoming damped as they approach the distal arterioles. The arterioles regulate the distribution of blood flow to the various capillary beds before the blood is returned in a relatively steady stream to the heart. The changing velocity profiles across the various vessels are reflections of the hemodynamic characteristics of the cardiovascular system.

This chapter attempts to deal with the application of some of the concepts of fluid mechanics to the relationship between pressure and volume flow in a vessel segment. A more detailed account can be found in *McDonald's Blood Flow in Arteries* [1].

Fluid flow

A fluid is a substance which cannot permanently withstand a shearing stress and a true liquid is an incompressible fluid. Two main types of fluid flow are recognized. The first is the orderly flow of neighboring layers of fluid moving past each other in a smooth manner. Each element of fluid follows a *streamline* path which does not cross over or become entangled with other streamlines. The second is characterized by an irregular erratic complex *turbulent* motion which occurs when the fluid exceeds a critical velocity. The term turbulence is often used incorrectly in vascular literature to describe any nonstreamline flow.

Steady flow in rigid tubes

Under the ideal circumstances of steady, fully developed streamline flow, in a cylindrical tube, particles moving at identical velocities are arranged in concentric *laminae*. Those particles immediately adjacent to the wall have zero velocity while those in the centre of the flow stream move more rapidly (Figure 1.1). In any longitudinal section that passes through the central axis of the tube, the velocities have a parabolic flow profile (Figure 1.2a).

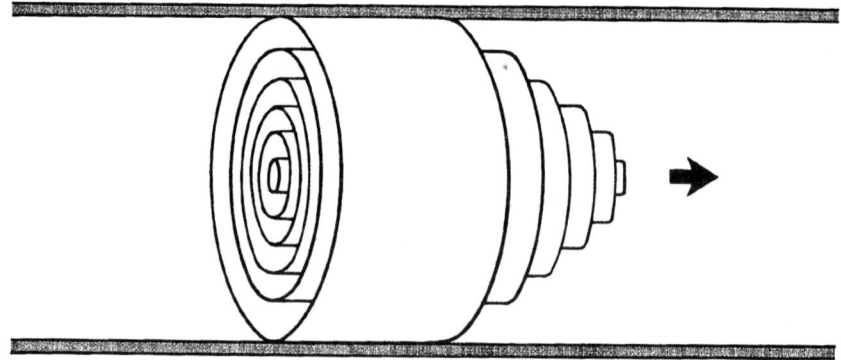

Figure 1.1. Laminar flow in a tube with circular cross-section. Concentric cylinders of fluid layers flow over each other with velocity increasing with distance from the vessel wall.

Pressure flow relationship

Pressure is one of the main determinants of the rate of flow, the driving force for flow is the pressure drop along the pipe. The flow, Q, is directly proportional to the difference between the inflow and outflow pressures P_i and P_o:

$$Q \propto P_i - P_o. \tag{1.1}$$

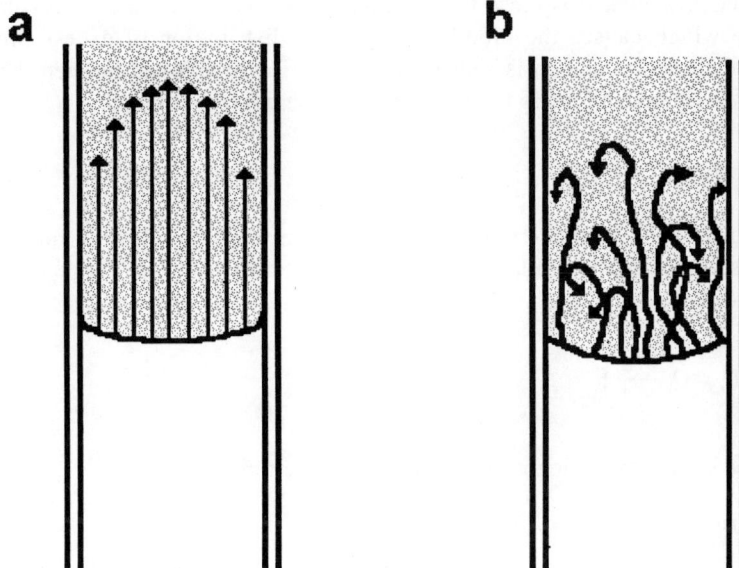

Figure 1.2. (a) Steady fully developed laminar flow showing streamline flow with a parabolic flow front; (b) Turbulent flow showing fluid moving irregularly in axial radial and circumferential directions.

For any given pressure difference between the two ends of a pipe the flow also depends on the dimensions of the pipe: the radius, r, and the length, l:

$$Q \propto r^4 / l. \tag{1.2}$$

Finally for a given pressure difference and for a cylindrical tube of given dimensions the flow varies as a function of the viscosity, η, of the fluid:

$$Q \propto 1/\eta. \tag{1.3}$$

In established steady flow of a Newtonian fluid in a long rigid cylindrical tube the relationship of all the above factors is characterized by the *Poiseuille* equation:

$$Q = \frac{\pi \Delta p r^4}{8 \eta l} \tag{1.4}$$

where Q = volume flow, Δp = the difference between the pressure at the beginning and at the end of the tube, r = the radius, η = the viscosity, l = the length and $\pi/8$ is the constant of proportionality.

The main force governing flow in the body is the pressure generated by the heart. The excess pressure at the root of the aorta fluctuates about an average of approximately 100 mmHg. This is much greater than the corresponding excess pressure in the vena cava (which is close to zero), and it is this arteriovenous pressure difference which causes the blood to flow. The distribution of excess pressure throughout the circulation is shown in Figure 1.3 where it can be seen that it is largely dissipated in forcing the blood through the microcirculation.

Flow resistance

Resistance to flow arises from viscous losses in the blood flowing through the vessel segment and is similar in concept to electrical resistance. If equation 1.4 is rearranged to give:

$$P_i - P_o = Q\left(\frac{8l\eta}{\pi r^4}\right) \tag{1.5}$$

it can be seen to be analogous to Ohms law in electricity:

$$U = IR \tag{1.6}$$

where U the electromotive force corresponds to $P_i - P_o$ the pressure difference, I the current corresponds to Q the flow, and R is the resistance. Thus the resistance to flow can be calculated as:

$$R = \frac{8l\eta}{\pi r^4}. \tag{1.7}$$

This means that the resistance to flow depends only on the dimension of the pipe and on the characteristics of the fluid. In an adult human being, for anatomical reasons, the length of the blood vessels are virtually constant and, although the viscosity of blood varies with the radius in small vessels, the mean viscosity can be regarded as constant. The biggest determinant of the resistance to flow in a given blood vessel is therefore its radius; decreasing the vessel radius by a factor of 2 increases the resistance to flow by a factor of 8. In the vascular bed the total resistance to flow is made up of the resistance in the arteries, arterioles, capillaries, venules and veins. From equation 5 the resistance is proportional to the pressure difference, the greatest upstream to downstream drop occurs in the arterioles (up to 60% of the total pressure drop), therefore the major component of resistance will originate in the arterioles [2]. The arterioles also have the greatest capacity for vasomotor control by activation of the circular smooth muscle cells in the vessel wall producing a change in vessel caliber.

Volume flow and velocity

It is important to differentiate between velocity and flow; velocity, $\overline{V}$, refers to the rate of displacement or the distance moved in unit time, while volume flow, Q, is

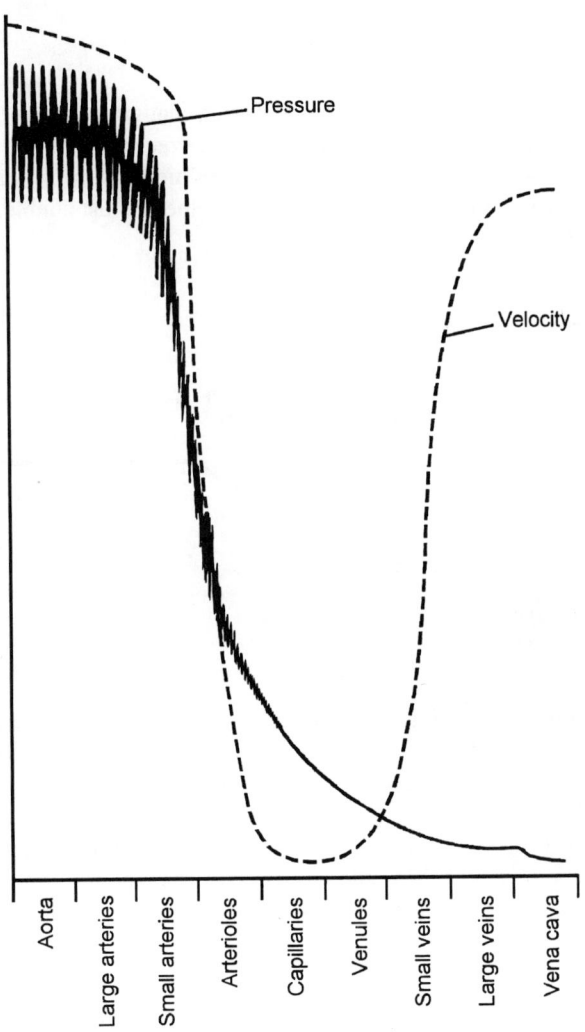

Figure 1.3. Excess pressure and flow velocity in the systemic circulation.

the volume of fluid moved in unit time. In a pipe of radius, r, they are related by the equation:

$$\bar{V} = Q/\pi r^2. \tag{1.8}$$

Since πr^2 is the cross-sectional area, A, of the vessel, the equation can be rewritten as:

$$\bar{V} = Q/A \text{ or } Q = \bar{V}A. \tag{1.9}$$

In Figure 1.4 the fluid is moving through a pipe of changing dimensions; provided the flow volume is constant the velocity will increase as the cross-section is reduced. For the same volume of incompressible fluid to pass from a tube with a cross-sectional area of 4 cm² to one of 2 cm² the velocity must double.

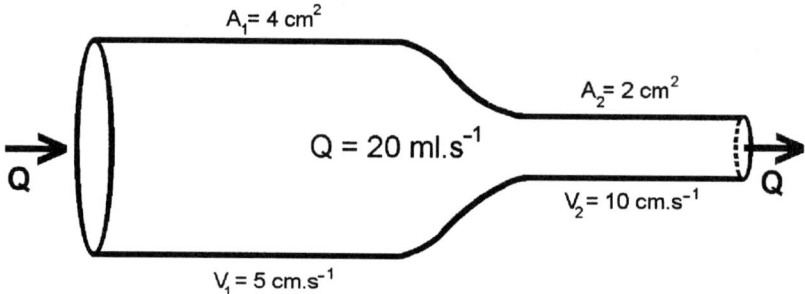

Figure 1.4. Fluid flow through a tube of changing cross-sectional area. Q = volume flow, A = cross sectional area, and V = velocity.

In the human the cross-sectional area of an individual artery, arteriole or capillary is less than that of the vessel from which it arose and the above discussion is valid. However the total cross-sectional area of groups of vessels, say the capillary beds compared to the arterioles, is large. Hence the velocity decreases progressively as the blood travels from the aorta into the large primary arterial branches, the smaller secondary branches, and the arterioles, reaching a minimum in the capillaries before gradually increasing as the blood passes into the venules, veins and the vena cava (Figure 1.3).

Viscosity

When two neighboring layers of fluid flow at different velocities a frictional force arises between them due to the viscosity of the fluid. Viscosity is that property of a fluid that indicates its internal friction. It is defined as the constant of proportionality between the stress applied τ, i.e. force per unit area, and the velocity gradient or shear rate dU/dY of the liquid laminar (Figure 1.5). The more viscous a fluid the

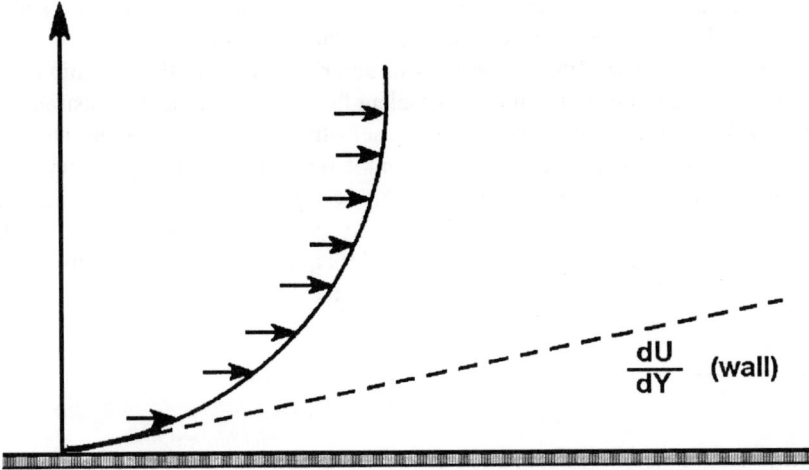

Figure 1.5. The shear stress on the vessel wall, τ, depends on velocity gradient at the wall dU/dY.

greater the force required to cause one layer to slide across another. Thus motor oils and syrup are more viscous than water and cooking oil.

A simple Newtonian fluid such as water is one in which the coefficient of viscosity is constant at all rates of shear. Blood is not a simple fluid but a suspension of solid elements, the cells, in a liquid, the plasma. The viscous friction in blood is therefore complex exhibiting anomalous properties. At low shear rates the apparent viscosity increases markedly whilst in small blood vessels, where the size of the cells is significant in comparison to the radius of the vessel, the apparent viscosity at higher shear rates is less than it is in large vessels [3]. Fortunately although blood with a normal hematocrit of 45% has a viscosity three to four times that of water it behaves approximately as a pure liquid provided that the blood vessels have a radius greater than 0.05 mm.

Disturbed and turbulent flow

In laminar flow fluid elements remain in one streamline or laminar as the fluid flows longitudinally along the pipe. We have seen that when the pressure difference along a segment of pipe of constant cross-sectional area increases then the velocity of the fluid flowing in the pipe increases. If the velocity is increased beyond a certain critical value the initial laminar flow is destabilized. Irregular motions of the fluid elements develop and radial mixing occurs, the velocity vectors of the individual fluid elements are randomly aimed in all directions and flow vortices form near the wall of the pipe (Figure 1.2b). The total velocity vector continues to point in the main direction of flow and the velocity profile is flat with a large velocity gradient near the vessel wall (Figure 1.13). Under conditions of turbulent flow frictional forces are high so a much greater pressure is required to force a given volume of fluid through the pipe; the pressure drop is proportional to the flow rate squared rather than the flow rate as is the situation with laminar flow.

Reynolds (1883) was the first person to describe precisely the condition under which the transition from laminar to turbulent flow occurred. He demonstrated that at higher flow rates the fluid becomes more sensitive to disturbances, until a critical point is reached where laminar flow cannot be maintained. He observed that the point at which this transformation occurs is dependent on the vessel diameter, $2r$ (r = radius), the mean velocity, $\bar{V}$, the density, ρ, and the viscosity of the fluid, η. These factors are expressed in the dimensionless quantity called Reynolds number, R_e, as the ratio of the inertial force to the viscosity:

$$R_e = \frac{\bar{V}2r\rho}{\eta} \qquad (1.10)$$

At Reynolds numbers less than 2000 the flow is usually laminar, for R_e greater than 3000 the flow will be turbulent. At Reynolds numbers approaching 2000, a disturbance is necessary to institute turbulence in a smooth pipe. The larger the Reynolds number the less disturbance is necessary to cause this turbulence [4]. Factors such as vessel curvature, changes in caliber, or damage to the inner wall may cause local turbulence to occur [5, 6]. The pulsatile nature of the flow encourages flow instabilities since at peak flow rates the critical Reynolds number (2000) is often exceeded. Eddies and vortices may occur, particularly at branch points. However the energy losses associated with these flow instabilities appear to be insignificant with respect to average flow rates. For this reason the appearance of eddies and vortices should be referred to as 'disturbed flow' rather than as turbulence [7]. The term disturbed flow describes the intermediate state between laminar flow and fully developed turbulence.

In normal pulsatile flow the deceleration phase after peak systole is the most unstable part of the pulse cycle; so whenever flow disturbances develop, they are first observed during this deceleration phase [8].

Effects of geometry on the flow profile

The velocity profile is flat in the initial portion of a segment of tube originating from a reservoir or as a branch of a tube with a larger diameter; a steady state parabolic velocity profile develops as the fluid flows along the distal segment. Curves, branches and constrictions in the tube will alter both the flow profile and the local pressure gradient.

Inlet effect

At the entrance to a tube all the fluid has the same velocity and it must travel some distance before a steady state velocity profile is achieved. On entering the tube the layer of fluid immediately in contact with the vessel wall will become stationary, the laminae close to this layer begin to slide on it and form a boundary layer. A large velocity gradient develops between the motionless fluid at the wall and adjacent moving fluid, i.e. there is a large shear stress at the wall. The shear stress varies from zero at the centre line to a maximum at the wall:

$$\tau = (4\bar{V}/r) \qquad (1.11)$$

where $\bar{V}$ is the average velocity and r is the tube radius. As the flow proceeds along the tube the effect of viscosity progressively modifies the velocity profile (Figure 1.6); the viscous drag exerted by the walls of the tube is transmitted to the centre of the tube as more of the fluid in the core becomes sheared and the boundary layer grows in thickness. A parabolic profile eventually develops and the shear stress at the wall falls to a constant value. The distance, L, required for the profile to achieve its fully developed state is known as the inlet length and is given by:

$$L = kr R_e \qquad (1.12)$$

where r is the radius of the tube, R_e the Reynolds number and $k = 0.08$ [9].

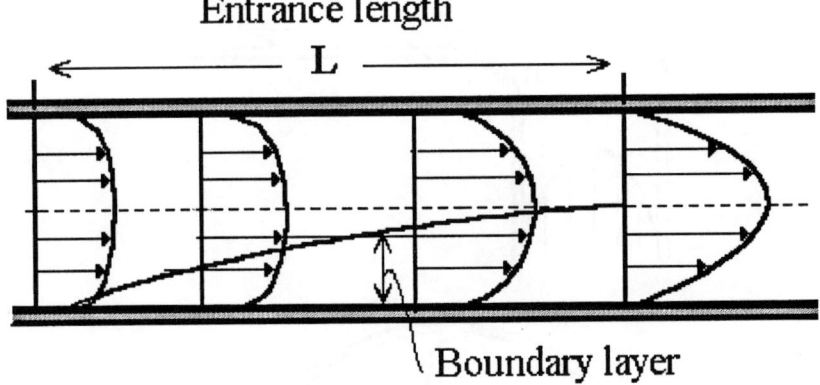

Figure 1.6. The development of steady state laminar flow in a tube with circular cross-section. The flat profile at the inlet is progressively modified as the boundary layer grows and Poiseuille flow is established at a distance L from the entrance.

Curved tubes

When fluid flow enters a curved section of pipe it experiences a centrifugal force, a change of direction of a fluid element implies an acceleration of the fluid in the direction of curvature. The change in flow pattern depends upon the shape of the velocity profile existing prior to entering the curve. In the case of steady fully developed flow, i.e. a parabolic flow front approaching a curve in a tube, there must be sufficient force or pressure gradient to deflect the faster moving fluid in the center stream around the bend in the tube. The slower moving fluid near the wall has less inertia and will be deflected more than the faster moving fluid. The fluid with the greatest velocity is displaced toward the outer wall of the curved tube and the velocity profile is skewed toward that wall (Figure 1.7a). The shear stress is therefore greatest on the outer wall and least on the inner wall. At the same time a transverse circulation or secondary motion is created near the walls and a vortex-like structure is superimposed on the flow in the axial direction. If the velocity profile entering a curved section of tube is flat then the profile becomes skewed in the opposite direction, i.e. towards the inner wall of the curve (Figure 1.7b) [10].

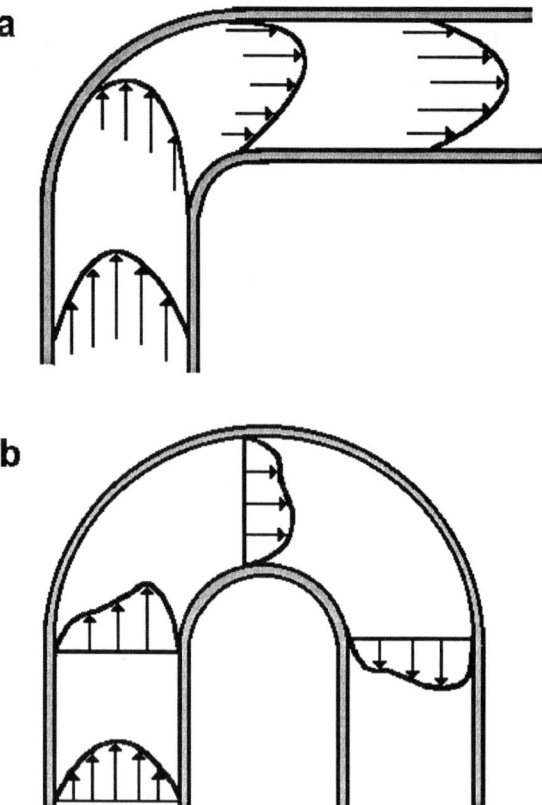

Figure 1.7. Schematic illustration of geometric effects on velocity profiles in a curved tube. (a) The faster center stream flow of the parabolic flow profile is displaced toward the outer wall; (b) A flat profile is skewed toward the inner wall of the vessel.

Bifurcations

The details of steady flow in a bifurcation are much more complicated but can be understood qualitatively using similar arguments to those above. The geometry of the bifurcation can range from a pure symmetric split to a tube branching off the main vessel at right angles. As the fast moving blood in the center approaches the flow divider, a pressure gradient must be set up large enough to deflect it into the daughter tubes. The flow will be split into two with the highest velocities, which were in the center stream of the parent vessel, being closest to the inner walls of the daughter tubes (Figure 1.8a). The slower moving fluid will be subjected to the same pressure gradient and a transverse secondary motion will be established in the regions close to the wall. A new boundary layer similar to that in the entry region is found on the flow divider. Hence the velocity gradient and shear stress can be very large compared to that experienced by the opposite outer wall. If the fluid velocity is great enough and the degree of curvature is large enough, the pressure gradient may cause flow separation and flow reversal at the outer wall of the bifurcation (Figure 1.8b). This will radically alter the velocity gradients and the distribution of the shear stress on the walls of the vessel. The total cross-sectional area of branched vessels usually exceeds that of the parent so the mean velocity and the Reynolds number will reduce, resulting in greater flow stability.

Constrictions

The effects of constrictions on flow is of particular importance in the circulation where arterial disease may cause significant obstruction to blood flow.

As fluid passes from a tube of larger diameter through one of smaller diameter, it must accelerate to a higher velocity in the narrow segment in order to maintain the same total flow. An additional pressure drop is also required to overcome the inertial forces. Investigations into flow and mathematical models have shown that at the site of a stenosis the blood flow accelerates while the lateral pressure decreases. Both experimental and clinical investigations indicate that it is necessary to have a marked stenosis with the lumen of the artery being reduced by as much as 80% before the mean resting flow rate is reduced [11, 12]. Up to this degree of narrowing, compensatory flow acceleration occurs at the site of stenosis; beyond this critical degree of stenosis there is a drop in pressure and a reduction in both the pulsatility of the flow wave form and the mean flow.

The stenotic resistance, R, is dependent upon the flow, Q, and the pressure difference across the stenosis Δp:

$$R = \frac{\Delta p}{Q}. \tag{1.13}$$

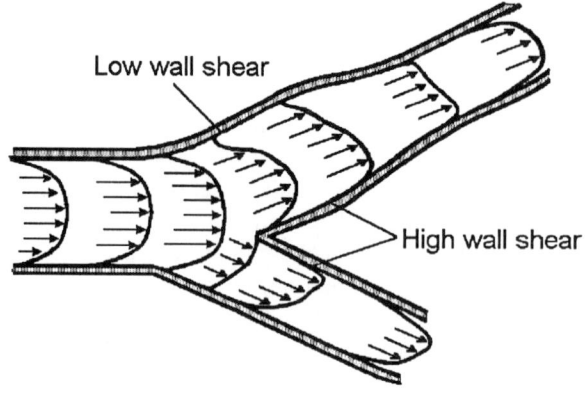

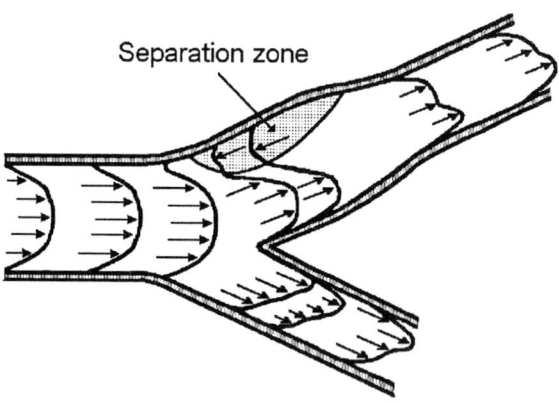

Figure 1.8. Schematic illustration of geometric effects on velocity profiles in a bifurcating tube. (a) The fastest fluid movement and the highest shear occurs on the walls of the flow divider, the shear is lowest on the outer walls; (b) Flow reversal and flow separation may occur near the outer wall.

Thus the effect of the stenosis increases as the flow increases. The resistance in the stenosis combined with the distal compliance in the artery act as a 'low pass filter' and differentially attenuate the higher frequencies of the incident pressure and flow waves. The blood velocity wave forms recorded from sites distal to severe narrowings are in general more damped than those recorded from undiseased arteries.

A post-stenotic increase in flow cross-section causes convective acceleration. The pressure drop required for convective acceleration is given by:

$$P_1 - P_2 = \frac{1}{2}\rho(v_2^2 - v_1^2). \tag{1.14}$$

where P is the pressure in the fluid, ρ is the density, v the velocity of flow, the subscript 1 denotes a position along the flow line prior to the stenosis and the subscript 2 denotes a position at the stenosis in the center of the flow jet. The equation is useful for calculating the pressure drop across an orifice such as a stenotic heart valve or septal defect. If the stenosis is very tight then the velocity v_1 prior to the stricture is very small compared to the velocity in the jet and equation 1.14 reduces to:

$$\Delta P \approx 4v_2^2. \tag{1.15}$$

Due to the increased flow velocity the intrastenotic Reynolds number can rise significantly in severe stenoses. This in turn can lead to disturbed flow and turbulence within the stenosis. The degree of flow disruption depends on the severity of the disease. Distal to the stenosis the maximum flow velocity may continue to be elevated and will be seen as a post-stenotic jet. Areas of flow separation and flow reversal can develop near the vessel wall (Figure 1.9). Since the flow enters the post-stenotic lumen at high velocities the post-stenotic Reynolds number can far exceed the intra-stenotic Reynolds number and cause marked turbulence to develop in the post-stenotic segments [13, 14]. Depending on the velocity and the degree of stenosis the flow disturbances may propagate distally extending down the arterial tree for several vessel diameters and well beyond the length occupied by one stroke volume [15]. If the stenosis is very tight the energy loss resulting from the pressure drop and the turbulence may cause a reduction in volume flow.

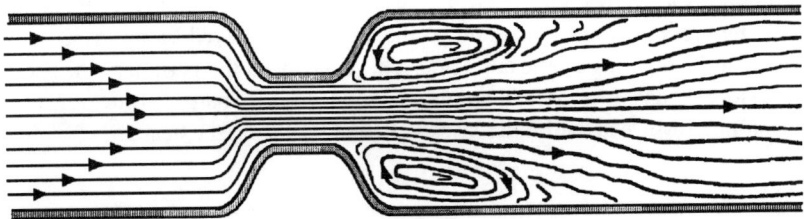

Figure 1.9. Schematic illustration of geometric effects on velocity profiles – in a diverging flow channel or post-stenosis. Proximal to and within the stenosis flow is laminar; distal to the stenosis zones of flow reversal develop with disturbed or turbulent flow extending along the vessel.

Pulsatile flow in elastic tubes

The physical principle of the steady flow of a Newtonian fluid through rigid pipes gives an adequate basic model for understanding the relationship between pressure gradient and flow and for predicting the flow profiles which will develop within arteries. However blood vessels have elastic walls and the flow is pulsatile; it is therefore important to consider the effect of these factors.

If a pulse of fluid is injected into an elastic tube, the local pressure will increase, distending the tube. The increased pressure will cause a pressure gradient resulting in a local acceleration of fluid into the next element of the tube. This process continues with the elastic properties of the wall providing the restoring force and the mass of fluid providing the inertia necessary for wave propagation. Thus the pressure pulse travels toward the periphery as a wave. The pulse wave will propagate with a speed c according to the Moens-Korteweg equation:

$$c = \sqrt{\rho\left(\frac{Eh}{D}\right)} \tag{1.16}$$

where ρ is the density of the fluid, E is Young's modulus of elasticity in the circumferential direction, h is the wall thickness and D is the diameter of the vessel. The terms contained within the bracket give a measure of the distensability of the vessel.

At the beginning of systole, pressure in the ventricle rises rapidly until it exceeds that in the aorta and causes the aortic valve to open; blood is ejected and the aortic pressure rises. During the early part of the ejection phase, ventricular pressure exceeds aortic pressure, but about halfway through ejection, the aortic pressure becomes dominant and an adverse pressure gradient develops across the aortic valve; this is maintained as both pressures start to fall. Thereafter the pressure in the ventricle falls rapidly as the heart relaxes, while the pressure in the aorta falls more slowly as the blood is forced out into the peripheral vessels. The closure of the aortic valve is marked by a notch (dicrotic notch) on the aortic pressure record.

The pressure pulse generated by ventricular contraction travels along the arterial system as a 'wave'. The transmission of the wave causes a propagation delay in the pressure and flow pulses as they travel toward the periphery. Typical pressure wave forms taken from the proximal, middle and distal portions of the descending aorta of a dog are shown in Figure 1.10. Examination of the pressure recordings shows that as the pressure wave moves down the aorta it is delayed by up to 60 ms, and because of the tapering of the aorta and reflections from the periphery the pressure wave also steepens, increases in amplitude and loses the sharp dicrotic notch. Thus the systolic pressure actually increases with distance from the heart.

Compliance

The elastic property of the arterial wall which enables an artery such as the aorta to accumulate energy by expanding and taking up a volume of blood during systole

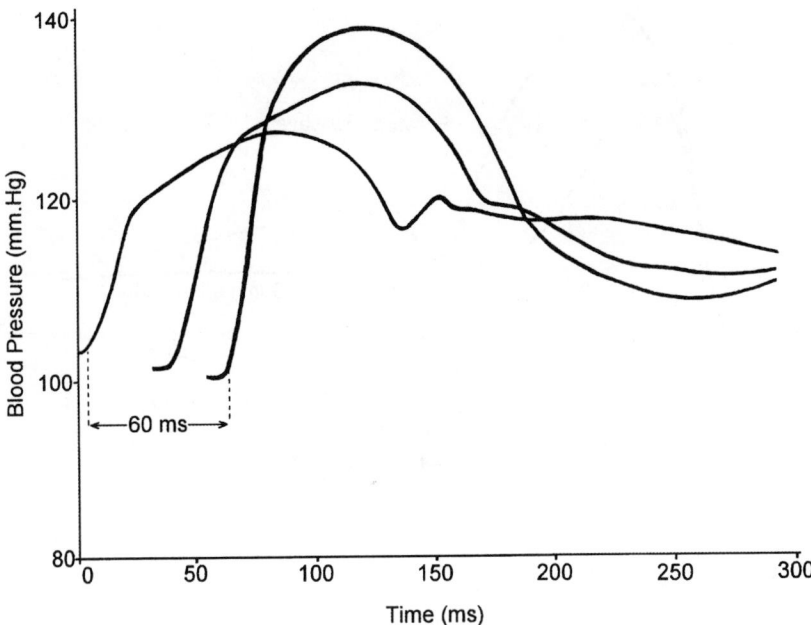

Figure 1.10. Pressure waveforms from the proximal, mid and distal portions of the aorta of a dog showing delay in the propagation of the pressure wave.

and discharge the energy and blood along the vessels during diastole is known as the *compliance, C*. It is inversely related to the elastic modulus and is defined as:

$$C = \frac{\Delta V}{\Delta P_a} \qquad (1.17)$$

where ΔV is the change in volume or the blood for any vessel segment and ΔP_a is the increase in pressure inside the vessel segment.

Vessel compliance decreases with age as increased rigidity is caused by progressive changes in the collagen and elastic content of the arterial walls. As compliance of the aorta decreases, the peak arterial pressure occurs progressively later in systole and the rapid ejection phase of systole is significantly prolonged.

The reflection of a transient pulse

An important factor in determining the shape and nature of the flow wave in arteries is wave reflection. A traveling wave such as the pulse wave will be reflected to some extent wherever there is a discontinuity in the system. The extreme cases are where the tube is completely blocked or opens into a large reservoir. In the circulation we are obviously dealing with intermediate conditions causing only partial reflections, but the terms 'closed' or 'open' are convenient to

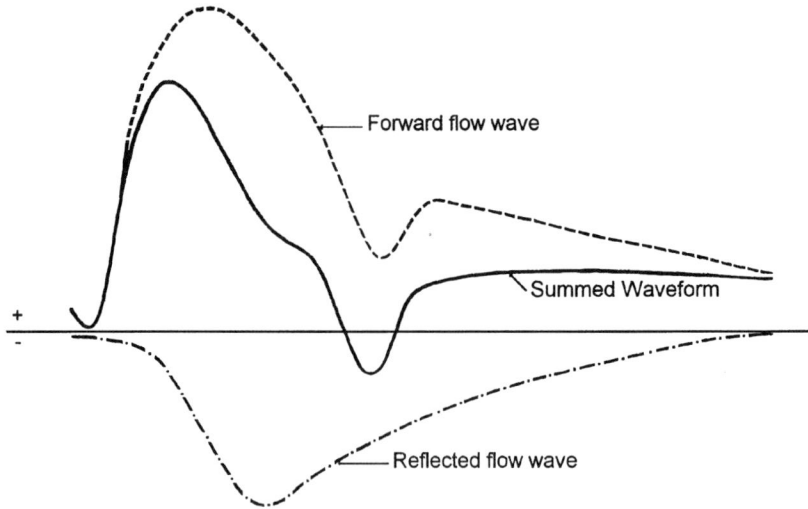

Figure 1.11. The influence of reflections on flow waveforms: --- is the forward waveform; -·-·- the reflected waveform; and ——— the summed waveform.

describe their character. The discontinuity may be a change in caliber, as at a point of branching, or merely a change in the elastic properties of the wall.

When the pulse reaches the end of the tube it is reflected. If the termination resistance is very high ('closed' end) a single positive flow pulse traveling toward the periphery will be reflected as a flow pulse opposite in sign to the input pulse. At the reflection site the forward and backward going flow pulses will tend to cancel one another out, while the associated pressure pulse at the same point will be augmented. Upstream from the reflecting site the actual flow will depend upon the sum of the forward and backward going pulses. If the backward going flow pulse arrives within the duration of the forward pulse, subtraction will occur; this may appear on the velocity curve as a notch or shelf (Figure 1.11).

Velocity profiles

In mammalian arteries flow profiles are seldom if ever completely parabolic. When flow is pulsatile, the velocity profile may closely approximate to a parabola during peak systole, but over much of the cardiac cycle, the profile is flattened. Since blood near the wall moves more slowly than that of the center stream the direction of flow near the wall is more sensitive to variations in the pressure gradient than the flow in the central laminae. Consequently when flow reversal begins, it starts at the wall, whilst it continues to flow in a forward direction at the center of the stream. Figure 1.12 shows a series of velocity profiles across an artery. These are seen to vary markedly throughout the cardiac cycle. As the pulse rate increases, there is no time for the development of a parabolic profile and the profile becomes flattened (plug flow). In large blood vessels such as the aorta, the profile may be quite blunt

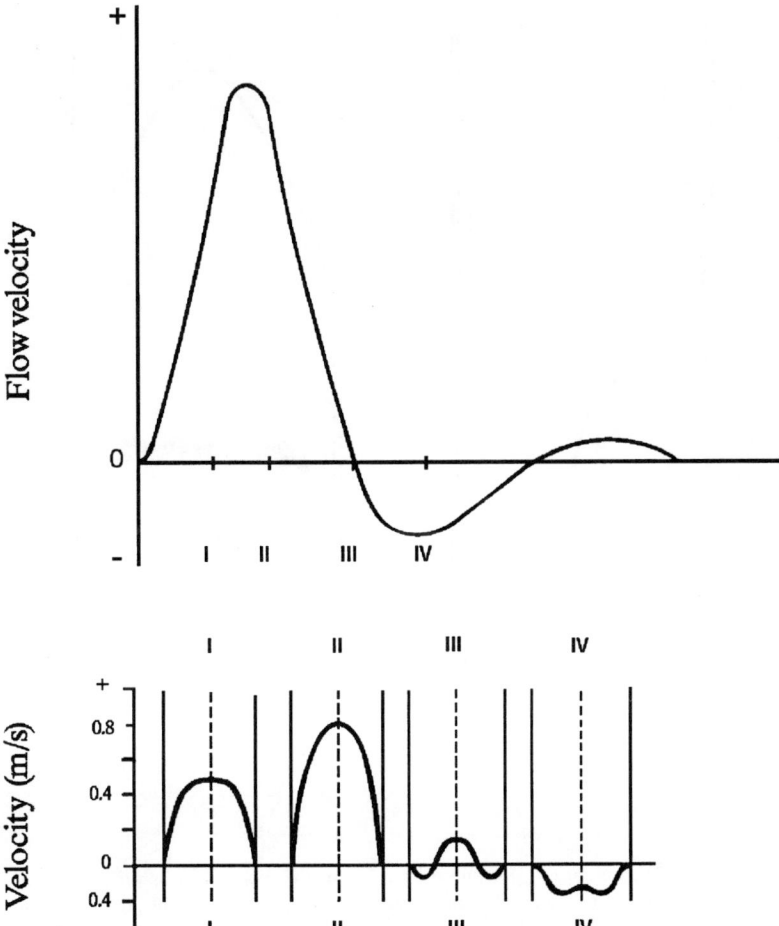

Figure 1.12. Variations in the blood velocity across an artery at various times in a cardiac cycle.

and skewed with the high velocities developing lateral to the central axis. Turbulent flow also produces a blunt profile. In Figure 1.13 examples of velocity profiles are shown schematically for a range of blood vessels. They all differ significantly from those associated with Poiseuille flow.

The flow velocities in the veins are much less pulsatile than those found in the arteries. The driving force is dominated by the muscular pump and by intra-thoracic and intra-abdominal pressure changes caused by breathing. Acceleration is low and the velocity profile is parabolic.

References

1. Nichols WW, O'Rouke MFO. McDonald's Blood flow in arteries, theoretical experimental and clinical principles. 3rd ed. London: Edward Arnold, 1990.

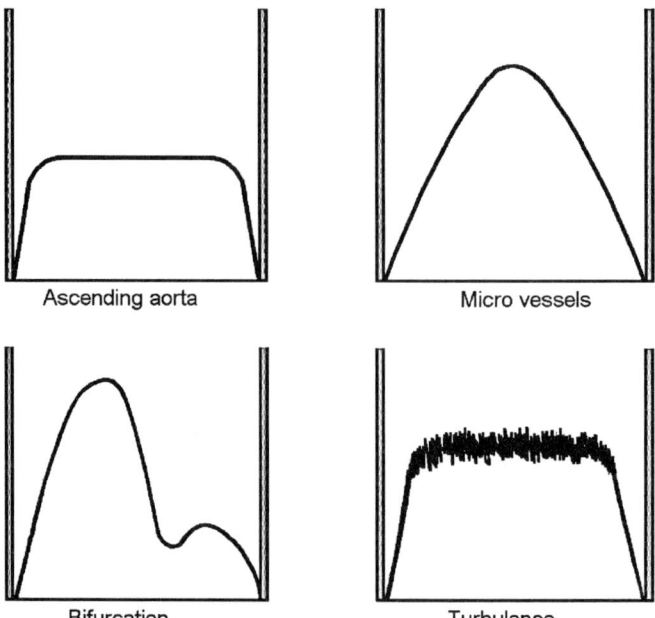

Figure 1.13. Examples of velocity profiles in the systemic circulation.

2. Zweifach BW, Lipowsky HH. Pressure-flow relations in blood and lymph microcirculation. In: Renkins EM, Michel CC (eds), The cardiovascular system. Handbook of physiology, Bethesda: American Physiology Society, 1984;4:251–307.
3. Chien S, Usami S, Skalak R. Blood flow in small tubes. In: Renkins EM, Michel CC (eds), The cardiovascular system. Handbook of physiology: Bethesda: American Physiology Society, 1984;4:217–49.
4. Whitemore RL. Rheology of the circulation. New York: Pergamon Press, 1968.
5. Winter DC, Nerem RM. Turbulence in pulsatile flows. Ann Biomed Eng 1984; 12:357–69.
6. Yongchareon W, Young DF. Initiation of turbulence in models of arterial stenosis. J Biomech 1976;12:185–96.
7. Attinger EO, Sugawara H, Navarro A, Anne A. Pulsatile flow patterns in distensible tubes. Circ Res 1966;18:447–56.
8. Ling SC, Atabek HB, Fry DL, Patel DJ, Janicki JS. Application of heat-film velocity and shear probes to haemodynamic studies. Circ Res 1968:23:789–801.
9. Chang CC, Atabek HB. The inlet length for oscillatory flow and its effects on the determination of the rate of flow in arteries. Phys Med Biol 1961;6:303–17.
10. Caro CG, Pedley TJ, Schroter RC, Seed WA. The mechanics of the circulation. London: Oxford University Press, 1978.
11. May AG, Van den Berg L, De Weese JA, Rob CG. Critical arterial stenosis. Surgery 1963;54:250–9.
12. Shipley RE, Gregg DE. The effect of external constriction of a blood vessel on blood flow. Am J Physiol 1994;141:289–96.

13. Khalifa AMA, Giddens DP. Analysis of disorder in pulsatile flows with application to poststenotic blood velocity measurement in dogs. J Biomech 1978;11:129–41.
14. Wille SO, Walloe L. Pulsatile pressure and flow in arterial stenoses simulated in a mathematical model. J Biomech Eng 1981;3:17–24.
15. Clark C. The propagation of turbulence produced by a stenosis. In: Taylor DEM, Stevens AL, (eds), Blood flow theory and practice. London: Academic Press, 1982:39–62.

2. Pathology of atherosclerosis

SIMON TROTTER and MUFEED ALI

Atherosclerosis represents one of the most important causes of morbidity and mortality in developed countries. Historically, many theories have been proposed to explain the pathogenesis of atheroma but the response to injury hypothesis proposed by Ross in 1976 and later amplified by the same author [1] has clarified our understanding of the disease. A fundamental aspect of this theory was that endothelial injury initiated atherosclerosis. Since Ross's initial hypothesis, the advent of new techniques in cellular biology and immunology has immensely widened our understanding of the pathogenesis of atherosclerosis.

Epidemiological considerations

The epidemiology of atherosclerosis presents a difficult subject, because firstly, epidemiological data have been gathered from studies of ischemic heart disease, and secondly, many of the factors implicated form a heterogeneous group, making it difficult to identify precise determinants of pathogenesis. Some of the most important factors that have consistently been shown to accelerate atherosclerosis are discussed below.

Major risk factors

Age and sex

Fully developed atherosclerosis is rare before the fourth decade and the incidence rises with age. Bierman and Ross [2] highlighted the fact that this may be due to increasing adiposity, blood glucose and blood pressure with age.

Many epidemiological studies have emphasized that developed atherosclerotic lesions are rare in premenopausal women, but, after the menopause, the incidence increases with age. This finding suggests that female sex hormones may restrain development of the disease, which may be mediated through high-density lipoprotein (HDL); the levels of HDL are raised with increasing doses of estrogen [3].

Race

There are considerable differences in the geographical incidence of atheroma. Whilst manifestly prevalent in the western world, the disease is rare in Asia and the Far East. These differences do not appear to be dependent upon race *per se* as an early important study showed that Japanese immigrating to America showed a higher incidence of ischemic heart disease than their fellows in Japan [4]. It thus seems likely that environmental factors are particularly relevant.

Hyperlipidemia

The contribution of hyperlipidemia to atherosclerosis is irrefutable, but the severity of the disease is dependent on the lipoprotein fraction that is raised. The HDL that is often raised in athletes appears to protect these subjects from atherosclerosis [5]. Conversely, subjects who have a raised value of low-density lipoprotein (LDL), for example in hereditary familial hyperlipidemia or in systemic illnesses such as glomerulonephritis or myxedema, are especially vulnerable to develop atherosclerotic disease. This carrier protein migrates freely through the intima but does not appear to initiate atherosclerosis. Goldstein proposed that LDL was acetylated to form an oxidized moiety and that this resulted in vigorous macrophage uptake by means of a 'scavenger' receptor [6]. Subsequent work showed that this chemical modification could be effected by various cells including smooth muscle and endothelial cells [7]. Furthermore, the oxidized lipoprotein is cytotoxic and thus aggravates cellular injury [8].

Hypertension

Although hypertension is not essential for the development of atherosclerosis, its presence has been found to accelerate atherogenesis. In the Framingham study, patients with hypertension (> 160/95 mmHg) had a twofold increase in ischemic heart disease [9].

Cigarette smoking

There is clear epidemiological evidence from a number of studies, including the Framingham report, that cigarette smoking is associated with ischemic heart disease. Necropsy studies have endorsed this, showing that atherosclerosis is more prevalent in smokers than in non-smokers [10]. The mechanism of these changes probably involves direct damage to the endothelium.

Diabetes mellitus

Diabetes mellitus represents an important risk factor for the evolution of atherosclerosis. Whilst some diabetics are hypercholesterolemic, some have normal cholesterol and the mechanism of atherogenesis in these patients is unclear.

Evolution of atherosclerosis

The fatty streak

The earliest lesion of atherosclerosis is the fatty streak, which macroscopically presents as linear streaks or dots which lie almost flush with the intimal surface of the vessel. The lesion is widespread and is seen in all ages from early childhood. Microscopically, the streak consists of intimal macrophages that have ingested lipid substances, predominantly cholesterol ester [11]. There is evidence that advanced atherosclerotic plaques evolve from these streaks, as these plaques are observed at sites where atheroma is frequent [12]. Nevertheless, fatty streaks are also seen in other regions which have a low incidence of atherosclerosis, suggesting that not all fatty streaks progress to atherosclerosis [11].

The atherosclerotic plaque

The atherosclerotic plaque is a focal lesion, seen in arteries ranging from approximately 3 mm in external diameter up to the aorta, presenting as a raised excrescence (Figures 2.1 and 2.2). The involvement is idiosyncratic – some vessels, such as the internal mammary artery and the arcuate arteries of the kidney, are seldom affected; others, such as the aorta, show frequent involvement. Its prevalence increases with age but appears to remain stable after 60 years, apart from cerebral atherosclerosis which continues to progress [13]. Complications such as

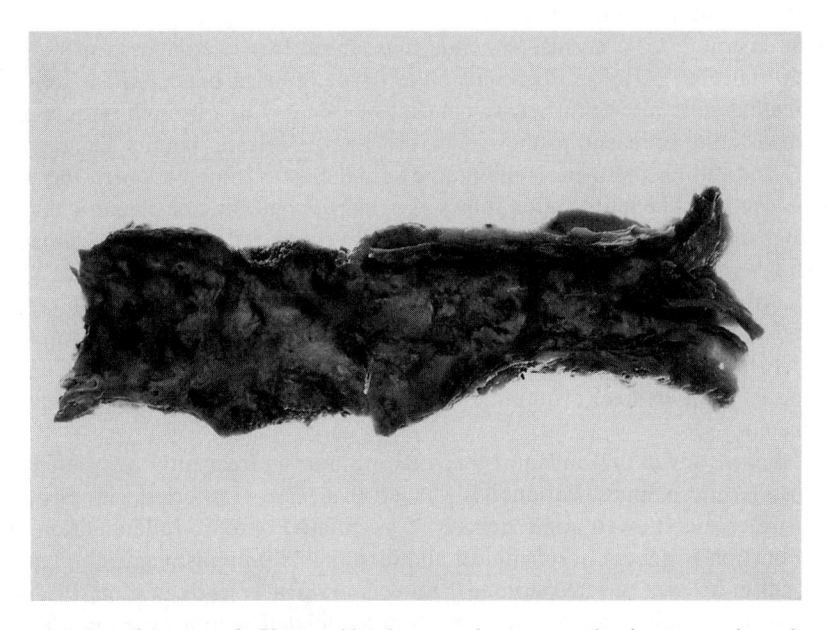

Figure 2.1. Part of the aorta of a 73-year-old male removed at necropsy showing severe atherosclerosis.

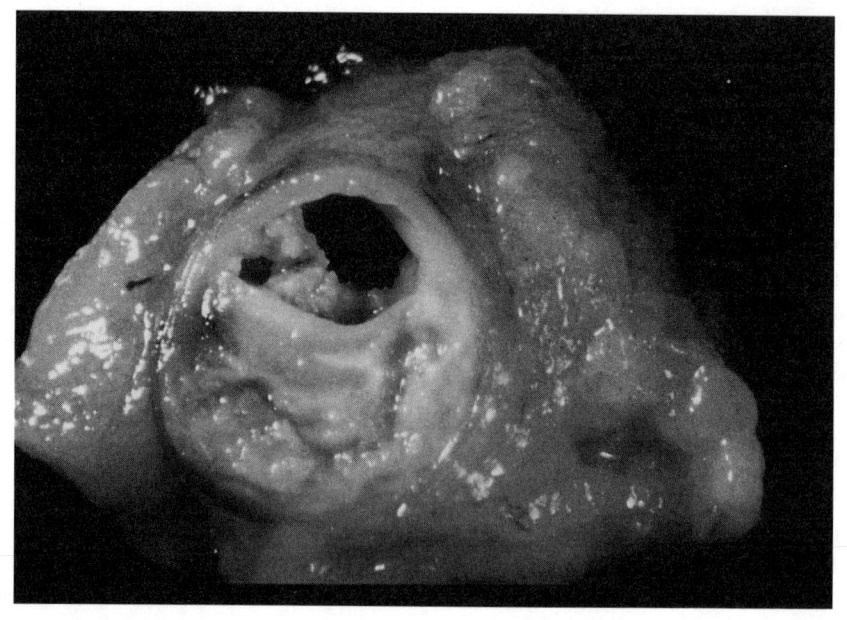

Figure 2.2. An eccentric atheromatous plaque in a coronary artery of a 62-year-old male, significantly narrowing the lumen. (Reproduced by kind permission of Dr A.G. Nicholson.)

ulceration, hemorrhage, thrombosis and aneurysmal dilation of the vessel are a major cause of morbidity and mortality.

The histology of a normal systemic muscular artery is composed of an outer adventitial coat of loose fibroconnective tissue, and an inner intimal lining of endothelial cells resting on scanty connective tissue with a smooth muscle collar between them representing the media. An internal elastic lamina separates the media and intima and there is often an external elastic lamina between the media and adventitia. The intima often shows age-related concentric or eccentric thickening by loose fibroelastic tissue: this should not be confused with atherosclerosis.

An atherosclerotic plaque varies histologically but essentially consists of a lipid core surrounded by foam cells. The cap of the plaque is formed by collagen and smooth muscle cells. Some plaques show obliteration of their lipid cores and consist almost entirely of fibrous tissue with just a few foam cells (Figure 2.3). The plaque is often erosive, disrupting the internal elastic lamina and extending into the media.

A chronic adventitial inflammatory cell infiltrate is frequently associated with atherosclerotic plaques. Parums [14] found that 92% of arteries with advanced atherosclerosis showed some degree of associated chronic inflammation. The inflammation is generally subclinical and identifiable only histologically, but, occasionally, it leads to retroperitoneal fibrosis or, if it extends into the media, to aneurysm formation. Such cases are often associated with a raised erythrocyte sedimentation rate. The cause of the inflammation appears to be an immune

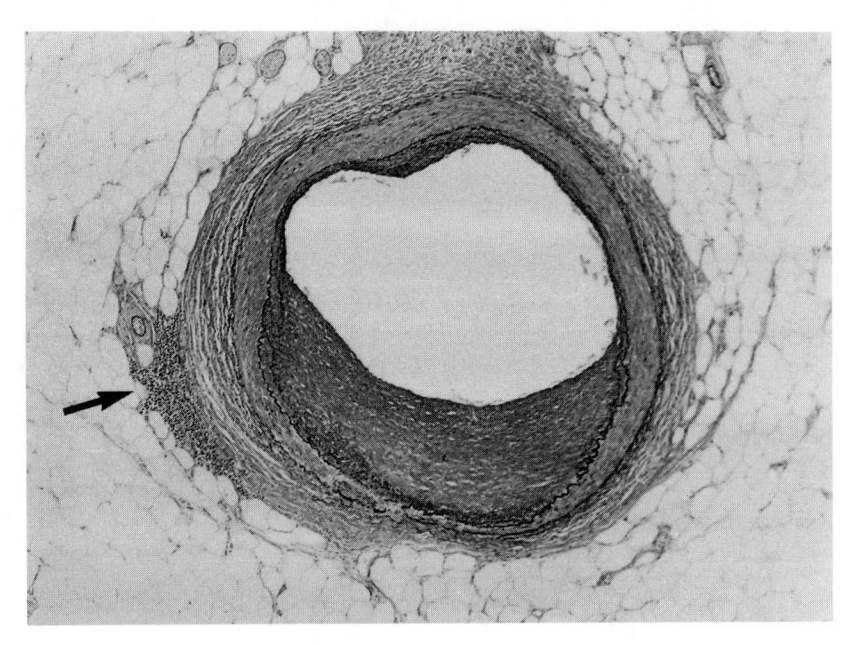

Figure 2.3. Histology of an atheromatous plaque in a coronary artery of a 53-year-old man. The plaque is predominantly composed of collagen. Note the small focal collection of perivascular lymphocytes (arrowed).

reaction to leakage of atherosclerotic material, as serum antibodies to oxidized LDL and ceroid have been detected in patients showing periaortitis [15].

Cellular mechanisms of atherogenesis

These are shown diagrammatically in Figure 2.4 and are discussed below.

Monocytes

Our understanding of the pathogenesis of atherosclerosis has been assisted by studies in animals. These enable the evolution of the disease to be studied through sequential observation and have shown that the blood monocyte is unquestionably relevant to the evolution of the atherosclerotic plaque as well as the fatty streak. Animal models [16, 17] and necropsy studies in man [18] have consistently shown that blood monocytes adhere to intact endothelium and enter the intima early in atherosclerosis eventually to become macrophages [19]. Several factors such as oxidized LDL may promote this process [20].

The adhesion of the monocytes appears to be focal and largely confined to the areas of the arterial tree that are prone to atherosclerosis for reasons that are still unclear. One theory suggests that endothelial cells are activated [21]; the causes of this are not completely understood but a variety of growth factors have been

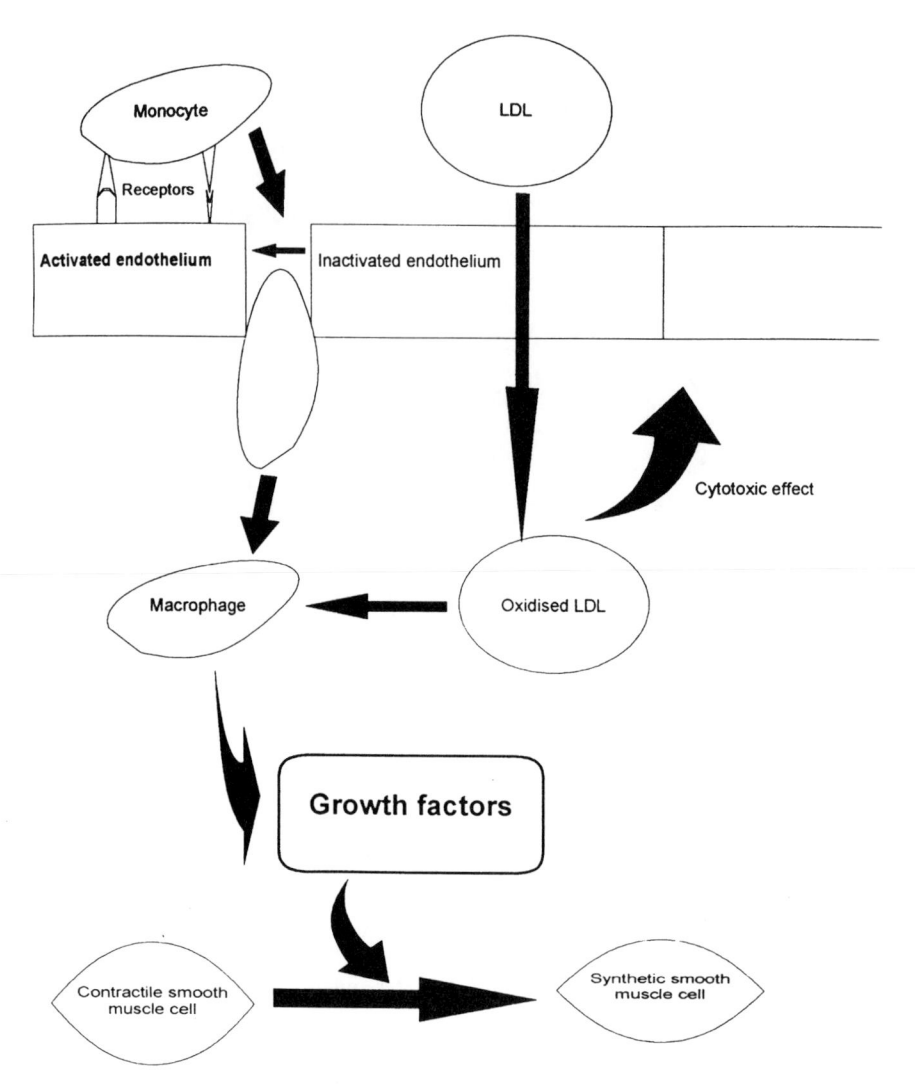

Figure 2.4. Simplified diagram showing some of the mechanisms involved in atherogenesis.

implicated [22]. The adhesion of the monocyte to the endothelial wall results from the interaction of surface proteins expressed by activated endothelial cells and receptors on monocytes. Many adhesion molecules such as VCAM-1 and ICAM-1 have been identified on the endothelial wall [23].

Smooth muscle cells

Smooth muscle cells are present in both fatty streaks and established atheromatous plaques [24], but there are ultrastructural differences between those in the media and those in an atheromatous plaque. The smooth muscle cells within an atheromatous plaque are termed synthetic as they show a distinctive increase in rough endoplasmic reticulum and Golgi bodies [25]. The alteration in the cytostructure is thought to be due to growth factors and other agents that alter the cell's metabolic and proliferative profiles [26].

Lymphocytes

Studies examining the cellular composition of the fibrous cap show that activated T lymphocytes are present [27]. One of the most important secretory products of these cells is the potent growth inhibitor, γ-interferon. This cytokine has been found to inhibit smooth muscle cell proliferation [28] and to suppress the 'scavenger' receptor gene on the macrophage [29], preventing lipid phagocytosis and transformation into a foam cell. Exciting animal studies have demonstrated that injections of γ-interferon after balloon angioplasty, reduced restenosis [30].

Pathological–radiological correlation of atherosclerotic plaques

The radiological identification of a plaque is often difficult. Erosion of the media by an intimal atheromatous lesion often results in an increase of the vessel diameter, obscuring the true extent of the atheromatous disease. It was pointed out that an angiogram can only indicate focal narrowing of an artery [31]; nevertheless, the radiological appearance of a plaque at angiography may be helpful in assessing the clinical outcome. Ambrose *et al.* [32] examined the angiographic morphology of plaques that had narrowed the lumen of coronary arteries by 50% or more. These were divided into concentric plaques, where there was symmetric narrowing, and eccentric plaques. The latter were subdivided into a type I lesion which was asymmetric and showed smooth borders and a broad neck, and a type II lesion which showed irregular borders and a narrow neck. The type II eccentric lesion was more frequent in patients with unstable angina, whereas concentric and type I lesions were more prevalent in sufferers from stable angina. Necropsy studies have shown that type II lesions were associated with plaque rupture or hemorrhage with organizing, partially occlusive, or recanalized thrombus [33]. Pathological studies have also permitted detailed analysis of plaques in coronary arteries. Davies and Thomas [34] found that plaques that show a preponderance of lipid are weaker and therefore more likely to fracture, particularly those that show an eccentrically placed lipid pool, possibly because the unbuttressed plaque cap is vulnerable to stress [35]. However, those plaques that are rich in collagen are more likely to be associated with significant stenosis. Eccentric atheromatous plaques in a coronary artery allow the unaffected segment of the vessel to contract whereas this will not occur with a concentric plaque. Plaques that are not angiographically visible are more likely to be eccentric than concentric and the degree of eccentricity appears to be inversely proportional to the degree of stenosis [31].

Atherosclerotic plaque rupture

Rupture of an atherosclerotic plaque and subsequent thrombosis are important developments and often result in grave clinical sequelae. The inexorable association between plaque fissuring and thrombosis, particularly in coronary arteries, has been firmly established by angiographic and pathological studies [34].

Regression of an atheromatous plaque

Early reports on the regression of atheroma were based on necropsy studies. These showed that atherosclerosis regressed following severe debilitating conditions such as occur in warfare, cancer or tuberculosis [36]. Angiography has enabled atherosclerotic regression to be evaluated, but difficulties remain because criteria are loose and discrepancies exist between angiographic and pathological findings. It seems likely in the past that angiographic accounts of regression may have been due to lysis of overlying thrombus [36]. Nevertheless, it has been established that vigorous treatment with lipid lowering drugs has reversed occlusive atherosclerotic lesions [37].

References

1. Ross R. The pathogenesis of atherosclerosis – an update. N Engl J Med 1986;314:488–500.
2. Bierman EL, Ross R. Ageing and atherosclerosis. In: Paoletti R, Gotto AM, (eds), Atherosclerosis Reviews 2. New York: Raven Press, 1977:79–81.
3. Bradley DD, Wingerd J, Pettiti DB, Krauss RM, Ramcharan S. Serum high density lipoprotein in women using oral contraceptives, estrogens and progestins. N Engl J Med 1978;229:17–20.
4. Keys A, Kimura N, Kusakawa A, Bronte-Stewart B, Larsen N, Keys MA. Lessons in serum cholesterol in Japan, Hawaii, and Los Angeles. Ann Intern Med 1958;48:83–94.
5. Miller GJ, Miller NE. Plasma high density lipoprotein concentration and development of ischaemic heart disease. Lancet 1975;1:16–9.
6. Goldstein JL, Ho YK, Basu SK, Brown MS. Binding site on macrophages that mediates uptake and degradation of acetylated low density lipoprotein producing massive cholesterol deposition. Proc Natl Acad Sci USA 1979;76:333–7.
7. Witztum JL. Role of oxidised low density lipoprotein in atherogenesis. Br Heart J 1993;69 (Suppl):12–8.
8. Morel DW, DiCorleto PE, Chisholm GM. Endothelial and smooth muscle cells alter low density lipoprotein in vitro by free radical oxidation. Arteriosclerosis 1984;4:357–64.
9. Kannel WB, Schwartz MD, McNamara PM. Blood pressure and risk of coronary heart disease: The Framingham study. Dis of Chest 1969;56:43–52.
10. Strong JP, Richards ML. Cigarette smoking and smoking in autopsied men. Atherosclerosis 1976;23:451–76.
11. Stary HC. Evolution and progression of atherosclerotic lesions in coronary arteries of children and young adults. Arteriosclerosis 1989;9 (Suppl 1):19–32.
12. Robertson WB, Geer JC, Strong JP, McGill HC, Jr. The fate of the fatty streak. Exp Mol Pathol 1963;2 (Suppl 1):28–39.
13. Weber G, Bianciardi G, Bussani R *et al*. Atherosclerosis and aging. A morphometric study on arterial lesions of elderly and very elderly necropsy subjects. Arch Pathol Lab Med 1988;112:1066–70.
14. Parums DV. The spectrum of chronic periaortitis. Histopathology 1990;16:423–31.

15. Parums DV, Brown DL, Mitchinson MJ. Serum antibodies to oxidized low-density lipoprotein and ceroid in chronic periaortitis. Arch Pathol Lab Med 1990;114:383–7.
16. Faggiotto A, Ross R, Harker L. Studies of hypercholesteraemia in the nonhuman primate I. Changes that lead to fatty streak formation. Arteriosclerosis 1984;4:323–40.
17. Faggiotto A, Ross R. Studies of hypercholesteraemia in the nonhuman primate. II. Fatty streak conversion to fibrous plaque. Arteriosclerosis 1984;4:341–56.
18. Aqel NM, Ball RY, Waldmann H, Mitchinson MJ. Identification of macrophages and smooth muscle cells in human atherosclerosis using monoclonal antibodies. J Pathol 1985;146:197–204.
19. Aqel NM, Ball RY, Waldmann H, Mitchinson MJ. Monocytic origin of foam cells in human atherosclerotic plaques. Atherosclerosis 1984;53:265–71.
20. Yla-Herttuala S, Palinski W, Rosenfeld ME et al. Evidence for the presence of oxidatively modified low density lipoprotein in atherosclerotic lesions of rabbit and man. J Clin Invest 1989;84:1086–95.
21. DiCorleto PE, Chisolm GM. Participation of the endothelium in the development of the atherosclerotic plaque. Prog Lipid Res 1986;25:365–74.
22. Faruqi RM, DiCorleto PE. Mechanisms of monocyte recruitment and accumulation. Br Heart J 1993;69 (Suppl):19–29.
23. van der Wal AC, Das PK, Tigges AJ, Becker AE. Adhesion molecules on the endothelium and mononuclear cells in human atherosclerotic lesions. Am J Pathol 1992;141:1427–33.
24. Stary HC, Blankenhorn DH, Chandler AB et al. A definition of the intima of human arteries and of its atherosclerosis-prone regions. A report from the Committee on Vascular Lesions of the Council on Arteriosclerosis, American Heart Association. Arterioscler Thromb 1992;12:120–34.
25. Campbell GR, Campbell JH, Manderson JA, Horrigan S, Rennick RE. Arterial smooth muscle. A multifunctional mesenchymal cell. Arch Pathol Lab Med 1988;112:977–86.
26. Raines EW, Ross R. Smooth muscle cells and the pathogenesis of the lesions of atherosclerosis. Br Heart J 1993;69 (Suppl):30–7.
27. Hansson GK, Holm J, Jonasson L. Detection of activated T lymphocytes in the human atherosclerotic plaque. Am J Pathol 1989;135:169–75.
28. Hansson GK, Jonasson L, Holm J, Clowes MM, Clowes AW. Gamma-interferon regulates vascular smooth muscle proliferation and Ia antigen expression in vivo and in vitro. Circ Res 1988;63:712–9.
29. Geng YJ, Hansson GK. Interferon-gamma inhibits scavenger receptor expression and foam cell formation in human monocyte-derived macrophages. J Clin Invest 1992;89:1322–30.
30. Hansson GK, Holm J. Interferon-gamma inhibits arterial stenosis after injury. Circulation 1991;84:1266–72.
31. Davies MJ, Woolf N. Atherosclerosis: what it is and why does it occur? Br Heart J 1993;69 (Suppl):3–11.
32. Ambrose JA, Winters SL, Stern A et al. Angiographic morphology and the pathogenesis of unstable angina pectoris. J Am Coll Cardiol 1985;5:609–16.
33. Levin DC, Fallon JT. Significance of the angiographic morphology of localised coronary stenoses: histopathological correlations. Circulation 1982;66:316–20.
34. Davies MJ, Thomas AC. Plaque fissuring – the cause of acute myocardial infarction, sudden ischaemic death and crescendo angina. Br Heart J 1985;53:363–73.
35. Richardson PD, Davies MJ, Born GV. Influence of plaque configuration and stress distribution on fissuring of coronary atherosclerotic plaques. Lancet 1989;2:941–4.
36. Armstrong ML, Heistad DD, Megan MB, Lopez JA, Harrison DG. Reversibility of atherosclerosis. Cardiovasc Clin 1990;20:113–26.
37. Kane JP, Malloy MJ, Ports TA, Phillips NR, Diehl JC, Havel RJ. Regression of coronary atherosclerosis during treatment of familial hypercholesterolemia with combined drug regimens. JAMA 1990;264:3007–12.

3. Thrombosis and thromboembolism

MICHAEL SCHACHTER

Thrombosis is of enormous importance in human disease. It may occur at any point in the circulation, from the lumen of the left ventricle to the capillary microcirculation. The effects may vary from a transient, very localized and essentially harmless interruption of blood flow to catastrophic infarction of the brain or myocardium or fatal circulatory obstruction at the pulmonary trunk. The specific pathologies are described in detail in other chapters, but some idea of the range of possible events is given by the following, far from comprehensive, list:

- intracardiac mural thrombus following myocardial infarction;
- intra-atrial thrombus during atrial fibrillation leading to emboli (especially cerebrovascular);
- coronary artery thrombosis associated with atherosclerosis and causing myocardial infarction;
- thrombosis in the cerebrovascular circulation (carotid arterioles) causing stroke;
- thrombosis of iliac or femoral arteries, complicating atherosclerosis and endangering whole lower limb;
- thrombosis in deep veins of leg or pelvis, possibly giving rise to pulmonary emboli; and
- disseminated intravascular coagulation in the microcirculation, causing depletion of platelets and clotting factors.

Although all thrombi consist of fibrin and circulating cells the precise composition is influenced by hemodynamic factors, so that arterial and venous thrombi are significantly different. Arterial thrombi tend to consist mainly of platelet aggregates with a low fibrin content, while venous thrombi have much more fibrin and fewer platelets, with a considerable number of entrapped red cells.

The remainder of this chapter will deal in general terms with factors promoting, or indeed preventing, thromboembolism and with therapeutic approaches in outline. Specific details will be found in the appropriate chapters throughout this book.

Pathogenetic factors in thrombosis

Thromboembolic events can be accounted for in terms of the disturbed balance between factors acting to prevent thrombosis and those making it more likely.

The known thrombogenic factors include:

- damaged or absent endothelial cells;
- activation of platelets by: circulating factors; mechanical obstacles such as prosthetic heart valves; or exposure to subendothelial collagen;
- overactivity of coagulation pathways;
- underactivity of fibrinolytic mechanisms; and
- stasis.

The contrary antithrombotic mechanisms include:

- intact endothelial layer;
- endogenous anticoagulants;
- degradation of clotting factors by the liver;
- active fibrinolysis; and
- uninterrupted and non-turbulent blood flow.

Clearly many of these mechanisms are actually mirror images of each other and can conveniently be considered under single overall headings.

The endothelium

The normal endothelium is non-thrombogenic. It does not permit platelet activation and adhesion, does not activate circulating coagulation factors and promotes fibrinolysis. Endothelial cells can, however, become thrombogenic without gross destruction. A large number of factors are known to cause endothelial damage of varying extent. Among the most clinically relevant are the following:

- hyperlipidemia (particularly increased low-density lipoproteins and lipoprotein (a));
- hypertension (and other causes of increased shear stress);
- smoking;
- ischemia/reperfusion (and oxygen free radicals);
- endotoxin;
- inflammatory cell mediated damage (for instance, in vasculitis);
- homocysteinemia; and
- iatrogenic damage (notably angioplasty).

The intact non-activated endothelial cell has an array of mechanisms which directly inhibit all aspects of thrombogenesis. These include:

- proteoglycans, containing heparan sulfate, which inhibits the coagulation cascade after interaction with antithrombin III (see below);
- thrombomodulin, which effectively inactivates thrombin;
- plasminogen activators (specifically tissue plasminogen activator) which trigger fibrinolysis; and
- prostacyclin and nitric oxide, which inhibit platelet activation, including adhesion, as well as promoting vasodilation.

Damaged endothelium will be deficient in most or all of these respects. If the endothelial layer is actually missing then there is the additional problem that subendothelial collagen, von Willebrand factor and fibronectin are exposed to the circulation. Platelet membrane receptors can interact with these proteins so that adhesion occurs. However, this does not usually lead to thrombosis in the presence of normal flow patterns within the vessel lumen.

The platelet

Platelet activation occurs as a result of many stimuli in the local micro-environment in the vasculature. Under normal circumstances this is a self-limiting process without detectable consequences and it is obviously of vital importance in the regulation of hemostasis. Despite the apparent, and entirely misleading, simplicity of the platelet, it is now clear that its activation is an extremely complex process. There are several interrelated components:

- adhesion;
- shape change;
- release reaction; and
- aggregation.

Adhesion can occur in response to various endogenous and artificial surfaces, but the typical substrate is one of the adhesive glycoproteins of the endothelium, most notably collagen but also including von Willebrand factor and fibronectin. The interaction is mediated by specific receptors on the surface of the platelet. *Shape change*, during which the platelet becomes spherical with protruding pseudopodia, is initiated by most agonists (thromboxane A_2, serotonin, adenosine diphosphate (ADP), thrombin, platelet activating factor) but not all (epinephrine). It is usually the earliest response of the platelet to stimulation and does not require any additional factors beyond the agonist itself. *Aggregation* is usually preceded by shape change but requires the presence of fibrinogen, which is bound to a specific platelet membrane receptor known as glycoprotein IIb/IIIa. This process, like the *release* reaction, is to some extent modified by a reinforcement mechanism. Several agonists, including thrombin, collagen and epinephrine, can activate the enzyme phospholipase A_2 in platelets, causing release of arachidonic acid which is then converted to thromboxane A_2 (TXA_2), itself a potent aggregant.

Such 'strong' agonists cause release of both types of platelet storage granules. Dense granules contain ADP, serotonin and calcium but the α-granules are much more complex, containing a remarkable range of proteins including platelet factor 4, von Willebrand factor and fibrinogen, but also growth modulators such as platelet-derived growth factor and transforming growth factor. 'Weak' agonists, like ADP, lead to the release of only dense granules.

The activated platelet is also pro-coagulant, through several mechanisms. It has binding sites for activated coagulation factor X (Xa), which is thereby protected from inactivation. Activated platelets can also directly activate factors XI and XII. In fact, most reactions of the coagulation cascades (see below) require the proximity of the platelet cell membrane, with the important exception of the final interaction between thrombin and fibrinogen.

The coagulation system

Blood coagulation is a complex cascade culminating in the generation of a fibrin clot. A much simplified overview is shown in Figure 3.1. Each step, whereby a pro-enzyme is converted to an active enzyme by another enzyme, clearly gives great scope for amplification and the maximization of response to a given stimulus. Although the distinction between the intrinsic and extrinsic pathways is almost always made, it is likely that this is of limited relevance *in vivo*. It is now generally thought that factor VIIa/tissue factor is usually responsible for initial generation of

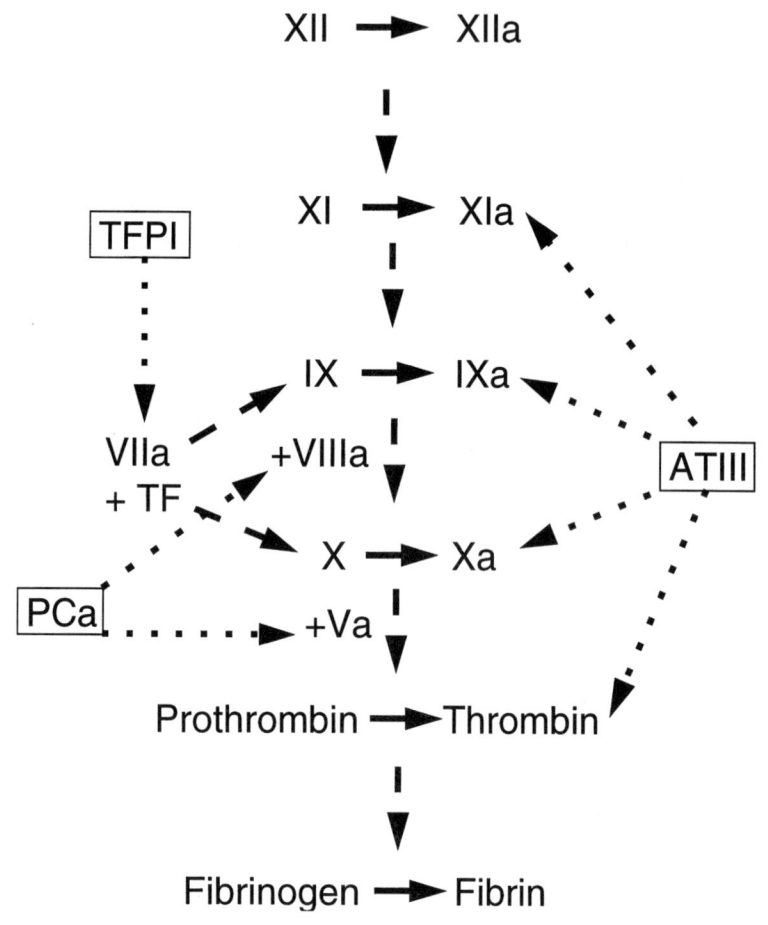

Figure 3.1. Schematic representation of the coagulation cascade. TFPI: tissue factor pathway inhibitor; PCa: activated protein C; ATIII: antithrombin III. Note that protein S is an essential cofactor for protein C activity.

factor Xa and hence thrombin, but the so-called intrinsic pathways, via factor IX, may need to be recruited for effective (even if sometimes inappropriate) hemostasis. The cascades are modulated by numerous feedback loops, both negative and positive, but this is beyond the scope of this chapter. Tissue factor is released by activated endothelial cells and by monocytes/macrophages. As the figure indicates, several endogenous anticoagulants inhibit the activation of the pathways at several points. The liver also rapidly clears activated coagulation factors from the circulation.

The fibrinolytic system

It is usual to consider the normal physiologic state of circulating blood as a dynamic equilibrium between coagulation and fibrinolysis. Like the coagulation system, fibrinolysis is the end result of an enzymatic cascade. Although somewhat less complex than coagulation it is proving to have far more components than was originally thought. The ultimate product of the pathway is the proteolytic enzyme plasmin, which degrades fibrin in thrombi. The enzyme is derived from an inactive precursor, plasminogen, which is bound to fibrin and actually forms an integral part of the thrombus. Tissue plasminogen activator (t-PA), itself a protease synthesized and stored by endothelial cells, converts plasminogen to plasmin. It has a high affinity for fibrin, thereby helping to ensure that fibrinolysis is appropriately localized. As might be expected, fibrinolysis is regulated by other mechanisms. The two most significant are α_2-antiplasmin and plasminogen activator inhibitor-1 (PAI-1). The former is itself activated by plasmin, to which it binds, forming an inactive complex. PAI-1, released by both endothelial cells and activated platelets, inactivates t-PA. A schematic diagram of the fibrinolytic pathway is shown in Figure 3.2.

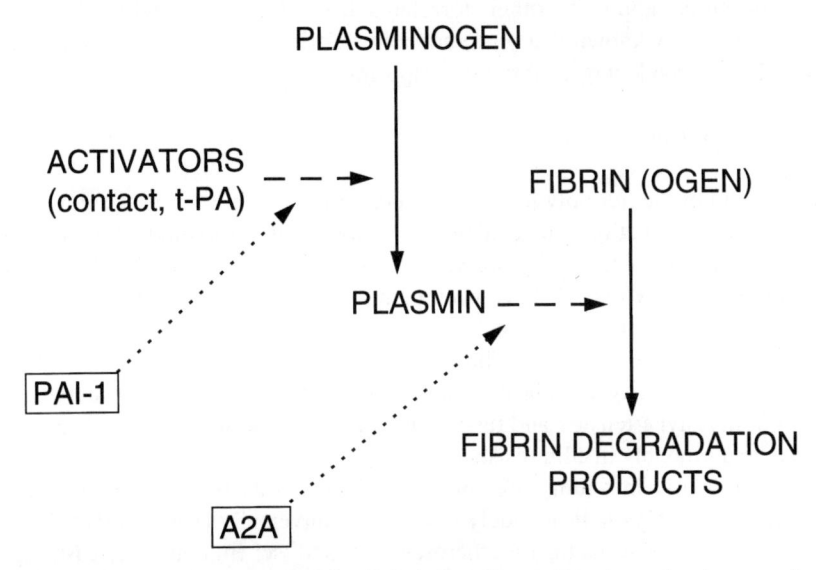

Figure 3.2. Schematic representation of the fibrinolytic pathway. t-PA: tissue plasminogen activator; PAI-1: plasminogen activator inhibitor-1; A2A: α2-antiplasmin.

Thrombosis and atherosclerosis

Although many important instances of thromboembolic disease are associated with mechanical flow disturbances (e.g. atrial fibrillation, deep vein thrombosis), most events occur in atherosclerotic arteries. It is now clear that there are strong links between atheroma and abnormalities of the hemostatic systems. Some of these connections will be considered in this section.

Fibrinogen

It is now well-established that an increased level of fibrinogen constitutes a strong independent risk factor for cardiovascular disease including coronary artery disease, claudication and stroke. This involves multiple mechanisms, apart from the likelihood of increased fibrin deposition, notably increased viscosity and enhanced platelet reactivity. Fibrinogen can be considered as an acute-phase inflammatory protein which is increased by numerous stimuli. These include smoking, diabetes, obesity and virtually any chronic inflammatory or infective state. Serum cholesterol and triglyceride concentration are also correlated with fibrinogen levels.

Factor VII

As Figure 3.1 clearly illustrates, factor VII has a pivotal position in the coagulation cascade. Most epidemiological studies suggest a positive association between plasma levels of activated factor VII and the incidence of coronary artery disease. Partly because measurement of the activated factor is technically difficult there is less information about its other correlates than is the case with fibrinogen. However, it is now known that postprandial hypertriglyceridemia is an activator of factor VII, independent of dietary fat composition.

Fibrinolytic system

Underactivity of the fibrinolytic system can contribute to thombosis as significantly as overactive coagulation. The evidence on this issue is surprisingly contradictory. Most positive studies linking depressed fibrinolysis and increased levels of PAI-1 with coronary artery disease have been composed of relatively young men and it has been suggested that such impaired activity promotes atherogenesis by permitting greater fibrin deposition. There does appear to be a positive correlation between PAI-1 activity and plasma insulin levels, and some have considered associated obesity, hypertension and raised triglycerides to be secondary to hyperinsulinemia (and probably insulin resistance).

One particularly intriguing possible association is that between lipoprotein (a) (Lp(a)) and fibrinolysis. It is widely though not universally accepted that a raised level of Lp(a) is a risk factor for atherosclerosis and ischemic heart disease. Lp(a) consists essentially of a particle of LDL, which is of course cholesterol-rich, linked to another apoprotein, apoprotein (a). This has a high degree of structural homology with plasminogen and it has been proposed that Lp(a) is therefore capable of acting as an inhibitor of plasmin generation by competing for plasminogen binding sites.

The platelet

There is considerable evidence that platelets are hyperreactive to many stimuli in patients with atherosclerosis and occlusive arterial disease. The mechanisms, however, are unclear. One possibility is that high plasma cholesterol levels directly influence the structure of the platelet cell membrane and increase the response to agonists, for instance by enhancing intracellular calcium release. Other studies have shown that *in vitro* LDL, particularly if partly oxidized, can directly activate platelets in a manner resembling conventional agonists. It is open to question whether this is relevant *in vivo*, where large quantities of possible functional antagonists are present, in particular HDL and albumin. Less controversially, it is recognized that relatively high platelet counts, even within the 'normal' range, can predispose to thrombosis. Another generally accepted risk factor for inappropriate platelet activation is the increased shear to which platelets are exposed in areas of plaque and stenosis.

The vessel wall

As previously described, the vessel wall is normally anti-thrombogenic. In atherosclerosis this may be altered in several respects. In particular, nitric oxide synthesis is impaired early in the development of atheroma, thereby impairing both endothelium-dependent vasodilatation and inhibition of platelet adhesion and aggregation. By contrast, prostacyclin production is undiminished and may even increase in parallel with thromboxane synthesis. The vessel wall, including endothelial and smooth muscle cells and macrophages, also shows localized areas of tissue factor expression associated with atheromatous lesions.

Approaches to therapy

Detailed description of the therapeutics of thromboembolic disease is obviously beyond the scope of this chapter. Broadly, antithrombotic drugs are divided into three major categories:

– agents which interfere with the coagulation pathways;
– agents which prevent platelet activation; and
– agents which remove or deplete circulating fibrinogen.

In addition, there is the growing class of thrombolytic agents which dissolve pre-existing thrombi, such as streptokinase and recombinant t-PA. These will not be discussed further in this chapter.

Anticoagulant drugs

The classic anticoagulant drugs are *warfarin* and related coumarin derivatives, and the *heparins*. Warfarin-like drugs are essentially vitamin K antagonists which prevent the conversion of vitamin K to the form required for the carboxylation and hence activation of coagulation factors VII, IX, X and prothrombin. There is therefore a delay before anticoagulation is fully established, since preexisting factors have to be depleted. Heparin (a glycosaminoglycan which can exist in molecular weights ranging from 3000 to 30 000) acts much more rapidly. For activity it must combine with the endogenous anticoagulant antithrombin III, forming a complex which potently antagonizes thrombin as well as well as activated factor X. The antithrombin effect also reduces platelet activation. Other glycosaminoglycans, such as *sulodexide*, have also been investigated as possible antithrombotic agents. Efforts are in progress to supplement these agents with novel therapeutic approaches, which will be considered briefly below.

Thrombin antagonists, or *antithrombins* are being developed as alternatives to heparin. *Hirudin*, the peptide anticoagulant of leeches, has been very extensively studied over the last 30 years. It is a specific and potent inhibitor of thrombin which, unlike heparin, does not require a co-factor (antithrombin III). Also unlike heparin it can inactivate clot-bound thrombin. Early clinical trials produced a high incidence of hemorrhage and it is now recognized that the doses were considerably higher than those required for antithrombotic effect. It seems likely that this problem can be overcome and hirudin can become therapeutically useful. Several smaller peptide analogues of hirudin, such as *hirulog*, *hirugen* and *argobatran* have been synthesized but it is unclear whether these have any advantage compared to the native peptide. *Thrombin receptor antagonist peptides* are also under development. It should be noted for all these agents that they do not affect thrombin generation.

In view of this possible weakness it may be advantageous to inhibit the coagulation cascade at an earlier point. *Factor Xa antagonists* are one approach to this problem. Two approaches appear promising. The recombinant *tick anticoagulant peptide* may be superior in antithrombotic activity to both heparin and hirudin and has little immunogenicity. It is, however, very expensive at present. A *synthetic pentasaccharide* has been produced which corresponds to the antithrombin III binding site on heparin. It acts by potentiation of the action of antithrombin III in antagonizing activated factor X. In this case there is no clear evidence that it is significantly superior to heparin.

Antiplatelet drugs

Aspirin remains by far the most widely used antiplatelet drug. Due to its vast accumulated experience, proven efficacy and minimal cost this is unlikely to change in the foreseeable future. It is an irreversible inhibitor of platelet cyclooxygenase/prostaglandin synthase, thereby preventing the formation of thromboxane A_2 and of other less potent aggregant prostanoids. *Sulfinpyrazone*, which has a similar mechanism of action, has also been used as an antiplatelet drug but with more severe toxicity and at greater cost. Aspirin itself is not universally tolerated, mostly because of gastrointestinal or hypersensitivity reactions, and there are undoubted limits to its efficacy. In view of the importance of this type of therapy there has been great interest in alternative drugs. Some of these are described below.

Inhibitors of ADP-induced platelet activation, the pro-drugs *ticlopidine* and *clopidogrel*, are already in clinical use in some countries. They inhibit binding of fibrinogen to the platelet membrane glycoprotein IIb/IIIa, which is triggered by ADP released from the platelets themselves, and represents a final common pathway of platelet aggregation. The precise mechanism of the interaction is not known but the drugs do *not* bind to the glycoprotein itself. Their efficacy is similar to that of aspirin but there has been considerable caution in the use of ticlopidine because of bone marrow toxicity: it is believed that clopidogrel does not have this property.

Direct *IIa/IIIb antagonists* are also now available. The first of these to be introduced are monoclonal antibodies, such as *abciximab*, which has already been tested in post-coronary angioplasty restenosis where it reduced the incidence of several end-points but also increased bleeding. *Synthetic peptides* and *non-peptide mimetics* have also been designed which compete with fibrinogen for the IIa/IIIb binding site.

Given the importance of thromboxane A_2 in amplifying platelet responses, it is not surprising that compounds have been developed which are *thromboxane synthase inhibitors, thromboxane receptor antagonists*, or both. Such an approach should also spare endothelial prostacyclin synthesis. Clinical results with specific inhibitors and antagonists have so far been disappointing. Drugs with dual activity, such as *ridogrel*, may prove more useful.

Stable analogues of prostacyclin for intravenous (*iloprost*) and more recently oral use (*cicaprost*) are effective antiaggregants which also possess vasodilator activity. Though this hemodynamic effect can sometimes be undesirable, particularly if it leads to hypotension, it might also be helpful in minimizing local ischemia. The actual clinical value of this remains controversial.

Summary and prospects

Our understanding of thrombosis has expanded almost beyond recognition in the last decade. In parallel with this techniques of both prophylaxis and treatment have greatly improved. Even so, thrombotic disease remains one of the world's major causes of morbidity and mortality, indeed in many developed countries it is the leading cause of the latter. There is therefore clearly room for great improvement and this is realized by researchers whether of clinical or basic science interests, in academia or in industry. As the previous section indicates there is great interest in the improvement of antithrombotic therapy although replacements for standard drugs are still a rather remote prospect. This will certainly change in the next decade, particularly as we gain greater insight into the relationship between thromboembolic disease and atherogenesis.

Further reading

As can readily be imagined the primary literature in this area is enormous. Even a very sparing selection of references would be longer than the text of this chapter and this does not seem necessary or desirable for a book directed at angiologists. The following is therefore a list of recent books, reviews and key articles which will in turn give access to many thousands of references for the interested reader.

References

Baillières Clinical Haematology (Thrombophilia) 1994;7(3).
British Medical Bulletin (Thrombosis) 1994;50(4).
Broze GJ. Tissue factor pathway inhibitor and the revised theory of coagulation. Annu Rev Med 1995;46:103–12.
Colman RW, Hirsch J, Marder VJ, Salzman EW (eds), Hemostasis and thrombosis; basic principles and clinical practice. 3rd edition. Philadelphia: JB Lippincott, 1994 (esp. chapter 57).
Genest J, Cohn JS. Clustering of cardiovascular risk factors: targeting high-risk individuals. Am J Cardiol 1995;76:8A–20A.
Mitropoulos KA. Lipoprotein metabolism and thrombosis. Curr Opin Lipidol 1994;5:227–35.
Verstraete M, Zoldhelyi P. Novel antithrombotic drugs in development. Drugs 1995;49:856–84.
Wennmalm A. Endothelial nitric oxide and cardiovascular disease. J Intern Med 1994:235:317–27.

4. Hemorheology and hemorheological mechanisms
MICHAEL RAMPLING

Hemorheology is the study of the flow properties of blood. At its heart lies the concept of viscosity which is the rheological parameter most commonly used in discussing resistance to flow. The essential concept is generally understood qualitatively, for example it is common knowledge that it is more difficult to pour or stir treacle than water because the former is the more viscous. For the rheologist, however, such a qualitative feel for viscosity is not enough and an ability to quantify it is essential.

Viscosity

To introduce the reader to the quantitation and rheological effects of viscosity a simplified situation will first be considered of a liquid flowing through a uniform, horizontal cylindrical tube. It will be assumed that the flow rate is low so that streamlined conditions obtain (the significance of which will be explained later) and that the liquid is a Newtonian one. That it is Newtonian simply means that its viscosity is constant and unaffected by the size of the tube through which it is flowing or by the flow rate.

In order to make the liquid flow a driving pressure is required, and it is assumed to be generated by the apparatus illustrated in Figure 4.1. The pressure is governed by the depth of liquid in the reservoir which, by the arrangement of the apparatus, is constant. The system comes to equilibrium such that the rate of flow through the tube is also constant. What actually happens is that the liquid has, for some short distance into the tube, a flattened velocity profile, but this quickly disappears until an effectively constant parabolic profile obtains (Figure 4.1). In such flow the velocity of the liquid at the wall of the tube is zero, but it increases steadily toward the center of the tube. Consider now that the radius of the tube is r_{max} and the velocity at the centre is v_{max}; if at any radial position, r, the velocity is v_r, then it can be shown [1] that the relationship between v_r and r is:

$$v_r/v_{max} = 1 - (r/r_{max})^2. \tag{4.1}$$

This means that the annuli of liquid flow past one another at different rates, which illustrates another important rheological concept, shear rate (τ). It is defined, at any

A.-M. Salmasi and A. Strano (eds), Angiology in Practice, 41–52.
© 1996 Kluwer Academic Publishers. Printed in Great Britain.

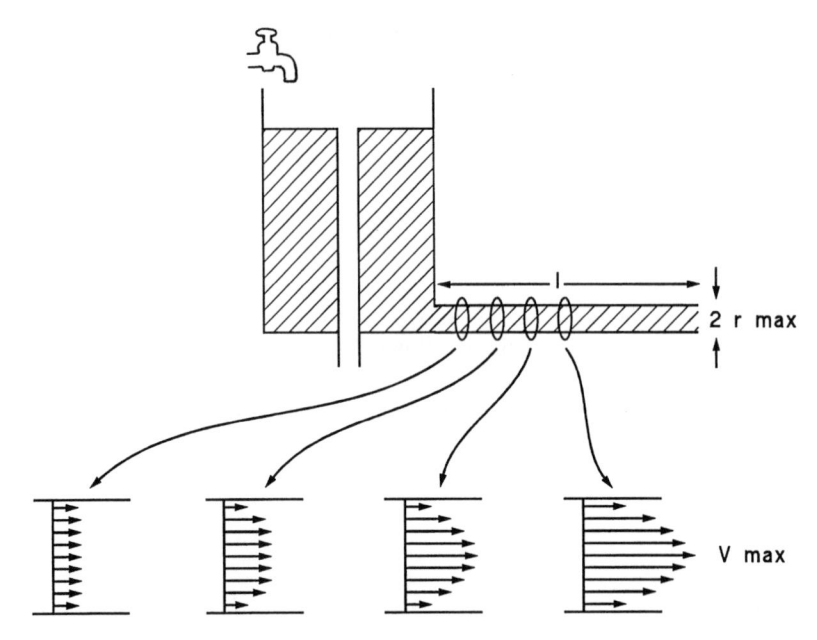

Figure 4.1. A device for generating Poiseuille flow. The flattened velocity profile (bottom left) quickly develops into a parabolic one (bottom right).

point, as the rate of change of velocity of the liquid with radial distance, or to put this mathematically:

$$\tau = dv/dr. \tag{4.2}$$

Hence the shear rate is maximal at the wall of the tube and minimal (zero) at the center. Shear rate, being a ratio of velocity to length, has the units of reciprocal seconds or s^{-1}.

It is important to note that, in spite of a constant driving force acting on the liquid, the system comes to equilibrium with a constant flow rate. This implies that there must be an equal opposing force along the line of flow acting against that generated by the driving pressure. This opposing force is derived from a form of fluid friction that acts between the annuli of liquid as they flow past one another at the rate determined by the shear rate. This opposing force, when expressed per unit area of any flowing annulus, is called the shear stress, γ. The viscosity (η) is then defined as the ratio of shear stress to shear rate at any point in the liquid:

$$\eta = \gamma/\tau. \tag{4.3}$$

The units are Pascal.seconds or Pa.s. It should be noted that for a Newtonian liquid equation 4.3 necessitates that the shear stress is always directly proportional to the shear rate.

In the circumstance of the above example it is possible to derive [1] an equation (usually called Poiseuille's equation) relating the volume rate of flow (dQ/dt) through the tube to its dimensions (length l, radius r_{max}), the driving pressure (P) and the viscosity of the liquid (η):

$$dQ/dt = (\pi P r_{max}^4)/(8l\eta). \tag{4.4}$$

This equation is useful because it allows the rate of flow of a Newtonian liquid of known viscosity through a cylindrical tube of known dimensions to be predicted for any driving pressure. Alternatively, if a Newtonian liquid is driven by a known pressure through a tube of known dimensions and the flow rate measured then equation 4.4 allows the viscosity to be determined. This is the basis of a range of instruments for measuring viscosity known as capillary viscometers, and is relevant here as they are commonly used clinically for measuring plasma viscosity.

Flow resistance in single and multiple tubes

Poiseuille's equation (equation 4.4) can be rewritten, by analogy with the well-known Ohm's Law equation of electrical theory, as:

$$dQ/dt = P/R \tag{4.5}$$

where R is the flow resistance and is given by:

$$R = (8/\pi)(\eta)(l/r_{max}^4) \tag{4.6}$$

and this can be simplified to:

$$R = (8/\pi)(R_{viscous})(R_{geometric}) \tag{4.7}$$

i.e. the viscous and geometric resistance terms can be separated.

Even in more complex geometries of tubes, of various sizes, in series or parallel arrangements, the viscous and geometric resistances can still be separated as shown in equation 4.7 [2]. This illustrates the importance of viscosity as a parameter determining flow resistance, and why it is such a fundamental concept in rheology.

Turbulent and streamlined flow

It was assumed in the above example that the flow was streamlined. What this means is that the flowing annuli slide past one another with no significant lateral movement of the liquid. If the flow rate is progressively increased this smoothness eventually breaks down and chaotic motion starts, with lateral mixing; this is turbulent flow and is less efficient than streamlined. In practice, conditions *in vivo* are such that there is normally very little turbulence, except briefly during systole in the larger arteries. This is relevant because the equation describing turbulent flow is considerably more complex than that for streamlined flow (i.e. Poiseuille's equation), but clearly it is unnecessary to consider it further here.

Plasma viscosity

Studies of plasma have shown that to a good approximation most samples are Newtonian, i.e. for a given sample the viscosity is constant except for a small temperature coefficient, this being close to that of water: a 2.4% decrease for each °C rise in temperature between about 20 and 40°C [3, 4]. The value for plasma viscosity usually given for healthy subjects is 1.25±0.10 mPa.s at 37°C, with no sex difference and only a small increase with age. The reason it is greater than that of water (0.7 mPa.s at 37°C) is the presence of plasma proteins. However, these vary in their influence, so although albumin constitutes some 60% of the protein pool it is responsible for only about 35% of the difference in viscosity between water and plasma. Fibrinogen on the other hand constitutes a mere 4% or so of the protein pool but contributes some 20% to the viscosity effect [5]. This variability in the effect of the proteins depends on their size and asymmetry; fibrinogen being one of the largest and most asymmetric has the greatest effect. Hence the viscosity of a plasma sample is very sensitive to the prevailing concentration of fibrinogen, for example, doubling it from the normal value of 3 g/L increases plasma viscosity by some 20%. The sensitivity to the concentrations of the larger proteins means that plasma viscosity varies in sympathy with the severity of a wide range of clinical conditions [5]. Of particular relevance here are the elevations that are commonly found in conditions of cardiovascular significance, such as diabetes and hypertension [6] and hypercholesterolemia [7] and its appearance as a risk factor for ischemic heart disease [8]. It is also a potent index of conditions such as Waldenström's macroglobulinemia, where it can increase by as much as 20-fold [9]. These findings have led to plasma viscosity being proposed as a general nonspecific index of pathology to replace the older erythrocyte sedimentation rate test [3].

Blood is a non-Newtonian liquid

It was explained above that Newtonian liquids are characterized by the direct proportionality between the shear stress and shear rate that they experience during flow, i.e.:

$$\gamma \: \alpha \: \tau \tag{4.8}$$

and that this is why their viscosity is constant. It is also the reason why it is possible to generate Poiseuille's equation as a general description of flow of all

Newtonian liquids under streamlined conditions. The problem with blood is that equation 4.8 does not obtain, rather there is a more complex relation between shear stress and shear rate [1]. This means that the viscosity of blood is not constant but depends on the shear rate it experiences. Thus capillary viscometry is inadequate when investigating blood because the viscosity effectively varies across the bore of the capillary and what is measured is some shear-rate-averaged value. The problem is that the shear rate profile across the tube is not known and is impossible to predict unless the viscosity: shear rate relation of the blood is already known. What is required when investigating blood is a means of obtaining viscosity measurements at a unique shear rate, then to be able to change the shear rate and repeat the measurement, and to continue the process until the full viscosity: shear rate relationship is obtained. Only with this data is the blood fully rheologically characterized.

Hemorheologists usually obtain such data by making use of viscometers based on the bob-in-cup or cone-on-plate principles (see Figure 4.2). In these devices the blood is placed in the gap between the bob and cup or between the cone and plate. The arrangement of the system necessitates that when the cup or plate is rotated an approximately constant shear rate is generated across the blood sample, depending on the geometry of the system and the rate of rotation [1]. The rotation causes the blood to move and imposes a stress on the bob or the cone which is sensed by the suspensory system. With this data the viscosity of the blood at that shear rate can be

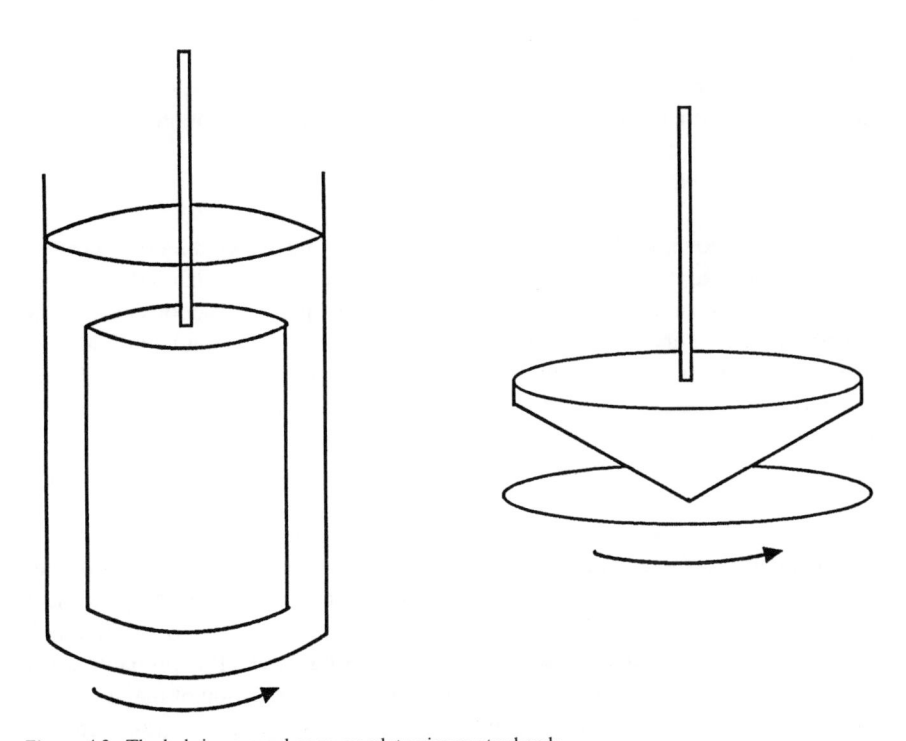

Figure 4.2. The bob-in-cup and cone-on-plate viscometer heads.

calculated. The measurement is then repeated at another rotational speed (and hence shear rate) and the viscosity redetermined; this is repeated until the required range of shear rates has been covered. Typical data generated in this way from a normal blood sample are shown in Figure 4.3a; it can be seen that the viscosity falls continuously as the shear rate increases, a phenomenon referred to as shear thinning. Replotting the same data on a double logarithmic plot simplifies it to reasonable bilinearity (Figure 4.3b).

Factors affecting blood viscosity

Shear rate

There are two principle causes of the shear thinning phenomenon just described, one responsible for the rapid low shear rate fall and the other for the slower high shear rate fall. To take the former first; at low shear rate the fall is due to the presence of plasma proteins which induces weak erythrocyte aggregation. This aggregation is of a peculiar form known as rouleaux and illustrated in Figure 4.3b, where the cells are seen to adhere face to face. The presence of these large aggregates at low shear produces a high viscometric drag and gives blood a high viscosity. As the shear rate increases the weak adhesive forces are overcome, the aggregates are disrupted, decrease in size, their drag is reduced and the viscosity falls. This is progressive until the system is effectively monodispersed at the point marked X on Figure 4.3b. The continuing small fall beyond X at high shear rate is due to the cells deforming into streamlined shapes as the shear rate increases, thus their viscometric drag is further reduced and the viscosity of the system continues to fall.

Rouleaux formation

As discussed above, rouleaux formation is a factor that affects blood viscosity at low shear rate and is caused by plasma proteins; it is now clear that only the larger proteins are rouleaugenic. Experiments using purified protein fractions have shown that fibrinogen is the most effective, followed by IgM, α_2-macroglobulin and IgG [10]. The effectiveness of fibrinogen in influencing low shear rate viscosity through rouleaux formation is illustrated Figure 4.4. This sensitivity is relevant because of the large variability of fibrinogen concentration in many pathologies.

While the quantitative relationships between the concentrations of plasma proteins and low shear rate blood viscosity are reasonably well established, a new problem is beginning to show itself: the inherent rouleaugenicity of red cells is variable. Until fairly recently it was assumed that in this respect all red cells were the same, but it is now evident that this is not the case and that erythrocytes from different subjects and within a given subject vary in their aggregability [11]. Nevertheless, it is still unclear what causes these differences. It is probably due to subtle variations in the cellular glycocalyx. Certainly degradation of the glycocalyx with trypsin or chymotrypsin dramatically increases cellular aggregation [12].

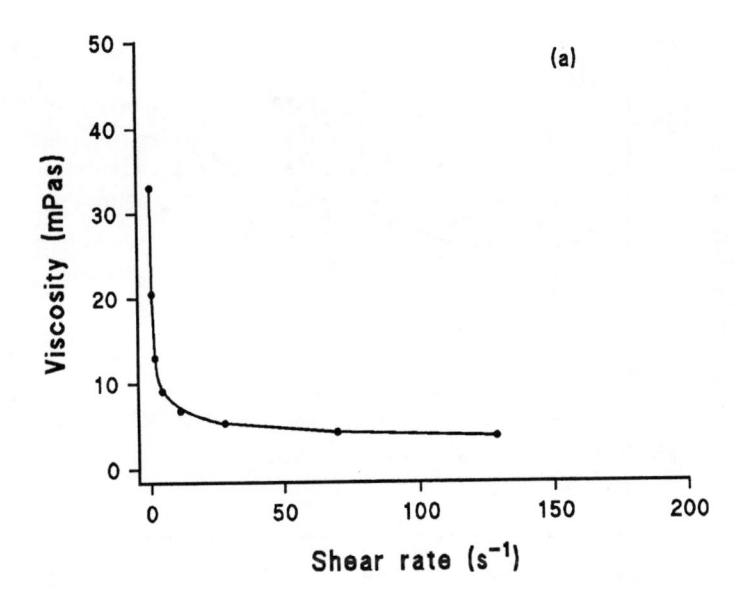

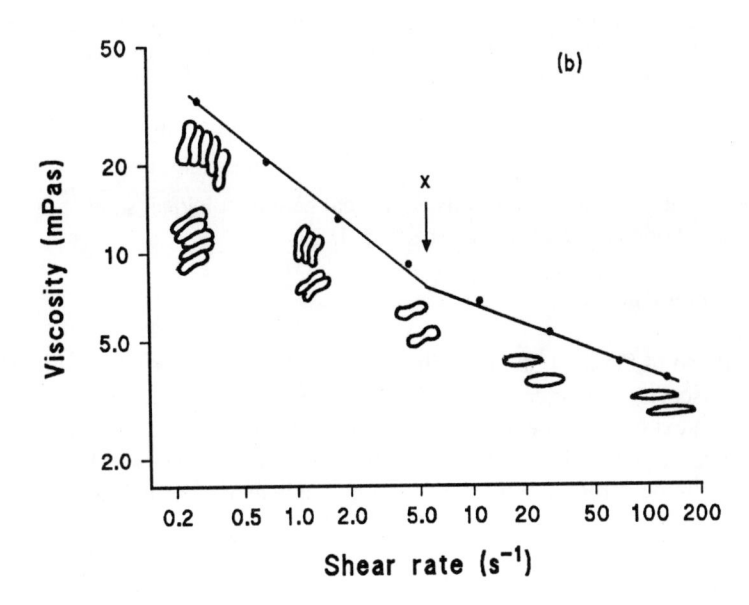

Figure 4.3. (a) The viscosity:shear rate relationship for a normal blood sample; (b) The same data plotted on log:log axes and illustrating the presence of rouleaux formation and red cell deformation.

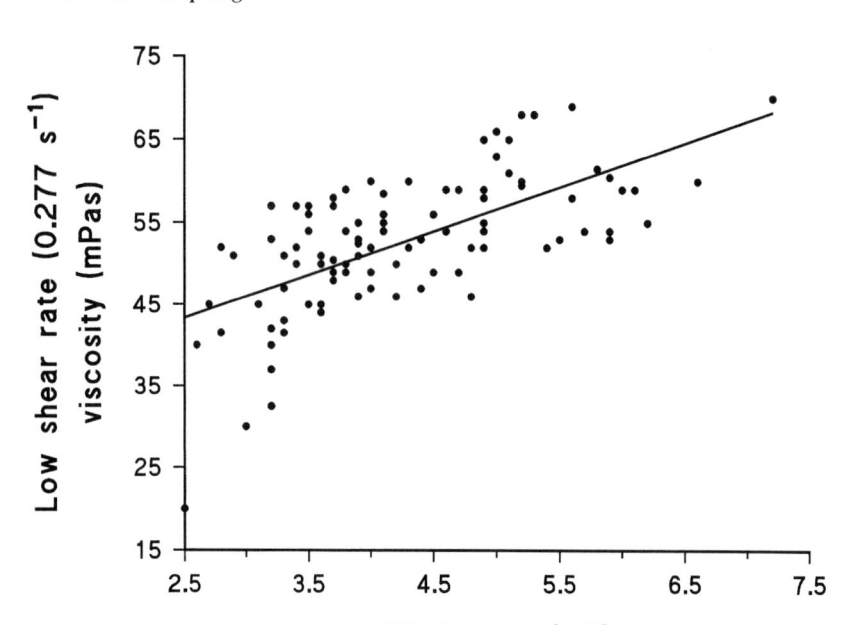

Figure 4.4. The relationship between low shear rate viscosity and fibrinogen concentration for a series of diabetic subjects. In each case the effect of hematocrit was removed by adjusting it to a standard of 45% by adding or subtracting autologous plasma.

Whether these variations in the cells are of real hemorheological significance or just a rheological oddity has yet to be ascertained.

Red cell deformability

As illustrated in Figure 4.3b, the ability of the red cell to deform contributes to the peculiar viscosity characteristics of blood. However, it is of little importance in the present context because the degree to which red cell deformability changes in most pathologies is too small to affect substantially the bulk viscosity of blood. Only in cases of extreme deformability change, for example deoxygenated sickle cells, does it have a significant effect.

Plasma viscosity

The sensitivity of plasma viscosity to protein concentration has been discussed above. This is of relevance to the viscosity of whole blood because any elevation in plasma viscosity almost inevitably leads to a rise in blood viscosity. The relationship is a simple one in that to a reasonable approximation they are proportional, for example an increase of 10% in plasma viscosity will of itself (ignoring protein-induced rouleaux formation) increase blood viscosity by about 10%.

Hematocrit

Hematocrit is the most potent of the factors affecting blood viscosity and the relationship between them is a relatively simple one over the normal range of hematocrits:

$$\log \eta = k_1 + k_2 H \tag{4.9}$$

where η is the viscosity of the blood, H the hematocrit and k_1 and k_2 are two shear rate dependent constants. This is illustrated in Figure 4.5. Thus, to a reasonable approximation, a change in hematocrit from 40 to 50% gives a viscosity increase of about 20% at a high shear rate of 100 s^{-1}, while at a low shear rate of 0.1 s^{-1} the increase is about 100%.

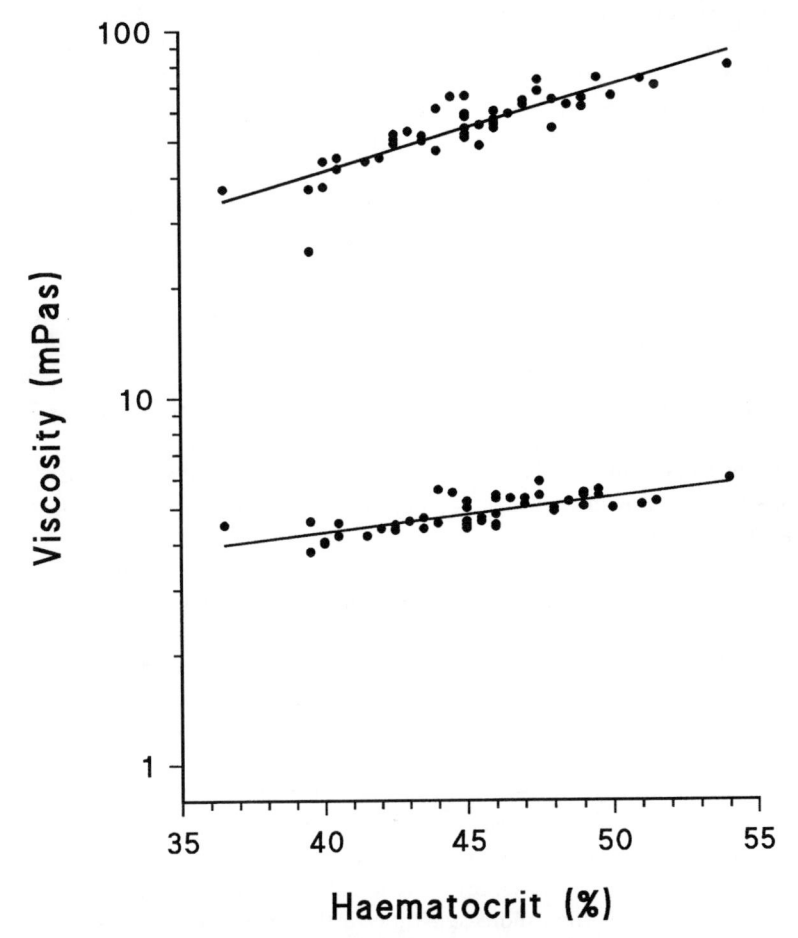

Figure 4.5. The relation between blood viscosity and hematocrit for a series of normal males. The upper line was measured at low shear rate (0.1 s^{-1}) and the lower line at high shear rate (100 s^{-1})

Temperature

Like any normal liquid, the viscosity of blood is temperature dependent, with a coefficient very similar to that of plasma and water (see above). Only in some unusual cases does it vary significantly from this, e.g. Raynaud's phenomenon [13]. Because of the tight control of body temperature, the temperature effect is not of great significance.

Large vessel flow

As shown above, the rate of flow of blood in large vessels depends on the geometric and viscous resistances. The geometric resistance depends on the state of dilatation of the vasculature and is not the subject of this chapter. The viscous resistance, however, depends on the averaged viscosity over the cross-sectional area of the vessel. Because blood viscosity varies with shear rate and because shear rate varies from 0 at the center of any vessel to between 100 and 800 s^{-1} at the wall of the vessel [14], the effective viscous resistance will be the viscosity averaged over this range of shear rates. Thus any factor increasing viscosity, such as elevated plasma viscosity, rouleaux formation, fibrinogen concentration or hematocrit will increase viscous resistance. Furthermore, because of the shear thinning property of blood, if the average shear rate falls viscous resistance will again rise.

Microvascular flow

What has been said above is valid for large vessel flow where the blood can be approximated to a continuous liquid and viscosity is a reasonable concept. However, the concept breaks down in the microcirculatory vessels where the radii become of similar size to the flowing cells, and blood is obviously a particulate suspension. At this level the rheological terms need to be considered individually. Another problem here is that the theory of flow is as yet poorly developed. However, experimental studies at this level allow some recognition of the importance of the rheological factors to microvascular flow. Thus, plasma viscosity is known to be a potent determining factor [15]. Hematocrit would also be expected to influence resistance at this level, but it is now clear that hematocrit is lower in the microvessels than in the systemic circulation [16], and thus makes a smaller contribution here to resistance. Another relevant red cell factor is rouleaux formation. The data here, however, are conflicting. There is evidence from tissue perfusion studies [17] that increasing rouleaux formation leads to reduced microvascular flow. However, there are other data from *in vitro* model systems [18] suggesting that it may enhance or reduce flow depending on vesssel orientation and flow rate.

Flow at this level is also more sensitive to the mechanical properties of the flowing cells. Thus it is here that the changes in the deformability of the red cell are considered to be relevant [19]. Finally, there are the leukocytes. They have no role to play in large vessel flow because of their low number concentration (1:700) compared with the erythrocytes, but at the microcirculatory level the situation is very different. This is due to: their deformability being some three orders of magnitude less than that of the red cell [20]; the great variability of their concentration in disease; and their ability to adhere to vascular endothelium, thereby partially occluding the lumen [14].

In vivo studies

There is now substantial evidence showing that hemorheological manipulation can alter both whole organ and whole body hemodynamics in line with the ideas developed above. There is space here only to touch on this. Thus, hemodilution and hemoconcentration have been shown to influence hemodynamics in the mesentery of the cat [21], changes in red cell deformability to affect pulmonary flow in the rat [22] and fibrinogen to alter myocardial flow in the rat [23]. In man, Dormandy [24] showed hemodilution to increase blood flow in the leg and Thomas *et al.* [25] demonstrated that it increases cerebral flow. Studies of patients undergoing therapeutic hemodilution have shown it to increase cardiac output and improve regional blood flow in adults [26] and in babies suffering from hyperviscosity syndrome [27]. Plasmapheresis in patients suffering from paraproteinemias leads to great improvement in hemodynamics associated with the alteration induced in the plasma viscosity [9]. These and other studies make it clear that alterations in the rheological properties of blood can have significant influences on hemodynamics *in vivo*.

References

1. Whitmore RL. Rheology of the circulation. Oxford: Pergamon Press, 1968.
2. Rampling MW. Effects of blood rheology on cardiac output. In: Salmasi AM, Iskandrian AS (eds), Cardiac output and regional blood flow in health and disease. Dordrecht: Kluwer, 1993:107–24.
3. Lowe GDO. Should plasma viscosity replace the ESR? Br J Haematol 1994;86:6–11.
4. International Committee for Standardisation in Haematology. Recommendation for the selected method for the measurement of plasma viscosity. J Clin Path 1984;37:1147–52.
5. Harkness J. The viscosity of human blood plasma; its measurement in health and disease. Biorheology 1971;8:171–93.
6. Rampling MW, Feher MD, Sever PS, Elkeles RS. Hemorheological disturbances in non-insulin-dependent diabetes and the effects of concomitant hypertension. Clin Hemorheol 1989;9:101–7.
7. Jay RH, Rampling MW, Betteridge DJ. Abnormalities of blood rheology in familial hyperchoesterolaemia: effects of treatment. Atherosclerosis 1990;85:249–56.
8. Yarnell JWG, Baker IA, Sweetman PM *et al*. Fibrinogen, viscosity, and white blood cell count are major risk factors for ischemic heart disease. Circulation 1991;83:836–43.
9. Somer T. Rheology of paraproteinaemias and plasma hyperviscosity syndrome. Bailliere's Clinical Haematology 1987;1:695–723.
10. Rampling MW. Red cell aggregation and yield stress. In: Lowe GDO (ed.), Clinical blood rheology. Vol I. Boca Raton: CRC Press, 1988:46–64.
11. Nash GB, Wemby RB, Sowemimo-Coker SO, Meiselman HJ. Influence of cellular properties on red cell aggregation. Clin Hemorheol 1987;7:93–108.

12. Rampling MW, Pearson MJ. Enzymatic degradation of the red cell surface and its effect on rouleaux formation. Clin Hemorheol 1994;14:531–8.
13. Goyle KB, Dormandy JA. Abnormal blood viscosity in Raynaud's phenomenon. Lancet 1976;i:1317–20.
14. Usami S. Physiological significance of blood rheology. Biorheology 1982;19:29–46.
15. Pries AP, Neuhaus D, Gaehtgens P. Blood viscosity in tube flow: dependence on diameter and haematocrit. Am J Physiol 1992;263:H1770–8.
16. Lipinsky HH, Usami S, Chien S. *In vivo* measurement of 'apparent viscosity' and microvessel haematocrit in the mesentery of the cat. Microvasc Res 1980;19:297–319.
17. Vicaut E, Hou X. *In vivo* effects of red cell aggregation on microcirculation in rat skeletal muscle. In: Stoltz JF (ed.), Hémorhéologie et agrégation érythocytaire. Vol 4. Cashan, Editione Médicale Internationale, 1994:131–5.
18. Alonso C, Pries AP, Gaehtgens P. Red blood cell aggregation and its effects on blood flow in the microcirculation. In: Stoltz JF (ed.), Hémorhéologie et agrégation érythocytaire. Vol 4. Cashan, Editione Medicale Internationale, 1994: 119–29.
19. Stuart J. Rheology of the haemolytic anaemias. In: Lowe GDO (ed.), Clinical blood rheology. Vol II. Boca Raton: CRC Press, 1988:43–65.
20. Chien S. White blood cell rheology. In: Lowe GDO (ed.), Clinical blood rheology. Vol I. Boca Raton: CRC Press, 1988:87–110.
21. Lipinsky HH, Farrel JC. Microvascular hemodynamics during systemic hemodilution and hemoconcentration. Am J Physiol 1986;250:H908–22.
22. Doyle MP, Galey WR, Walker BR. Reduced erythrocyte deformability alters pulmonary hemodynamics. J Appl Physiol 1989;67:2593–9.
23. Baskurt O, Edremitilioglu M. Myocardial tissue hematocrit: existence of a transmural gradient and alterations after fibrinogen infusions. Clin Hemorheol 1995;15:97–105.
24. Dormandy JA. Influence of blood viscosity on blood flow and the effects of low molecular weight dextran. Br Med J 1971;4:716–9.
25. Thomas DS, de Boulay GH, Marshall J. Cerebral blood flow in polycythaemia. Lancet 1977;ii:161–3.
26. Lowe GDO. Rheological therapy. In: Lowe GDO (ed.), Clinical blood rheology. Vol II. Boca Raton: CRC Press, 1988:1–23.
27. Maertzdorf WJ, Tangelder GJ, Slaaf DW, Blanco CE. Effects of partial plasma exchange transfusion on cerebral blood flow velocity in polycythaemic preterm, term and small for date newborn infants. Eur J Pediatr 1989;148:774–8.

5. The role of vascular endothelium in the modulation of coronary vasomotor tone

JUAN CARLOS KASKI

The vascular endothelium forms the biological interface between circulating blood and the various tissues of the body. For many decades, the vascular endothelium was considered to be a simple diffusion barrier. In recent years, however, *in vivo* and *in vitro* investigations have shown that the endothelium is a multifunctional organ, essential to vascular physiology [1]. The functions of the vascular endothelium are multiple and include: a selective permeability barrier, the expression of cytokines and growth regulatory agents, the modulation of vasomotor tone, and hemostatic balance. The endothelium also acts as a transducer of biomechanical forces. In the past 20 years, research and clinical studies have shed light on the role of the vascular endothelium in atherogenesis [2] and modulation of coronary blood flow [1]. The integrity of the endothelium is of extreme importance for vascular physiology, and it has become apparent that injury to the endothelium, whether local or generalized, results in endothelial dysfunction. This may be expressed as an imbalance of the thrombotic/thrombolytic equilibrium, abnormal vasomotion, increased monocyte adhesiveness and abnormal responses to biomechanical forces. It is not difficult to understand that due to its anatomic location, the vascular endothelium defines the intra and extravascular compartments and has the possibility of interacting dynamically with both circulating blood elements and underlying vascular smooth muscle cells. The endothelium senses biochemical signals that originate from the blood cells and reacts to these stimuli by releasing soluble products which affect the function of the cardiovascular system.

This chapter will focus on the role of the vascular endothelium in the modulation of coronary vasomotion.

The endothelium and coronary vasomotion

The modulation of vasomotor tone has been, for many years, considered to be dependent on the autonomic nervous system and several circulating hormones. It was not until 1980 that the 'obligatory' role of the endothelium in modulation of vascular tone became apparent. The pioneering work of Furchgott and Zawadzki [3] signalled a new era in the understanding of the pathophysiological role of this structure. These investigators described the essential role of the endothelium for modulation of the responses of the vascular smooth muscle to diverse stimuli. The original study by Furchgott and Zawadzki demonstrated that the vascular relaxation induced by acetylcholine was dependent on the presence of the endothelium; this provided evidence for the existence of an endothelium-derived relaxing factor. The original report by Furchgott and Zawadzki was followed by a multitude of studies which confirmed and expanded the observation of these investigators. For many years, the nature of the vasodilator substance produced by the intact endothelium remained unknown. Authors referred to this agent as 'endothelium-derived relaxing factor' (EDRF) [4]. In 1987 Moncada et al. [5] convincingly demonstrated that EDRF was nitric oxide [NO], a finding that represented a major breakthrough in the knowledge of vascular pathology. The elucidation of the chemical nature of EDRF triggered a large series of investigations which further contributed to the understanding of the role of the vascular endothelium in modulation of vasomotor tone.

Soon after the biochemical characterization of EDRF, the metabolic pathways that lead to formation of NO by the vascular endothelium were identified [6]. NO is synthesized from the terminal guanido nitrogen of L-arginine by the enzyme NO synthase (NOS) [6, 7]. NOS is a family of enzymes with three major isoforms, neuronal NOS (nNOS), endothelial NOS (eNOS) and inducible NOS (iNOS). nNOS and eNOS are calcium/calmodulin-dependent and are usually constitutively present in cerebellar neurons and in endothelial cells [7]. iNOS is independent of ionic calcium and its expression is induced in various types of cells, including vascular smooth muscle cells and myocytes. The availability of substances that block the production of NO by the endothelial cell has contributed to the fast advance of our knowledge in this area [8]. NO production can be inhibited by a number of L-arginine analogs substituted at one or both of the guanidino nitrogens, such as N^G-monomethyl-L-arginine (L-NMMA), N^G-nitro-L-arginine (L-NNA) and N^G-nitro-L-arginine methylester (L-NAME): all of these act through the inhibition of NOS [8].

The endothelium plays a key role in maintaining the vasoconstrictor/vasodilator balance of the cardiovascular system [1, 9]. In order to keep this balance, a series of constrictor and dilator substances are produced by the vascular endothelium, which modulate the function of the underlying vascular smooth muscle [10]. These substances also interact with other products of the vascular endothelium such as procoagulant substances and adhesion molecules [11]. The modulatory function of the endothelium is influenced by growth factors and cytokines also produced by the endothelial cell [11].

The intact, normal, vascular endothelium is a nonthrombogenic structure. This is mainly due to the balanced production by the endothelial cells of anticoagulant and thrombogenic agents. Prostacyclin, a potent inhibitor of platelet aggregation [12], protein C-thrombomodulin and tissue plasminogen activator 'compete' against the thrombogenic effects of platelet activating factor and tissue factor, among others, which are also produced by the endothelium [13, 14]. Factor V and plasminogen activator inhibitor-1 also exert prothrombotic effects. It is thus clear that the endothelium is capable of playing antagonistic roles, such as favouring and preventing thrombosis and exerting vasoconstrictor actions as well as potent vasodilator effects. Which of these antagonistic forces prevail at particular points in time will depend on the status of the endothelium and the characteristics of the stimuli acting on the vascular endothelium.

Endothelium-derived vasorelaxation

The endothelium can elicit vascular smooth muscle relaxations when stimulated by neurotransmitters, hormones, substances derived from platelets, circulating blood shear forces and components of the coagulation system. As mentioned previously the mediator of these responses is a diffusible substance with a half-life of a few seconds, the so-called endothelium-derived relaxing factor, which has recently been identified as the free radical nitric oxide [5]. NO is formed from L-arginine by oxidation of its guanidine-nitrogen terminal [6]. The catalyzing enzyme NO synthase is constitutively expressed and exists in several isoforms in endothelial cells, platelets, macrophages, vascular smooth muscle cells, and the brain [7].

Release of EDRF was observed under basal conditions as well as after stimulation with acetylcholine, thrombin, substance P, bradykinin, hypoxia, and increase in blood flow [1]. NO acts intracellularly by increasing levels of cyclic guanosine monophosphate which results in vasorelaxation. Other important actions of NO are inhibition of adhesion and activation of neutrophils and platelets as well as inactivation of oxygen free radicals [15–17]. NO synthesized in endothelial cells is released both intraluminally to inhibit leukocyte adhesion and to suppress platelet adhesion and activation, and abluminally to modulate vascular tone. Results from studies using NOS inhibitors, have shown a continuous basal release of NO from the vascular endothelium which produces a background vasodilator tone. Inhibition of NO synthesis with L-NMMA induces an endothelium-dependent constriction [6] of rabbit aortic rings and an increase in coronary perfusion pressure in the isolated rabbit heart [18]. Administration of L-arginine analogs induces an increase in blood pressure and decrease in coronary flow in various animal species including rabbit [9], guinea-pig and dog. In humans, infusion of L-NMMA into the brachial artery or coronary arteries also induces vasoconstriction [19]. Experimental studies recently reported indicate that mice lacking the gene for NOS are hypertensive, further supporting the notion that eNOS mediates baseline vasodilation [20].

Certain plasma proteins such as albumin may act as circulating reservoirs of NO. In platelets, an increase of intracellular $3'5'$-GMP is associated with reduced adhesion and aggregation [12]. Platelets release substances, such as adenosine diphosphate and triphosphate as well as serotonin, which activate the release of NO and prostacyclin from the endothelium [17]. Furthermore, thrombin also stimulates the formation of NO by the endothelium. Therefore, at vascular sites where platelets and the coagulation mechanisms are activated, the normal intact endothellal cells release NO which in turn causes vasodilation and platelet inhibition, preventing abnormal vasoconstriction and formation of thrombus. In addition to NO, prostacyclin is released by endothelial cells in response to stimuli such as shear stress, hypoxia, and several other substances that also release NO. Prostacyclin increases cyclic $3',5'$-adenosine monophosphate in smooth muscle and platelets [12, 21]. NO and prostacyclin synergistically inhibit platelet aggregation [21].

In the coronary circulation, not all endothelium-dependent relaxations are prevented by inhibitors of the L-arginine pathway. These NO-independent relaxations are even more prominent in intramyocardial vessels. Because vascular smooth muscle cells become hyperpolarized, a factor of yet unknown chemical structure has been proposed [10, 22, 23]. Indirect evidence suggests that it may be a product of the cytochrome P450 pathway, but C-type natriuretic peptide may also be a candidate [23].

The mechanism by which hyperpolarization causes relaxation is controversial. The most direct and obvious explanation is that hyperpolarization of the smooth muscle cell membrane inhibits the opening of voltage-dependent calcium channels, allows calcium sequestration and removal mechanisms to lower intracellular calcium, and leads to relaxation. Although this mechanism may operate in some blood vessels under some conditions, it does not fully explain the mechanism of relaxation [23].

In situations in which endothelium-dependent relaxations resistant to prostanoid and nitric oxide synthesis inhibitors are blocked by potassium channel antagonists or elevated potassium, hyperpolarization may be implicated in causing the relaxation. However, some studies suggest that the degree to which hyperpolarization contributes to relaxation may be small or nonexistent [23].

Endothelium-derived vasoconstriction

Soon after the discovery of endothelium-derived relaxing factors, it became clear that endothelial cells also can mediate contraction. Endothelium-derived contracting factors include the 21-amino acid peptide endothelin, vasoconstrictor prostanoids such as thromboxane A_2 and prostaglandin H_2, as well as components of the renin–angiotensin system.

Endothelin

Early studies demonstrated that the vasoconstrictor substance found in the culture medium of endothelial cells and called 'EDCF' was a peptide. In 1988, this peptide was purified and sequenced by Yanagisawa et al. [24] and was subsequently named endothelin-1 (ET-1). ET-1 is synthesized as a prepropeptide which is proteolytically cleaved to produce the 38 (human) or 39 (porcine) amino acid intermediate big ET-1. Big ET-1 is subsequently transformed by the endothelin converting enzyme (ECE) to the 21-amino acid ET-1. Analysis of human genomic sequences revealed that there are three different genes for ET, encoding three distinct ET peptides: ET-1, ET-2 and ET-3 [25]. All three ET isoforms have 21 amino acid residues. ET isoforms are produced in a variety of tissues and cell types. However, only ET-1 is produced by the endothelium. Although ET-1 was originally thought to be produced solely by endothelial cells, it has subsequently been shown to be produced by other cells such as vascular smooth muscle cells, cardiomyocytes, macrophages and bone marrow mast cells.

Several growth factors and cytokines such as TGFβ, TFNα and interleukin-1 have been shown to promote ET gene expression. ET-1 production can be inhibited by the NO donors nitroprusside and nitroglycerin and by atrial natriuretic peptide via a cGMP-dependent mechanism. ET-1 is mainly released abluminally and only a small proportion of the peptide enters the circulation. Thus circulating plasma levels of ET-1 are low. ET-1 acts primarily in a paraautocrine way. Enhanced plasma levels indicating release of ET-like immunoreactivity have been described in several cardiovascular pathophysiological conditions in both experimental animals and patients. Among these are unstable angina [26], myocardial infarction [27], congestive heart failure [28], atherosclerosis [29] and septic shock [30].

Two ET receptor subtypes, ET_A and ET_B have been cloned and characterized in mammalians [31, 32]. The ET_A receptor shows higher affinity for ET-1 and ET-2 than for ET-3, while the ET_B receptor has equal affinity for the three ET isoforms. Endothelial cells express only ET_B messenger RNA (mRNA) but vascular smooth muscle cells express both ET_A and ET_B mRNA. Both ET_A and ET_B receptors are present in human myocardium and coronary artery, but ET_A receptors predominate [33].

Constrictor mechanisms of endothelin

Activation of ET_A and ET_B receptors located on smooth muscle induces G-protein-mediated activation of phospholipase C, which in turn leads to rapid formation of inositol triphosphate and accumulation of diacylglycerol. This increases cytosolic free Ca^{2+} concentration by both mobilizing intracellular Ca^{2+} and enhancing the influx of extracellular Ca^{2+}, which induces contraction of the vascular smooth muscle [34]. Conversely, activation of endothelial ET_B receptors causes vasodilation through the release of NO and/or PGI_2 leading to formation of cGMP or cAMP, respectively, in the vascular smooth muscle.

Of relevance to modulation of coronary vasomotor tone, ET not only exerts direct vasoconstrictor effects but it has been shown that at subthreshold concentrations it also potentiates contractile responses to other vasoconstrictor substances such as norepinephrine and serotonin [35]. Thus, even small amounts of locally produced ET may act as a modulator of vascular tone. ET-1 administered exogenously is a potent vasoconstrictor of large and small coronary arteries and leads to myocardial ischemia in animal models.

Endothelial dysfunction and coronary risk factors – clinical assessment

When the endothelium becomes activated or injured, 'dysfunction' develops. Different stimuli may cause endothelial activation or dysfunction and these include hypoxia, viral infection, oxidized lipoproteins, oxygen free radical production, inflammation, etc. Endothelial cell activation or damage can be responsible for the initial stages of coronary atherosclerosis [36]. An activated endothelium will show prothrombotic activity [37], favour the release of cytokines [11], the expression of adhesion molecules [11, 38] and the production and release of diverse growth factors [11]. In the presence of endothelial damage, platelet aggregation will not be antagonized, leading to thrombus formation; abnormal vasoconstrictor may also develop. This may result in atheromatous plaque formation or growth, and myocardial ischemia.

In recent years it has become apparent that endothelial dysfunction may be responsible for a variety of cardiovascular syndromes and this is currently the subject of intense clinical research. Tests of endothelial function, using acetylcholine, substance P or sympathetic stimulation are now currently used in clinical practice with the aim of identifying early functional alterations of the vascular endothelium. In the clinical arena, these tests are useful to identify individuals who are more likely to develop rapidly progressing forms of coronary atherosclerosis and heart transplant rejection [39]. The observation that risk factors for coronary artery disease such as hypertension, diabetes, hyperlipidemia and smoking are associated with a generalized dysfunction of the vascular endothelium has lead to the development of noninvasive tests which, in the not too distant future may be useful for the detection of early endothelial dysfunction and the evaluation of different therapeutic agents. Acetylcholine, which exerts its vasodilatory action through the release of nitric oxide via the endothelial cell, has been the most widely used agent to assess the functional integrity of the endothelium, both experimentally and clinically. Other agents, such as substance P and serotonin, which also have a vasodilator effect in the presence of an intact endothelium, have been used. The vast majority of experimental and clinical studies have shown an inverse relationship between coronary atherosclerosis and endothelium dependent vasodilation [40–42]. Even early atherosclerotic changes may impair the function of the vascular endothelium. In humans, impaired endothelium dependent vasodilation has been observed even in the absence of angiographic coronary artery disease in patients with hypercholesterolemia [43]. Cholesterol lowering treatment has been shown to improve coronary endothelium dependent vasorelaxation [44].

It is likely that oxidized low density lipoproteins (LDL) are a major determinant of the alteration of endothelium dependent relaxations observed in patients with hyperlipidemia. In animal experiments, the presence of atherosclerosis and hypercholesterolemia is associated with a reduction of biologically active nitric oxide [45]. The administration of exogenous L-arginine has been shown to restore the abnormal endothelium dependent relaxation even in the presence of oxidized LDL. This suggests the possibility of a reduced availability of intracellular L-arginine for the formation of nitric oxide in this condition. Of interest is the observation that in experimental hypercholesterolemic rabbit aorta the overall production of nitric oxide is not reduced but markedly increased. NO, however, becomes inactivated by superoxide radicals produced by the endothelium.

Not only can a reduction in the availability of biologically active NO be responsible for the abnormal endothelial responses to vasodilating agents but also the increased production of constrictor peptides such as endothelin. Indeed, in the presence of hyperlipidemia and atherosclerosis, the production of endothelin is increased [46]. Again, it has been suggested that endothelin production in hyperlipidemic experimental models is triggered by oxidized LDL [47]. Oxidized LDL increases endothelin gene expression and stimulates the release of endothelin from pig vascular endothelial cells. As suggested by Luscher and Noll [47], oxidation of low density lipoproteins is a crucial process for the release of endothelin from atherosclerotic vessels. Vascular smooth muscle cells activated during the atherosclerostic process also produce endothelin. It has been shown that growth factors such as platelet-derived growth factor and transforming growth factor beta can stimulate the production of endothelin [48]. Of particular interest is the observation by Zeiher et al. [49] that complex coronary artery stenoses in patients with unstable angina have a high content of endothelin-1. These findings suggest that vascular endothelin may contribute to abnormal coronary vasomotion in patients with unstable angina. Endothelin may thus contribute to increased coronary vasoconstriction in atherosclerotic patients. Moreover, Kaski et al. [50] have recently observed that plasma endothelin-1 levels are increased in patients with microvascular angina (chest pain and normal coronary arteriograms). These findings indicate that endothelin may also play a role in the genesis of microvascular dysfunction, even in the absence of angiographic coronary artery disease.

The contribution of endothelial dysfunction to abnormal vasoconstriction in the presence of coronary artery disease is well established. However the role of a dysfunctional endothelium in the genesis of variant angina pectoris is more controversial. Kaski et al. [51] have observed that in patients with Prinzmetal's variant angina coronary artery spasm can be provoked by a variety of stimuli that act through different vascular receptors. It has also been shown that an abnormal reactivity of the vascular smooth muscle is a key element in the pathogenesis of human coronary artery spasm. The fact that coronary artery spasm usually develops at sites of atheroma has led to the hypothesis that endothelial dysfunction may be responsible for coronary artery spasm in patients. However, coronary artery spasm may also occur in the absence of atheroma, even when coronary artery disease is assessed with intravascular ultrasound or in post-mortem specimens. Moreover, coronary artery spasm as seen in variant angina patients is a rare entity, whereas coronary atherosclerosis can be found almost universally in adult humans. Toyooka et al. [52] reported that endothelin concentration is increased in the coronary sinus of patients with coronary artery spasm. Endothelin-1, being a potent coronary vasoconstrictor is a potential trigger of coronary artery spasm. However, the fact that endothelin usually acts mainly in the microvessels and also has a very prolonged vasoconstrictor effect makes it an unlikely cause of coronary spasm. Indeed, epicardial coronary artery spasm in variant angina develops rapidly and tends to resolve spontaneously within minutes. The possibility exists, however, that endothelin exerts its 'spasmogenic' action by facilitating the effects of other constrictor agents [35].

Future directions

Many questions remain open to further investigation regarding the mechanisms responsible for the endothelium-dependent vasodilation and contraction. Clinical application of tests of endothelial function may help to identify early stages of endothelial dysfunction and provide the basis for rational patient management [53–55].

References

1. Lüscher TF, Vanhoutte PM. The endothelium: modulator of cardiovascular function. Boca Raton: CRC Press, 1990.
2. Ross R. The pathogenesis of atherosclerosis: a perspective for the 1990s. Nature 1993;362:801.
3. Furchgott RF, Zawadzki JV. The obligatory role of endothelial cells in the relaxation of arterial smooth muscle by acetylcholine. Nature 1980;299:373.
4. Moncada S, Palmer RMJ. Gryglewski RJ. Mechanism of action of some inhibitors of endothelium-derived relaxing factor. Proc Natl Acad Sci USA. 1986;83:9164–9168.
5. Moncada S, Herman AG, Vanhoutte PM. Endothelium-derived relaxing factor is identified as nitric oxide. Trends Pharmacol Sci 1987;8:365–368.
6. Palmer RM, Ashton DS, Moncada S. Vascular endothelial cells synthesize nitric oxide from L-arginine. Nature 1988;333:664.
7. Bredt DS, Hwang PM, Snyder SH. Localization of nitric oxide synthase indicating a neural role for nitric oxide. Nature 1990;347:768.
8. Rees DD, Palmer RM, Schulz R et al. Characterization of three inhibitors of endothelial nitric oxide synthase in vitro and in vivo. Br J Pharmacol 1990;101:746.
9. Rees DD, Palmer RMJ, Moncada S. Role of endothelium-derived nitric oxide in the regulation of blood pressure. Proc Natl Acad Sci 1989;86:3375.
10. Vanhoutte PM. Other endothelium-derived vasoactive factors. Circulation 1993;87 (Suppl V):V9–17.
11. DiCorleto PE, Hassid A. Growth factor production by endothelial cells. In Ryan U (ed.). Endothelial cells. Boca Raton: CRC Press, 1990;51.
12. Moncada S, Vane VR. Pharmacology and endogenous roles of prostaglandin endoperoxides, thromboxane A2 and prostacyclin. Pharmacol Rev 1979;30:293.
13. Gimbrone MA Jr (ed). Vascular endothelium in hemostasis and thrombosis. Edinburgh: Churchill Livingstone, 1986.
14. Gimbrone MA Jr. Vascular endothelium: nature's blood-compatible container. Ann N Y Acad Sci 1987;516:5–11.
15. Wright CE, Rees DD, Moncada S. Protective and pathological roles of nitric oxide in endotoxin shock. Cardiovasc Res 1992;26:48.
16. Rapoport RM, Draznin MB, Murad F. Endothelium-dependent relaxation in rat aorta may be mediated through cyclic GMP-dependent protein phosphorylation. Nature 1983;306:174.
17. Cohen RA, Shepherd JT, Vanhoutte PM. Inhibitory role of the endothelium in the response of isolated coronary arteries to platelets. Science 1983;221:273.
18. Amezcua JL, Palmer RMJ, de Souza BM and Moncada S. Nitric oxide synthesized from L-arginine regulates vascular tone in the coronary circulation of the rabbit. Br J Pharmacol 1989;97:1119–24.
19. Vallance P, Collier J and Moncada S. Effects of endothelium-derived nitric oxide on peripheral arteriolar tone in man. Lancet 1989;ii:997–1000.
20. Huang PL, Huang ZH, Mashimo H et al. Hypertension in mice lacking the gene for endothelial nitric oxide synthase. Nature 1995;377:239–42.
21. Radomski MW, Palmer RM, Moncada S. Comparative pharmacology of endothelium-derived relaxing factor, nitric oxide and prostacyclin in platelets. Br J Pharmacol 1987;92:181.

22. Vanhoutte PM. The end of the quest? Nature 1987;327:459–60.
23. Cohen RA, Vanhoutte PM. Endothelium dependent hyperpolarization: beyond NO and cGMP. Circulation 1995;92:3337–49.
24. Yanagisawa M, Kurihara H, Kimura S et al. A novel potent vasoconstrictor peptide produced by vascular endothelial cells. Nature 1988;332:411.
25. Inoue A, Yanagisawa M, Kimura S et al. The human endothelin family, three structurally and pharmacologically distinct isopeptides predicted by three separate genes. Proc Natl Acad Sci USA 1989;86:2863–7.
26. Wieczorek I, Haynes WG, Webb D, Ludlans CA, Fox KAA. Raised plasma endothelin in unstable angina and non Q wave myocardial infarction: relation to cardiovascular outcome. Br Heart J 1994; 72:436–41.
27. Stewart DJ, Kubac G, Costello KB, Cernacek P. Increased plasma endothelin-1 in the early hours of acute myocardial infarction. J Am Coll Cardiol 1991;18:38–43.
28. Stewart DJ. Endothelin in cardiopulmonary disease: factor paracrine vs neurohumoral. Eur Heart J 1993; 14 (Suppl 1):48–54.
29. Lerman A, Edwards BS, Hallett JW et al. Circulating and tissue endothelin immunoreactivity in advanced atherosclerosis. New Engl J Med 1991;325:997.
30. Pernow J, Hemsén A, Hallén A, Lundberg JM. Release of endothelin-like immunoreactivity in relation to neuropeptide Y and noradrenaline during endotoxin shock and asphyxia in the pig. Acta Physiol Scand 1990;140:311–22.
31. Arai H, Hori S, Aramori I et al. Cloning and expression of a cDNA encoding an endothelin receptor. Nature 1990;348:730.
32. Sakurai T, Yanagisawa M, Takuwa Y et al. Cloning of a cDNA encoding a non-isopeptide-selective subtype of the endothelin receptor. Nature 1990;348:732.
33. Davenport AP, Oreilly G, Kuc RE. Endothelin ET(a) and ET(b) mRNA and receptors expressed by smooth muscle in the human vasculature: majority of the ET(a) sub-type. Br J Pharmacol 1995;114:1110–6.
34. Rubanyi GM and Vanhoutte PM. Superoxide anions and hyperoxia inactivate endothelium-derived relaxing factor. Am J Physiol 1986;250:H822–H827.
35. Yang Z, Richard V, Von SL et al. Threshold concentrations of endothelin-1 potentiate contractions to norepinephrine and serotonin in human arteries. A new mechanism of vasospasm? Circulation 1990;82:188.
36. DiCorleto PE, Chisolm GM. Participation of the endothelium in the development of the atherosclerotic plaque. Prog Lipid Res 1986;25:365–74.
37. Gimbrone MA Jr, Bevilacqua MP. Vascular endothelium: functional modulation at the blood interface. In: Simionescu N, Simionescu M, (eds), Endothelial cell biology in health and disease. New York: Plenum Press, 1988;255–73.
38. Pober JS, Cotran RC. Cytokines and endothelial cell biology. Physiol Rev 1990;70:427–51.
39. Fish RD, Nabel EG, Selwyn AP et al. Responses of coronary arteries of cardiac transplant patients to acetylocholine. J. Clin Invest 1998;81:21–31.
40. Gimbrone MA Jr. Endothelial dysfunction and atherosclerosis. J Card Surg 1989; 4:180–3.
41. Panza JA, Quyyumi AA, Brush JJ et al. Abnormal endothelium-dependent vascular relaxation in patients with essential hypertension. N Engl J Med 1990;323:22.
42. Ludmer PL, Selwyn AP, Shook TL et al. Paradoxical vasoconstriction induced by acetylcholine in atherosclerotic coronary arteries. N Engl J Med 1986;315:1046.
43. Zeiher AM, Drexler H, Saurbier B et al. Endothelium-mediated coronary blood flow modulation in humans. Effects of age, atherosclerosis, hypercholesterolemia, and hypertension. J Clin Invest 1993;92:652.
44. Anderson TJ, Meredith IT, Yeung AC, Frei B, Selwyn AP, Ganz P. The effect of cholesterol-lowering and antioxidant therapy on endothelium-dependent coronary vasomotion (see comments). N Engl J Med 1995; 332:488–93.
45. Tanner FC, Noll G, Boulanger CM et al. Oxidized low density lipoproteins inhibit relaxations of porcine coronary arteries. Role of scavenger receptor and endothelium-derived nitric oxide. Circulation 1991;83:2012.

46. Winkles JA, Alberts GF, Brogi E et al. Endothelin-1 and endothelin receptor mRNA expression in normal and atherosclerotic human arteries. Biochem Biophys Res Commun 1993;191:1081.
47. Luscher TF, Noll G. The endothelium in coronary vascular control. In: Braunwald E (ed.), Heart disease update 3. WB Saunders Company, 1995:1–12.
48. Kurihara H, Yoshizumi M, Sugiyama T et al. Transforming growth factor beta stimulates the expression of endothelin mRNA by vascular endothelial cells. Biochem Biophys Res Commun. 1989; 159:1435–40.
49. Zeiher AM, Ihling C, Pistorius K et al. Increased tissue endothelin immunoreactivity in atherosclerotic lesions associated with acute coronary syndromes. Lancet 1994;344:1405.
50. Kaski JC, Elliott PM, Salomone O et al. Concentration of circulating plasma endothelin in patients with angina and normal coronary angiograms. Br Heart J 1995; 74:620–4.
51. Kaski JC, Crea F, Meran D et al. Local coronary supersensitivity to diverse vasoconstrictive stimuli in patients with variant angina. Circulation 1986; 74:1255–65.
52. Toyo-oka T, Aizawa T, Suzuki N et al. Increased plasma level of endothelin-1 and coronary spasm induction in patients with vasospastic angina pectoris. Circulation 1991;83:476.
53. Drexler H, Zeiher AM, Meinzer K et al. Correction of endothelial dysfunction in coronary microcirculation of hypercholesterolaemic patients by L-arginine. Lancet 1991;338:1546.
54. Clozel M, Breu V, Burri K et al. Pathophysiologic role of endothelin revealed by the first orally active endothelin receptor antagonist. Nature 1993;365:759.
55. Celermajer DS, Sorensen KE, Gooch VM et al. Non-invasive detection of endothelial dysfunction in children and adults at risk of atherosclerosis. Lancet 1992;340:1111–15.

6. Cerebrovascular flow dynamics and pathophysiology

SUSAN B. SHERRIFF

The brain has a very high demand for oxygen and glucose and the most common cause of neurological deficit is cerebrovascular disease or accident. An abrupt incident of vascular insufficiency lasting more than a few minutes results in necrosis or *infarction* of the brain and is called an *ischemic stroke*. A bleed into or immediately adjacent to the brain is called a *hemorrhagic stroke* and usually results from the spontaneous rupture of small penetrating arteries. Other vascular problems include aneurysms and congenital malformations such as arteriovenous anastomoses. Aneurysms, balloon-like swellings of the arterial wall, are most commonly found in the anterior half of the circle of Willis and cause neurological deficit by compressing brain structures or by rupture. Arteriovenous malformations increase in size with age, have a low resistance, and can cause neurological deficit either by stealing blood from adjacent tissue or by rupturing. However, in most industrialized countries, ischemic conditions caused by embolic and thrombotic events account for around 70% of all cerebrovascular disease [1] and will be the focus of this chapter.

The etiology of transient ischemic attacks (TIAs) and ischemic stroke is explained by two hypotheses: the embolic theory and the hemodynamic concept. In the former, emboli emanating from irregular atherosclerotic plaques, often located in the extracranial carotid arteries, are carried along in the bloodstream and occlude the distal circulation of the brain; in the latter, a critical stenosis produces symptoms by reducing cerebral blood flow.

Blood supply to the brain

Familiarity with the intracranial and extracranial vasculature is essential in order to understand both hemodynamic changes and clinical neurological manifestations produced by cerebrovascular disease. The arterial supply to the brain is derived from two pairs of vessels, the internal carotid arteries and the vertebral arteries (Figure 6.1); the main trunks arise from the aortic arch and, except for the origins and proximal portions of these trunk vessels, the arterial supply is symmetrical. Venous drainage occurs through a system of superficial and deep veins which empty via the dural venous sinuses into the internal jugular vein.

64   Susan B. Sherriff

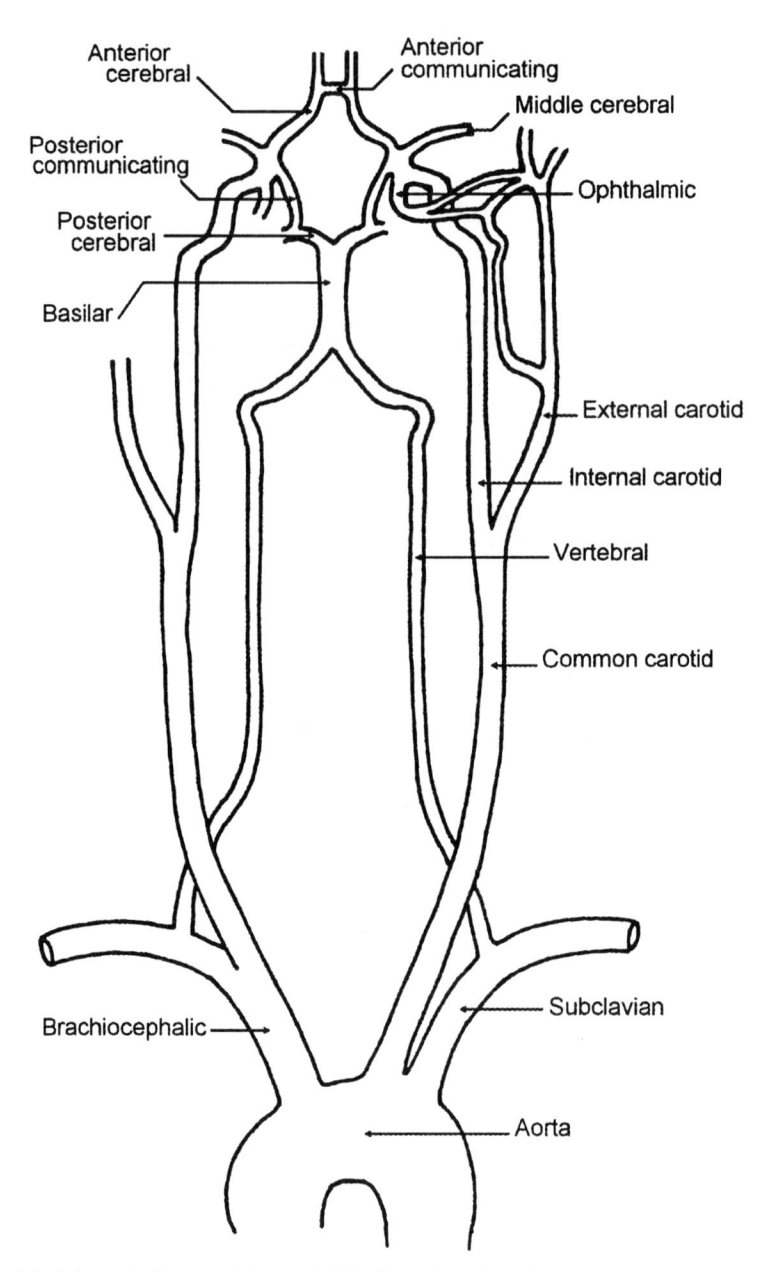

Figure 6.1. Schematic diagram of the arterial blood supply to the brain.

On the right side the brachiocephalic artery arises from the aorta and after a short distance divides to supply the arm, via the subclavian artery, and the head, via the common carotid artery. On the left the subclavian and common carotid artery originate independently from the aortic arch. Each common carotid artery passes obliquely upwards behind the supraclavicular joint to the level of the upper border of the thyroid cartilage where it divides into an internal carotid artery and an external carotid artery. At its point of division the vessel shows a dilatation, termed the carotid bulb, which usually involves the proximal part of the internal carotid artery.

The external carotid artery supplies blood to the structures of the face scalp and neck and via its numerous branches provides an important collateral pathway to the brain. The internal carotid artery supplies the greater part of the cerebral hemisphere, the eye and its accessory organs and sends branches to the forehead and nose. It ascends to the base of the skull without giving off any branches, enters the skull through the canal of the temporal bone, curves anteriorly medially and then posteriorly to pierce the dura mater at the medial side of the anterior clinoid process. At this point the internal carotid artery gives off the ophthalmic artery which enters the optic foramen inferior to the optic nerve. The internal carotid then gives off two small branches, the anterior choroidal artery and the posterior communicating artery, before dividing into the middle cerebral and anterior cerebral arteries.

Although the subclavian arteries primarily supply the upper limb they also give rise to the vertebral arteries which ascend through the foramina in the transverse processes of the upper six cervical vertebrae, wind behind the lateral mass of the atlas, enter the skull through the foramen magnum and at the lower border of the pons join with the vessel of the opposite side to form the basilar artery. This in turn divides to form the posterior cerebral arteries and supplies structures in the posterior portion of the cranial cavity.

Communication between the vertebral and carotid artery systems is accommodated by the circle of Willis which lies at the base of the brain. The arteries of the circle of Willis branch into a network of arteries that supply the surface of the brain. They also give rise to many very small thin walled branches, the penetrating arteries, which supply the deep structures of the brain.

Collateral circulation

Collateral circulation is a term used to describe blood flow in the subsidiary vascular channels that are present throughout the circulatory network and which provide a secondary defence mechanism against failure of the primary vessels. The brain is protected by a number of extracranial and intracranial collateral system, the main ones being:

- anastomoses between the major extracranial arteries;
- anastomotic connections between the external carotid artery and the intracranial system via the ophthalmic artery;
- the intracranial system of the circle of Willis; and
- the intracerebral leptomeningeal anastomoses of Heubner [2].

In chapter 1 we showed that blood flow, Q, is a function of the pressure gradient, ΔP, and the resistance, R:

$$P_i - P_o = Q\left(\frac{8l\eta}{\pi r^4}\right) \text{ i.e. } Q = \frac{\Delta P}{R}.$$

The pressure differential across the site of an obstruction is the most significant factor in the opening of collateral channels. The distal decrease in blood pressure is transmitted throughout the territory of the next major branch of the obstructed primary artery; this lowered blood pressure induces the opening of anastomotic channels between the branch arteries and adjacent arteries, retrograde flow into the branch artery and then into the obstructed artery occurs, and blood flow is maintained. The total vascular resistance in the cerebrovascular system is a combination of the resistance in the main extracerebral conducting vessels and the resistance in the penetrating intracerebral vessels. When an artery in the cerebral circulation is severely obstructed or occluded and the pressure in the artery distal to the obstruction is decreased, a compensatory autoregulatory dilation of the intracerebral arteries occurs with a resultant reduction in the resistance of the peripheral bed. If an artery from another source is in anatomical continuity with the distal low resistance zone then blood flow through this collateral artery will increase.

The rich anastomotic channels between the carotid and vertebral arteries provide a powerful collateral system but the potential for collateral blood flow sharply decreases in the more distal segments of the cerebral circulation. Hence, the more distal the occlusion the more liable it is to cause dysfunction or infarction. The most important intracranial anastomoses are those of the circle of Willis. Ordinarily there is little flow from one side to the other or between the posterior and anterior segments. However in the case of either basilar or internal carotid artery occlusion the posterior communicating arteries may become extremely important conduits for collateral blood flow; in addition circulation across the midline may occur via the proximal portions of the anterior cerebral arteries and the anterior communicating artery. Like all anastomoses the circle of Willis is of potential rather than actual value because it does not open up rapidly.

The parenchymal arteries of the intracerebral circulation are essentially end arteries. The collateral blood supply is therefore poor and depends almost entirely on the network of leptomeningeal anastomoses on the surface of the brain. The adequacy of this system depends on the number and vascular tone of the anastomotic channels, the viscosity of the blood, and the perfusion pressure; the perfusion pressure being a function of intracranial pressure and systemic blood pressure.

The provision of anastomotic conduits together with changes in pressure gradient across the anastomotic connections allows blood to be diverted from a region of normal perfusion to a region of ischemia. These diversions occur in both the extracranial and the intracerebral circulations. The diversion, known as a 'steal', may result in adverse symptoms in the original non-ischemic region [3].

Hemodynamics and atherogenesis

The mechanics of pulsatile flow in arteries has been discussed in chapter 1. There is a strong belief, apparently first advanced by Rindfleich in 1872, that there is an association between the distribution of atherosclerosis in arteries and the local arterial blood pressure and flow [4–7].

The forces that can deform the elastic walls of arteries include the pressure and shear stress exerted by the blood, the tension developed by the smooth muscle of the wall, and the tethering imposed by surrounding tissue. Wall shear appears to influence the dimensions of the arteries [8] and the orientation morphology structure and metabolism of endothelial cells [9–11]. Wall shear also influences transintimal transport and at high levels can cause endothelial damage [12, 13]. As was discussed in chapter 1 the velocity field in arteries is complex; this produces complicated movements of the blood cells and determines their interaction with the vessel wall, particularly in respect of platelets and sites where the vessel wall is abnormal [14]. At low shear rates the erythrocytes and platelets aggregate; in laminar flow this aggregation occurs in the centre of the vessel, and dissaggregation of the erythrocytes occurs as they move into an area of high shear close to the vessel wall [15]. However aggregates of platelets do not dissaggregate as they move close to the vessel wall but may be mechanically damaged and become even more adhesive [16].

The growth of atherosclerotic plaques occurs at certain favoured sites in the vascular tree and is related to the uneven distribution of hemodynamic stresses. Areas of predilection include the inner wall of a curved segment [17], and the proximal lip of a branch [4]. The flow region adjacent to these sites is generally a region of low wall shear stress in which the flow may be separated or turbulent; pulsatile flow provokes marked oscillations in the direction of wall shear, and the residence time of blood products and toxins increases. Such flow conditions exist on the outer wall of the carotid bulb. Lesions also develop in regions of relatively high wall shear such as those along the medial walls of bifurcations, at the flow divider [17].

Atherosclerotic plaque development

The arterial wall consists of three concentric layers: the intima, the media and the adventitia (Figure 6.2). The intima is a single row of endothelial cells lying on a thin musculo-elastic lamella. The cells form a continuous permeable barrier between the blood in the vessel and the arterial wall and provide a blood compatible surface that minimizes the probability of coagulation and blood cell adherence. Progressive intimal thickening occurs with growth and is of particular note in areas such as bends and bifurcations where hemodynamic forces produce mechanical stress [18]. Loss of endothelial continuity compromises thromboresistance and contributes to the development of atherosclerotic plaque. The media is the arterial muscle; it is elastic in the subclavian and common carotid arteries and muscular in the other cerebral arteries. If the smooth muscle cells in the media are subjected to hemodynamic stress they may proliferate and migrate into the intima [19]. The adventitia is a layer of loose connective tissue containing fibroblasts and adipose tissue and penetrated by small vessels, the vasa vasorum.

Atherosclerosis is the most common cause of occlusive disease in the cerebrovascular system. It affects both large elastic and medium-sized muscular arteries and is defined by the World Health Organization as 'a variable combination of

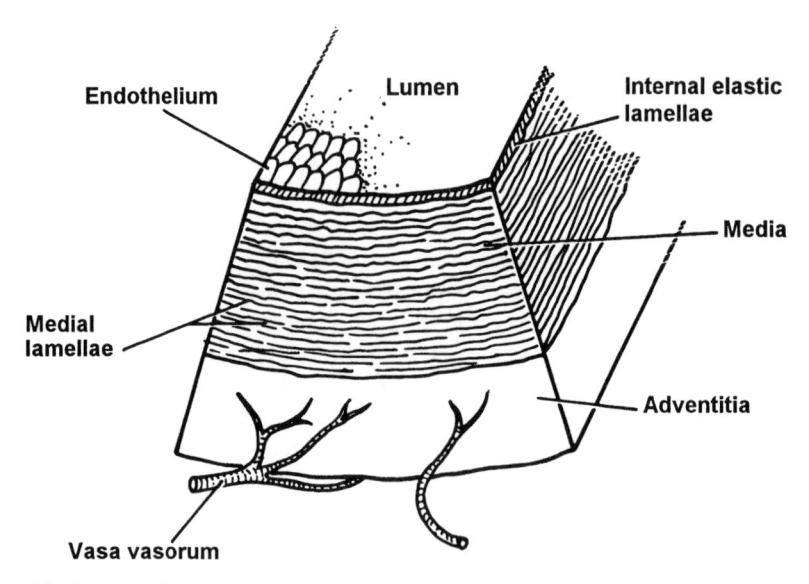

Figure 6.2. Structure of the arterial wall.

intimal changes consisting of the focal accumulation of lipids, complex carbohydrates, blood and blood products, fibrous tissue and calcium deposits, and associated with changes in the media' [20]. A necessary precursor of atherosclerosis is the presence of nodular irregularly distributed yellow fatty streaks involving the intima of the vessel. The initial pathological finding appears to begin as an abnormal infiltration of lipid into the intimal cells; this may progress to an uncomplicated fibrous plaque, which can regress or remain static [21]; or it may develop into a complicated atheromatous lesion. Uncomplicated plaques are located in the intima of the artery and consist of a central acellular lipid core, containing cholesterol and cell debris, separated from the lumen by a fibrous cap. The media underlying the plaque is usually thinned and richly vascularized by ingrowth from the vasa vasorum. Complicated atheromatous plaques are characterized by the occurrence of one or more events (Figure 6.3): subintimal necrosis; calcification; loss of intimal continuity, or ulceration; intraluminal thrombus formation; and hemorrhage into the plaque.

Calcification

Calcification appears as small aggregates or as a large well-defined plate in the fibrous rim of the atherosclerotic plaque. Calcification is present in most advanced lesions and together with a hemorrhage beneath the plate may result in stenosis [22]. However, although calcification is considered to be a complication of atherosclerosis it is less likely to provoke cerebral ischemic events than a soft plaque [23].

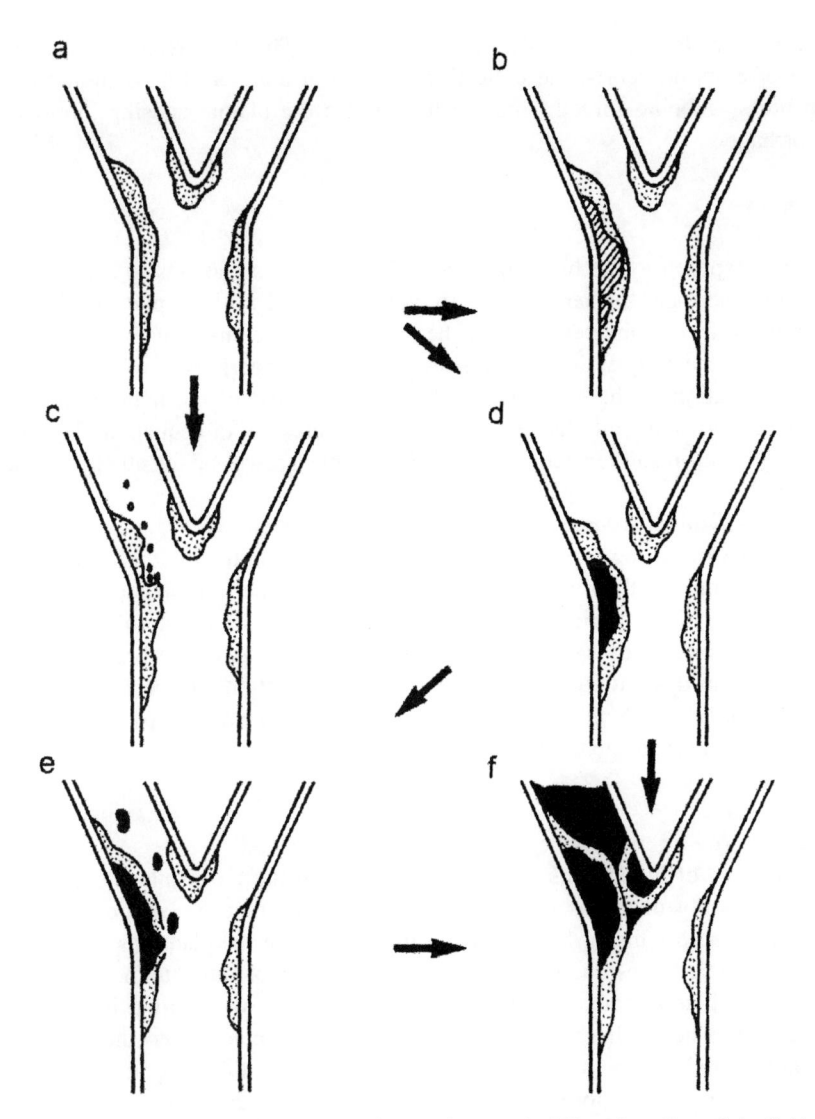

Figure 6.3. Carotid plaque development: (a) fibrous plaque at the bifurcation; (b) acellular lipid core, containing cholesterol and cell debris, separated from the lumen by a fibrous cap; (c) loss of intimal continuity causing ulceration, aggregation of fibrin and platelets on the roughened surface and possible fibrinoplatelet emboli; (d) hemorrhage into the plaque; (e) subintimal necrosis and release of fragments of thrombus; (f) total occlusion.

Ulceration

If the fibrous cap covering a plaque is broken, ulceration results; the cause is obscure although several explanations have been proposed including hemorrhage, inflammation and mechanical stress. The ulcer erodes down into the fibrous plaque and lipid core thus exposing it to the bloodstream. This then results in the emergence of embolic debris, the collection of a fibrin platelet plug, or blood under high pressure being forced from the lumen into the plaque causing intraplaque hemorrhage.

Thrombus

Collagen exposed to the blood by loss of intima causes platelets to adhere to the roughened surface, further platelets to aggregate, and a fibrinoplatelet plug or a thrombus to form. Three events may then take place: the thrombus becomes incorporated into the plaque, the surface slowly heals with overgrowth of fibrous tissue and regeneration of the endothelium; the whole or part of the material becomes dislodged, forms an embolus and causes distal occlusion; or sequential deposition of platelets, fibrin and red cells occurs, the thrombus grows and eventually occludes the vessel.

The most widely accepted hypothesis for the pathogenesis of transient ischemic attacks (TIA) resulting from involvement of structures in the internal carotid territory is the embolic theory [24, 25]. Embolization of the intraplaque hemorrhage debris, or the friable fibrin platelet plug, or the release of cholesterol and calcium from an ulcerated area within a plaque may fall on areas of the brain and cause transient brain dysfunction; or they may lead to infarction and permanent neurological changes by heaping further insult on a brain already poorly perfused secondary to a severe stenotic carotid plaque.

Hemorrhage

Large masses of blood cells can accumulate within the raised plaque. There are two theories postulated as to how this happens. The first explanation is that as blood flows across the surface of the protruding plaque the plaque is subjected to increasing shear forces; these mechanical stresses are transmitted to the neovascular base of the plaque causing rupture of the delicate newly grown intimal vasa vasorum. The hemorrhage then causes bulging of the plaque into the lumen, increasing arterial obstruction, ulceration and secondary to this, thrombosis [26, 27]. The second and now more accepted theory is that rupture of the vasa vasorum cannot produce significant accumulation of blood inside the plaque; instead the hemodynamic forces on the plaque, particularly at the shoulder, cause the fibrous cap to fracture, blood from within the vessel lumen enters the plaque through the fissure in the cap and intramural hemorrhage results [28].

Several investigators have demonstrated that intraplaque hemorrhage is frequently present in plaques harvested from the carotid territory at surgery [22, 26, 27, 29]. The observations of these workers suggest that intraplaque hemorrhage may occur at any time in the history of a carotid plaque but that they occur with greater frequency when the stenosis compromises the arterial lumen by more than 40%. Some hemorrhages lead to sudden changes in the stenosis, causing a reduction in blood flow to the brain to below the critical level for adequate perfusion.

Stenoses

In clinical terms stenoses can be divided into two groups: those that reduce the total blood flow, and those that do not [30]. A hemodynamically or pressure significant stenosis is one where the lumen narrowing is such that further small decrements in luminal area result in an abrupt reduction in pressure and flow distal to the stenosis. In the carotid system it is thought that this 'critical' stenosis occurs when there is a reduction in inter-lumen diameter of 50%, corresponding to a cross-sectional decrease of 75% [31, 32]. This degree of narrowing is the basis for the hemodynamic theory of transient ischemic attacks [33]; however, provided an adequate collateral system exists, a flow or pressure reducing lesion of 50% diameter loss is unlikely to be the sole cause of a transient ischemic attack. Significant compromise in blood flow is more likely to occur when the degree of stenosis exceeds 75% of the vessel diameter.

Atherosclerosis may involve the origins of the common carotid, vertebral and subclavian arteries [34] but the carotid bifurcation, and in particular the origin of the internal carotid and that portion of the common carotid adjacent to it, is the site in the extracranial vessels most frequently involved [35] and is thought to be the source of a major proportion of all strokes [36, 37]. The intracranial lesions having the greatest impact on brain dysfunction are those involving the middle cerebral, basilar or internal carotid arteries.

References

1. Kannel WB. Epidemiology of cerebrovascular disease. In: Ross Russel RW (ed.), Cerebral arterial disease. Edinburgh: Churchill Livingstone, 1976;1–23.
2. Van der Eecken HM, Adams RD. The anatomy and functional significance of the meningeal arterial anastamoses of the human brain. J Neuropath Exp Neurol 1953;12:132–57.
3. Toole JF, McGraw CP. The steal syndromes. Annu Rev Med 1975;26:321–9.
4. Caro CG, Fitzgerald JM, Schroter RC. Arterial wall shear and distribution of early atheroma in man. Nature 1969;223:1159–60.
5. Gessner FB. Haemodynamic theories of atherogenesis. Circ Res 1973;23:259–66.
6. Zarins CK, Giddens DP, Bharadvaj BK, Sottiurai VS, Mabon RF, Glagov S. Carotid bifurcation atherosclerosis: quantitative correlation of plaque localization with flow velocity profiles and wall shear stress. Circ Res 1983;53:502–14.
7. Ku DN, Giddens DP, Zarins CK, Glagov S. Pulsatile flow and arteriosclerosis in the human carotid bifurcation. Positive correlation between plaque location and low and oscillating shear stress. Arteriosclerosis 1983;5:293–302.
8. Kamiya A, Tagawa T. Adaptive regulation of wall shear stress to flow change in the canine carotid artery. Am J Physiol 1980;239:H14–21.
9. Dewey CF. Effects of fluid flow on living vascular cells. J Biomech Eng 1984;106:31–5
10. Nerem RM, Levesque MJ. The case for fluid dynamics as a localizing factor in atherogenesis. In Schetter G, Nerem RM, Schmid-Schonbein H, Morl H, Diehm C, (eds). Fluid dynamics as a localizing factor for atherosclerosis. Berlin: Springer-Verlag 1983.
11. Frangos JA, Eskin SG, McIntyre LV, Ives CL. Flow effects on prostacyclin production by cultured human endothelial cells. Science 1985;227:1477–9.
12. Fry DL. Certain histological and chemical responses of the vascular interface to acutely induced mechanical stress in the aorta of the dog. Circ Res 1969;24:93–108.

13. Stehbens WE. Fluid dynamic approaches to atherosclerosis. In: Schetter G, Nerem RM, Schmid-Schonbein H, Morl H, Diehm C (eds), Fluid dynamics as a localizing factor for atherosclerosis. Berlin: Springer-Verlag, 1983.
14. Born GVR. Haemodynamic influences on platelets in haemostasis and thrombosis. In: Schettler G, Nerem RM, Schmid-Schonbein H, Morl H, Diehm C (eds), Fluid Dynamics as a localizing factor for atherosclerosis. Berlin: Springer-Verlag, 1983.
15. Schmid-Schonbein H. Factors promoting and preventing the fluidity of blood. In: Effros RM, Schmid-Schonbein H, Ditzel J (eds), Microcirculation. New York: Academic Press, 1981:249–66.
16. Wood JH, Kee DB Jr. Hemorrheology of the cerebral circulation in stroke. Stroke 1985;16:765–72.
17. Texon M, Imparato AM, Helpern M. The role of vascular dynamics in the development of atherosclerosis. JAMA 1965;194:1226–30.
18. Robertson JH. Stress zones in foetal arteries. J Clin Pathol 1960;13:133–9.
19. Ross R. Smooth muscle cells and atherosclerosis. In: Moore S, (ed.), Vascular injury and atherosclerosis. New York: Marcel Dekker, 1981:53–7.
20. World Health Organisation Study Group. Classification of atherosclerotic lesions. WHO Tech Rep Ser 1958;143:1–20.
21. Hennerici M, Rautenberg W, Trockel U, Kladetzky RG. Spontaneous progression and regression of small carotid atheroma. Lancet 1985;1415–9.
22. Persson AV, Robichaux WT, Silverman M. The natural history of carotid plaque development. Arch Surg 1983;118:1048–52.
23. Johnson JM, Kennelly MM, Decesare D, Morgan S, Sparron A. Natural history of asymptomatic carotid plaque. Arch Surg 1985;120:1010–2.
24. Fields WS. Selection of patients with ischaemic cerebrovascular disease for arterial surgery. World J Surg 1979;3:147–54.
25. Thiele BL, Young IV, Chikos PM, Hirsch JH, Strandness DE. Correlation of arteriographic findings with symptoms in patients with cerebrovascular disease. Neurology 1980;30:1041–6.
26. Imparato AM, Riles TS, Gorstein F. The carotid bifurcation plaque: pathologic findings associated with cerebral ischaemia. Stroke 1979;10:238–42.
27. Lusby RJ, Ferrell LD, Ehrenfeld WK. Carotid plaque haemorrhage: its role in the production of cerebral ischaemia. Arch Surg 1982;117:1479–88.
28. Capron L. Extra and intracranial atherosclerosis. In: Vinken PJ, Bruyn GW, Klawans HL (eds), Handbook of clinical neurology. Toole JF, co-editor. Vascular disease, part 1. Amsterdam: Elsevier Science, 1988;53:91–106.
29. Dixon S, Pais SO, Raviola C. Natural history of nonstenotic asymptomatic ulcerative lesions of the carotid artery. A further analysis. Arch Surg 1982;117:1493–8.
30. Strandness DE, Sumner DS. Haemodynamics for surgeons. New York: Grune and Stratton, 1977.
31. Berguer R, Hwang NHC. Critical arterial stenosis: a theoretical and experimental solution. Ann Surg 1974;180:39–50.
32. De Weese JA, May A, Lipchik EO, Rob CG. Anatomic and hemodynamic correlations in carotid artery stenosis. Stroke 1970;1:149–57.
33. Eastcott HHG, Pickering GW, Rob GC. Reconstruction of the internal carotid artery in a patient with intermittent attacks of hemiplegia. Lancet 1954;2:994–9.
34. Wylie EJ, Ehrenfeld WK. Extracranial occlusive cerebrovascular disease, diagnosis and management. Philadelphia: Saunders, 1970.
35. Health D, Smith P, Harris P, Winson M. The atherosclerotic human carotid sinus. J Pathol 1973;110:49–58.
36. Thompson JE, Talkington CM. Carotid surgery for cerebral ischemia. Surg Clin N Am 1979;59:539–53.
37. Ammar AD, Wilson RL, Travers H, Lin JJ, Farha SJ, Chang FC. Intraplaque haemorrhage: its significance in cerebrovascular disease. Am J Surg 1984;148:840–3.

7. Stroke epidemiology and risk factors

MUNTHER I. ALDOORI, PETER A. GAINES and JONATHAN D. BEARD

Stroke is one of the most devastating of human illnesses and the most common life-threatening neurological disease [1]. Although stroke is more often disabling than lethal, it is still the third most common cause of death in the Western world after coronary heart disease and cancer [2, 3]. According to a consensus statement on stroke, 'Every five minutes someone in the United Kingdom has a stroke' [4]. Stroke patients occupy around 10% of bed-days in the NHS and account for about 5% of health-care expenditure [5]. At 12 months after stroke onset, about 25% of patients will be dead and a further 30% will be reliant on the help of others for at least some of their activities of daily life [6]. The mortality from stroke has been declining worldwide over the last 30 years. In the UK the overall mortality from stroke fell about 20% between 1976 and 1986 but it is still double that in the USA [4]. The decline in mortality is most probably multifactorial, but has occurred in tandem with a reduced incidence of death from rheumatic and coronary heart disease and the improved control of hypertension [7]. The decline in mortality seems to be slowing, and stroke will remain a major health problem for the foreseeable future [5].

Epidemiology of stroke

Epidemiology is defined as 'the study of the distribution and determinants of disease frequency' in the human population [8]. Stroke epidemiology has lagged behind coronary heart disease due to the diversity in stroke pathology (atherothrombotic, embolic and hemorrhagic) (Tables 7.1 and 7.2) and because in the majority of previous cohort studies, stroke was diagnosed clinically and rarely confirmed by CT scanning. The reported incidence of stroke may not be accurate for a number of reasons. Low post-mortem rate resulted in both over and under reporting of stroke mortality in death certificates, even in the Framingham study [9]. Sudden death is rarely caused by stroke and when it is, it is more likely to be due to intracranial hemorrhage than infarction. Whether some patients who died suddenly were certified as stroke rather than coronary death is unclear [1]. On the other hand late mortality from stroke might be attributed to other causes such as pneumonia.

A.-M. Salmasi and A. Strano (eds), Angiology in Practice, 73–86.
© 1996 Kluwer Academic Publishers. Printed in Great Britain.

Table 7.1. First time stroke diagnosed by CT scan.

Types of stroke	
Ischemic (thromboembolic)	80%
Intracerebral hemorrhage	10%
Subarachnoid hemorrhage	5%
Uncertain cause	5%

(Oxfordshire Community Stroke Programme 1981–1986 [63].)

Incidence of mortality for stroke patients

The Oxford prospective community study showed that in the UK the incidence of stroke is about 2 per 1000 per annum. About 100 000 patients have a first stroke every year [6]. Interestingly, the incidence of stroke in the Oxford Study is more or less similar to the incidence of stroke in other industrial countries using similar prospective community based studies [1]. The incidence of all three main types of stroke (thromboembolic, primary intracerebral hemorrhage and subarachnoid hemorrhage) increases with age [1]. About half of strokes occur above the age of 75 and only a quarter occur below the age of 65 [1]. There is evidence that the mortality associated with stroke is declining [7]. The reasons for decreasing stroke mortality could be related to decreasing incidence and/or improved prognosis. Recent studies showed that this is probably due to improved survival rather than a decline in incidence [10, 11].

Racial, socio-economical and geographical variation

Black people have a higher incidence of stroke and mortality than caucasians. Age adjusted incidence rates were 1.5 times higher for black men and 2.3 times higher for black women, while age adjusted stroke mortality for blacks was nearly double that for whites [8]. The Northern Manhattan stroke study in 1995 showed that intracranial atherosclerosis was more frequent in blacks and Hispanics, while the proportion of extracranial atherosclerotic strokes was not different to that in white residents. Patients with intracranial disease were significantly younger and had an increased frequency of hypercholesterolemia and insulin-dependent diabetes [12]. Orientals have been known to have a low rate of coronary heart disease and a high prevalence of stroke. This is usually attributed to the high incidence of hypertension and the low level of blood lipids which were associated with hemorrhagic stroke. It is now well established that infarction, not hemorrhage is the most frequent stroke mechanism in Japanese and accounts for two-thirds of stroke events in Japan and in Japanese people in Hawaii [8]. However, intracerebral hemorrhage is still higher in the Japanese than in the American whites or blacks.

Stroke mortality is greater in deprived than in affluent areas, and among the unemployed [13], and in lower compared with higher social classes [14]. Geographical variations in mortality from ischemic heart disease and stroke in

Table 7.2. Cause of ischemic strokes.

Atheromatous thromboembolism of cerebral vessels	50%
Lamunar infarct	25%
Embolization from the heart	5%
Miscellaneous	5%

(Oxfordshire Community Stroke Programme 1981–1986 [69].)

England and Wales have persisted for decades but are poorly explained [15]. Baker *et al.*, working in Southampton, introduce the fetal origin hypothesis, which states that 'retardation in intrauterine growth increases the risk for adult diseases, such as diabetes mellitus, cardiovascular diseases and hypertension' [16]. Barker and Osmond [17] showed that poor maternal and infant health are associated with increased mortality from stroke some time later. The same group reported a high ratio of placental weight to fetal weight (placental ratio) at birth and linked this with essential hypertension [17]. Recent studies have not supported the hypothesis that higher placental ratios are a marker of poor maternal nutrition [18]. Perry *et al.* [18] showed that placental ratio was similar in European, Asian and Afro-Caribbean women despite the evidence of poor nutrition among pregnant Asian Women in Birmingham. The placental ratio was increased due to obesity. Other factors influence placental weight such as maternal diabetes, maternal smoking and gestational age [16]. If the fetal theory is correct, twins should have higher mortality from cardiovascular diseases. Twins are on average more than 900 g lighter than single children at birth. Christensen *et al.* [19] showed no difference in mortality among twins and the general population. Barker *et al.* [20] suggested that the low mortality from stroke in Greater London could be attributed to the migration of relatively well nourished young women into domestic service in the capital earlier this century, who later gave birth to babies who were healthier than those of mothers who had not migrated.

A recent study [21] showed a low risk of fatal stroke among non-immigrants in Greater London which also occurred among these people who migrated to London during 1939–1971. This shows that the low mortality from stroke in Greater London cannot be fully explained by better fetal development of infants born in London to selectively healthy domestic workers who migrated from the countryside in the early part of this century, as has been previously hypothesized by Barker *et al.* [20].

Seasonal and diurnal variation

Stroke mortality (and probably incidence) is higher in winter than summer [22]. This could be related to higher blood pressures in winter and also to increased associated stroke complications such as pneumonia in winter [23]. It has been shown that ischemic stroke frequently occurs in the morning (usually one or two hours after waking) [24] while hemorrhagic stroke is more likely to occur during strenuous activities [25].

Risk factors and stroke prevention

Epidemiological studies have elucidated the major risk factors for stroke. The importance of a particular risk factor to an individual is expressed in terms of the relative risk (the risk of disease occurrence in a group of individuals exposed to the factor compared with the incidence in individuals not exposed), and the absolute risk (the incidence of disease in those exposed to the risk factor minus the incidence in those not exposed). The importance of particular risk to the community depends not only on the relative and absolute risks but also the occurrence of the risk factor in the community; this is expressed as the population attributable risk which estimates the proportion of stroke in a community resulting from the effects of a particular risk factor [1, 5]. For example, the relative risk of stroke for patients with rheumatic atrial fibrillation is very high, but as rheumatic heart disease is now very rare, this is thus a very rare cause of stroke in developed countries. On the other hand mild hypertension does not carry a high relative risk but is very common and therefore has a high population attributable risk.

Major modifiable risk factors

Hypertension

Hypertension is the paramount risk factor for stroke. Patients with blood pressure less than 140/90 mmHg are considered normotensive. Mildly hypertensive patients are those with a blood pressure between 140/90 and 160/95 mm/Hg. Elevated levels of both systolic and diastolic blood pressure have been shown to be associated with increased risk of stroke in many studies [5], and hypertension represents the single most important risk factor for stroke after age [5].

Recent review of nine prospective studies including more than 418 000 patients with a mean follow-up of ten years showed that the risk of stroke increased in an exponential manner as diastolic blood pressure increased in the range 70–110 mmHg. A 7.5 mmHg rise in diastolic blood pressure, within the range of 70–110 mmHg was associated with a doubling of the risk of stroke [26]. The relationship with systolic blood pressure is similar and possibly stronger [15]. Even isolated systolic blood pressure is associated with increased risk [27]. A striking beneficial effect of blood pressure reduction on stroke incidence in isolated systolic hypertension has been reported [28]. Recent randomized, controlled trials in the drug treatment of mild diastolic hypertension (95–110 mmHg) confirmed that, over an average treatment of 2 years, an average reduction of 6 mmHg in diastolic pressure resulted in a relative reduction of 40% in the risk of stroke and in a 5% reduction in the risk of coronary heart disease [29]. The risk of stroke is related to the level of blood pressure throughout its range with no critical cut-off value of systolic or diastolic below which there is no association with stroke. Hypertension increases stroke risk, probably by increasing the extent and severity of atheroma [30] and because of the prevalence of microvascular disease in small penetrating arteries within the brain [31]. Hypertension is more common in patients with TIAs than in the normal population but it is not clear whether controlling hypertension reduces the incidence of TIAs.

Cigarette smoking

It is now generally accepted that cigarette smoking increases the risk of atherothrombotic stroke and subarachnoid hemorrhage, but the relationship between cigarette smoking and primary intracerebral hemorrhage is less well established [1]. Analysis of the Framingham Heart Study cohort of 4255 men and women showed that after 26 years follow-up, cigarette smoking was a risk factor for stroke in both normotensive and hypertensive subjects, in women as well as men. Furthermore, the risk of stroke increased with the increasing number of cigarettes smoked. Stroke risk decreased significantly two years after cessation of smoking and reached the non-smoker level by five years [32]. A similar association was reported in the prospective Honolulu Heart Program Study. After 12 years follow-up of 7872 Hawaiian men of Japanese ancestry, cigarette smokers had two to three times the risk of thromboembolic or hemorrhagic stroke than non-smokers [33].

Shinton and Beevers in [34], in a meta-analysis of 32 separate studies, showed that cigarette smoking was an independently significant contributor to stroke incidence in both sexes and at all ages. The overall relative risk (RR) of stroke associated with cigarette smoking was 1.5 (95% confidence interval 1.4 to 1.6). The risk of stroke is far greater in younger people (< 55 years, RR = 2.9; 55–74 years RR = 1.8; and > 75 years RR = 1.1). The greatest relative risk [2.9] was of subarachnoid hemorrhage, followed by cerebral infarction (1.9). Smoking has been related to the extent of extracranial carotid disease in patients selected for angiography and in those studied by ultrasound scanning [35, 36]. Spagnoli *et al.* performed a study of carotid plaque morphology and showed that in smokers the plaques were frequently complicated by mural thrombi [37]. Other studies showed that only current smoking was associated with increased risk for stroke [38, 39]. Donnan *et al.* [40] showed that passive smoking is associated with a slight increase in the risk of stroke.

Hyperlipidemia

Law *et al.* [41] combined data from 10 large cohort studies covering nearly half a million men. A 10% lowering of plasma cholesterol concentration was associated with a 25% difference in coronary heart disease.

The relationship between cholesterol, lipid fractions and stroke is less clear cut, but there is almost certainly some interaction [42]. A recently published overview, based on 10 prospective studies, found a significant association between plasma cholesterol > 5.7 mmol/L and risk of cerebrovascular disease [43]. The Copenhagen City Heart Study showed that the risk of ischemic stroke was increased only with plasma cholesterol concentrations > 8 mmol/L [44].

Data from a prospective study of more than 350 000 men (90% white) who were screened as part of the Multiple Risk Factor Intervention Trial (MRFIT), demonstrated that deaths caused by stroke showed a U-shaped relation with total serum cholesterol concentration. The highest mortality was in those with a concentration < 4.2 mmol/L (hemorrhagic stroke) and > 7.74 mmol/L (ischemic stroke) [45]. For those who died from intracranial hemorrhage, the death was significant only in people with diastolic blood pressure above 90 mmHg. The relationship between low total serum cholesterol and increased incidence of intracerebral hemorrhage was initially observed in the Japanese, who generally had a lower serum cholesterol level than the European Standard. However, this link has been observed in oriental populations other than the Hawaiian and Japanese. Recent cohort studies from Norway [46] and Finland [47] showed that controlling hypertension, cessation of smoking and lowering cholesterol all reduced mortality from stroke.

There are fears that lowering blood cholesterol concentrations may increase the risks of non-cardiovascular death. Marmot [42] suggested that lowering cholesterol concentrations may not be effective and may even be harmful in anyone other than men at high risk. Recent cohort studies of 7735 men aged 40–59 years followed up for 14.8 years (range 13.5–6 years) have shown that the association between the excess risk of cancer and other non-cardiovascular disease and lower blood cholesterol concentrations (< 4.8 mmol) was produced by the existence of preclinical cancer, chronic ill health, smoking and heavy alcohol drinking. The excess of death in men with lower cholesterol levels occurred in the first five years of follow-up and became non-significant with longer follow-up. Non-cancer mortality was related to respiratory and liver disease which most probably resulted from smoking and excessive alcohol drinking respectively [48, 49].

Risk factors with potential for modification but uncertain benefit

Truncal obesity

The relationship between obesity and coronary heart disease is controversial. Recent studies have suggested that the pattern of obesity is important, with central obesity and abdominal deposition of fat more strongly associated with atherosclerosis [50]. The adverse effect of obesity on health is probably mediated through elevated blood pressure, impaired glucose tolerance and other factors such as hypercholesterolemia [51]. In the Whitehall Study of 17,753 men aged 40 to 64 years the risk of death for overweight men was more apparent in younger subjects and non-smokers[52].

Alcohol consumption

Mild to moderate consumption of alcohol is associated with a reduced incidence of coronary heart disease [1]. Available evidence indicates an adverse effect of heavy alcohol consumption on stroke incidence [53, 54]. Cardiac rhythm disturbances (especially atrial fibrillation) occur with alcohol intoxication [15]. Stroke, both thrombotic and subarachnoid hemorrhage, can be precipitated by acute alcohol intoxication in young people [55, 56]. In the Honolulu Heart Program, alcohol consumption was an independent risk factor for both subarachnoid and intracerebral hemorrhage, but not for thromboembolic stroke [57]. In summary the role of recent heavy alcohol consumption as a risk factor of ischemic stroke is unclear.

Physical activity

In a study of 17 000 former Harvard students those who were more physically active had about half the risk of fatal coronary heart disease and one-third the mortality rate of their least active fellow alumni. Vigorous exercise may exert a beneficial influence on the risk factors for atherosclerosis by reducing blood pressure, body weight, pulse rate and low density lipoprotein cholesterol and by improving glucose tolerance and increasing high density lipoprotein cholesterol [58].

Impaired glucose tolerance

The Whitehall study showed that a blood glucose concentration > 5.4 mmol/L two hours after a 50-g oral glucose load was independently associated with risk of stroke [59]. Data from the Framingham study suggest that both men and women of all ages with glucose intolerance have approximately double the risk of ischemic stroke than people with normal glucose tolerance [8].

Raised hematocrit and serum fibrinogen

The relationship between increasing hematocrit and risk of stroke is weak and confounded by cigarette smoking, blood pressure and plasma fibrinogen [60]. Increased concentration of red cells in combination with high blood fibrinogen levels increases blood viscosity. A number of epidemiological studies have shown a substantial and significant independent impact of fibrinogen on the incidence of coronary heart disease and stroke. The association is attenuated by cigarette smoking and other confounding variables [43]. At least part of the adverse vascular effect of smoking is mediated by increasing fibrinogen level in the circulation [61]. However, it is far from clear that raised fibrinogen is causally related to stroke. There is also a suggestion that mild elevation of the hematocrit is associated with good outcome [62].

Risk factors not easily modified

Age

Age is the strongest risk factor for atherothrombotic and hemorrhagic stroke including their subtypes. Two-thirds of strokes occur above the age of 75. Age is also a risk factor for transient ischemic attacks (TIAs) [63].

Sex

There is only a slight excess of stroke in males which is most prominent in middle age. A similar pattern is found for TIAs [64].

Diabetes mellitus

This is a predisposing factor for atherosclerosis in general, but has also strong association with cerebral infarction. It doubles the risk of stroke compared with non-diabetic patients and carries a higher mortality. It is not clear whether strict control of diabetes reduces the risk of stroke [63].

Cardiac disorders

Acute myocardial infarction is a causal factor for stroke [1]. Anterior wall infarcts are more likely to lead to stroke than transmural infarcts at other sites [65]. Embolization of a mural thrombus is a more likely cause than coincidental atheroma in the coronary and cerebral circulation in the same patient [65]. Silent myocardial infarction, non-Q wave infarct and angina pectoris are associated with an increased risk of stroke.

Left ventricular hypertrophy

Left ventricular hypertrophy (LVH) is an independent risk factor for myocardial infarction and death in men and women with hypertension and in asymptomatic subjects with normal blood pressure [66]. Asymptomatic LVH increases with age and the risk of cerebral infarction is increased by more than four-fold in men and six-fold in women with abnormal ECG pattern [8]. Such patients are at a high risk of mortality including cardiac death [66].

Atrial fibrillation

Atrial fibrillation is the most frequent potential cardiac source of embolism to the brain [1]. It is the most common cardiac arrhythmia in the elderly and is associated with a 5.6-fold increase in stroke incidence [8]. Some of the association between atrial fibrillation and stroke incidence may be coincidental as atrial fibrillation can be caused by coronary and hypertensive heart disease, both conditions being associated with stroke by mechanisms other than embolization [67].

Peripheral vascular disease

Claudicants are at risk of both myocardial infarction and stroke. The relative risk of stroke mortality among claudicants is about three times higher than in non-claudicants [68].

Other important risk factors

Transient ischemic attacks

A TIA is defined as an acute loss of focal cerebral or monocular function with symptoms lasting < 24 hours which, after adequate investigation, is presumed to be due to embolic or thrombotic vascular disease [1]. This definition is widely accepted by clinicians and it includes amaurosis fugax (transient monocular blindness) which has a more favorable prognosis than hemispheric TIAs [70]. There is little difference between TIAs and minor stroke as they have similar pathology, pathogenesis, prognosis and subsequent risk of major stroke, myocardial infarction and death [70]. It is difficult to determine the exact incidence of TIAs as they can be unrecognized by physicians and unreported by patients. Community based studies suggest that the annual incidence of TIAs is around 5 per 1000 [64]. The risk of stroke is higher during the first year after TIA (a figure of 11.6–13% has been reported [64]. The annual risk of stroke is estimated at 6% for the first five years [64]. The risk of stroke and/or death (including myocardial infarction) is approximately 10% per annum after a TIA.

Asymptomatic carotid stenosis

It has been estimated that about 4% of the general population over the age of 50 years have carotid murmurs [71]. Carotid murmurs were thought to be an indicator of diffuse vascular atherosclerosis with a relation to myocardial infarction and death [72, 73]. Two-thirds of the patients with carotid murmurs have detectable carotid stenosis by non-invasive testing [74]. Previous angiographic studies showed that about half the patients had at least 50% stenosis of the internal carotid artery [75]. Non-invasive duplex scanning studies showed that asymptomatic patients with severe (> 75% luminal reduction) carotid stenosis had an annual stroke rate of 5% [76] two-thirds of the strokes being ipsilateral to the stenosed carotid artery. There is evidence that soft, non-calcified, echolucent atheromatous plaques may be more likely to cause a stroke whereas calcified or fibrous echodense plaques on ultrasound are thought to be stable and of less sinister significance [77].

Contraceptive pill

Prospective cohort studies have suggested that women on the contraceptive pill have an attributable risk for a fatal stroke of two and for non-fatal strokes, up to five times that for women not on the contraceptive pill [78]. It has been reported that taking the oral contraceptive pill tripled the risk of strokes in young women (including hemorrhagic strokes) [79]. The danger of the contraceptive pill is greater in women above the age of 35 who smoke cigarettes and suffer from hypertension [80]. The modern oral contraceptives with lower estrogen content probably carry a lower risk of stroke [81]. Three studies are currently examining whether the risk of vascular disease in women taking the newer oral contraceptive pill (the so-called

Table 7.3. Risk factors for stroke.

Major modifiable risk factors:
  Hypertension
  Cigarette smoking
  Hyperlipidemia

There is potential for modification, but uncertain benefit:
  Truncal obesity
  Alcohol consumption
  Physical activity
  Impaired glucose tolerance
  Raised hematocrit and serum fibrinogen

Risk factors not easy to modify:
  Age, sex and genetic factors
  Diabetes mellitus
  Cardiac disorders

Other important risk factors:
  Transient ischemic attacks
  Asymptomatic carotid stenosis

Minor modifiable risk factors:
  Contraceptive pills
  Deficiency of fresh fruit and vegetables
  Excessive salt intake
  Snoring etc.

third generation progestogens, desogestrel and gestodene) differs from that in women taking slightly older pills containing predominantly the progestogen levonorgestrel. The expectation was that they would probably have a lower risk of myocardial infarction and stroke. Unfortunately the unpublished data suggest that they might be associated with an increased risk of venous thromboembolism (15 per 100 000) [82, 83].

Summary

The most important, modifiable risk factors for stroke are hypertension, smoking and hyperlipidemia. By controlling these factors the risk of stroke can be reduced (Table 7.3).

References

1. Warlow C. Disorders of cerebral circulation. In: Walton J, (ed.), Brain's diseases of the nervous system. Oxford: Oxford University Press, 1993:197–210.
2. Yatsu FM, Fisher M. Atherosclerosis: Current concepts on pathogenesis and interventional therapy. Ann Neurol 1989;26:3.

3. Oxford Community Stroke Project 1983. Incidence of stroke in Oxfordshire: First year's experience of a community stroke register. Br Med J 1988;287:713–6.
4. Shaper AG, Phillips AN, Pocock SJ, Walker M, Macfarlawe PW. Risk factors for stroke in middle aged British men. Br Med J 1991;302:111–5.
5. Dunbabin D, Sandercock P. Stroke prevention. Hosp Update 1992;July:540–5.
6. Bamford J, Sandercock P, Dennis M, Burn J, Warlow CP. A prospective study of acute cerebrovascular disease in the community. The Oxfordshire Community Stroke Project 1981–1986. 1. Methodology, demography and incident cases of first ever stroke. J Neurol Neurosurg Psychiat 1988;51:1373.
7. Whisanant JP. The decline of stroke. Stroke 1984;15:160–8.
8. Wolf AP, Cobb JL, D'Agustine RB. Epidemiology of stroke. In: Barnett HJ, Bennett MS, Mohr JP, Yatsu FM (eds), Stroke: Pathopysiology, diagnosis and management. New York: Churchill Livingstone, 1992:3–27.
9. Crowin LI, Wolf PA, Kannel WB, McNamara PM. Accuracy of death certification of stroke. The Framingham Study. Stroke 1982;13:818.
10. Modan B, Wagener DK. Some epidemiological aspects of stroke: Mortality/morbidity trends, age, sex, race, socioeconomic status. Stroke 1992;23(9):1230–6.
11. Harmsen P, Tsipogianni A, Wilhelmsen L. Stroke incidence rates were unchanged while fatality rates declined, during 1971–1987 in Goteborg, Sweden. Stroke 1992;23(10):1410–5.
12. Sacco RL, Kargman DE, Gu Q, Zamanillo MC. Race – ethnicity and determinants of intra-cranial atherosclerotic cerebral infarction. The Northern Manhatten Stroke Study. Stroke 1995;26(1):14–20.
13. Franks PJ, Adamson C, Bulpitt PF, Bulpitt CJ. Stroke death and unemployment in London. J Epidemiol C Health 1991;45:16.
14. Acheson RM, Williams DRR. Does consumption of fruit and vegetables protect against stroke? Lancet 1983;1:1191.
15. Shaper AG, Phillips AN, Pocock SJ, Walker M, Macfarlane PW. Risk factors for stroke in middle aged British men. Br Med J 1991;302:111.
16. Pameth N, Sugger M. Early origin of coronary heart disease (the 'Barker Hypothesis'). Hypothesis, no matter how intriguing, needs rigorous attempts at refutation. Br Med J 1995;310:411–2.
17. Barker DJP, Osmond C. Death rates from stroke in England and Wales predicated from post maternal mortality. Br Med J 1987;295:83–6.
18. Perry I, Beevers DG, Whincup PH, Bareford D. Predictors of ratio of placental weight to fetal weight in multiethnic community. Br Med J 1995;310:436–8.
19. Christensen K, Vaupel JW, Holm NV, Yashin AI. Mortality among twins after age 6: Fetal origins hypothesis versus twin method. Br Med J 1995;310:432–5.
20. Barker DJP, Osmond C, Pannett B. Why Londoners have low death rates from ischaemic heart disease and stroke. Br Med J 1992;305:551–4.
21. Strachan DP, Leon DA, Dodgeon B. Mortality from cardiovascular disease among interregional migrants in England and Wales. Br Med J 1995;310:423–7.
22. Haberman S, Capildeo R, Rose FC. Sex differences in the incidence of cerebrovascular disease. J Epidemiol Commun Health 1981;35:45.
23. Shin Kawa A, Veda K, Hasuo Y, Kiyohara Y, Fujishima A. Seasonal variation in stroke incidence in Hisayama, Japan. Stroke 1990;21(9):1262–7.
24. Argentino C, Toni D, Rasura M. Circadian variation in the frequency of ischaemic stroke. Stroke 1990;21(3):387–9.
25. Wroe SJ, Sandercock P, Bemford J. Diurnal variation in the incidence of stroke. The Oxfordshire Community Stroke Project. Br Med J 1992;304:155.
26. McMahon S, Peto R, Cutler J et al. Blood pressure, stroke and coronary heart disease. Part 1. Lancet 1990;335:765–74.
27. Rowe JW. Systolic hypertension in the elderly. N Engl J Med 1983;309:1246.
28. Collins R, Peto R, MacMahon S et al. Blood pressure, stroke and coronary heart disease. Part II. Lancet 1990;335:827–38.

29. SHEP Cooperative Research Group Prevention of Stroke by antihypertensive drug treatment in older person with isolated systolic hypertension: final results of the Systolic Hypertension in the Elderly Persons (SHEP). JAMA 1991;265:3255.
30. Hormer D, Ingall TJ, Baker HL et al. Serum lipids and lipoproteins are less powerfull predictors of extracranial carotid artery atherosclerosis than are cigarette smoking and hypertension. Mayo Clinic Proc 1991;66:259.
31. Russell RWR. Observations are intracerebral aneurysms. Brain 1963;86:425.
32. Wolf PA, D'Agustino RB, Kannel WB et al. Cigarette smoking as a risk factor for stroke. The Framingham Study. JAMA 1988;259:1025–9.
33. Abott RD, Yin Y, Reed DM, Yano K. Risk of stroke in male cigarette smokers. N Engl J Med 1986;315:717–20.
34. Shinton R, Beevers G. Meta-analysis of relation between cigarette smoking and stroke. Br Med J 1989;298:789–794.
35. Whisnant JP, Homer D, Ingall TJ et al. Duration of cigarette smoking is the strongest predictor of severe extracranial carotid artery atherosclerosis. Stroke 1990;21:707–14.
36. Dempsey RJ, Moore SW. Amount of smoking independently predicts carotid artery atherosclerosis severity. Stroke 1992;23:693–6.
37. Spagnoli LG, Mauiello A, Palmier G, Santeusanio G, Amante A, Taurino M. Relationship between risk factors and morphological patterns of human carotid atherosclerotic plaques. A multivariant discriminant analysis. Atherosclerosis 1994;108:39–60.
38. Robbins AS, Manson JE, Lee IM, Satterfield S, Henneken CH. Cigarette smoking and stroke in a cohort of US male physicians. Ann Intern Med 1994;120:458–62.
39. Lakier JB. Smoking and cardiovascular disease (Review). Am J Med 1992;93(1A):85–125.
40. Donnan GA, McNeil JJ, Adena MA et al. Smoking as a risk factor for cerebral ischaemia Lancet 1989;2:643.
41. Law MR, Wald NJ, Wu T, Hackshaw A, Bailey A. Systemic under-estimation of association between serum cholesterol concentration and ischaemic heart disease in observational studies: Data from BUPA studies. Br Med J 1994;308:363–6.
42. Marmot M. Cholesterol papers. Lowering population cholesterol concentration probably is not harmful. Br Med J 1994;308:351–2.
43. Quiziblash N, Duffy SW, Warlow C, Mann J. Lipids are risk factors for ischaemic stroke: Overview and review. Cerebrovasc Dis 1992;2:127–36.
44. Lindenstrom E, Boysen G, Nyboe J. Influence of total cholesterol, high density lipoprotein cholesterol and triglycerides on risk of cerebrovascular disease. The Copenhagen City Heart Study. Br Med J 1994;309:11–5.
45. Iso H, Jacobs DR, Wentworth D, Neaton JD, Cohen JD. Serum cholesterol level and six year mortality from stroke in 350,977 men screened for the multiple risk factor intervention trial. N Engl J Med 1989;320:904–9.
46. Hahelm LL, Holme I, Hjermann I, Leren P. Risk factors of stroke incidence and mortality. A 12-year follow up of the Oslo Study. Stroke 1993;24:1484–9.
47. Sirti C, Vartiainen E, Torppa Tuomileto J, Puska P. Trends in cerebrovascular mortality and in its risk factors in Finland during the last 20 years. Health Rep 1994;6(1):196–206.
48. Jacobs D, Blackburn H, Higgins M et al. Report of the conference on low cholesterol. Mortality associations. Circulation 1993;86:1046–60.
49. Wannamethee G, Shaper AG, Whincup PH, Walker M. Low serum total cholesterol concentration and mortality in middle age British men. Br Med J 1995;311:409–13.
50. Folsom AR, Prineas RJ, Kaye SA, Munger RG. Incidence of hypertension and stroke in relation to body fat distribution and other risk factors in older women. Stroke 1990;21:701.
51. Vanltallie TB. The perils of obesity in middle aged women. N Engl J Med 1990;322:928.
52. Shinton R, Shipley M, Rose G. Overweight and stroke in the Whitehall Study. J Epidemiol Comm Health – London 1991;45:138–42.
53. Stampfer MJ, Colditz GA, Willett WC et al. A prospective study of moderate alcohol consumption and the risk of coronary disease and stroke in women. N Engl J Med 1988;319:267.
54. Gorellck PB. The status of alcohol as a risk factor for stroke. Stroke 1989;12:1607.

55. Ettinger PO, Wu CF, De La Cruz C *et al.* Arrhythmias and 'holiday heart'. Alcohol associated cardiac rhythm disorders. Am Heart J 1985;95:55.
56. Hillbom M, Kaste M. Does ethanol intoxication promote brian infarction in young adults? Lancet 1978;21:181.
57. Hillbom M, Haapaniemi H, Juvela S, Palomaki H, Numminen H, Kaste M. Recent alcohol consumption cigarette smoking and cerebral infarction in young adults. Stroke 1995;26:40–5.
58. Paffenbarger RS, Wing Al, Hyde RT. Physical activity as an index of heart attack risk in college alumni. Am J Epidemiol 1978;108:161.
59. Fuller JH, Shipley MJ, Rose G, Jarrett RJ, Keen H. Mortality from coronary heart disease and stroke in relation to degree of glycaemia: The Whitehall Study. Br Med J 1983; 287:867–70.
60. Welin L, Svardsudd K, Wilhelmsen L *et al.* Analysis of risk factors for stroke in cohort of men born in 1913. N Engl J Med 1987;317:521.
61. Wilhelmsen L, Svardsudd K, Korban-Bengsten K *et al.* Fibrinogen as risk factor for stroke and myocardial infarction. N Engl J Med 1984;311:501.
62. Wade JPH, Taylor W, Barnett HJM, Hachinski VC. Haemoglobin concentration and the prognosis in severe cerebrovascular occlusive disease. Stroke 1987;18:68–71.
63. Bamford J, Sanderock P, Denis M *et al.* A prospective study of acute cerebrovascular disease in the community. The Oxfordshire Community Stroke Program 1981–1986. 2. Incidence, case fatality rates and overall outcome at one year of cerebral infarction, primary intracerebral and subarachnoid haemorrhage. J Neurol Neurosurg Psychiat 1990;53:16.
64. Dennis M, Bamford J, Sanderock P, Warlow C. Incidence of transient ischaemic attacks in Oxfordshire England. Stroke 1989;20:333–9.
65. Buchan AM, Barrnett HJM. Ischaemic stroke. In: Swash M, Oxbury J, (eds), Clinical Neurology. Edinburgh: Churchill Livingstone, 1991:924–52.
66. Chambers J. Left ventricular hypertrophy. An underappreciated coronary risk factor. Br Med J 1995;311:273–4.
67. Davies PH, Dambrosia JM, Schoenberg BS *et al.* Risk factors for ischaemic stroke. A prospective study in Rochester, Minnesota. Ann Neurol 1987;22:319.
68. Smith GD, Shipley MI, Rose G. Intermittent claudication, heart disease risk factors and mortality. The Whitehall Study. Circulation 1990;82:1925.
69. Sanderock PAG, Warlow CP, Jones LN *et al.* Predisposing factors for cerebral infarction: The Oxfordshire Community Stroke Project. Br Med J 1989;289:751.
70. Dennis MS, Bamford JM, Sanderock PAG, Warlow CP. A comparison of risk factors and prognosis for transient ischaemic attacks and minor strokes. The Oxfordshire Community Stroke Project. Stroke 1989;20:1494–9.
71. Wolf PA, Kannel WB, Solire P, McNamara P. Asymptomatic carotid bruit and risk of stroke. JAMA 1981;245:1442–4.
72. Hennerici M, Salsbomer HB, Hefter H, Lammerts D, Rautenberg W. Natural history of asymptomatic extra-cranial arterial disease. Brain 1987;110:777–91.
73. Aldoori MI, Benveniste GL, Baird RN, Horrocks M. Asymptomatic carotid murmur – ultrasonic factors influencing outcome. Br J Surg 1987;74:496–8.
74. Chambers BR, Norris JW. Clinical significance of asymptomatic neck bruits. Neurology 1985;35:742–5.
75. Riles TS, Liberman A, Kopelman I, Imparto AM. Symptoms, stenosis and bruit. Arch Surg 1981;116:218–20.
76. Bogousslavsky J, Despland PA, Regli F. Asymptomatic tight stenosis of the internal carotid artery: Long-term prognosis. Neurology 1986;36:861–3.
77. Langsfield M, Gray-Weale AC, Lusby RJ. J Vasc Surg 1990;9:548–70.
78. Stampfer MJ, Willett WC, Colditz GA *et al.* A prospective study of post use of oral contraceptive agents and risk of cardiovascular disease. N Engl J Med 1988;319:1313.
79. Stadel BV. Oral contraceptives and cardiovascular disease. N Engl J Med 1981;288:672.
80. Meade TW, Greenburg G, Thompson SG. Progestogens and cardiovascular reactions associated with oral contraceptives and a comparison of the safety of 50 and 30 mg estrogen preparations. Br Med J 280:1157.

81. Vassey MP, Villard-Mackintosh L, McPherson K, Yeates D. Mortality among oral contraceptive users: 20 years follow-up of women in cohort study. Br Med J 1989;299:1487.
82. Guillebaud J. Advising women on which pill to take. The informed user should be the chooser. Br Med J 1995;311:1111–2.
83. MacRae K, Kay C. Third generation oral contraceptive pills. Is the scare over the increased risk of thrombosis justified. Br Med J 1995;311:1112.

8. The investigation of extracranial carotid disease

PETER A. GAINES, TIMOTHY J. HODGSON, MUNTHER I. ALDOORI and JONATHAN D. BEARD

Ultrasound

Duplex sonography combines the ability to real time image the carotid artery and accurately sample the vessel using pulsed Doppler. The flow information is presented graphically as velocity vs. time (Figure 8.1). It has become possible to color encode the velocity information and superimpose this upon the 2D gray-scale

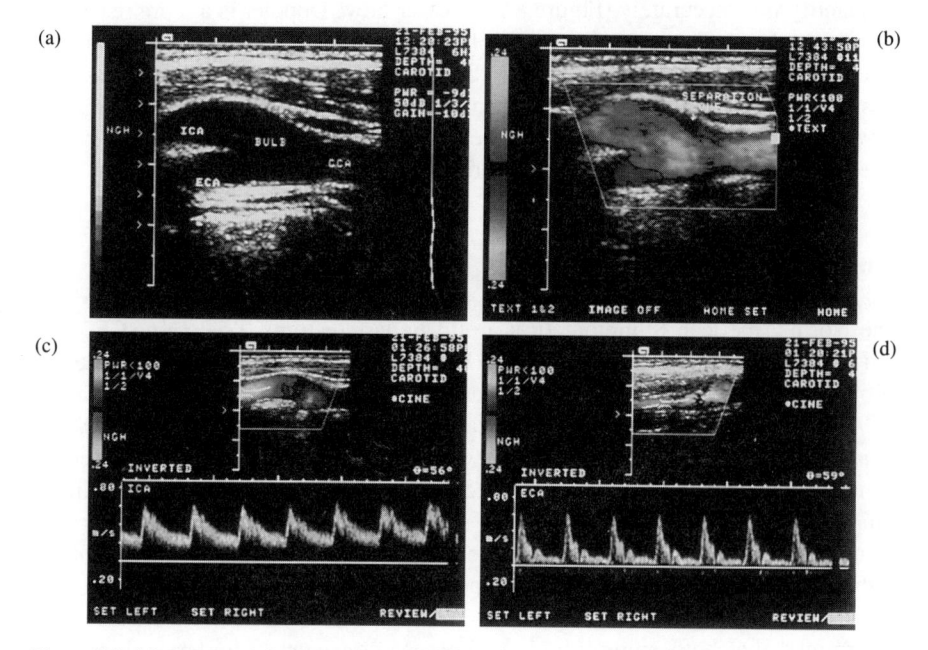

Figure 8.1. (a) shows a typical normal carotid bifurcation on conventional 2D gray-scale sonography (ICA: internal carotid artery; ECA: external carotid artery; CCA: common carotid artery); (b) is a typical color duplex image whereby the flow information has been color encoded and superimposed upon the conventional 2D image. Flow in the ICA is orange because it is toward the transducer; flow in the ECA is blue because it is away from the transducer; and there is an area in the bulb of reverse flow; (c) shows the typical low resistance flow pattern from the internal carotid artery; (d) shows a typical high resistance flow pattern of the external carotid artery.

A.-M. Salmasi and A. Strano (eds), Angiology in Practice, 87–95.
© 1996 Kluwer Academic Publishers. Printed in Great Britain.

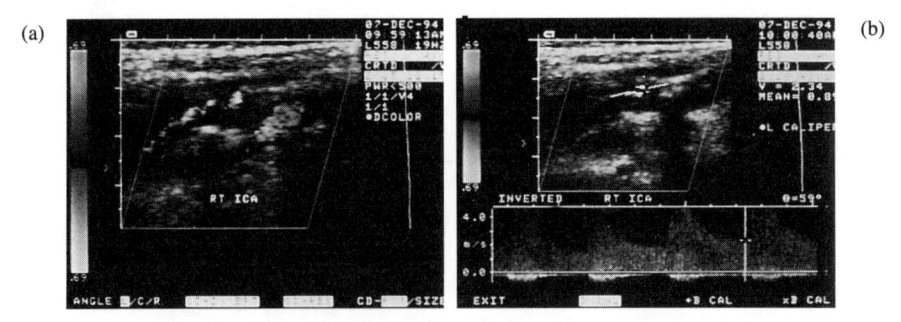

Figure 8.2. (a) shows markedly disturbed flow in the internal carotid artery around an echo-lucent plaque; (b) demonstrates high velocity disturbed flow at the point of sampling with a peak systolic velocity of greater than 4 m s^{-1} and an end diastolic velocity of greater than 2 m s^{-1}.

image – color flow Doppler. The color of each pixel displayed is the mean velocity and not peak velocity. It is standard practice that color flow Doppler is used quickly to locate and identify vessels and areas of turbulence; pulsed Doppler is then used to quantify flow accurately (Figure 8.2). 'Power flow' Doppler is a more recent development that analyzes the amplitude of the returning signal rather than frequency and direction. The signal is sensitive to flow, has a high signal to noise ratio and is less dependent upon the angle of insonation than pulsed or color flow Doppler. However, the image does not produce information on either peak velocity or direction of flow and is one of anatomy rather than function.

Symptomatic carotid atherosclerosis

The North American Symptomatic Carotid Endarterectomy Trial (NASCET) [1] and the European Carotid Surgery Trial (ECST) [2] have both confirmed the benefit of operating on symptomatic carotid disease when there is an internal carotid artery (ICA) stenosis of 70–99%. No benefit was found when the stenosis was < 30% and there is ongoing evaluation of the 30–69% group. Both trials determined the percent stenosis by angiographic criteria, although the methods of assessment were different. The NASCET compared the most severe stenosis demonstrated against the normal internal carotid artery above the lesion whereas the ECST compared the highest measurable stenosis against the perceived normal carotid bulb. Alexandrov [3] studied 45 complete endarterectomy specimens of severe carotid stenoses and determined that both angiographic techniques consistently underestimated the degree of stenosis, but the ECST technique was more accurate than the NASCET, and duplex was more accurate than both angiographic techniques. This is interesting but largely irrelevant since the diagnostic groups which return benefit from surgery were based on angiographic data. Incidentally, simple visual assessment of the percent stenosis was found to be more accurate than the techniques described in the surgical trials. Despite this the Reporting Committee on Standards for Non-Invasive Testing of the Society for Vascular Surgery, and the International Society for Cardiovascular Surgery [4] recommended the NASCET technique. Ultrasound

Table 8.1. Typical ultrasound criteria used to quantify carotid stenoses (after Strandness).

Percent stenosis	PSV (cm s^{-1})	EDV (cm s^{-1})	Spectral analysis
0	< 125		Normal
1–15	< 125		No flow reversal in bulb
16–49	< 125		Spectral broadening throughout systole
50–79	> 125		Marked spectral broadening
80–99	> 125	> 140	Marked spectral broadening
Occlusion	–	–	No flow

PSV: peak systolic velocity; EDV: end-diastolic velocity.

assessment of the carotid artery is very operator dependent but has several technical advantages over angiography. It is quicker (a complete examination taking 30–45 minutes), safer, cheaper and does not require ionizing radiation. Its accuracy in determining internal carotid artery stenoses compared to angiography has been extensively investigated prior to the two trials, but the subgroups of degrees of stenosis (typically 1–15%, 10–49%, 50–79%, 80–99%, occluded) (Table 8.1) were not those of the three bands of the surgical trials (0–30%, 30–69%, 70–99%). Work is now available to determine the ultrasound criteria for the surgical bands (Table 8.2). It is clear that ultrasound is not 100% accurate when compared against angiography and that the criteria for the diagnosis of the 70–99% stenosis group differs substantially between the units. This is probably a reflection upon different examination techniques, and between the different instruments used, and illustrates the requirement for in-house standardization of ultrasound criteria against angiography as the gold standard. Which parameters are used as a determinant of usefulness (sensitivity, specificity, positive predicted value, negative predicted value) will largely be down to the individual unit, and depend upon whether angiography is to be used to verify the data, and such local factors as angiographic complication rates, prevalence of disease, surgical complication rates, finance etc.

The diagnosis by ultrasound of internal carotid artery stenoses > 50% has a high sensitivity and negative predictive value and may be used as an accurate 'screening test' prior to angiography (see Table 8.2). For lesions < 50% the stenosis may not produce a change in PSV with only some spectral broadening, and therefore require another form of quantification if action is to be taken. Direct measurement of the stenosis using calipers on the 2D image has limitations because the plaque may be anechoic and the lumen may be obscured by vessel wall calcification. Color flow and power Doppler offer some help by filling the vessel with the color and depicting the anechoic plaque.

Complete occlusions are determined by lack of detectable flow and supporting features such as the diastolic flow in the common carotid artery approaching zero, increased velocity in the external carotid artery and a 'thump' at the stump of the ICA. Because of the high morbidity associated with severe critical (99%) stenoses, it is important to differentiate them from total occlusions. These severe stenoses may only have trickle flow (with velocities 2–4 cps) that is difficult to detect by ultrasound. Kirsch [8] has shown a 92.5% positive predicted value for detecting

Table 8.2. Contemporary published ultrasound criteria used to quantity carotid stenoses using NASCET groups.

Author	Percent stenosis	Criteria	Accuracy (%)	Sensitivity (%)	Specificity (%)	Positive predictive value (%)	Negative predictive value (%)
Faught et al. [5]	≥ 30	PSV > 120	89	77	98	96	86
	≥ 50	PSV > 130	97	97	97	93	99
	≥ 70	PSV > 210	93	89	94	75	78
	≥ 70	EDV > 100	80	77	85	89	70
	≥ 70	PSV > 210 and EDV > 100	95	81	98	89	96
	≥ 70	ICA:CCA PSV ratio > 4 (using Moneta criteria)		50			
Moneta et al. [6]	≥ 70	PSV > 325	88	83	91	80	92
	≥ 70	ICA:CCA PSV ratio > 4	88	91	87	76	96
	≥ 70	PSV > 265 (using Neale criteria)	86	90	85	73	95
Neale et al. [7]	≥ 70	PSV > 270	88	96	86		
	≥ 70	EDV > 110	93	91	93		
	≥ 70	PSV > 270 and EDV > 110	93	96	91		
	≥ 50	PSV > 125 and EDV < 140 (using Strandness criteria)	89	96	85	81	97

PSV: peak systolic velocity; EDV: end-diastolic velocity; ICA: internal carotid artery; CCA: common carotid artery.

these lesions (rising to 97% in the latter part of his study), but recommends that because of the high associated morbidity of missing these lesions that verification of a complete occlusion in a symptomatic patient should be obtained by selective angiography.

Other indications

It has been suggested that the morphology of plaque may have a relationship to the production of symptoms by distal embolization. Attempts have been made to categorize plaque according to ultrasound criteria into echolucent (Group 1), predominantly echolucent (Group 2), predominantly echogenic (Group 3) and purely echogenic (Group 4), and to predict the histology of the plaque by the identification of fibrous lesions, calcification, surface ulceration, and foci of lipid and intraplaque hemorrhage. The results have been extremely variable and further work is required to determine how such characterization relates to symptomatology [9].

The screening of post-endarterectomy sites for the development of recurrent stenoses is perfectly feasible with ultrasound, but since most carotid restenoses are asymptomatic the value of such a program is limited.

Ultrasound is of value in determining the nature of masses within the neck (lymph node, aneurysm, tortuous carotid brachiocephalic and subclavian vessels, carotid tumors), and in many centers is the screening investigation of choice.

The vertebral arteries are shown in 92–93% of cases, but the origin is difficult to visualize and this is where the majority of stenoses occur. The major value is probably in the determination of vertebral artery steals by the detection of reverse flow within the vertebral artery.

Angiographic assessment of extracranial vascular disease

Technique

Selective catheterization of the supra-aorta arteries is usually performed by percutaneous femoral puncture under local anesthesia. Modern non-ionic contrast agents are extremely safe and obviate the need for either general anesthesia or sedation in the vast majority of cases. Contemporary catheters have high torque providing quick assessment of the vessels, and are small allowing outpatient examination in most cases. The origin of the major vessels may be assessed by prior arch arteriography, or by the placement of the selective catheter close to the ostia. Images of the carotid bifurcation are often performed by selective catheterization of the common carotid artery and images are obtained of at least two complementary planes at right angles to each other (and often with images taken in four directions; AP, lateral and two obliques). Further views are usually routinely taken of the intracerebral circulation (at least AP and lateral). Conventional image acquisition required the direct exposure of radiographic film using a high-speed film changer. In the majority of large radiology departments digital subtraction angiography (DSA) is now available. The digitized information on a 512×512 or 1024×1024 matrix has high contrast resolution, is acquired instantaneously and may be retrieved almost real time, and can be manipulated. The DSA arteriogram uses less contrast agent and is quicker than conventional techniques. The intravenous administration of contrast agents directly into the vena cava or right atrium has not gained popularity because of the poor image quality.

Safety

The morbidity and mortality of angiography has a direct bearing on its acceptability particularly where it has a direct effect on the benefit of carotid endarterectomy for the management of cerebrovascular disease. Local groin complications, death and complications resulting from contrast agents are extremely rare. It is the cerebrovascular complications that are of major concern. When all patients having a cerebral arteriogram are reviewed the neurological complication rate of intra-

Table 8.3. Complications of cerebral angiography.

Author	Years	Study	All patients	Patients with cerebrovascular ischemia		
				All complications (%)	Temporary (%)	Permanent (%)
Hankey et al. [10]	1977–86	?	N/A	2.6	1.3	1.3
Heiserman et al. [11]	1992–93	Conventional	1% (0.5% temporary) (0.5% permanent)	3.1	1.6	1.6
Warnock et al. [12]	1989–91	IADSA	N/A	3.72	3.2	0.52
Grzyska et al. [13]	?	IADSA	0.54 (0.09% permanent)	0.80	0.52	0.26

IADSA: intra-arterial digital subtraction angiography; N/A: not applicable

arterial DSA is small, with approximately 0.5% of patients experienceing some form of cerebral ischemic episode (0.09% permanent, 0.45% temporary). However, for patients being assessed for carotid cerebrovascular disease the complication rate rises to 0.5%–1.5% (0.5%–3.2% temporary, 0.26%–1.6% permanent), see Table 8.3. The risk is probably highest in patients with previous CVA or significant stenosis, precisely the patients requiring assessment. The complication rate is only slightly reduced from that recorded using conventional diagnostic equipment. Whilst the size and quality of catheters has improved during the transition from conventional to DSA acquisition, most patients are still being assessed by selective arteriography, and from our own work it is probably the catheter manipulation in the vessel that causes cerebral embolization. Within our own institution the diagnostic arteriogram is performed entirely by arch arteriography without selective catheterization whenever possible.

Embolic cerebrovascular disease

The diagnostic criteria used in the NASCET and ECST trials have been based on the angiographic determination of diagnostic subgroups (see previously). Unfortunately, as discussed, this requires an invasive investigation that carries a definite risk. In addition the reliability of the technique in assigning patients to the subgroups of carotid stenosis has been questioned. Perhaps the best variability assessment was carried out by Chikos *et al.* [14]. They demonstrated, using selective non-DSA arteriography and an ECST type quantification, an intra-observer agreement in the diagnosis of ICA stenosis of > 0%, > 50%, or total occlusions of 95.9%, 90.4% and 96.8% respectively. The inter-observer agreement for the same arteriograms and diagnostic groups was 93%, 85.4% and 96.8% respectively. Similar variability in results between two observers (3% ± 5.2% using NASCET criteria, 4.5% ± 6.3% using ECST criteria) was recorded by Neale et al. [7]. Whilst these are perhaps acceptable, Chikos classified the arteriograms into five diagnostic groups (0%, 1–9%, 10–49%, 50–99%, 100% internal carotid artery stenoses) and observed that the intra-observer agreement fell to 83%, and the inter-observer agreement to 75%. It is likely that classification into the four subgroups of NASCET and ECST (0%–30%, 31%–70%, 71%–99%, 100% internal carotid artery stenoses) results in a slightly higher agreement, but there is still considerable variability. Despite this the surgical groups in both major surgical trials were defined by angiographic criteria, and ultrasound studies probably have about the same level of reproducibility [15].

Angiography may demonstrate tandem lesions away from the carotid bifurcation, although these probably do not have a significant adverse affect on surgical outcome [16]. Angiography is presently the diagnostic technique of choice in visualizing the vertebral system when posterior fossa symptoms are suspected.

Other uses

Angiography may be useful in confirming carotid body tumors. Arteriovenous malformations are probably best assessed as to their suitability for intervention by the use of angiography. By this technique the lesions can be classified into those suitable for embolization (high flow, fistulas) and the potential collateral pathways demonstrated.

Magnetic resonance angiography

The normal extra-cranial carotid artery may be satisfactorily imaged by magnetic resonance angiography (MRA) due to its rapid and laminar flow. The technique of MRA uses either the so-called time of flight (TOF) principle (or 'flow related enhancement') or phase contrast. This is discussed in detail in other texts [17] and will not be described further. Recent papers [18, 19] have suggested that MRA may be comparable to duplex ultrasound in the assessment of extra-cranial vascular disease.

Good quality MRA images require a high field strength system (1 or 1.5 Tesla), with presaturation bands eliminating confusing venous flow and appropriate post-processing software. In a cooperative patient without swallowing or respiratory artefacts it will be possible to obtain multi-angled projections of both carotid arteries using a TOF sequence in approximately 8 minutes. Rapid laminar flow will yield high quality representative images but in the presence of a stenosis several potential pitfalls must be recognized.

Laminar flow does not occur distal to stenoses of 50% or more, but undergoes turbulence and vortex formation causing an apparent drop-off in signal. As a result, the degree of stenosis appears to be exaggerated. In addition, loops within the proximal internal carotid artery (ICA) causing a change in the direction of flow may be interpreted as a stenosis or even occlusion. The maximum signal from a vessel is obtained when the vessel runs at 90° to the plane of imaging. A tortuous ICA will have no signal when it runs parallel to the plane [20].

The average length of carotid artery imaged using a standard TOF sequence is 10 to 12 cm. As a result, MRA may fail to detect stenoses particularly as the great vessels take origin from the aorta and close to the skull base, a problem also encountered with duplex ultrasound but not conventional angiography. MRA can increase the coverage by more imaging acquisitions but significantly increases both examination and post-processing time.

A recent publication [18] examined stenoses of > 70% at the carotid bifurcation. An accuracy of 94% was found when MRA was compared to conventional angiography and 88% when compared to duplex scanning. Overall, MRA was no more accurate than duplex and 10% of patients could not be assessed with MRA due to motion artefacts and claustrophobia. Overall, duplex imaging is a more cost-effective screening tool than MRA and remains the primary non-invasive assessment of carotid disease.

The role of MRA in other pathology of the neck, such as arteriovenous malformations (AVMs) and vascular tumors, is not established. The size and distribution of AVMs may be demonstrated but conventional angiography remains the investigation of choice in their pre-intervention assessment.

Spiral CT angiography

Spiral CT images a volume of tissue by using a constantly rotating gantry and a moving table. Intravenous contrast enhances the vessels and by using 3D and multiplanar reconstructions the vessels can be imaged and stenoses quantified.

The assessment of spiral CT angiography in the carotid vessels is in its infancy but Cumming and Morrow [21] present interesting data. Of 70 carotid bifurcations imaged using both spiral CT and angiography they correctly identified the 17 carotid stenoses of 70–99%. Of the remaining 46 arteries with stenoses less than 70% and the seven occluded internal carotid arteries, only one was placed incorrectly into the surgical group.

Although the area imaged is limited, the technique deserves further refinement and evaluation.

References

1. North American Symptomatic Carotid Endarterectomy Trial Collaborators. Beneficial effect of carotid endarterectomy in symptomatic patients with high-grade carotid stenosis. N Engl J Med 1991;325:445–53.
2. European Carotid Surgery Trialists Collaborative Group. MRC European Carotid Surgery Trial: Interim results for symptomatic patients with severe (70–99%) or with mild (1–29%) carotid stenosis. Lancet 1991;337:1235–42.
3. Alexandrov AV, Bladin CF, Maggisano R, Norris JW. Measuring carotid stenosis: Time for a reappraisal. Stroke 1993;24:1292–6.

4. Thiele BL, Jones AM, Hobson RW *et al.* Standards in the noninvasive cerebrovascular testing: Report from the Committee on Standards for Noninvasive Vascular Testing of the Society of Vascular Surgery and the North American Chapter of the International Society of Cardiovascular Surgery. J Vasc Surg 1992; 15:495–503.
5. Faught WE, Mattos MA, van Bemmelen PS *et al.* Color-flow duplex scanning of carotid arteries: New velocity criteria based on receiver operator characteristic analysis for threshold stenoses used in the symptomatic and asymptomatic carotid trials. J Vasc Surg 1994;19:818–28.
6. Moneta GL, Edwards M, Chitwood RW *et al.* Correlation of North American symptomatic carotid endarterectomy trial (NASCET) angiographic definition of 70% to 99% internal carotid artery stenosis with duplex scanning. J Vasc Surg 1993;17:152–9.
7. Neale ML, Chambers JL, Kelly AT *et al.* Reappraisal of duplex criteria to assess significant carotid stenosis with special reference to reports from the North American Symptomatic Carotid Endarterectomy Trial and the European Carotid Surgery Trial. J Vasc Surg 1994;20:642–9.
8. Kirsch JD, Wagner LR, James WE *et al.* Carotid artery occlusion: Positive predictive value of duplex sonography compared with arteriography. J Vasc Surg 1994;19:642–9.
9. Hayward JK, Davies AH, Lamont PM. Carotid plaque morphology: A review. Eur J Vasc Endovasc Surg 1995;9:368–74.
10. Hankey JG, Warlow CP, Molyneux AJ. Complications of cerebral angiography for patients with mild carotid territory ischaemia being considered for carotid endarterectomy. J Neurol Neurosurg Psychiat 1990;53:542–8.
11. Heiserman JE, Dean BL, Hodak JA *et al.* Neurological complications of cerebral angiography. Am J Neuroradiol 1994;15:1401–7.
12. Warnock NG, Bergvall U, Powell T. Complications of intra-arterial digital subtraction angiography in patients investigated for cerebral vascular disease. Br J Radiol 1993;66:855–8.
13. Grzyska U, Freitag J, Zeumer H. Selective cerebral intra-arterial DSA: complication rate and control of risk factors. Neuroradiology 1990;32:296–9.
14. Chikos PM, Fisher LD, Hirsch JH *et al.* Observer variability in evaluating carotid artery stenosis. Stroke 1983;14:885–92.
15. Polak JF, Dobkin GR, O'Leary DH, Wang A-M, Cutler SS. Internal carotid artery stenosis: Accuracy and reproducibility of color-Doppler-assisted duplex imaging. Radiology 1989;173:793–8.
16. Schuler JJ, Flanigan DP, Tim LT *et al.* The effect of carotid syphon stenosis on stroke rate, death, and relief of symptoms following elective carotid endarterectomy. Surgery 1983;92:1058–65.
17. Edelman RR, Hesselink JR. Clinical management resonance imaging. WB Saunders, 1990:147–79.
18. Turnipseed WD, Kennell TW, Turski PA *et al.* Magnetic resonance angiography and duplex imaging: noninvasive tests for selecting symptomatic carotid endarterectomy candidates. Surgery 1993;114:643–9.
19. Anderson CM, Saloner D, Lee RE *et al.* Assessment of carotid artery stenosis by MR angiography: Comparison with X-ray angiography and color-coded Doppler ultrasound. Am J Neuroradiol 1992;13:989–1003.
20. Patel MR, Klufas RA, Kim D *et al.* MR angiography of the carotid bifurcation: artifacts and limitations. Am J Roentgenol 1994;162:1431–7.
21. Cumming JM, Morrow IM. Carotid artery stenoses: A prospective comparison of CT angiography and conventional angiography. Am J Radiol 1994;163:517–23.

9. Management of extracranial carotid disease

JONATHAN D. BEARD, MUNTHER I. ALDOORI and PETER A. GAINES

Indications for intervention

The first part of this chapter deals with the interventional indications for carotid artery disease based on the results of the recently published North American and European trials. The management of asymptomatic patients and those with acute stroke is also discussed.

Symptomatic stenosis

Before the advent of the North American Symptomatic Carotid Surgery Trial (NASCET) [1] and the European Carotid Surgery Trial (ECST) [2] the indications for carotid endarterectomy varied widely from surgeon to surgeon and country to country. In both studies, patients with a recent non-disabling carotid territory ischemic stroke, transient ischemic attack (TIA) or retinal infarct, and an ipsilateral carotid stenosis on angiography were randomized to surgery. Fifty North American centers participated in the NASCET trial and 80 European centers in the ECST trial. All patients received best medical care including antiplatelet therapy and correction of risk factors. Patients in both trials were stratified into high grade stenosis (70–99%) and medium grade stenosis (30–69%). The ECST trial also included a low grade stenosis group (0–29%). The management of patients with symptomatic carotid artery stenosis is summarized in Figure 9.1.

Severe stenosis
The conclusions of both trials were similar in that patients with a severe stenosis benefited significantly from carotid endarterectomy. In the NASCET trial there were 659 patients in the severe stenosis group. After 2 years, the risk of major or

Mild stenosis	Moderate stenosis	Severe stenosis	Occlusion
(0–29%)	(30–69%)	(70–99%)	(100%)
↓	↓	↓	↓
Antiplatelet therapy	Consider entry into trial	Carotid endarterectomy	No operation

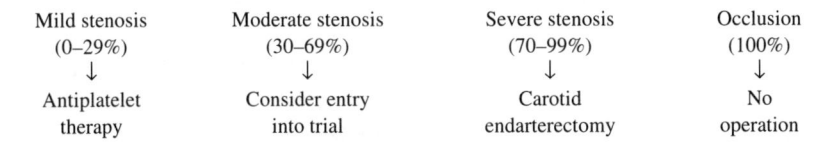

Figure 9.1. Management of patients with symptomatic carotid artery stenosis.

A.-M. Salmasi and A. Strano (eds), Angiology in Practice, 97–108.
© 1996 Kluwer Academic Publishers. Printed in Great Britain.

fatal ipsilateral stroke in the medically treated group was 13.1% compared to 2.5% in those receiving surgery. The figures for the ECST Trial at 3 years were 21.9% versus 12.3% respectively for the 778 patients in this group. The highest risk of stroke in the surgery group was in the perioperative period and varied considerably from surgeon to surgeon. In the medical group the risks diminished after the first year. This suggests that surgery for severe stenosis should not be delayed and that the operation should be performed by an experienced surgeon with acceptable results (< 4% death or disabling stroke within 30 days).

Mild/moderate stenosis
For the 374 patients with a mild stenosis (0–29%) in the ECST, those treated medically had little risk of ipsilateral stroke and so the benefits of surgery were outweighed by the early risks. Patients with moderate stenosis (30–69%) made up about half of the total number in both trials. For this group, no conclusions could be drawn regarding the risk-benefit of surgery and recruitment into a combined study is continuing. However, it is likely that patients with stenoses at the upper end of the moderate range will benefit from surgery, especially those with continued symptoms despite antiplatelet therapy. Determination of plaque morphology might also be important as those heterogenous or ulcerated plaques appear to be at higher risk of stroke [3].

Asymptomatic stenosis

Some patients with carotid artery stenosis proceed to death or disabling stroke without less severe warning symptoms. Although endarterectomy for asymptomatic carotid stenosis (ACS) has been advocated, there is no clear evidence of benefit. Between 5% and 10% of the population over 65 years of age [4] and between 20% and 30% of hospital patients with ischemic heart or peripheral vascular disease [5] have a carotid artery stenosis of more than 50%. A policy of screening and surgery to detect and treat ACS would, therefore, have major public health implications.

The results of randomized trials of surgery versus medical treatment for high grade (> 70%) ACS have been inconclusive. The Mayo Clinic Trial [6] was terminated after only 71 patients had been entered because an excess number of patients in the surgical group had myocardial infarctions. The CASANOVA German Trial [7] and Veterans Administration Trial (8) were both inconclusive. Although the risk of stroke was lower in the surgery groups, both trials decided that the numbers of patients required to detect a significant reduction was beyond the scope of any contemporary clinical trial, and that meta-analysis would be required. The results of two current trials – the Asymptomatic Carotid Artery Study (ACAS) in the USA [9], and the Asymptomatic Carotid Surgery Trial (ACST) in Europe [10] may help to clarify the situation. However, on current evidence population screening is not justified and endarterectomy for ACS should only be performed in the context of a randomized clinical trial.

Coronary artery bypass surgery

High grade (> 70%) ACS is present in 2–4% of patients undergoing coronary artery bypass grafting (CABG) with a peroperative stroke risk of 9% compared to < 3% for all patients undergoing CABG [11]. However, there is little evidence that the additional risks of a carotid endarterectomy are justified if the patient is asymptomatic. For patients with a symptomatic high grade stenosis, the question is whether the endarterectomy should be done as a staged or synchronous procedure. The advantage of a synchronous procedure is that it avoids the myocardial ischemia that may be caused if the carotid endarterectomy is performed first [11].

Acute Stroke

Emergency endarterectomy used to be recommended by some surgeons for patients with a severe carotid stenosis and a progressing stroke or crescendo TIAs [12]. However, most neurologists and surgeons now believe that surgery should be delayed for 4–6 weeks after a CT-confirmed infarct, accepting the risk of new strokes during this time that may occur in up to 21% of cases [13]. The rationale for this delay is due to the concern that surgery may convert an 'ischemic' into a 'hemorrhagic' infarct [14]. The Joint Study of Extracranial Arterial Occlusion also documented the uselessness of emergency revascularization of patients with acute stroke and carotid occlusion [15]. More recently, good results for small series of selected patients with acute stroke have been reported [16].

Interventional techniques

This section concentrates on the various controversies surrounding carotid endarterectomy. The main issues concern the anesthetic, the surgical technique, use of a shunt, patch closure, and the introduction of balloon angioplasty. Much attention has been focused on these aspects because of the need for a low operative mortality and morbidity to guarantee benefit from the operation.

Anesthetic

Local anesthesia (LA) has been used for carotid surgery since the 1960s and some surgeons are of the opinion that only by having the patient awake and alert can the surgeon determine the safety of temporary occlusion of the carotid artery and then decide whether the patient needs a shunt or not [17]. It has also been suggested that LA is cheaper, quicker, and less stressful for the patient. However, if the procedure is prolonged due to technical difficulties the patient may become agitated, which adds to the surgeon's stress. The majority of surgeons opt for general anesthesia (GA), quoting the advantages of better airway control, reduced cebrebral metabolic demand, and easier dissection.

There are many reports of equally good results with both forms of anesthetic but only one randomized trial of 114 patients performed at Malmö Hospital, Sweden [18]. Not surprisingly for a study of this size, there were no differences in stroke or mortality. There was definite evidence of anxiety in the LA group, including angina attacks prior to induction and agitation with higher levels of blood pressure and plasma norepinephrine during surgery. Other studies have noted a longer intensive care unit stay after GA due to more problems with postoperative hypertension [19]. However, no such differences were noted in the randomized study.

Postoperatively it is important that all patients are monitored in an intensive care or high dependency unit because of labile blood pressure. Correction of a severe carotid stenosis may result in cerebral hyperperfusion due to defective vascular autoregulation [20]. Cerebral hyperperfusion is blood pressure dependent and failure to control it may result in cerebral edema, fits, and intracranial hemorrhage.

Standard endarterectomy

Conventional endarterectomy is performed under light GA. The head is turned away from the site of operation and placed on a rubber ring with the neck extended. An oblique incision is made along the anterior border of the sternocleidomastoid muscle [21]. The carotid bifurcation is exposed by ligating and dividing the overlying anterior facial veins allowing lateral displacement of the internal jugular vein. The common carotid (CCA), internal carotid (ICA), and external carotid (ECA) branches are controlled with slings after infiltration of the carotid sinus area with 1% lidocaine to prevent reflex hypotension and bradycardia. The distal ICA is freed for 1 cm beyond the distal end of the plaque. It is vital that manipulation of the arteries is minimized during dissection to prevent embolization. It is important to avoid damage to the mandibular branch of the facial nerve, vagus, hypoglossal, and superior laryngeal nerves due to excessive dissection and traction. The transverse branch of the cervical plexus is usually divided leading to anesthesia medial to the incision. High dissections near the base of the skull risk damage to the glossopharyngeal nerve and subsequent difficulty in swallowing [22].

After systemic anticoagulation with 5000 units of heparin IV, soft clamps are applied to the CCA and ICA and the ECA branches occluded with slings or bulldog clamps. A linear arteriotomy is made from the CCA into the ICA beyond the distal end of the plaque. If a shunt is to be used it is usually inserted at this time (Figure 9.2). The appropriate endarterectomy plane is entered with a fine dissector and the plaque dissected from the CCA, ECA origin and proximal ICA. The distal end of the plaque normally feathers off smoothly but occasionally it requires securing with 2 or 3 interrupted 6/0 polyester or polypropylene sutures to prevent dissection. Small pieces of loose plaque can be identified by flushing with saline and picked out with forceps. The arteriotomy is then closed with a running suture of 6/0 prolene or patched. Flow is restored to the ECA first, allowing any debris or air to be flushed into it rather than up the ICA.

Reversal of anticoagulation is usually unnecessary and may increase the risk of acute thrombosis. Long-term antiplatelet therapy is usually continued after surgery as there is some evidence of a reduction in early postoperative neurological events

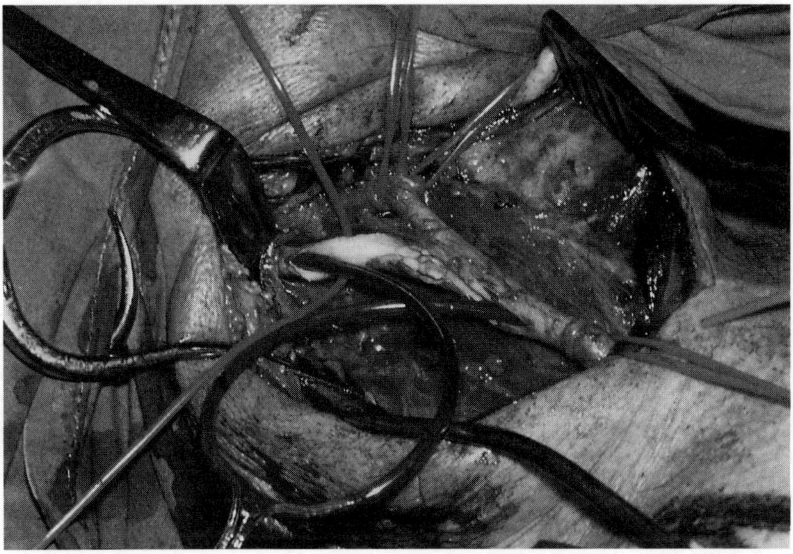

Figure 9.2. Carotid endarterectomy. The carotid bifurcation has been exposed and the vessels controlled with slings. A longitudinal arteriotomy has been performed and the stenosis at the origin of the ICA can be seen. A Pruitt–Inahara shunt has been inserted to maintain cerebral perfusion during the endarterectomy.

and improved long-term survival [23]. There is no evidence that anticoagulation confers any additional benefit.

Eversion endarterectomy

Eversion endarterectomy by transection of the CCA was first mentioned by De Bakey in 1959. However, assessment of the distal intima was uncertain and tortuosity of the ICA could not be corrected. Eversion endarterectomy of the ICA has recently been described [24]. In this technique, the origin of the ICA is transected and reimplanted after eversion endarterectomy of the ICA and conventional endarterectomy of the CCA and ECA. The ICA is then reimplanted permitting correction of any tortuosity. The postoperative restenosis rate may also be reduced. This method is only suitable if the disease is confined to the origin of the ICA.

Patch angioplasty

Significant carotid artery restenosis (> 50%) may affect between 10–20% of patients within 2–5 years of surgery [25]. Postoperative occlusion occurs in about 2% of cases, often resulting in stroke and, in the longer term, 1–2% of patients will have recurrent symptoms due to carotid restenosis. The four randomized studies of patch angioplasty have all shown a benefit over simple closure in terms of a reduction in the incidence of postoperative neurological events and restenosis rate assessed by duplex ultrasound [26]. However, use of a patch increases clamping time by 15–30 minutes and there is a risk of rupture with vein and infection with prosthetic patches. Many surgeons therefore employ a policy of selectively patching only small caliber vessels (< 5 mm).

Shunting

Proponents of carotid shunting argue that its routine use allows time for a more thorough endarterectomy because of continued cerebral perfusion and that the need for intraoperative monitoring is reduced. Those who do not use shunts claim that there is a risk of embolization of air or atheromatous debris and that intimal damage can occur during shunt insertion [27]. Many surgeons advocate the selective use of a shunt based upon the results of intraoperative monitoring [28]. The most commonly used shunts are the Javid shunt which gives better flow rates and the Pruitt–Inahara shunt which is more flexible [29].

Despite numerous reports of good results with and without a shunt there have been very few randomized studies. One such German study of 503 carotid endarterectomies found no difference in postoperative stroke or death [30]. However, neuromonitoring was employed and 10 patients with severe EEG changes randomized to no shunt were shunted.

Balloon angioplasty and stenting

Percutaneous transluminal balloon angioplasty is a well established procedure for the treatment of peripheral arterial disease. However, it has only recently been used to treat carotid artery stenosis. Technically it should produce good results in view of the short stenosis but adequacy of dilatation is not the main concern. The chief worry is cerebral embolization as it has been estimated that up to 80% of neurological defects related to conventional carotid endarterectomy are due to embolization [31].

In Sheffield we have treated 54 patients with symptomatic stenoses > 70% of the CCA or ICA. All were treated by balloon dilatation via a femoral approach under LA and 4 patients also received a Palmaz stent (Figure 9.3). In all cases there was evidence of cerebral embolization on TCD monitoring. Seven (13%) had a temporary neurological deficit that resolved by 30 days and 2 (3.7%) had a permanent deficit. Patients have been followed up to 2 years and there has been no symptomatic recurrence. Similar results have been reported by other centers but the numbers are small. The low rate of significant neurological deficits despite cerebral embolization might be due to the short period of carotid occlusion during angioplasty (15 s).

Theron *et al.* [32] have developed a coaxial catheter system which incorporates a temporary occlusion balloon distal to the dilating balloon. It is claimed that this reduces cerebral embolization but the system is rather cumbersome to use. Stents also have the potential to reduce embolization and possibly improve the restenosis rate but any such benefit needs to be properly demonstrated.

Carotid angioplasty also has the advantage of a shorter hospital stay, and lack of morbidity associated with a cervical incision. However, all patients treated by this technique should be part of a randomized trial. The CAVATAS study in the UK is presently randomizing patients with symptomatic severe carotid stenosis to surgery or angioplasty and the results are awaited with interest.

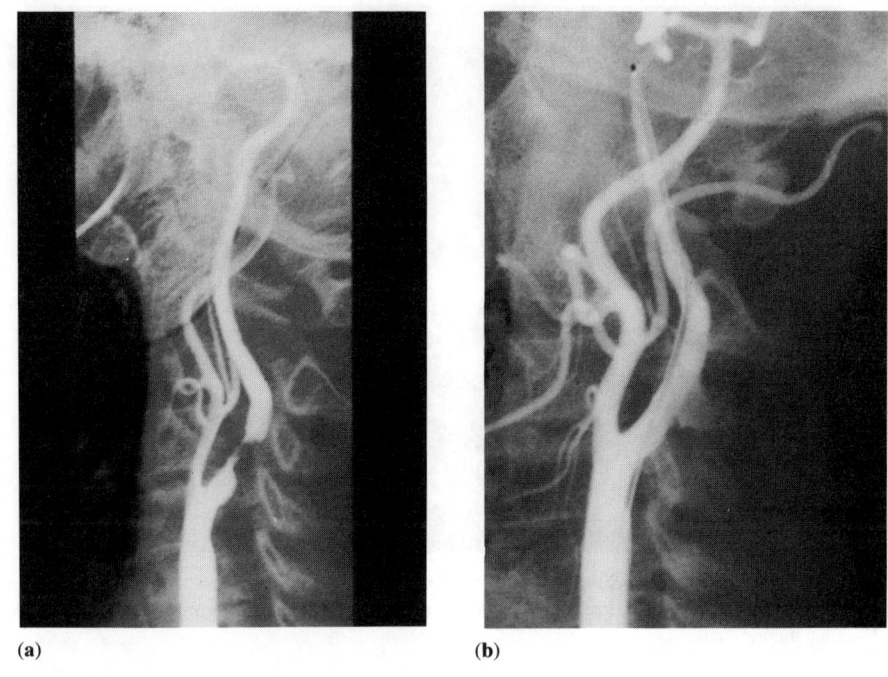

Figure 9.3. Carotid arteriogram showing a 90% stenosis at the origin of the ICA (a) and a smooth vessel with no residual stenosis after balloon angioplasty (b).

Operative measurements

Carotid endarterectomy is an operation that demands careful measurement and monitoring throughout. Such measurement has several roles which can be divided into three categories:

1. Assessment of the need for a shunt.
2. Cerebral monitoring.
3. Quality control.

Some methods of measurement can cover all three aspects whereas others are more limited in their application. Apart from measurement of stump pressures, most methods of cerebral monitoring can be used to assess the need for a shunt.

Measurement of the ICA stump back pressure above the clamp, prior to endarterectomy, was one of the first methods used to decide on the need for a shunt [33]. However, its accuracy in predicting those patients at risk of stroke during carotid cross clamping has been recently questioned and many surgeons prefer to use a method that permits continued assessment throughout the operation.

Cerebral monitoring

Cerebral ischemia has been estimated to occur in 4–33% of patients undergoing surgery. Those at highest risk include patients with cerebral infarcts and

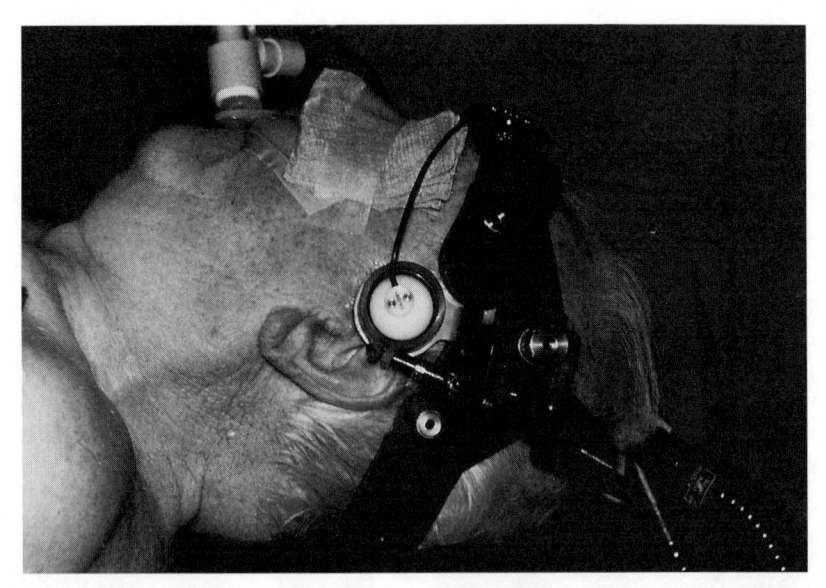

Figure 9.4. Transcranial Doppler monitoring of the middle cerebral artery blood flow velocity during carotid endarterectomy. A low frequency (2.5 MHz) pulsed-wave ultrasound beam is directed through the thin temporal bone.

contralateral carotid artery occlusion. The aim of cerebral monitoring is to detect and correct cerebral ischemia before permanent neurological damage is caused. There are three categories of cerebral monitoring:

1. Carotid or cerebral artery blood flow.
2. Cerebral tissue perfusion.
3. Neurological activity and function.

In general the simpler methods of blood flow measurement are easiest to perform and interpret. The exception is the highest form of neurological function monitoring, i.e. the awake patient under LA.

Although carotid or shunt blood flow can be measured with a flow meter, like back pressures it may bear little relation to intracerebral arterial flow which is also affected by the completeness of the Circle of Willis and collateral supply. Transcranial Doppler (TCD) is probably the most versatile and practical of all available methods as it can also be used preoperatively to assess cerebral blood flow reserve and postoperatively to detect hyperperfusion [34]. TCD employs a low frequency (2.5 MHz) pulsed wave ultrasound beam directed through the thin temporal bone (Figure 9.4). This permits insonation of most of the Circle of Willis and, in particular, the middle cerebral artery (MCA). The quality of the signal depends on the thickness of the cranium and is inadequate in 5–10% of patients. A fall in MCA blood flow velocity on carotid clamping is usually regarded as an indication for shunting. In addition, TCD can detect air or particulate emboli which can

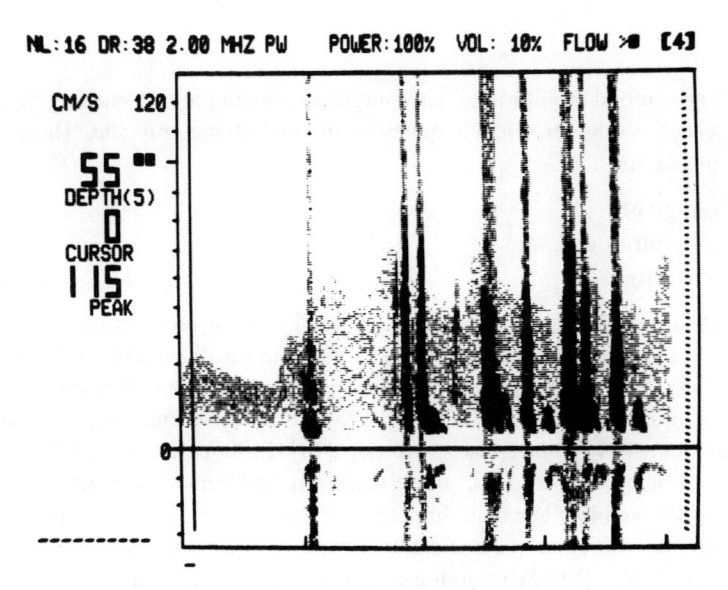

Figure 9.5. Transcranial Doppler signal from the MCA showing multiple 'spikes' due to air emboli at the time of restoration of carotid flow after completion of the endarterectomy.

alert the surgeon to technical problems (Figure 9.5). Measurement of cerebral tissue perfusion can be performed by either isotopic clearance or infrared spectroscopic techniques. Isotopic methods [35] use intravenously administered ^{133}Xenon to measure two-dimensional cerebral blood flow (CBF) using detectors placed over each hemisphere or ^{99}Technetium-hexamethyl propylene amine oxime to measure three-dimensional CBF using single photon emission computed tomography (SPECT). Near infrared spectroscopy (NIRS) depends on the absorption of near infrared light, transmitted through the skull into the cerebral hemispheres, by the chromophores oxyhemoglobin (HbO_2), deoxyhemoglobin (Hb) and oxidized cytochrome ($Cyt-O_2$). Changes in cerebral hemoglobin oxygenation have been shown to correlate closely with MCAV measured with TCD [36]. The disadvantage of both of these techniques at present is the costly equipment required which means that their use is mainly confined to research.

Conventional EEG, both unprocessed or converted to frequency spectra, has been used to monitor neurological activity [37]. A greater than 50% increase in theta or delta activity or a decrease in alpha or beta activity indicates cerebral dysfunction. The main problem with EEG is interpretation and somatosensory electrical potentials (SEPs) are claimed to have a lower false positive rate for detecting ischemia [38]. SEP is based on the amplitude of the electrical potential produced by the somatosensory cortex in response to sensory stimulation of the median nerve at the wrist. In general, cortical SEPs are too small to be seen in the raw data and signal averaging must be employed. This adds a time delay and both EEG and SEP activity are also affected by most general anesthetic agents.

Quality control

As well as cerebral monitoring, many surgeons also employ an imaging modality as a final check on the technical adquacy of the endarterectomy site. These imaging modalities include:

1. Arteriography.
2. Duplex ultrasound.
3. Angioscopy.

Completion angiography following peripheral arterial reconstruction is standard practice but many surgeons reject its use following carotid endarterectomy as being unnecessary, potentially misleading and possibly dangerous. However, some surgeons have used it routinely for many years to detect intimal flaps, thrombus, or residual stenosis without apparent mishap [39]. Intraoperative duplex has the advantage of being able to detect these technical problems in various planes and is also noninvasive [40]. The main limitation of this technique has been the size of the probes and the difficulty of sterilization, but smaller sterilizable probes are now becoming available. Duplex scanning is also useful to check on the patency of the carotid if the patient develops postoperative neurological symptoms [41]. Angioscopy can be used to directly inspect the lumen of the carotid artery immediately prior to closure and clamp release [42]. However, the equipment is expensive and because of the magnification, minor defects that do not require correction are often seen.

References

1. North American Symptomatic Carotid Endarterectomy Trial Collaborators. Beneficial effect of carotid endarterectomy in symptomatic patients with high-grade stenosis. N Engl J Med 1991;325:445–53.
2. European Carotid Surgery Trialists' Collaborative Group. MRC European carotid surgery trial: Interim results for symptomatic patients with severe (70–99%) or with mild (0–29%) carotid stenosis. Lancet 1991;337:1235–43.
3. Holdsworth RJ, McCollum PT, Bryce JS, Harrison DK. Symptoms, stenosis and carotid plaque morphology. Is plaque morphology relevant? Eur J Vasc Endovasc Surg 1995;9:80–5.
4. Ricci S, Flamini F, Coloni MG. Prevalence of internal carotid artery stenosis in subjects older than 49 years: A population study. Cerebrovasc Dis 1991;1:16–9.
5. Klop RBJ, Eikelboon BC, Taks ACJM. Screening of the internal carotid arteries in patients with peripheral vascular disease by colour-flow duplex scanning. Eur J Vasc Surg 1991;5:41–5.
6. Mayo Asymptomatic Carotid Endarterectomy Study Group. Effectiveness of CEA for asymptomatic carotid artery stenosis; design of a clinical trial. Mayo Clinic Proc 1989;64:897–904.
7. The CASANOVA Study Group. Carotid surgery versus medical therapy in asymptomatic carotid stenosis. Stroke 1991;22:1229–35.
8. Hobson RW II, Weiss DG, Fields WS and the VA Cooperative Study Group. Efficacy of carotid endarterectomy for asymptomatic carotid stenosis. N Engl J Med 1993;328:221–7.
9. Asymptomatic Carotid Atherosclerosis Study Group (ACAS). Study design for randomised prospective trial of carotid endarterectomy for symptomatic atherosclerosis. Stroke 1989;20:844.
10. Halliday AW for the Steering Committee and for the Collaborators. The asymptomatic carotid surgery trial (ACST). Rationale and design. Eur J Vasc Surg 1994;8:703–10.

11. Bernstein EF. Staged versus simultaneous carotid endarterectomy in patients undergoing cardiac surgery. J Vasc Surg 1992;15:870–1.
12. Goldstone J, Moore WS. A new look at emergency carotid surgery operations for the treatment of cerebrovascular insufficiency. Stroke 1978;9:599–602.
13. Dosik SM, Whalen RC, Gale SS. Carotid endarterectomy in the stroke patient: CT to determine timing. J Vasc Surg 1985;2:214–9.
14. Wylie EJ, Hein MF, Adams JE. Intracranial haemorrhage following surgical revascularization for treatment of acute strokes. J Neurosurg 1964;2:212–5.
15. Blaisdell WF, Clauss RH, Goldbraith JG, Imparato AM, Wylie EJ. Joint study of extracranial arterial occlusion: A review of surgical considerations. J Am Med Assoc 1979;209:1889–95.
16. Cuming R, Perkin GD, Greenhalgh RM. Urgent carotid surgery. In: Greenhalgh RM, Hollier LH (eds), Emergency vascular surgery. London: Saunders, 1992.
17. Spencer F, Eiseman B. Technique of carotid endarterectomy. Surg Gynecol Obstet 1962;115:115–7.
18. Forsell C, Takolander R, Bagqvist D, Johansson A. Local versus general anaesthesia in carotid surgery. A prospective, randomised study. Eur J Vasc Surg 1989;3:503–9.
19. Godin M, Bell W, Schwedler M, Kastain M. Cost effectiveness of regional anaesthesia in carotid endarterectomy. Ann Surg 1989;55:656–9.
20. Jorgensen LG, Shroeder TV. Defective cerebrovascular regulation after carotid endarterectomy. Eur J Vasc Surg 1993;7:370–9.
21. Thompson JE. Carotid endarterectomy. In: Greenhalgh RM (ed), Vascular surgical techniques, an atlas. 2nd ed. London: Saunders, 1989:83–8.
22. Forsell C, Bergqvist D, Bergentz SE. Peripheral nerve injuries in carotid artery surgery. In: Greenhalgh TM, Hollier LH (eds), Surgery for stroke. London: Saunders, 1993:217–34.
23. Kretschmer G, Bischof G, Pratschner T et al. Antiplatelet or anticoagulant therapy after carotid endarterectomy: Results of a trial and an analysis supported by postdata matching. In: Greenhalgh RM, Hollier LH (eds), Surgery for stroke. London: Saunders, 1993:319–27.
24. Kasprzat P, Raithel D. Evasion carotid endarterectomy. Technique and early results. J Cardiovasc Surg 1989;30:49.
25. Baker WH, Hayes AC, Mahler D, Littooy FN. Durability of carotid endarterectomy. Surgery 1983;94:112–5.
26. Ranaboldo CJ, Barros D'Sa AAB, Bell PRF, Chant ADB, Perry PM for the Joint Vascular Research Group. Randomized controlled trial of patch angioplasty for carotid endarterectomy. Br J Surg 1993;80:1528–30.
27. Halsey JH. Risks and benefits of shunting in carotid endarterectomy. Stroke 1992; 23:1583–7.
28. Sundt TM. The ischemic tolerance of neural tissue and the need for monitoring and selective shunting during carotid endarterectomy. Stroke 1983;14:93–8.
29. Beard JD. Blood flow in carotid shunts. In: Greenhalgh RM, Hollier LH (eds), Surgery for stroke. London: Saunders, 1993:167–82.
30. Sandmann W, Willeke F, Kolvenbach R, Benecke R, Godehardt E. Shunting and neuromonitoring: A prospective randomised study. In: Greenhalgh RM, Hollier LH (eds) Surgery for stroke. London: Saunders, 1993:287–96.
31. Krul JMJ, van Gÿn J, Ackerstaff RGA, Eikelboon BC, Theodorides T. Vermeulen FE. Site and pathogenesis of infarcts associated with carotid endarterectomy. Stroke 1989;20:324–8.
32. Theron J, Courtheoux P, Alachkar F, Bouvard G, Maiza D. A new triple coaxial catheter system for carotid angioplasty with cerebral protection. AJNR 1990,11: 869–74.
33. Hunter GC, Sieffert G, Malone JM, Moore WS. The accuracy of carotid back pressure as an index of shunt requirement. Stroke 1982;13:319–26.
34. Naylor AR, Bell PRF, Ruckley CV. Monitoring and cerebral protection during carotid endarterectomy. Br J Surg 1992;79:735–41.
35. Algotsson L. Ryding E, Rehncrona S, Messeter K. Cerebral blood flow during carotid endarterectomy determined by three dimensional SPECT measurement; relation to peroperative risk assessment. Eur J Vasc Surg 1993;7:46–53.
36. Mason PF, Dyson EH, Sellars V, Beard JD. The assessment of cerebral oxygenation during carotid endarterectomy utilizing near infrared spectroscopy. Eur J Vasc Surg 1994;8:590–4.

37. Ahn SS, Jordon SE, Nuwer MR, Marcus DR, Moore WS. Computed electroencephalographic topographic brain mapping. A new and accurate monitor of cerebral circulation and function for patients having carotid endarterectomy. J Vasc Surg 1988;8:247–54.
38. Lam AM, Manninen PH, Ferguson GG, Nantau W. Monitoring electrophysiologic function during carotid endarterectomy. A comparison of somatosensory evoked potentials and conventional electroencephalogram. Anaesthesiology 1991;75:15–21.
39. Blaisdell FW. Routine operative arteriography following carotid endarterectomy. Surgery 1978;83:114–5.
40. Schwartz PA, Petersen GL, Noland KA, Howes JF, Naunheim KS. Intraoperative duplex scanning after carotid artery reconstruction: A valuable tool. J Vasc Surg 1988;7:620–4.
41. Cuming R, Blair SD, Powell JT, Greenhalgh RM. The use of duplex scanning to diagnose perioperative carotid occlusions. Eur J Vasc Surg 1994;8:142–7.
42. Raithel D, Kasprzak P. Angioscopy after carotid endarterectomy. Ann Chir Gynaecol 1992;81:192–5.

10. Hemodynamics of coronary flow in normal and abnormal states

MARIO MARIANI and ALBERTO BALBARINI

The main function of coronary circulation is to ensure a constant and adequate blood flow in order to meet myocardial metabolic requirements. In basal conditions 100 g of myocardium requires a blood flow of about 60–90 ml/min: 80–100 ml/min/100 g in the left ventricle and 50–70 ml/min/100 g in the right ventricle. However, depending on the hemodynamic parameters, metabolic requirements and coronary flow can vary greatly.

The principal factors regulating coronary flow are expressed by the following equation:

$$\text{Coronary flow} = \frac{\text{Perfusion gradient}}{\text{Coronary resistance}}$$

The mechanisms involved in coronary resistance regulation, such as myogenic, nervous, metabolic, and endothelial factors provide a continuous match between oxygen demand and offer. These mechanisms will be extensively examined throughout the text.

Since specific myocardial regions are subjected to variable hemodynamic load and perfusion conditions, they show different tendencies to develop ischemia in pathological conditions. Therefore extreme tachycardia, aortic stenosis or hypotension are more likely to induce subendocardial than subepicardial ischemia.

Finally, the hemodynamic effects of fixed and dynamic stenoses of epicardial coronary arteries on coronary circulation will be examined.

Factors influencing myocardial oxygen consumption

Myocardial oxygen consumption is about 10–15 ml oxygen/100 g tissue. In the non-beating heart it decreases to about 10% (1.5 ml/100 g) of normal values, which is the amount required to maintain basal metabolic processes [1] (see Figure 10.1). Membrane electrical activities account for less than 0.5% of the total oxygen consumption [2]. Most myocardial oxygen consumption occurs in contractile activity and is influenced by many hemodynamic parameters (see Table 10.1). In particular, myocardial oxygen requirements are highly correlated with the level of systolic

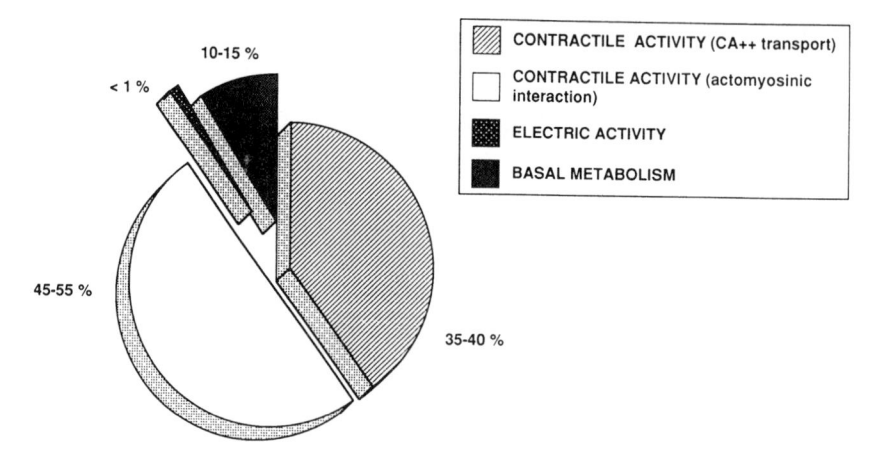

Figure 10.1. Pie chart of myocardial energetic metabolism: values, expressed in percentage, refer to contractile activity, basal metabolism and membrane electrical activities. Contractile energetic requirements also include active Ca^{++} ion transport through the sarcoplasmic reticulum membrane and sarcolemma as well as actomyosinic ATPase activity.

Table 10.1. Main factors determining myocardial oxygen consumption.

Inotropism	Fenn effect
Hemodynamic load	Membrane ionic pumps
Heart rate	Basal metabolism

tension and with the time during which this tension is maintained (expressed as the integral of tension over time, or 'tension time index') [3].

Isotonic work (stroke volume) also influences myocardial energetic consumption, even if to a less extent. Experimental data show an excellent correlation between oxygen consumption and the pressure–volume loop area of the left ventricle [4–6]. The load applied to myocardial fibers during systole does not only depend on intraventricular pressure, but also on the cavity radium and on the left ventricle wall thickness, according to the well known equation:

$$\text{Wall stress} = \frac{\text{Intracavitary pressure} \times \text{Radius}}{\text{Wall thickness}}$$

Oxygen consumption is directly dependent on wall stress rather than on intraventricular pressure; for this reason factors modifying left ventricular dimensions can influence oxygen myocardial consumption without varying the pressure.

Contractility is another important factor which influences myocardial metabolic requirements. In healthy hearts, positive inotropic agents such as cardiac glycosides, β-agonists and phosphodiesterase inhibitors cause an increase in oxygen myocardial consumption, while negative inotropic agents such as β-blockers, Ca-antagonists and procainamide reduce it independently from the effect on muscular tension [7, 8]. On the contrary, it is important to stress that in failing hearts these positive inotropic agents cause a reduction in ventricular dimensions and therefore

TELEDIASTOLE   TELESYSTOLE

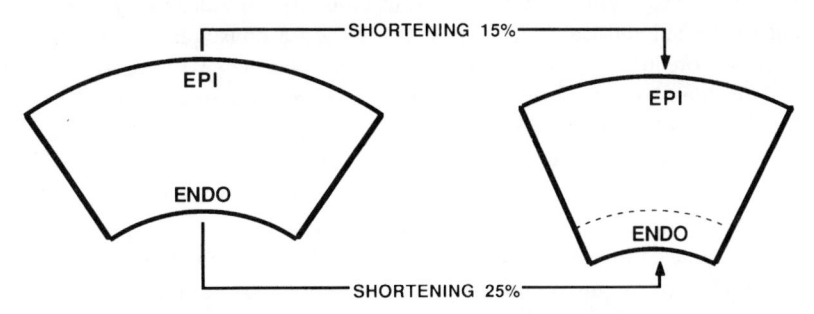

Figure 10.2. Subendocardial and subepicardial layer percentage shortening during systole. The subendocardial layer, for geometric reasons (wall thickening with a subsequent shift of subendocardial layer toward the central ventricular cavity), presents a greater systolic shortening with respect to the subepicardial layer.

in muscular tension. Such afterload reduction counterbalances the effect on contractility and can decrease oxygen consumption. Heart rate variations can also influence oxygen consumption, modifying the frequency of systolic activation per unit of time and myocardial contractility [3, 9].

Finally, oxygen consumption is not the same in all the myocardium. In particular, energetic requirements are lower in the right ventricular free wall which is subjected to a lower pressure-load in systole than the left ventricle. Similarly, subendocardial layers consume more oxygen than subepicardial ones due to higher wall stress values and percentage shortening occurring at this level (see Figure 10.2).

Coronary flow regulation

Many complex mechanisms are involved in coronary flow regulation. As in every other vascular system, coronary flow is directly proportional to the perfusion pressure gradient and inversely proportional to vascular resistance. However, coronary circulation has peculiar characteristics in comparison to other vascular systems, since the coronary perfusion gradient, influenced by intracavitary pressure, is not the same in every myocardial district and changes in relation to the various phases of the cardiac cycle. In fact, the branches of epicardial coronary arteries cross the ventricular walls and are therefore influenced by intramyocardial pressure. As a consequence, the actual coronary perfusion gradient is not represented by the difference in pressure between the aorta and the right atrium, but by the difference between aortic and intramyocardial pressure which is strictly dependent on intraventricular pressure. For this reason myocardial perfusion is highest in protodiastole, it decreases progressively during diastase and end-diastole and falls abruptly, until stopping in isometric systole when intramyocardial pressure is equal to that of the aorta. These coronary flow systodiastolic variations are particularly evident near the subendocardial layers, where wall stress is greater than in the subepicardial ones, so that the reduction in coronary flow during systole is more evident in the subendocardial layers [10, 11]. As a consequence, the subendocardium is more prone to contract an 'oxygen debt' when subjected to greater stress. This 'debt' must be 'paid' for during diastole utilizing a part of coronary reserve. Studies of regional perfusion have in fact demonstrated that in basal conditions, regional coronary flow in diastole is greater in subendocardial layers than in subepicardial ones, due to higher vasodilatation in the subendocardium [12].

From the above data, one can easily understand why the endocardium is more susceptible to ischemia. Higher systolic wall tension and lower systolic perfusion increase metabolic requirements and cause the subendocardium to be highly dependent on diastolic flow for its oxygen supply. Furthermore, it is important to note that in the left ventricle, coronary perfusion occurs mainly in diastole (80% in diastole and 20% in systole) while in the right ventricle, blood flow is continuous since its muscle is thinner and wall stress is lower than in the left ventricle.

Many physiological conditions can favor and/or induce subendocardial ischemia (see Table 10.2). Among these it is important to point out that aortic stenosis determines an increase in ventricular afterload and therefore an increase in oxygen myocardial consumption. Simultaneously, left ventricular concentric hypertrophy causes a reduction in left ventricular compliance and consequently an increase in end-diastolic left ventricular pressure with a reduction in the diastolic perfusion gradient. Aortic incompetence is another condition where a reduction in diastolic aortic pressure occurs, along with an increase in left ventricular diastolic pressure which is accompanied by a marked reduction in the diastolic perfusion gradient. In the case of aortic stenosis and incompetence, subendocardial ischemia can be present even in the absence of coronary disease (hemodynamic angina). However, while patients with aortic stenosis usually experience angina during exercise (caused by an excessive increase in oxygen demand), patients with aortic incompetence often experience angina at rest, due to a progressive reduction in the coronary perfusion gradient during diastole. Other physiopathological conditions such as tachycardia, severe hypotension or hypertension, severe anemia, fever, and hyperthyroidism can induce subendocardial ischemia. Left ventricular dilation can also induce subendocardial ischemia due to an increase in afterload, as well as an increase in left ventricular end-diastolic pressure with a subsequent reduction in the coronary perfusion gradient.

Table 10.2. Factors favoring subendocardial ischemia.

Tachycardia	Severe hypotension
Aortic stenosis	Fever
Aortic incompetence	Hyperthyroidism
Myocardial hypertrophy	Anemia
Arterial hypertension	

Coronary resistance regulation

As mentioned above, coronary flow must be able to adapt continuously to widely variable myocardial metabolic requirements. For example, during exercise, coronary flow increases its basal value by a factor of 4 or 5 in order to meet increased metabolic and oxygen requirements. The only way to obtain more oxygen is to increase the blood flow, keeping in mind that oxygen tissue extraction in basal conditions is already high (70%) and can only increase up to 80%. Coronary resistance modulation is the principle mechanism through which coronary flow can increase or decrease. The vasodilation capacity of a coronary arterial district, called 'coronary reserve', is fundamental in determining the functional capacity of a myocardial region and of the whole ventricle.

Coronary reserve is generally measured as the ratio between whole or regional coronary flow during maximum vasodilation and in basal conditions. Since this parameter is greatly influenced by many variables such as hemodynamic load, metabolic requirements, and heart rate, the concept of 'relative coronary reserve' has been proposed instead of 'regional coronary reserve'. The former is defined as the relationship between maximum coronary flow in a district under study and maximum coronary flow in a district supplied by normal coronary arteries.

The following sections will examine the main nervous, myogenic, metabolic, and endothelial mechanisms involved in coronary resistance regulation (see Figure 10.3).

The autonomic nervous system

The sympathetic and parasympathetic nervous systems extensively innervate coronary arteries [13]. Sympathetic stimulation determines complex direct and indirect vasomotor coronary effects. A coronary vasoconstriction [14] is probably mediated

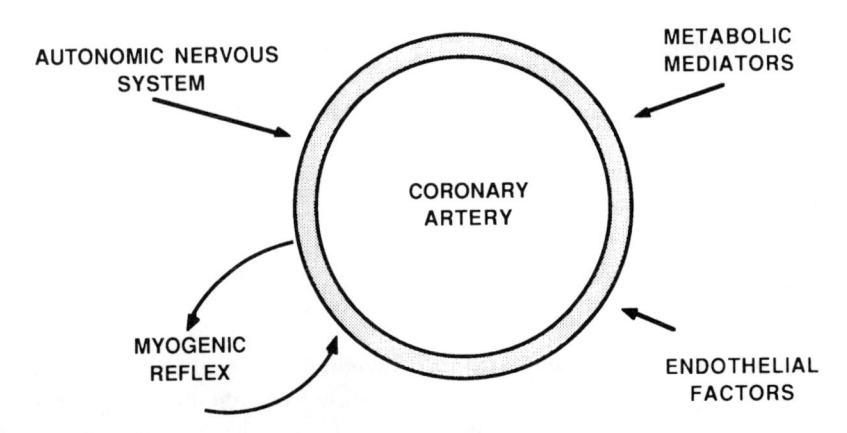

Figure 10.3. Main regulatory mechanisms of coronary vasomotor tone.

by α-1 and α-2 receptors [15] when their positive inotropic and chronotropic effects are blocked, for example, by β-blockers. Similarly, an increase in coronary resistance occurs when α-1 receptors are activated by the infusion of metoxamine [16]. Furthermore, experimental evidence indicates that a coronary vasoconstrictor α-adrenergic tone is present in basal conditions. In fact, α-blocker infusion in anesthetized dogs determines a significant reduction in coronary resistance [17], whereas the stimulation or inhibition of β-1 and β-2 receptors determines a coronary vasodilation or vasoconstriction, respectively [16].

However, the real importance of β-adrenergic tone in coronary resistance regulation is still not known. Rather than acting directly on coronary arterial wall receptors, the effect of β-agonists and β-blockers on coronary tone are mainly indirect, mediated by changes in myocardial energy metabolism. [18]. Parasympathetic stimulation induces coronary vasodilation via the release of acetylcholine, which can be blocked by atropine [13]. As will be discussed later, the effects of acetylcholine are complex, partly due to a endothelium mediated vasodilating effect, and to a direct vasoconstricting effect on smooth muscular cells [19, 20]. Finally, the renin–angiotensin tissue and plasma system can also influence coronary vasomotor tone, since angiotensin II, locally produced or present in the circulation, is able to determine a coronary vasoconstriction by activating the phosphatidyl-inositol system.

Myogenic factors

A contractile reaction is induced by an increase in intraluminal pressure which in turn stretches the smooth muscle cells [21]. This myogenic mechanism, also defined as the 'Bayliss reflex' has a homeostatic purpose, in that it tends to maintain the blood flow constant. However, the importance of the myogenic reflex on coronary resistance regulation is still not completely clear and seems to play only a secondary role [13].

Metabolic control

As stated previously, the main function of coronary circulation is to ensure an adequate supply of energy metabolites to the myocardium. Therefore, it is not surprising that metabolic factors play a major role in coronary resistance regulation.

Many substances such as hydrogen, potassium, calcium ions and carbon dioxide are released by hypoperfused myocardial cells and accumulate in the interstitial space [22]. Although each of these substances may have a vasomotor effect, most experimental results indicate that adenosine is by far the most important in coronary resistance regulation [23–25].

Adenosine is a purine with a strong vasodilating effect derived from the catabolism of purine nucleotides [24]. Its release by cardiomyocytes, however, depends on their energetic condition [23]. In fact, if the ATP hydrolysis rate exceeds the ATP resynthesis rate, intracellular AMP concentration increases, resulting in an increased production of adenosine by the enzyme 5'-nucleotidase. Since adenosine can cross the sarcolemma, it accumulates in the interstitial space and acts on specific receptors located in coronary smooth muscle and endothelial cells. It then leaves the myocardial interstice, either washed out unchanged by blood flow, or catabolized by hypoxanthine deaminase and xanthine dehydrogenase enzymes [26]. Thus, the vasodilating effect of adenosine is an important homeostatic mechanism for the correct regulation of oxygen myocardial supply. This mechanism ensures an increase in regional coronary flow each time there is a decrease in cellular energetic charge and vice versa.

Recent experimental data furthermore indicate that vascular coronary reactivity to adenosine differs in various physiopathological conditions [27]. A lower sensitivity to the vasodilating effect of adenosine in an isolated and perfused rat heart is evident during hypoxia in respect to control hearts. On the contrary, coronary circulation seems to be more sensitive to adenosine in comparison to the control hearts during postischemic reperfusion [27].

Endothelium factors

Recent experimental results have emphasized the importance of the endothelium in mediating the vasomotor effects of vasoactive substances and in controlling coronary resistance. Furchgott and Zawadski were the first to demonstrate that the integrity of the endothelium is necessary for substances such as ATP, ADP, acetylcholine, and histamine to have a vasodilating effect [19, 28]. In fact, vasoactive substances such as acetylcholine and serotonin have a vasodilating effect on intact coronary arteries and a vasoconstricting effect on coronary arteries with a damaged endothelium [28, 29]. Human coronary arteries with atherosclerotic disease also have a damaged endothelium and therefore react to acetylcholine or serotonin infusion by vasoconstricting [20, 29]. The reversal of vasoactive effects of some substances in the presence and in the absence of an intact endothelium is due to a direct vasoconstricting action on the smooth muscle cells of arterial media and simultaneously an indirect vasodilating action caused by the release of vasodilating substances from the endothelium (see Figure 10.4).

Among the many endothelial vasoactive substances which have recently been isolated and identified (some with a vasodilating and others with a vasoconstricting effect, see Figure 10.5), endothelium-derived relaxing factor (EDRF) seems to have a primary role in mediating the vasodilating effect of substances such as acetylcholine, histamine, and serotonin. An increase in coronary flow also seems to induce, through the increase in the endothelial 'shear stress', an EDRF-mediated vasodilation [30]. EDRF has recently been identified as a nitric oxide molecule (or as its derivative, nitrosothiol) [31]; it probably acts by stimulating the guanylate cyclase and therefore the synthesis of cGMP in smooth muscle cells. Moreover, the endothelium synthesizes and releases two vasodilating prostaglandins, PGE_2 and PGI_2, which probably play a role in modulating the vasoconstricting effects of α-

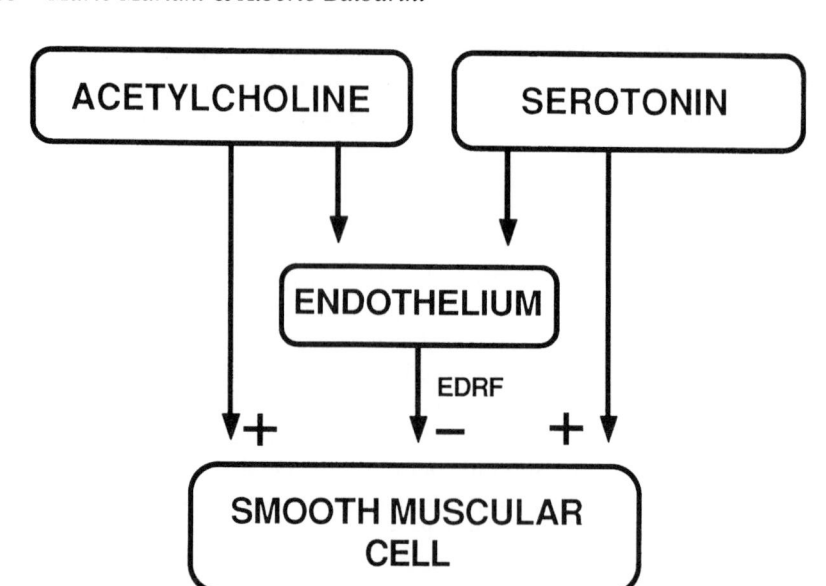

Figure 10.4. Acetylcholine and serotonin vasomotor effects. Both have a direct vasoconstricting effect on coronary smooth muscular cells and an indirect vasodilating effect mediated by EDRF (endothelium-derived relaxing factor) release.

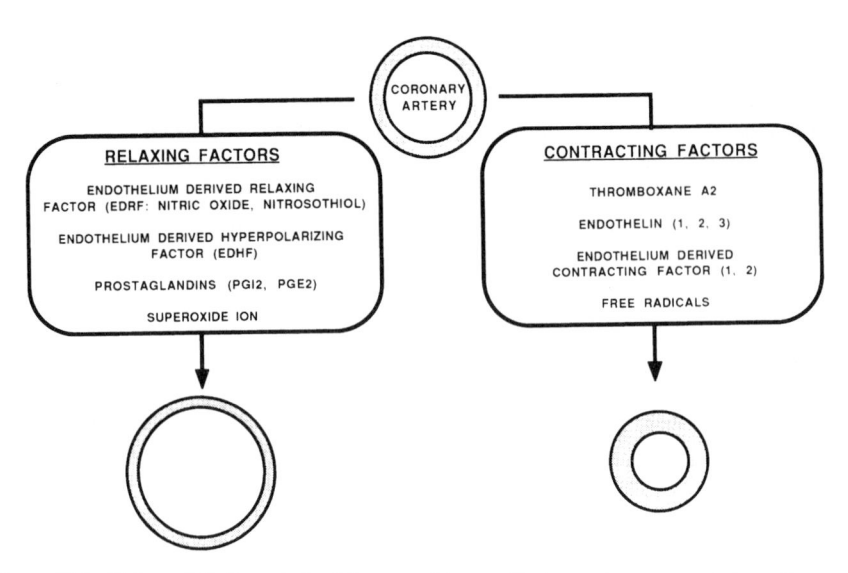

Figure 10.5. Main endothelium-derived factors with vasodilating and vasoconstricting effects on coronary circulation.

adrenergic stimulation. Their synthesis is inhibited by cyclooxygenase inhibitors, resulting in an increase in the α-mediated coronary vasoconstriction induced by a cold-pressor test [32].

Finally, the endothelium synthesizes vasoconstricting substances such as various peptides called endothelins. Three different isopeptides have been isolated (endothelin 1, 2, 3), each with a long and potent vasoconstricting effect [31]. Many substances such as thrombin, phorbol-ester, epinephrine, and the calcium ionophor A2318 can induce synthesis and release of endothelin 1. This vasoconstriction is probably due to the intracellular activation of the enzyme phospholipase C and the subsequent production of inositol triphosphate and diacylglycerol.

Recent experimental data also demonstrate a significant increase in the plasma levels of endothelin 1 in heart failure, along with a reduction in coronary reserve [33]. However, further studies are necessary to clarify the role of endothelins in coronary resistance control.

The hemodynamic effects of fixed or dynamic stenosis of epicardial coronary arteries

In physiological conditions, arteriolar resistance accounts for the largest part of coronary resistance, and can be reduced to about 20%, with a 4- to 5-fold increase in coronary flow (coronary reserve). The presence of a fixed stenosis in an epicardial coronary artery (caused, in most cases, by an atherosclerotic lesion of the intima), determines a resistance to flow in the epicardial district. The degree of resistance (and that of the pressure gradient) is determined by a coronary stenosis and is directly proportional to the length and inversely proportional to the fourth power of the radius of the stenotic vessel [34]. This increase in epicardial resistance is compensated (via the above mentioned control mechanisms), by a parallel reduction in arteriolar resistance so that coronary flow remains constant [35]. This leads to a reduction in coronary reserve so that any further increase in oxygen myocardial requirements cannot be matched by a parallel increase in coronary flow.

Thus, we can understand how a fixed coronary stenosis can induce the so-called 'secondary angina', which is characterized by myocardial ischemia and 'angor' during effort or other stress able to induce an increase in myocardial metabolic requirements. A coronary stenosis of between 50% and 90% results in a progressive reduction in coronary reserve with a consequent reduction in the effort angina threshold. If the stenosis is equal to or greater than 90%, the increase in epicardial resistance cannot be compensated by a reduction in arteriolar resistance. Consequently, there is a reduction in basal coronary flow and the appearance of myocardial ischemia at rest [36]. The hemodynamic effects of a fixed coronary stenosis often vary in time for several reasons. Platelet aggregates on the endothelial surface damaged by atherosclerotic plaque and/or vascular tone variations in the presence of an eccentric stenosis can induce significant changes in the degree of stenosis and consequently in the ischemic threshold. Furthermore, an increase in linear blood flow velocity in the narrow site of the vessel causes a further reduction in pressure (Venturi effect) and can result in a passive collapse of the artery [37]. This explains why 'fixed threshold angina' is relatively rare in comparison to 'variable threshold angina' and the frequent coexistence, in some patients, of angina under effort and at rest.

Coronary spasm

Coronary spasm is a temporary and localized size reduction in a coronary artery followed by sudden reduction in coronary flow and consequent myocardial ischemia that is not caused by an increase in oxygen myocardial consumption. This physiopathological condition is responsible for 'primary angina' or 'variant angina of Prinzmetal' [38]. Focal vasospasm often occurs in proximity to atherosclerotic plaques which alone do not cause a significant reduction in the artery diameter [39]. Therefore it has been hypothesized that the damaged endothelium produces less EDRF and, perhaps, more endothelin near an atherosclerotic plaque. Consequently, the vasodilating effects of vasoactive substances such as acetylcholine and serotonin are reversed [39, 40]. Moreover, the plaque's neovascularized tissue often favors the release of vasoconstricting substances such as serotonin, thromboxane A_2, thrombin, and leukotrienes [40]. Further data indicate that mastocytes [41] and magnesium ions [42, 43] may also play a role in the pathogenesis of coronary spasm.

References

1. McKeever, WP, Gregg DE, Canney PC. Oxygen uptake of the nonworking left ventricle. Circ Res 1958;6:612–23.
2. Klocke FJ, Braunwald E, Ross J Jr. Oxygen cost of electrical activation of the heart. Circ Res 1966;18:357–65.
3. Sarnoff SJ, Braunwald E, Welch GH Jr, Case RB, Stainsby WN, Macruz R. Hemodynamic determinants of the oxygen consumption of the heart with special reference to the tension time index. Am J Physiol 1958;192:148–56.
4. Rooke GA, Feigl EO. Work as a correlate of canine left ventricular oxygen consumption and the problem of catecholamine oxygen wasting. Circ Res 1982;50:273–86.
5. Suga H, Hisano R, Goto Y, Yamada O, Igarashi Y. Effect of positive inotropic agents on the relation between oxygen consumption and systolic pressure volume area in canine left ventricle. Circ Res 1983;53:306–18.
6. Suga H, Yamada O, Goto Y, Igarashi Y. Oxygen consumption and pressure–volume area of abnormal contractions in canine heart. Am J Physiol 1984;246:H154–60.
7. Braunwald E. Control of myocardial oxygen consumption: Physiologic and clinical considerations. Am J Cardiol 1971;27:416–32.
8. Graham TP Jr, Covell JW, Sonnenblick EH, Ross J Jr, Braunwald E. Control of myocardial oxygen consumption: Relative influence of contractile state and tension development. J Clin Invest 1968;47:375–85.
9. Boerth RC, Covell JW, Pool PE, Ross J Jr. Increased myocardial oxygen consumption and contractile state associated with increased heart rate in dogs. Circ Res 1969;24:725–34.
10. Marcus ML. The coronary circulation in health and disease. New York: McGraw-Hill, 1983:465.
11. Olsson RA, Bugni WJ. Coronary circulation. In: Fozzard HA, Haber E, Katz A, Jennings R, Morgan HE (eds.), The heart and the cardiovascular system. New York: Raven Press, 1986:987–1038.
12. Klocke FJ. Coronary blood flow in man. Prog Cardiovasc Dis 1976;19:117–20.

13. Berne RM, Rubio R. Coronary Circulation. In: Berne RM, Sperelakis N, Geiger SR (eds), Handbook of physiology; the cardiovascular system. Bethesda: American Physiological Society, 1979:897.
14. Rinkema LE, Thomas JX, Randall WC. Regional coronary vasoconstriction in response to stimulation of stellate ganglia. Am J Physiol 1982;243:H410–5.
15. Vatner SF. α-adrenergic tone in the coronary circulation of the conscious dog. Fed Proc 1984;43:2867–72.
16. Young MA, Vatner SF. Regulation of large coronary arteries. Circ Res 1986;59:579–96.
17. Macho P, Vatner SF. Effects of prazosin on coronary and left ventricular dynamics in conscious dogs. Circulation 1982;65:1186–92.
18. Vatner SF, Hintze TH. Mechanism of constriction of large coronary arteries by β-adrenergic receptor blockade. Circ Res 1983;53:389–400.
19. Furchgott RF. Role of endothelium in responses of vascular smooth muscle. Circ Res 1983;53:557–73.
20. Ludmer PL, Selwyn AP, Shook TL et al. Paradoxical vasoconstriction induced by acetylcholine in atherosclerotic coronary arteries. N Engl J Med 1986;315:1046–51.
21. Øien AH, Aukland K. A mathematical analysis of the myogenic hypothesis with special reference to autoregulation of renal blood flow. Circ Res 1983;52:241–52.
22. Marcus ML. Metabolic regulation of coronary blood flow. In: The coronary circulation in health and disease. New York: McGraw-Hill, 1983:85.
23. Sparks HV, Bardenheuer H. Regulation of adenosine formation by the heart. Circ Res 1986;58:193–201.
24. Rubio R, Berne RM. Release of adenosine by the normal myocardium in dogs and its relationship to the regulation of coronary resistance. Circ Res 1969;25:407–15.
25. Bardenheuer H, Schrader J. Supply-to-demand ratio for oxygen determines formation of adenosine by the heart. Am J Physiol 1986;250:H173–80.
26. Rubio R, Berne RM, Dobson JG. Sites of adenosine production in cardiac and skeletal muscle. Am J Physiol 1973;225:H938–53.
27. Zucchi R, Limbruno U, Poddighe R, Mariani M, Ronca G. The adenosine hypothesis revisited: Relationship between purine release and coronary flow in isolated rat heart. Cardiovasc Res 1989;23:125–31.
28. Furchgott RF, Zawadski JV. The obligatory role of endothelial cells in the relaxation of arterial smooth muscle by acetylcholine. Nature 1980;288:373–6.
29. Golino P, Piscione F, Willerson JT et al. Divergent effects of serotonin on coronary artery dimensions and blood flow in patients with coronary atherosclerosis and control patients. N Engl J Med 1991;324:641–8.
30. Hintze TH, Vatner SF. Reactive dilation of large coronary arteries in conscious dogs. Cir Res 1984;54:50–7.
31. Katusic ZS. Endothelium-derived vasoactive factors and coronary artery tone. Cardiologia 1990;35(suppl 1)12:423.
32. Neri Serneri GG, Gensini GF, Prisco D. Il ruolo delle prostaglandine nella cardiopatia ischemica. Cardiologia 1990;35(suppl 1)12:409.
33. Grenier O, Komajda M, Maistre G et al. Endothelin plasma concentration is increased in chronic congestive heart failure. Circulation 1990;82(4):III–381 (Abs. 1574).
34. Gould KL. Assessing coronary stenosis severity: A recurrent clinical need. J Am Coll Cardiol 1986;8:91–4.
35. Gould KL. Coronary artery stenosis. New York: Elsevier, 1991:323.
36. Klocke FJ. Measurements of coronary blood flow and degree of stenosis: Current clinical implications and continuing uncertainties. J Am Coll Cardiol 1983;1:31–41.
37. Epstein SE, Cannon RO, Talbot TL. Hemodynamic principles in the control of coronary blood flow. Am J Cardiol 1985;56:4E–10E.
38. Printzmetal M, Kennamer R, Merliss R, Wada T, Bor N. A variant form of angina pectoris. Am J Med 1959;27:375–88.
39. Ganz P, Alexander RW. New insights into the cellular mechanisms of vasospasm. Am J Cardiol 1985;56:11E–15E.

40. McFadden EP, Clarke JG, Davies GJ, Kaski JC, Haider AW, Maseri A. Effect of intracoronary serotonin on coronary vessels in patients with stable angina and patients with variant angina. N Engl J Med 1991;324:648–54.
41. Forman MB, Oates JA, Robertson D, Roberston RM, Roberts LJ, Virmani R. Increased adventitial mastcells in a patient with coronary spasm. N Engl J Med 1985;313:1138–41.
42. Cohen L, Kitzes R. Prompt termination and/or prevention of cold-pressor-stimulus-induced vasoconstriction of different vascular beds by magnesium sulfate in patients with Printzmetal's angina. Magnesium 1986;5:144.
43. Miyagi H, Yasue H, Okumura K, Ogawa H, Goto K, Oshima S. Effect of magnesium on anginal attack induced by hyperventilation in patients with variant angina. Circulation 1989;79:597–602.

11. The pathology and pathophysiology of coronary artery disease

IAN COX and ROBERT CROOK

Atherosclerosis is by far the most common and clinically important condition to affect the coronary arteries, causing 127,000 deaths due to myocardial infarction in the United Kingdom each year. Consequently, the terms coronary artery disease and coronary atherosclerosis are often used synonymously although a variety of other pathological processes may affect the coronaries. This chapter will concentrate on the pathophysiology of coronary atherosclerosis with particular emphasis on the relationship between the natural history of atherosclerotic disease progression and the evolution of clinical disease. The pathophysiology of other forms of coronary disease will not be covered.

Coronary atherosclerotic disease

Coronary atherosclerosis is characterized by focal intimal plaques in the large and medium sized epicardial coronary arteries which may cause obstruction to coronary blood flow. Myocardial ischemia due to coronary atherosclerotic disease presents as a spectrum of clinical syndromes including the following:

- chronic stable angina pectoris;
- Prinzmetal's variant angina;
- unstable angina;
- myocardial infarction;
- sudden cardiac death;
- chronic cardiac failure; and
- cardiac arrhythmia.

The symptomatology, investigation, and treatment of these conditions will be discussed in detail elsewhere.

The authors thank Dr J.C. Kaski and Dr M.R. Chester for their assistance during the preparation of this chapter.

The pathophysiology of coronary atherosclerotic disease

The coronary circulation consists of a branching network of epicardial arteries which divide into numerous smaller intramyocardial vessels penetrating the substance of the myocardium. Human coronary arteries function as regional end arteries, and under normal circumstances anastomotic flow between regions is strictly limited [1]. Under resting conditions a relatively high fixed percentage of oxygen is extracted from coronary arterial blood and changes in oxygen release produce little additional benefit. Consequently, myocardial oxygen delivery is largely dependent on coronary blood flow.

Regulation of coronary blood flow is primarily achieved by variations in the vasomotor tone of the coronary resistance vessels, in particular the small intramyocardial arteries and arterioles (ranging in diameter from 0.1 to 0.5 mm). These vessels are responsive to a variety of neural and humoral influences and when maximally dilated can produce a several-fold increase in coronary blood flow [2]. The ratio between coronary flow under basal conditions and maximal coronary flow after vasodilation is termed the coronary flow reserve. In the presence of a flow restricting stenosis in an epicardial coronary artery, the smaller distal vessels dilate in an adaptive response to minimize flow restriction due to the upstream stenosis. Hemodynamic studies have shown that this mechanism is largely exhausted by the time a stenosis has produced a reduction in luminal cross-sectional area of approximately 75% (equivalent to a 50% reduction in luminal diameter) [3, 4]. At this stage the coronary flow reserve is reduced to near zero and local flow can only be increased by augmenting perfusion pressure. Under these circumstances any increase in myocardial oxygen demand above basal levels is liable to provoke ischemia. Such critical flow limitation is usually associated with anginal symptoms characterized by a predictable pattern of chest pain occuring during exertion or emotional excitement and relieved by rest. Such ischemia due to obstructive coronary disease may be further compounded by factors which increase myocardial oxygen demand (notably increases in heart rate or systemic blood pressure) or conditions resulting in either a reduction of the coronary artery perfusion pressure or increased coronary vasomotor tone.

Coronary artery vasomotion and vasospasm

Coronary vasomotor tone, associated with the activity of medial smooth muscle cells, plays an important role in the normal autoregulation of coronary blood flow. In the presence of atherosclerotic disease the normal regulation of vasomotor tone is disturbed [5–7] with impaired release of endothelial-derived mediators such as nitric oxide and endothelin. In the presence of a critical flow-limiting stenosis relatively minor changes in tone can have dramatic effects on perfusion and thus contribute adversely in the evolution of ischemia. The significance of changes in vasomotor tone is variable between different atherosclerotic stenoses (see below) and such dynamic changes may explain the diurnal and day-to-day variations in anginal threshold which are experienced by some patients [8]. Reduction of vasomotor tone may, in part, explain how coronary vasodilator drugs exert their beneficial effect in some patients with angina [9].

A small minority of patients manifest episodes of severe focal coronary artery spasm even at sites of relatively mild atherosclerotic stenoses [10]. Such episodes of primarily vasospastic flow restriction produce characteristic anginal chest pain which, in contrast to typical angina, often occur at rest. This variant form of angina may also occur in the absence of angiographic coronary disease although the presence of subangiographic atheroma may be a contributory factor in some cases.

Coronary steal

The mechanism of coronary steal may also play a significant role in the evolution of ischemia due to coronary atherosclerosis. The basis of this mechanism lies in the fact that a coronary circuit subtended by a critically stenotic artery will be maximally or near maximally dilated even under basal conditions (see above). Subsequent vasodilation in other parallel coronary circuits increases flow to those territories but may reduce the overall perfusion pressure. This results in a selective redistribution of flow away from the stenotic territory. The coronary steal phenomenon is exploited during clinical isotope perfusion studies where vasodilators such as dipyridamole are used to identify territories which are liable to reversible ischemia.

Consequences of myocardial ischemia

Ischemic reduction in myocardial oxygen supply restricts aerobic metabolism in myocardial cells and production of high energy phosphates through mitochondrial oxidative phosphorylation falls dramatically. This impairs the interaction of contractile proteins and results in reduced myocardial systolic contraction. Diastolic relaxation is also impaired causing the left ventricle to stiffen and left ventricular end diastolic pressure to rise. The elevated pressure is transmitted to the pulmonary vasculature resulting in pulmonary congestion and dyspnea. Ischemia also causes local accumulation of metabolites e.g. lactate, kinins, serotonin, and adenosine. It is suspected that one or more of these compounds activates peripheral pain receptors resulting in the characteristic chest pain known as angina pectoris. Ischemic abnormalities of myocyte membrane ion transport and accumulation of local metabolites may also act to promote cardiac arrhythmia. If frequent or prolonged, ischemia can result in permanent damage to myocardial cells (see below under myocardial infarction).

Pathogenesis of coronary atherosclerosis

Detailed discussion of the pathogenesis of atherosclerosis was provided in Chapter 2 and this topic will only be summarized briefly here. Coronary atherosclerosis is characterized by the accumulation of lipid, macrophages, and smooth muscle cells in focal intimal plaques. Mechanical shear stresses, biochemical abnormalities and immunological factors may all contribute to the initial endothelial 'injury' which is believed to trigger atherogenesis [11, 12]. Local endothelial dysfunction allows accumulation of low density lipoprotein (LDL) which is subsequently oxidized and taken up by macrophages to produce lipid-laden foam cells. Release of a host of cytokines such as platelet-derived growth factor (PDGF) and transforming growth factor-β (TGF-β) promote further accumulation of macrophages as well as smooth muscle cell migration and proliferation.

Postmortem studies have revealed that the evolution of coronary atherosclerosis usually begins in the second or third decade of life [13, 14]. The earliest macroscopically visible signs of atherosclerosis are flat, lipid-rich lesions called fatty streaks. Fatty streaks do not give rise to clinical symptoms but may develop into larger raised intimal lesions termed fibrolipid plaques [14]. Mature fibrolipid plaques consist of a cap of subendothelial fibromuscular tissue and a necrotic core containing tissue debris and extracellular lipid. Large fibrolipid plaques cause obstruction of the arterial lumen and the natural history of fibrolipid plaque progression is intimately associated with the evolution of clinical syndromes associated with coronary atherosclerosis.

Composition of atherosclerotic plaques

The composition of plaque appears to be an important determinant of plaque stability and subsequent stenosis progression (see plaque rupture below). Individual fibrolipid plaques contain variable proportions of lipid, fibrous tissue, and calcium [15]. In some cases, discrete collections of semifluid cholesterol and cholesterol esters also form large local collections or 'pools' within the intimal plaque [16]. These intimal pools result from the death of lipid-laden macrophages, a process sometimes referred to as atheronecrosis [17]. Most patients appear to have a mixture of fibrous and lipid plaques although in individual patients either type may predominate. The factors which contribute to these variations in plaque composition are poorly understood.

Calcification occurs commonly in atherosclerotic plaques. In a recent intravascular ultrasound study, in patients undergoing coronary angioplasty, significant calcification was demonstrated in approximately three-quarters of target lesions [18]. The distribution of calcium within such lesions is variable. In some cases small foci of calcification are scattered throughout the lesion whereas in other cases calcium deposition appears to adopt a more laminar configuration which may involve superficial and/or deep plaque. The factors contributing to variations in calcification are not well understood but this may have considerable influence on the physical properties of plaque particularly in the context of transluminal angioplasty [19].

Circumferential distribution of plaque

The distribution of plaque around the vessel's circumference may divided into eccentric and concentric patterns [15]. Eccentric lesions (Figure 11.1b) are characterized by a nonuniform distribution of plaque and the presence of an arc of normal or near normal arterial wall. Concentric lesions (Figure 11.1a) are characterized by an even distribution of plaque around the whole vessel circumference with no unaffected sections. Intravascular ultrasound studies have demonstrated a ratio of eccentric to concentric plaque of around four to one [20]. Similar proportions have also been demonstrated in postmortem series [21] although figures vary according to patient selection. In contrast, angiographic studies have suggested a much lower rate of lesion eccentricity, highlighting the limitations of angiography in regard to the assessment of plaque distribution (see below).

The morphological difference between concentric and eccentric lesions has important functional significance. The media beneath atheromatous plaques becomes grossly atrophic [22] and consequently the majority of medial muscle is lost in concentric lesions. Concentric lesions therefore exhibit a marked reduction in vasomotion and result in stenoses of largely fixed severity. In contrast, eccentric plaques often retain an arc of normal medial muscle giving rise to a greater potential for vasomotor reactivity [23, 24]. Alterations in vasomotor tone can exert a greater influence on the lumen diameter in such eccentric lesions [25]. Similarly, as an atheromatous stenosis progresses, the likelihood of retaining a disease-free segment of vessel wall diminishes and consequently the most severe stenoses tend to have fixed stenotic properties.

The circumferential distribution of plaque also has considerable significance in the context of transluminal coronary angioplasty. In particular, balloon angioplasty may be less successful in the presence of an eccentric lesion due to the presence of a compliant arc of normal arterial wall which may allow considerable dilation followed by elastic recoil without plaque disruption [26]. The distribution of plaque can also have a significant influence on the success of new device angioplasty including directional atherectomy and rotablator techniques [19, 20].

Longitudinal distribution of coronary atherosclerosis

Angiographic studies have demonstrated that clinically significant stenosing plaques may be located anywhere within the three major epicardial coronary arteries but tend to predominate within the first two centimeters of the left anterior descending and left circumflex arteries and the proximal and distal thirds of the right coronary artery. However, postmortem findings suggest that coronary atheroma is often present in a more diffuse pattern of distribution than is apparent at angiography [27, 28]. The discrepancy between angiographic and pathological findings illustrates the insensitivity of angiographic techniques for detecting low grade atheromatous changes. This is partly due to the phenomenon of adaptive remodelling which refers to local compensatory enlargement of diseased coronary segments [29, 30]. This mechanism acts to preserve the luminal dimensions and can prevent luminal encroachment by plaque volumes up to 40% of the total vessel cross-sectional area. Recent work with intravascular ultrasound has helped to substantiate the importance of this mechanism *in vivo* [31, 32]. Intravascular ultrasound studies of patients undergoing transluminal angioplasty have also demonstrated that angiographically normal reference segments contain an average plaque burden

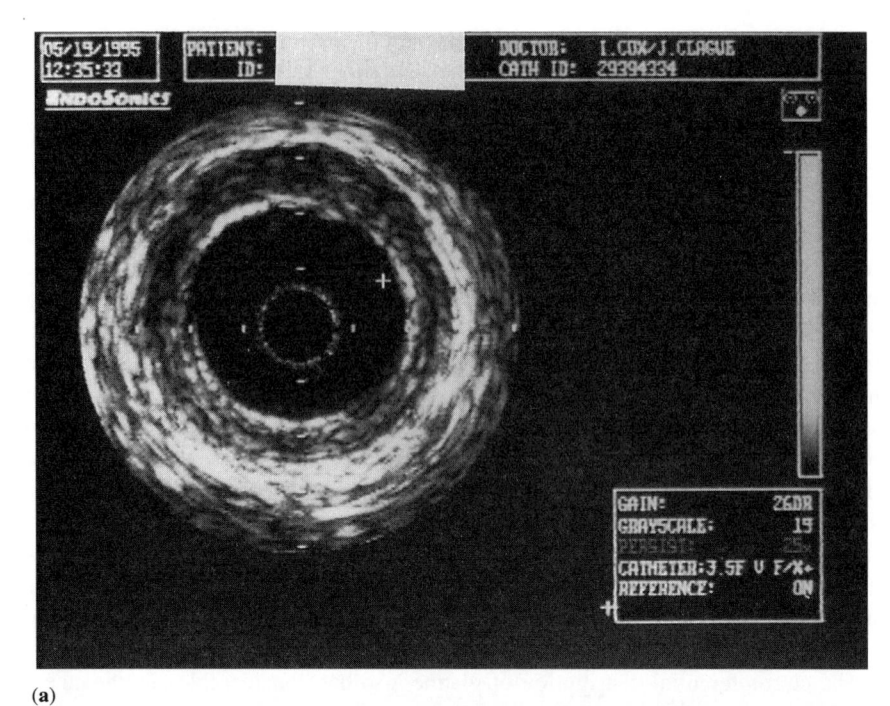

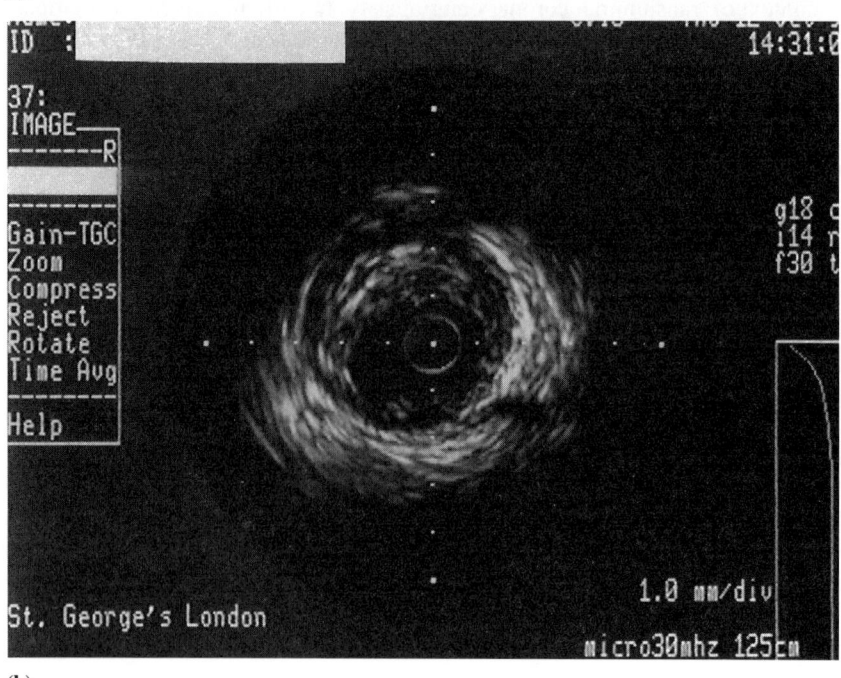

Figure 11.1. Intravascular ultrasound pictures demonstrating: (a) concentric and (b) eccentric distributions of atherosclerotic plaque.

equivalent to 35–40% of the measured vessel cross-sectional area [33, 34]. Similarly, significant atherosclerotic disease has been demonstrated by the same technique in 90% of angiographically normal or near normal left main coronary arteries in angioplasty patients [35]. These studies have helped to highlight once again the diffuse nature of atheromatous changes in patients with coronary atherosclerosis.

Adaptive mechanisms which reduce the ischemic impact of coronary stenoses

The hemodynamic impact of atherosclerotic lesions is reduced by a number of adaptive mechanisms which operate in the coronary system. Post-stenotic vasodilation and adaptive remodeling have already been described above. The ischemic stimulus produced by the presence of a chronic severe stenosis in a particular artery can also stimulate the development of collateral vessels from other regional arteries as can be clearly demonstrated at angiography. Such collaterals can considerabley reduce the ischemic impact of a stenosis, increasing the threshold of myocardial demand necessary to precipitate ischemia. Collaterals may also prevent or limit the extent of infarction when such a stenosis progresses to occlusion. In one pathological study 65% of patients with stable angina but no evidence of healed infarction had chronically occluded coronary segments [15]. Angiographic studies have similarly demonstrated that occlusion of significant stenoses can occur in both stable and unstable angina patients without accompanying acute coronary events [36, 37]. However, collateralization is rarely able to match the perfusion provided by the disease-free native artery and consequently ischemia under stress is rarely eliminated entirely by this mechanism.

Plaque disruption

Plaque rupture results from fissuring of the fibrous cap leading to exposure of subendothelial collagen and necrotic plaque contents to the arterial lumen (Figure 11.2). This process can lead to sudden changes in plaque geometry and histopathological evidence suggests that this event represents the common pathological substrate underlying the evolution of acute ischemic coronary syndromes including myocardial infarction, unstable angina, and sudden cardiac death [38, 39]. Exposure of the extracellular matrix (in particular tissue factor) triggers platelet adhesion, aggregation, and activation. Platelet activation leads to the release of active mediators (including thromboxane A_2, serotonin, and ADP) which trigger further platelet activation and activation of the coagulation cascade [40, 41]. Local endothelial dysfunction also contributes to thrombosis by reducing the secretion of inhibitory substances such as thrombomodulin and prostacyclin. Local thrombus may have both intraplaque and intraluminal components and may lead to total occlusion of the affected vessel and in some cases myocardial infarction. Microembolization of thrombotic fragments to distal intramyocardial vessels may also result in myocardial damage [42, 43].

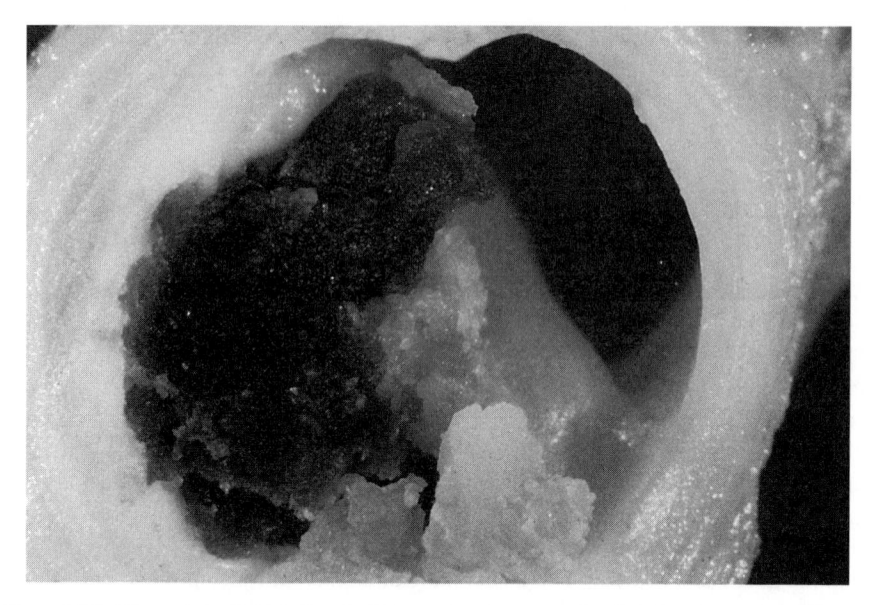

Figure 11.2. Histopathological section of a human coronary artery showing plaque rupture and thrombosis (provided by Professor M.J. Davies).

Transient local vasoconstriction exacerbates distal ischemia following plaque disruption. This may be triggered by vasoactive substances released from aggregating platelets, such as serotonin and thromboxane A_2, or because the damaged endothelium does not produce normal vasodilatory substances such as nitric oxide and prostacyclin. Superimposed thrombosis and vasoconstriction after plaque rupture explain the pathological finding that stable and unstable angina differ primarily in terms of intact versus disrupted plaque surface rather than in terms of severity of atherosclerotic stenoses [44–46].

Factors triggering plaque disruption

The pathogenetic mechanisms which trigger plaque rupture are not fully understood although it appears that rupture may depend more on plaque composition than on plaque size [47, 48]. Plaques are more likely to rupture if they have a large 'soft' lipid core [49], low collagen content [50] and a thin fibrous cap [51]. Plaques with a high proportion of macrophages compared to smooth muscle cells also appear prone to rupture [52]. The shoulder region is particularly vulnerable to rupture [53] at the site where the cap is infiltrated by activated mast cells [54, 55]. Histological examination of atherectomy specimens have also demonstrated a higher incidence of macrophage rich areas in patients with unstable angina and non-Q-wave myocardial infarction when compared to chronic stable angina [56]. These findings are consistent with the hypothesis that release of lytic enzymes (including matrix metalloproteinases such as collagenase and elastase) by activated macrophages may be an important trigger to plaque rupture [57].

Extrinsic factors including arterial wall tension and shear forces associated with coronary blood flow also play a role in plaque rupture. Such external forces may act on the surface of a vulnerable plaque to trigger rupture. Fissures frequently occur at the junction of the fibrous cap with adjacent normal arterial wall, a location associated with high circumferential stress/shear forces [53]. Consequently, acute rises in arterial blood pressure, tachycardia, and local vasospasm may all contribute to plaque rupture. Symptomatic onset of acute coronary syndromes during episodes of exertion is well recognized and may be related to these factors [58, 59]. In this context it is also interesting to note that the peak time of onset for acute myocardial infarction is between 9 and 11 a.m., a period associated with a surge in blood pressure and heightened platelet reactivity [60].

As stated above substantial plaque rupture associated with dramatic changes in plaque geometry may result in vessel occlusion or a dramatic increase in stenosis. However, more minor episodes of plaque disruption may have less dramatic effects and occur without acute ischemia [61, 62]. Postmortem studies have revealed evidence of silent plaque disruption in up to 9% of normal individuals, 22% of patients with diabetes or hypertension [61], and over 50% of patients with coronary artery disease [63]. These findings support the suggestion that plaque rupture is a far more common event in patients with coronary atherosclerosis than suggested by the incidence of acute coronary syndromes. Plaques which rupture without causing vessel occlusion can subsequently reseal incorporating associated thrombus. This leads to a significant increase in the size of the plaque and increased lumenal stenosis. Plaque rupture occurring as a dynamic and repetitive process appears to play a central role in atherosclerotic disease progression. Further insight into the role of plaque rupture in coronary disease progression has been gained from serial angiographic studies.

Insights on coronary disease progression from angiographic studies

The limitations of serial angiographic studies are well recognized and have already been mentioned in earlier sections. However, such studies have provided important information about the natural history of coronary atherosclerosis. Plaque growth secondary to rupture, thrombosis, and healing correlates well with the unpredictable, nonlinear progression of coronary artery disease demonstrated by serial angiographic studies [64, 65]. This pattern of progression is characterized by variable periods of apparent stability interspersed by episodes of rapid disease progression. The majority of clinical events are associated with rapid disease progression at angiography [66–68] although such episodes can also occur silently i.e. unheralded by an obvious change in the patient's symptoms [37, 69–71]. A previous history of an acute coronary syndrome is also associated with an increased incidence of subsequent rapid disease progression [70, 72, 73].

In terms of the total angiographic plaque burden the incidence of rapid disease progression is relatively rare. Thus, events occurring at a small number of vulnerable segments appear to be responsible for clinically significant disease progression whilst the vast bulk of the atheroma remains essentially stable. It is important to recognize that rapid disease progression often occurs at previously normal or mildly stenotic sites [66] and consequently that plaque rupture at such sites is frequently responsible for the genesis of acute coronary syndromes [74–76]. This may account for the failure of previous studies to demonstrate a long-term prognostic benefit from the selective treatment of individual severe coronary stenoses by transluminal coronary angioplasty [77].

Angiographic lesion morphology also appears to be associated with plaque activity and disease progression. Angiographic stenoses can be classified as 'complex' (characterized by irregular borders, overhanging edges, or thrombus, see Figure 11.3) or 'smooth' (characterized by the absence of complex features) [78]. Complex lesions are thought to represent the angiographic counterpart of plaque disruption [15, 39, 79] and are frequently seen at angiography following acute coronary events [66, 73–75, 79–80]. Complex stenoses may also develop unheralded by acute coronary syndromes [71] consistent with episodes of silent plaque disruption as discussed above. Regardless of the circumstances of their evolution, lesions with complex morphology appear to identify a subgroup of stenoses associated with disease progression [74, 75, 81–83] and adverse clinical outcomes [69, 73, 80, 81, 84–86].

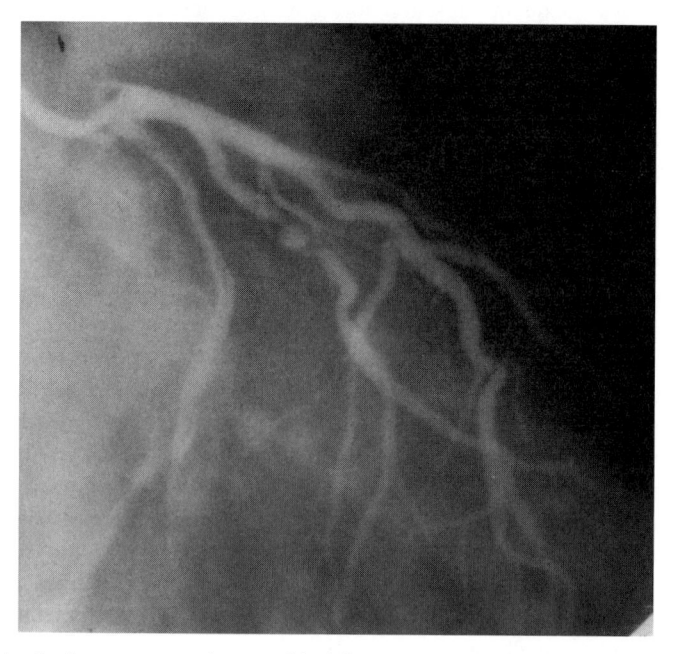

Figure 11.3. A selective coronary angiogram of the left coronary system (right anterior oblique projection) depicting a complex coronary stenosis in the first diagonal branch of the left anterior descending artery.

Myocardial infarction

Myocardial infarction is characterized by necrosis of myocardial tissue secondary to a prolonged ischemic insult. This process can be subdivided into two major groups according to the extent of necrosis within the myocardial wall. Transmural myocardial infarction is characterized by full or nearly full thickness necrosis of the ventricular wall usually in the distribution of a single coronary artery. The pathological basis of regional, transmural infarction is believed to be acute plaque rupture and superimposed occlusive thrombus [87]. Postmortem studies have confirmed the presence of thrombotic arterial occlusion in more than 90% of cases of full thickness myocardial infarction [88, 89] and the majority of these occlusive thrombi appear to be associated with evidence of acute plaque disruption [90]. Angiography performed on living patients at 4 hours after the acute onset myocardial infarction confirms complete coronary occlusion in 90% of cases [91–93]. The incidence of acute occlusion falls to around 60–70% if angiography is delayed until 12–24 hours after onset of infarction indicating either spontaneous clot lysis or relaxation of local vasospasm [94]. The importance of thrombosis in infarction has also been supported by the numerous studies which have shown that flow can be restored by thrombolytic therapy administered early after the onset of pain [95]. Furthermore, angiography following successful thrombolytic therapy often reveals the presence of an underlying stenosis with complex morphological features consistent with the presence of local plaque disruption [74, 75]. A small number of fatal infarcts due to occlusive coronary thrombosis appear to occur in the absence of plaque fissuring, primarily at sites of high-grade stenosis in smaller epicardial arteries [90]. In the remaining 10% of cases, regional transmural myocardial infarction has been documented in the absence of atherosclerotic thrombotic occlusion. Severe vasospasm, usually in relation to a stenosed segment but very occasionally in the absence of stenosing atherosclerosis, may be responsible for infarction in such cases.

Subendocardial (nontransmural) infarction consists of an area of ischemic necrosis limited to the inner one-third to one-half of the ventricular wall. The subendocardium is the myocardial zone most vulnerable to ischemia, partly because it is subjected to the highest pressure from the ventricular chamber but also because it is located furthest from the main epicardial vessels and is supplied by small arteries that pass through layers of contracting myocardium [96]. Subendocardial infarcts are often confined to the territory of a single coronary artery as with transmural infarction. Such cases are also usually associated with plaque disruption although the incidence of total vessel occlusion is far less than in transmural infarcts [97]. This may reflect early lysis of an occluding thrombus leading to transient vessel occlusion of insufficient duration to cause full thickness infarction. Where a thrombotic occlusion is present, the failure to progress to full thickness infarction may also be due to the presence of extensive distal collaterals [98]. Subendocardial infarction may also present in a more diffuse pattern, extending beyond the perfusion territory of a single coronary. This pattern of infarction is usually seen in patients with extensive coronary atherosclerosis following a hypotensive episode resulting in global reduction in coronary perfusion pressure.

Factors contributing to infarct size

Infarct size is of critical prognostic significance after acute infarction. A variety of factors contribute to the extent of tissue that succumbs to infarction secondary to thrombotic occlusion of a coronary artery. These factors include the site and duration of occlusion, the extent of distal collateralization of the ischemic territory and the metabolic/oxygen demands of the at risk myocardium during the period of occlusion. Further extension of infarction may also occur some time after the initial thrombotic event. Retrograde propagation of thrombus and proximal vasospasm may contribute to extension of the infarcted territory in such cases. Reduction in total coronary perfusion due to the establishment of a low cardiac output state secondary to myocardial damage or arrhythmia can also contribute adversely to ischemic damage.

Ischemic preconditioning

Ischemic preconditioning represents a further important factor which may modify the response of myocardial tissue to an ischemic insult. Ischemic preconditioning was first described in canine hearts [99] and refers to the phenomenon whereby a transient ischemic insult, insufficient to cause permanent injury, results in increased tolerance to subsequent episodes of more prolonged ischemia. The initial period of ischemia must be followed by at least one minute, but not more than 120 minutes, of reperfusion and will give a variable degree of protection for up to 90 minutes [100]. Preconditioning has been demonstrated in isolated human muscle using right atrial trabeculae suspended in organ baths [101]. During intermittent cross-clamp fibrillation, the resultant fall in myocardial ATP concentration can be dramatically reduced by the use of two preceding sequences of three-minute periods of ischemia [102]. Ischemic preconditioning may also explain the apparent protection conferred by previous angina on in-hospital outcome after myocardial infarction seen in the subgroup analysis of the Thrombolysis in Myocardial Infarction (TIMI) 4 study [103]. Studies in which reversible ischemia was induced by stress testing, atrial pacing, and percutaneous transluminal coronary angioplasty provide further indirect evidence of preconditioning *in vivo* [104].

Various theories have been postulated as to the cellular mechanism of ischemic preconditioning. Adenosine, formed from the breakdown of ATP, appears to play a central role in preconditioning. Adenosine A_1 receptor antagonists have been shown to abolish preconditioning [105] and blockade of ATP sensitive potassium channels (linked to A_1 receptors) prevents preconditioning in dogs [106]. Trials to evaluate the possible cardioprotective properties of potassium channel openers are currently being undertaken.

Sudden cardiac death

Temporal definitions of sudden cardiac death (SCD) vary but one widely accepted form states that SCD is death due to cardiac causes which occurs within six hours of the onset of symptoms. Postmortem studies have revealed that coronary atheroma is the cause of death in around 70% of such cases [107]. Forty percent of all deaths due to coronary atherosclerosis occur suddenly in this way although up to 50% of patients dying suddenly due to coronary atheroma have no preceding history of coronary disease.

The majority of cases of SCD due to atheroma appear to be due to fatal ventricular arrhythmia triggered by acute myocardial ischemia. However, the exact pathogenetic events underlying this mechanism remains the subject of some controversy. Postmortem studies have shown the presence of angiographically complex lesions with plaque fissuring and thrombosis in more than 90% of sudden ischemic cardiac deaths [108–110]. Likewise, a study in which angiography was performed shortly after resuscitation in patients with 'failed' SCD showed a 72% incidence of total vessel occlusion [111]. Other series of SCD survivors have also shown that infarction can only be documented in a minority of cases [112], confirming that sudden ischemic cardiac death is not necessarily associated with acute myocardial infarction. Sudden cardiac death may also occur in patients with established severe coronary atherosclerosis in the absence of any obvious acute thrombotic event [113]. Such cases probably result from reentrant ventricular arrhythmia arising in areas of chronic ischemic damage secondary to previous infarction [114].

Conclusion

Postmortem and angiographic studies have provided important insights into the evolution and natural history of coronary atherosclerosis. Future advances in treatment and prevention will depend on a greater understanding of the pathology and pathophysiology of this complex and multifactorial disease. Techniques such as intravascular ultrasound, vascular biology, and molecular genetics provide exciting prospects for further progress in this area.

References

1. Schaper W. Natural defence mechanisms during ischaemia. Eur Heart J 1983;4:73–8.
2. Poole-Wilson PA. Haemodynamic and metabolic consequences of angina and myocardial infarction. In: Fox KM,. (ed.), Ischaemic heart disease. Lancaster: MTP Press 1987:123.
3. Higgins D, Santamore WP, Walinsky P, Nemir P. Haemodynamics of human arterial stenosis. Int J Cardiol 1985;87:177–92.
4. Klocke FJ. Measurement of coronary blood flow and degree of stenosis: Current clinical implications and continuing uncertainties. J Am Coll Cardiol 1983;1:31–41.
5. Ludmer PL, Selwyn AP, Shook TI et al. Paradoxical vasoconstriction induced by acetylcholine in atherosclerotic coronary arteries. N Engl J Med 1986;315:1046–51.
6. Kawachi Y, Tomoiki H, Marvoka Y et al. Selective hypercontraction caused by ergonovine in canine coronary artery under conditions of induced atherosclerosis. Circulation 1984;69:441–50.
7. Heistad DD, Armstrong ML, Marcul ML, Piegorş DJ, Mark AL. Augmented responses to vasoconstrictor stimuli in hypercholesterolaemic and atherosclerotic monkeys. Circ Res 1984;54:711–8.
8. Maseri A, Davies G, Hackett D, Kaski JC. Coronary artery spasm and vasoconstriction. The case for a distinction. Circulation 1990;81:1983–91.

9. Kaski JC, Tousoulis D, Haider AW, Gavrielides S, Crea F, Maseri A. Reactivity of eccentric and concentric coronary stenoses in patients with chronic stable angina. J Am Coll Cardiol 1991;17:627–33.
10. Maseri A, Severi S, Nes MD et al. Variant angina: One aspect of a continuous spectrum of vasospastic myocardial ischaemia. Pathogenetic mechanisms, estimated incidence, clinical and coronary arteriographic findings in 138 patients. Am J Cardiol 1978;42:1019–35.
11. Ross R, Glomset JA. Atherosclerosis and the arterial smooth muscle cell. Proliferation of smooth muscle is a key event in the genesis of the lesions of atherosclerosis. Science 1973;180:1332–9.
12. Ross R. The pathogenesis of atherosclerosis – An update. N Engl J Med 1986;314:488–500.
13. Enos WF, Beyer JC, Holmes RH. Pathogenesis of coronary artery disease in American soldiers killed in Korea. J Am Med Assoc 1955;158:912–4.
14. Stary HC. Evolution and progression of atherosclerotic lesions in coronary arteries of children and young adults. Arteriosclerosis 1989;9:19–32.
15. Hangartner JRW, Charleston AJ, Davies MJ, Thomas AC. Morphological characteristics of clinically significant coronary artery stenoses in stable angina. Br Heart J 1986;56:501–8.
16. Lundberg B. Chemical composition and physical state of lipid deposits in atherosclerosis. Atherosclerosis 1985;56:93–110.
17. Mitchinson MJ, Ball RY. Macrophages and atherogenesis. Lancet 1987;2:146–8.
18. Mintz GS, Doueck P, Pichard AD et al. Target lesion calcification in coronary artery disease: An intravascular ultrasound study. J Am Coll Cardiol 1992;201:149–55.
19. Mintz G, Pichard A, Kovach JA et al. Impact of preintervention intravascular ultrasound on transcatheter treatment strategies in coronary artery disease. Am J Cardiol 1994;73:423–30.
20. Fitzgerald PJ, Yock PG. Mechanisms and outcomes of angioplasty and atherectomy assessed by intravascular ultrasound. J Clin Ultrasound 1993;21:579–88.
21. Waller B. The eccentric coronary atherosclerotic plaque: Morphological observations and clinical relevance. Clin Cardiol 1989;12:14–20.
22. Isner JM, Donaldson RF, Fortin AH, Tischler A, Clarke RH. Attenuation of the media of coronary arteries in advanced atherosclerosis. Am J Cardiol 1986;58:937–9.
23. Brown BG. Coronary vasospasm: Observations linking the clinical spectrum of ischaemic heart disease to the dynamic pathology of coronary atherosclerosis. Arch Int Med 1981;141:716–22.
24. Brown B, Bolson EL, Dodge HT. Dynamic mechanisms in human coronary stenosis. Circulation 1984;70:917–22.
25. Saner HE, Gobel FL, Salomonowitz E, Erlien DA, Edwards JE. The disease free wall in coronary atherosclerosis: Its relation to the degree of obstruction. J Am Coll Cardiol 1985;6:1096–9.
26. Honye J, Mahon DJ, Jain A et al. Morphological effects of coronary balloon angioplasty *in vivo* assessed by intravascular ultrasound imaging. Circulation 1992;85:1012–25.
27. Arnett EN, Isner JM, Redwood DR et al. Coronary artery narrowing in coronary heart disease: comparison of cineangiographic and necropsy findings. Ann Int Med 1979;91:350–6.
28. Vlodaver Z, Frech R, van Tassel RA, Edwards JE. Correlation of antemortem coronary angiogram and postmortem specimens. Circulation 1973;47:162–8.
29. Glagov S, Weisenberg E, Zarins CK, Stankunavicius R, Kolettis GJ. Compensatory enlargement of human atherosclerotic coronary arteries. N Engl J Med 1987;316:1371–5.
30. Zarins CK, Weisenberg E, Kolettis G, Stankunavicius R, Glagov S. Differential enlargement of artery segments in response to enlarging atherosclerotic plaques. J Vasc Surg 1988;7:386–94.
31. Ge J, Erbel R, Zamorano J et al. Coronary artery remodelling in atherosclerotic disease: An intravascular ultrasound study *in vivo*. Coronary Artery Dis 1993;4:981–6.
32. Hermiller JB, Tenaglia AN, Kisslo KB et al. *In vivo* validation of compensatory enlargement of atherosclerotic coronary arteries. Am J Cardiol 1993;71:665–8.
33. Hodgson JM, Reddy KG, Suneja R, Nair RN, Lesnefsky EJ, Sheehan HM. Intracoronary ultrasound imaging: Correlation of plaque morphology with angiography, clinical syndrome and procedural results in patients undergoing coronary angioplasty. J Am Coll Cardiol 1993;21:35–44.
34. Tobis JM, Mallery J, Gessert J et al. Intravascular ultrasound cross-sectional arterial imaging before and after balloon angioplasty *in vitro*. Circulation 1989;80:873–882.

35. Hermiller J, Buller C, Tenaglia A *et al.* Unrecognised left main coronary artery disease in patients undergoing interventional procedures. Am J Cardiol 1993;71:173–8.
36. Danchin N, Oswald T, Voiriot P, Juilliere Y, Cherrier F. Significance of spontaneous obstruction of high degree coronary artery stenoses between diagnostic angiography and later percutaneous transluminal coronary angioplasty. Am J Cardiol 1989;63:660–2.
37. Waters D, Craven TE, Lesperance J. Prognostic significance of progression of coronary atherosclerosis. Circulation 1993;87:1067–75.
38. Davies MJ, Thomas A. Thrombosis and acute coronary lesions in sudden cardiac ischaemic death. N Engl J Med 1984;310:1137–40.
39. Davies MJ, Thomas AC. Plaque fissuring – the cause of acute myocardial infarction, sudden ischaemic death and crescendo angina. Br Heart J 1985;53:363–73.
40. Buja LM, Willerson JT. Relationship of ischaemic heart disease to sudden death. J For Sci 1991;36:25–33.
41. Willerson JT, Eidt JF, McNatt J *et al.* Role of thromboxane and serotonin as mediators in the development of spontaneous alterations in coronary blood flow and neointimal proliferation in canine models with chronic coronary artery stenoses and endothelial injury. J Am Coll Cardiol 1991;17:101B–110B.
42. Davies MJ, Thomas AC, Knapman PA, Hangartener JR. Intramyocardial platelet aggregation in unstable angina and sudden ischaemic cardiac death. Circulation 1986;73:418–27.
43. Falk E. Unstable angina with fatal outcome: Dynamic coronary thrombosis leading to infarction and/or sudden death. Circulation 1985;71:699–708.
44. Alison HW, Russell RO, Mantle JA, Kouchoukos NT, Moraski RE, Rackley CE. Coronary anatomy and arteriography in patients with unstable angina. Am J Cardiol 1978;41:204–9.
45. Fuster V, Frye RL, Connolly DC *et al.* Angiographic patterns early in the onset of the coronary syndromes. Br Heart J 1975;37:1250–5.
46. Falk E. Morphologic features of unstable atherothrombotic plaques underlying acute coronary syndromes. Am J Cardiol 1989;63:114E–20E.
47. Fuster V, Badimon L, Badimon JJ, Chesebro JH. Mechanisms of disease: The pathogenesis of coronary artery disease and the acute coronary syndromes (first of two parts). N Engl J Med 1992;326:242–50.
48. Fuster V, Badimon L, Badimon JJ, Chesebro JH. Mechanisms of disease: The pathogenesis of coronary artery disease and the acute coronary syndromes (second of two parts). N Engl J Med 1992;326:310–8.
49. Gertz SD, Roberts WC. Haemodynamic shear force in rupture of coronary arterial atherosclerotic plaques. Am J Cardiol 1990;66:1368–72.
50. Burleigh MC, Briggs AD, Lendon CL, Davies MJ, Born GV, Richardson PD. Collagen types I and III, collagen content, GAGs and mechanical strength of human atherosclerotic plaque caps: Span wise variations. Atherosclerosis 1992;96:71–81.
51. Loree HM, Kamm RD, Stringfellow RG, Lee RT. Effects of fibrous cap thickness on peak circumferential thickness in model atherosclerotic vessels. Circ Res 1992;71:850–8.
52. Davies MJ, Richardson PD, Woolf N, Katz DR, Mann J. Risk of thrombosis in human atherosclerotic plaques: Role of extracellular lipid, macrophage, and smooth muscle cell content. Br Heart J 1993;69:377–81.
53. Richardson PD, Davies MJ, Born GVR. Influence of plaque configuration and stress distribution on fissuring of coronary atherosclerotic plaques. Lancet 1989;2:941–4.
54. van der Wal AC, Becker AE, van der Loos CM, Das PK. Site of intimal rupture or erosion of thrombosed coronary atherosclerotic plaques is characterized by an inflammatory process irrespective of the dominant plaque morphology. Circulation 1994;89:36–44.
55. Kaartinen M, Penttila A, Kovanen PT. Accumulation of activated mast cells in the shoulder region of human coronary atheroma, the predilection site of atheromatous rupture. Circulation 1994;90:1669–78.
56. Moreno PR, Falk E, Palacios IF, Newell JB, Fuster V, Fallon LT. Macrophage infiltration in acute coronary syndromes: Implications for acute plaque rupture. Circulation 1994;90:775–8.
57. Matrisian LM. The matrix degrading metalloproteinases. Bioassays 1992;14:455–63.

58. Ciampricotti R, Elgamal M. Exercise induced plaque rupture producing myocardial infarction. Int J Cardiol 1986;12:102–8.
59. Black A, Black MM, Gensini G. Exertion and acute coronary artery injury. Angiology 1975;26:759–83.
60. Muller JE, Toffler JH, Stone, PH et al. Circadian variation and triggers of onset of acute cardiovascular disease. Circulation 1989;79:733–43.
61. Davies MJ, Bland JM, Hangartener JRW, Angelini A, Thomas AC. Factors influencing the presence of absence of acute coronary artery thrombi in sudden ischaemic death. Eur Heart J 1989;10:203–8.
62. Falk E. Plaque rupture with severe pre-existing stenosis precipitating coronary thrombosis: Characteristics of coronary atherosclerotic plaques underlying fatal occlusive thrombi. Br Heart J 1983;50:127–34.
63. Frink RJ. Chronic ulcerated plaques: New insights into the pathogenesis of acute coronary disease. J Invasive Cardiol 1994;6:173–85.
64. Bruschke AVG, Kramer JR, Bal ET, Haque IU, Detrano RC, Goormastic M. The dynamics of progression of coronary atherosclerosis studied in 168 medically treated patients who underwent coronary arteriography three times. Am Heart J 1989;117:296–305.
65. Singh RN. Progression of coronary atherosclerosis. Clues to the pathogenesis from serial coronary angiography. Br Heart J 1984;52:451–61.
66. Ambrose JA, Winters SL, Arora RR. Angiographic evolution of coronary artery morphology in unstable angina. J Am Coll Cardiol 1986;7:472–8.
67. Ambrose JA, Tannenbaum MA, Alexopoulos D et al. Angiographic progression of coronary artery disease and the development of myocardial infarction. J Am Coll Cardiol 1988;12:56–62.
68. Kimbiris D, Iskandrian A, Saras H. Rapid progression of coronary stenosis in patients with unstable angina pectoris selected for coronary angioplasty. Cath Cardiovasc Diag 1984;10:101–14.
69. Kaski JC, Tousoulis D, Pereira W, Crea F, Maseri A. Progression of complex coronary artery stenosis in patients with angina pectoris: Its relation to clinical events. Cor Art Dis 1992;3:305–12.
70. Kaski JC, Chen L, Chester MR. Rapid angiographic coronary stenosis progression in patients with ischaemic heart disease. Circulation 1995 (in press).
71. Chester MR, Chen L, Kaski JC. Angiographic evidence for frequent 'silent' plaque disruption in patients with stable angina. J Am Coll Cardiol 1995;428A:812–3.
72. Chester MR, Chen L, Kaski JC. Indentification of patients at high risk for adverse coronary events whilst awaiting routine coronary angioplasty. Br Heart J 1995;73:216–22.
73. Chen L, Chester MR, Redwood S, Huang J, Leatham E, Kaski JC. Angiographic stenosis progression and coronary events in patients with 'stabilized' unstable angina. Circulation 1995;91:2319–24.
74. Ambrose JA, Winters SL, Arora RR et al. Coronary angiographic morphology in myocardial infarction: A link between the pathogenesis of unstable angina and myocardial infarction. J Am Coll Cardiol 1985;6:1233–8.
75. Ambrose JA, Winters SL, Stern A et al. Angiographic morphology and the pathogenesis of unstable angina pectoris. J Am Coll Cardiol 1985;5:609–16.
76. Hackett D, Davies G, Maseri A. Pre-existing coronary stenoses in patients with first myocardial infarction are not necessarily severe. Eur Heart J 1988;9:1317–23.
77. Parisi AF, Folland ED, Hartigan PA. Comparison of angioplasty with medical therapy in the treatment of single-vessel coronary artery disease. Veterans Affairs ACME Investigators. N Engl J Med 1992;326:10–6.
78. Levin D, Gardiner G. Complex and simple coronary artery stenoses: A new way to interpret coronary angiograms based on morphologic features of lesions. Radiology 1987;164:675–80.
79. Levin DC, Fallon JT. Significance of the angiographic morphology of localized coronary stenoses: Histopathologic correlations. Circulation 1982;66:316–20.
80. Davies SW, Marchant B, Lyons JP et al. Irregular coronary lesion morphology after thrombolysis predicts early clinical instability. J Am Coll Cardiol 1991;18:669–74.
81. Williams AE, Freeman MR, Chisholm RJ, Patt NL, Armstrong PW. Angiographic morphology in unstable angina pectoris. Am J Cardiol 1988;62:1024–7.

82. Moise A, Theroux P, Taeymans Y *et al.* Unstable angina and progression of coronary atherosclerosis. N Engl J Med 1983;309:685–9.
83. Nagatomo Y, Nakagawa S, Koiwaya Y, Tanaka K. Coronary angiographic ruptured atheromatous plaque as a predictor of future progression of stenosis. Am Heart J 1990;119:1224–53.
84. Ambrose JA. Prognostic implications of lesion irregularity on coronary angiography. J Am Coll Cardiol 1991;18:675–6.
85. Haft JI, Al-Zarka AM. The origin and fate of complex coronary lesions. Am Heart J 1991;121:1050–61.
86. Bugiardini R, Pozzati A, Borghi A. Angiographic morphology in unstable angina and its relation to transient myocardial ischemia and hospital outcome. Am J Cardiol 1991;67:460–4.
87. Maseri A, Chierchia S, Davies G. Pathophysiology of coronary occlusion in acute infarction. Circulation 1986;73:233–9.
88. Davies MJ, Woolf N, Robertson WB. Pathology of acute myocardial infarction with particular reference to occlusive thrombi. Br Heart J 1976;38:659–64.
89. Ridolphi RL, Hutchins GM. The relationship between coronary artery lesions and myocardial infarcts: Ulceration of atherosclerotic plaques precipitating coronary thrombosis. Am Heart J 1977;93:468–86.
90. Chandler AB. Mechanisms and frequency of thrombosis in the coronary circulation. Thromb Res 1974;4(Suppl):3–23.
91. DeWood MA, Spores J, Hensley GR *et al.* Coronary arteriographic findings in acute transmural myocardial infarction. Circulation 1983;68:139–49.
92. Stadius MI, Maynard C, Fritz JK *et al.* Coronary anatomy and left ventricular function in the first twelve hours of acute myocardial infarction. Circulation 1985;72:292–301.
93. Bertrand MF, Lefebvre JM, Laisne CL, Rousseau MF, Carre AG, Lekieffre JP. Coronary angiography in acute transmural myocardial infarction. Am Heart J 1979;97:61–9.
94. Hackett D, Davies G, Chierchia S, Maseri A. High frequency of intermittent coronary occlusion in acute myocardial infarction. Circulation 1986;74(Suppl. II):278 (Abstract).
95. Marder VJ, Sherry S. Thrombolytic therapy: Current status. N Engl J Med 1988;318:1512–85.
96. Hoffman JIE. Coronary physiology and pathophysiology. In: Fox KM (ed.), Ischaemic heart disease. Lancaster: MTP Press 1987:69.
97. DeWood MA, Spores J, Notske RN *et al.* Nontransmural (subendocardial) infarction in man: The prevalence of total coronary occlusion. Am J Cardiol, 1981;47:459 (Abstract).
98. Levine HD. Subendocardial infarction in retrospect: pathologic, cardiographic and ancillary features. Circulation 1985;72:790–800.
99. Murry CE, Jennings RB, Reimer KA. Preconditioning with ischaemia: A delay of lethal cell injury in ischaemic myocardium. Circulation 1986;74:1124–36.
100. Walker DM, Yellon DM. Ischaemic preconditioning – from mechanisms to exploitation. Cardiovasc Res 1992;26:734–9.
101. Walker DM, Walker JM, Pattison C, Pugsley C, Pugsley W, Yellon DM. Preconditioning protects isolated human muscle. Circulation 1993;88:1–138.
102. Yellon DM, Alkhulaifi AM, Pugsley WB. Preconditioning the human myocardium. Lancet 1993;342:276–7.
103. Kloner RA, Snook T, Przyklenk K *et al.* Previous angina alters in-hospital outcome in TIMI 4. A clinical correlate to preconditioning? Circulation 1995;91:37–47.
104. Lawson CS. Does ischaemic preconditioning occur in the human heart? Cardiovasc Res 1994;28:1461–6.
105. Cohen MV, Downey JM. Ischaemic preconditioning: Can the protection be bottled? Lancent 1993;342:6.
106. Gross GJ, Auchampach JA. Blockade of ATP sensitive potassium channels prevents myocardial preconditioning in dogs. Circulation 1992;88:1264–72.
107. Thomas A, Knapman P, Krikler D, Davies MJ. Community study of the causes of 'natural' sudden death. Br Med J 1988;297:1453–6.
108. Davies MJ, Thomas A. Thrombosis of acute coronary artery lesions in sudden cardiac ischaemic death. N Engl J Med 1984;310:1137–40.

109. Van Dantzig JM, Becker EF. Sudden cardiac death and acute pathology of coronary arteries. Eur Heart J 1986;7:987–91.
110. El Fawal MA, Berg GA, Wheatley DJ, Harland A. Sudden death in Glasgow: Nature and frequency of acute coronary lesions. Br Heart J 1987;57;420–6.
111. DeWood MA, Spores J, Notske RN *et al.* Coronary artery occlusion determined early after sudden cardiac death due to myocardial infarction. J Am Coll Cardiol 1985;5:401 (Abstract).
112. Cobb LA, Werner JA, Trobaugh GB. Sudden cardiac death: A decade's experience with out-of-hospital resuscitation. Modern concepts in cardiovascular disease. 1980;49:31–6.
113. Warnes CA, Roberts WC. Sudden coronary death: Comparison of patients with and without coronary thrombosis at necropsy. Am J Cardiol 1984;54:1206–11.
114. Davies MJ. Anatomic features in victims of sudden coronary death. Circulation 1992;85:I-19–24.

12. Epidemiology and risk factors of coronary artery disease

TIMOTHY J. BOWKER, MAHMOUD BARBIR AND CHARLES ILSLEY

Diseases of the coronary arteries are divided into two groups – congenital anomalies [1] and diseases resulting as sequelae of their luminal narrowing or occlusion. This chapter will concentrate on the latter, which in the majority of cases are secondary to the intramural deposition of atheroma and/or the intraluminal formation of thrombus.

Epidemiology is concerned with the study of disease occurrence in predefined populations. Such populations can be of any size (from a whole country to a single hospital's catchment population) provided that the denominator population in which the cases studied have arisen is known. This allows inferences to be made about the denominator population and generalizations to be made about, and comparisons to be made with, similar populations. These principles apply whether the study in question is a descriptive cross-sectional survey of blood pressure in a single general practice or a multicenter multinational randomized controlled trial of a new strategy for the management of acute myocardial infarction.

The role of epidemiology in the study of coronary artery disease is (as it is in most diseases) twofold, firstly descriptive and secondly analytic. Epidemiology's first role is to describe the frequency of coronary artery disease (cases per denominator population, in a defined time duration), not only as an absolute measure, but also in terms of its distribution – e.g. by gender, geographic place, age group, time period, etc. The last of these, time period, allows trends in coronary artery disease to be addressed. Epidemiology's second role is to test hypotheses about coronary disease, these hypotheses being either about its etiology or about its management.

Case definition and subject classification

The external validity of any study of coronary artery disease depends upon how the presence of the disease is defined. The internal validity depends upon the ability of the study's methodology to classify cases and non-cases (however defined) correctly.

Clinical manifestations (and/or the results of non-invasive cardiac tests), which are the usual consequences of occlusive coronary artery disease, are in many studies, and particularly in population-based studies, taken as a surrogate for the presence of coronary atheroma. However, such clinical manifestations (or test results) may cause the subject to be misclassified as having coronary atheroma. This may arise in one of two ways. Firstly, the clinical diagnosis of coronary artery disease, while meeting the definition set by the study (e.g. a positive Rose questionnaire) [2], may still be wrong, the patient's symptoms subsequently being shown to be non-cardiac (e.g. the chest pain was in fact esophageal). This type of misclassification can, of course, be in either direction, i.e. true cardiac pain could be misdiagnosed as esophageal, and misclassified as non-cardiac. Secondly, the clinical diagnosis of ischemic cardiac pain may in fact be correct, but the coronary arteries are normal on angiography, the subject falling into the unusual category labeled as 'syndrome X' [3, 4]. Both these instances of misclassification are issues of external validity and raise the question of what should be the 'gold standard' for measurement of the presence of coronary atheroma. In clinical practice the usual answer to this question is coronary angiography. (It is worth noting that there exists another constellation of features – non-insulin dependent diabetes mellitus, hypertension, and hyperlipidemia – which is also labeled syndrome X, but is in the field of metabolic medicine and endocrinology [5]. Indeed hyperinsulinemia may link the two [6]).

The final arbiter of the presence or absence of coronary atheroma is a postmortem examination. The information obtained from a postmortem examination, however, is that of structure but not of function. Indeed, the finding of mild or moderate coronary atheroma at postmortem may be coincidental and does not necessarily imply that there was antemortem myocardial ischemia. Nevertheless, unexpected deaths in apparently previously healthy individuals are often ascribed to ischemic heart disease when (even only mild) coronary atheroma is the only postmortem abnormality [7]. In an individual whose esophageal pain is misdiagnosed as cardiac (the first example of misclassification given in the previous paragraph), it might even be more complicated, if coincidentally the patient had some mild (but asymptomatic) coronary atheroma. The classification of such a case in practice, depends upon how much is known about the patient. With only the Rose questionnaire result, such a patient would be classified as a case of coronary artery disease. After the endoscopy and response to H_2 blockade, the patient would be classified as a non-case. But if in the following month the subject was killed in a car crash and the coroner's postmortem examination revealed the mild coronary atheroma, the conclusion would depend upon was to be measured – structure or function, preclinical disease or clinically manifest disease. It would be less easy to decide, however, if the coroner's postmortem examination followed the sudden unexpected death of the individual.

Few epidemiological studies (i.e. those with a known denominator population in which the cases have occurred) have the opportunity to classify all their subjects by postmortem findings. (Some are the International Atherosclerosis Project, and regional and national surveys of sudden death [8–11]). In practice, the variable manifestation of coronary disease means that epidemiological studies of the frequency of its occurrence and of its etiology require the use of clinical findings (and/or noninvasive cardiac tests) as surrogate markers for its presence, with the resultant problem of possible misclassification. Although this is a potential weakness of such epidemiological studies, it cannot be avoided. The strength of a properly designed and executed study is that misclassification should occur randomly in both directions, thereby avoiding bias and maintaining validity. In addition, such studies should allow the collection of information about other covariates, which may be important confounders or effect modifiers, and which can be adjusted for in the data analysis.

Descriptive studies

Disease frequency

Historical perspective and time trends
Depending upon the question addressed, different studies have attempted to measure the frequency of different precursors to, or manifestations of, atheromatous coronary artery disease (from birth and infant weight [12] to coronary angiography [13]). Historically, it was the deaths certified as due to ischemic heart disease and recorded annually by the England and Wales Registrar General that were the first measure of the disease's frequency in the United Kingdom. The change in the number of these death certifications (per unit population alive) with time became the first indication that atheromatous coronary artery disease was to become the most frequent cause of mortality in the United Kingdom (as well as in the rest of the Western world).

The majority of publications on ischemic heart disease trends in the United Kingdom have taken deaths certified as due to the appropriate International Classification of Diseases (ICD) ischemic heart disease codes [14] as their measure of the disease's frequency, some comparing the United Kingdom with other countries [15–17], whilst others have taken other manifestations of the disease, or its recognized risk factors [18], as their measure and have studied their temporal changes.

One potential drawback of studies based upon death certification data is that the accuracy of the diagnosis given as the cause of death on the certificate can be questioned, and such accuracy can vary not only from country to country, but also from one decade to the next. Thus observed (measured) differences in death rates either between countries or between time periods may be due at least in part to differences in death certification custom between countries or between time periods, rather than due entirely to a true difference or true change in the rate. Any true difference or change may be either enhanced or diminished by this effect.

In 1963 Campbell [19, 20] described trends in England and Wales mortality certified due to cardiac causes from 1876 to 1959. Cardiac mortality, having remained steady for 50 years, began to rise sharply in the early 1920s, more than doubling by 1959. Campbell felt this increase could have resulted from aging of the population (secondary to the control of infectious disease at the beginning of the century). England and Wales certified ischemic heart disease (IHD) mortality also began to rise in the 1920s, but geometrically rather than arithmetically. Because of a concomitant fall in deaths certified as due to myocardial degeneration and to other myocardial diseases over the same time period, Campbell felt that one possible explanation for the exponential rise in deaths certified due to IHD was diagnostic transfer, i.e. a change in the diagnostic fashion of those completing the death certificates. For example, deaths which early in the century were ascribed (presumably in the absence of postmortem evidence) to the ICD category 'myocardial degeneration' might later in the century have been certified as due to 'ischemic heart disease'. On the basis of this theory Campbell made predictions for cardiac mortality up to 1990, which have turned out to be underestimates (by 70%) of the observed value [21].

Later publications [15, 22–24] indicated that certified IHD mortality in middle-aged groups of both sexes in the UK continued to rise until 1972–74, after which rates reached a plateau. From 1950 to the mid-1970s the rise in UK IHD mortality rates may have been exaggerated by diagnostic transfer from myocardial degeneration in the older of these age groups [22, 25]. Some authors believe that a decline in United Kingdom IHD mortality began in 1973–74. While there is controversy as to whether this represented a trend or chance variation [26], subgroup analysis suggests the fall was real in certain age, social and regional groups [18, 27].

International comparisons
A comparison, made in 1990, between the USA and England and Wales certified IHD mortality rates [28] indicated that the USA's IHD mortality rates reached a peak synchronously in both sexes at the end of the 1960s, whereas IHD mortality rates in England and Wales males did not reach their peak until 10 years later, with England and Wales females lagging by at least a further five years. When at their peak, US age-specific absolute rates were up to 56% greater (8687 vs. 5551 per 100 000) than the respective England and Wales rates. By the late 1980s US female rates were similar to, and US male rates had fallen below, those of England and Wales. Cohort analysis showed a marked age effect with earlier onset in males in both countries, and a period effect occurring 10 years earlier in the USA. Both US sexes showed a gradual attenuation of age effect with each successive five-year birth cohort from 1889 to 1929, whereas such attenuation was barely detectable in England and Wales.

Exploration of the temporal changes in deaths certified to ischemic heart disease, hypertensive heart disease, and to the various descriptors of myocardial disease used in different ICD revisions (namely cardiomyopathy, heart failure, myocardial degeneration and myocardial insufficiency), suggested that in England and Wales true IHD mortality rate rises in the young and middle aged had in the past been exaggerated by diagnostic transfer in the elderly, and that this diagnostic transfer was liable to have been mainly from the ICD category of 'myocardial degeneration'. In the USA however, diagnostic transfer was likely to have been less pronounced, but both from the myocardial degeneration and from the hypertensive heart disease ICD categories [25].

Current cross-sectional comparisons of national IHD rates (based on centrally collected death certification data) yield a 'league table,' at the foot of which is Japan (with absolute rates of the order of 50 per 100 000 35–74-year-olds) and the 'southern' European countries of France, Spain, Portugal, and Italy (rates of 100–200 per 100 000 35–74-year-olds), and at the top of which are the 'northern' European countries of Scotland, Northern Ireland, and Finland (rates of 500–600 per 100 000). In the middle of the table are countries such as Australia and the USA with rates between 300 and 400 per 100 000. The exact order of the nations varies with time, depending upon the secular trend within each. Whereas some countries (e.g. Australia and the USA) display an established downward trend, in others – particularly those now at or near the top of the league table – the downward trend is either less pronounced (e.g. Scotland, England, and Wales) or non-existent (e.g. Hungary) [29].

Issues of study design and the 'ecological fallacy'
A distinction must be made between studies in which relationships between characteristics of a series of whole populations (or groups) is examined (so-called cross-population or cross-cultural studies) and those in which relationships between the characteristics of the individual subjects within one or more populations are examined (so-called within-population studies). (The international studies mentioned above are examples of the former, and subsequent cohort studies, such as the Framingham or Whitehall studies [30, 31], provide examples of the latter.) The reason for this is that, although there is some controversy, it is generally held that the results of the latter (within-population studies) can be more reliably interpreted than those of the former (cross-population studies). This is because some cross-population studies may be subject to what is termed the 'ecological fallacy', which is said to occur when an association detected by a cross-population study is no longer apparent when the same data are reanalysed as a within-population study, i.e. by individual, rather than by population grouping.

The principle is perhaps best illustrated by the original example given by Emile Durkheim who related the religious composition of four groups of Prussian provinces to their suicide rate in the mid 1880s [32]. The group of provinces with the highest suicide rate (28 per 100 000) was 95% protestant and the group with the lowest suicide rate (9 per 100 000) was only 30% protestant, with the two intermediary groups (with suicide rates of 17 and 22 per 100 000) falling on an almost straight line between the two extremes, being 48% and 78% protestant, respectively.

In 1969 a study of 8829 male civil servants in Israel grouped the subjects by place of birth (Africa, Asia, Israel, southern, eastern, and central Europe) and, by comparing the mean serum cholesterol of the six geographical groupings to their dietary saturated fatty acid intake, demonstrated a significant positive relationship ($r = 0.94$) between serum cholesterol and dietary saturated fat [33]. However in 1988, reanalysis [34] relating the serum cholesterol of each of the 8829 males to his own dietary intake, i.e. within the population rather than across its geographic subgroups, failed to demonstrate any relationship ($r = 0.03$) between serum cholesterol and dietary saturated fat. Although such examples of the ecological fallacy have been used to undermine their value, cross-population studies should not be discounted. The apparent paradox and methodological approaches [35] for adjusting for the hierarchical data generated by cross-population studies, have been well reviewed by Morgenstern [36] and by Elliott [37].

Disease markers and case frequencies
The clinical findings (and/or cardiac tests) which should be used as surrogate markers for the presence of atheromatous coronary artery disease will depend upon the question being addressed by the investigators. In terms of severity, atheromatous coronary disease provides a spectrum from fatty streaks or early fibrous plaques in apparently healthy asymptomatic individuals at one end, to death at the other – either acutely following thrombus formation upon a complicated plaque or less acutely with a scarred myocardium. At any point along the spectrum, the disease (be it clinically overt, or clinically covert and thus detectable only by special cardiac investigations) results in myocardial ischemia.

Efforts to measure the overall frequency of IHD in a community must attempt to measure more than just mortality. The frequency of individuals with acute myocardial infarction and its complications, with acute myocardial ischemia (without evidence of infarction) and with stable angina should also be measured. Some would argue that in order to measure the full burden of ischemic heart disease, perhaps even those individuals in whom the only evidence of disease is 'silent' myocardial ischemia (detected non-invasively, with or without angiographic confirmation of coronary disease) should be included in the numerator.

Covert preclinical disease

Attempts to measure covert preclinical disease have yielded prevalence estimates ranging from 0.9% to 34%, depending upon the cardiac investigations used and the population studied [38]. In centers using coronary angiography as their 'gold standard' (13, 39–42), prevalences ranged from 0.9 to 12%. In none of the latter was the study population representative of a geographically defined area. The two studies in which the study population was geographically representative [43, 44] were based on non-invasive tests only. In the study based on Holter ambulatory ECG monitoring alone [44], the prevalence of evidence of covert myocardial ischemia in overtly healthy individuals was 9.5%. In the study in which subjects first underwent ambulatory and exercise electrocardiography and then non-invasive myocardial imaging [43], the prevalence was 16% when based on electrocardiography alone, 14% when based upon non-invasive imaging alone and 6% when both electrocardiography and non-invasive imaging were required to be positive. This illustrates the importance of case and study population definition, and of the selection of surrogate markers to measure the presence of coronary disease.

In a small English national pilot study [11], ischemic heart disease was found to be the cause of 88% of sudden unexpected cardiac deaths occurring in apparently healthy individuals (the most abrupt way in which previously undiagnosed coronary disease can present), the occurrence rate of which was estimated to be about 1 per 10 000 in 16–64-year-olds.

When addressing the population burden of coronary disease, the distinction between preclinical and clinically overt disease is fundamental, as they differ entirely in terms of the strategy for, and the implications of, their subsequent management. Management of the former (preclinical disease) falls within the realm of primary prevention, which requires screening of, and possible use of potentially harmful strategies for an asymptomatic population. Supportive evidence is more difficult to collect [45] and moral and ethical issues are more complex than when addressing the management of clinically overt disease, which comprises symptom relief and secondary prevention. From an epidemiological viewpoint, it is useful to subdivide clinically overt disease into that which is presenting for the first time (new or incident cases) and that which was previously diagnosed or is recurrent (old or recurrent cases). Etiological questions are better addressed by studying the former (incident cases), whereas questions of management strategy can be addressed by studying either.

Clinically overt coronary disease

The frequencies of the different manifestations of non-fatal clinically overt coronary disease (stable angina, acute myocardial ischemia without evidence of infarction, acute myocardial infarction) has been measured in a number of geographically representative populations, at various times.

Estimates of the prevalence (i.e. incident and recurrent cases combined) of stable angina from surveys of representative samples of the 40–59-year-old population of the United Kingdom have varied from 4.8% in males [46] to 8.5% in (Scottish) females [47], and the annual incidence (i.e. frequency of incident cases only) of stable angina in southern England was recently measured as 0.83 per thousand 31–70-year-olds (1.13 per 1000 males and 0.53 per 1000 females) [48]. Combining data from this and the same authors' previous report [44] allows the 9.5% prevalence of covert myocardial ischemia in overtly healthy individuals (quoted in the previous section) to be converted into an occurrence rate of 0.15 per thousand 31–70-years-olds.

The initial population-based studies on the occurrence of new and recurrent acute cases of ischemic heart disease in various communities within the UK were performed over two decades ago, since when there have been radical changes in the management of the acute manifestations of coronary artery disease. These studies took the form of community based registers of new and recurrent episodes of definite myocardial infarction (plus or minus 'possible' or 'presumed' myocardial infarction) occurring in specified age-groups, periods and geographical areas (in those under 70 years of age during the 1960s in Edinburgh and in Oxford, and in those under 65 years during the 1970s in Tower Hamlets) [49–51]. These studies included sudden deaths occurring in the community, who never reached hospital. Myocardial infarction was classified as definite if there was unequivocal necropsy or ECG and enzyme evidence, or 'possible/presumed' if the evidence was equivocal or there had been no necropsy. Perhaps those classified as having had 'possible' myocardial infarctions would today be labelled as 'unstable angina', i.e. acute myocardial ischemia without evidence of infarction.

Age grouping varied between the studies. However the studies revealed an annual 'attack' rate of new and recurrent episodes of both definite and possible myocardial infarction which varied from 15.5 per 1000 males aged 40–69 years in Edinburgh, through 10 per 1000 males aged 45–64 years in Tower Hamlets to 6.2 per 1000 males aged 40–69 years in Oxford. The corresponding figures for females were 5.1 in Edinburgh, 2.7 in Tower Hamlets and 1.3 in Oxford. In the Tower Hamlets study 40% of cases had previously had angina and 35% had had prior myocardial infarctions (50% either angina or myocardial infarction). The equivalent figures in the Oxford study were 44% and 19% respectively. In Edinburgh 7.0 per 1000 males and 2.2 per 1000 females were classified as having had a first 'attack'. In the Tower Hamlets study 2 per 1000 males and 0.3 per 1000 females aged 45–64 years were classified as having had non-fatal 'possible' myocardial infarctions per annum, and so perhaps this represents the best estimate of the then occurrence of acute myocardial ischemia without evidence of infarction ('unstable angina'), though this would have included both first and recurrent episodes, and both diagnostic criteria and diagnostic fashion will have since changed.

Data from the third national survey on morbidity from general practice [52] performed in 1981/82 and published in 1986 were collected on 332 270 individuals registered with a sample of 48 general practices throughout England and Wales. Its results are tabulated by International Classification of Diseases, 9th revision (ICD 9) code groupings, gender and age group, and indicate that in the 45–64-year-old age group, 12.4 per 1000 males and 4.1 per 1000 females consulted their GP for a first or recurrent episode of ICD 9 code numbers 410 or 411, which are respectively 'acute myocardial infarction' and 'other acute and subacute forms of ischemic heart disease'. In the 45–64-year-old age group, 18.3 per 1000 males and 9.5 per 1000 females consulted their GP for a first or recurrent episode of part of ICD 9 code number 412 ('angina pectoris'). The other part of ICD 9 code number 412 was grouped with ICD 9 code number 413 ('other forms of chronic ischemic heart disease'), the first and recurrent episodes of this grouping having 11.3 per 1000 males and 4.7 per 1000 females amongst 45–64-year-olds.

The most recent and most geographically comprehensive study of both fatal and non-fatal myocardial infarction is the WHO MONICA project [53], which measured acute myocardial infarction and coronary deaths occurring in men and women aged 35 to 64 years in 41 geographically defined communities throughout 27 countries between 1985 and 1987. Male annual event rates covered a 12-fold range from 915 per 100 000 in North Karelia, Finland to 76 per 100 000 in Beijing. Female annual event rates covered an 8.5-fold range from 256 per 100 000 in Glasgow to 30 per 100 000 in Catalonia. These rates are consistent with the geographic distribution of certified IHD mortality statistics. The fact that they are considerably lower than the event rates measured in the UK in the late 1960s and early 1970s is consistent with the recent fall in certified IHD mortality, but may also be due to different age groupings or methodologies and perhaps to changing diagnostic accuracy and/or fashion.

Measurement of the population frequency of acute myocardial ischemia without evidence of infarction (which is often labeled as 'unstable angina') has received less attention, perhaps because of the lack of a generally accepted case definition. The Nottingham group have addressed this diagnostic category [54] and a UK pilot survey has made a preliminary estimate of its national occurrence rate in 40–69-year-olds as 3.9 per 1000 males and 1.9 per 1000 females for incident and recurrent cases combined (and 0.9 per 1000 males and 0.2 per 1000 females for incidence alone) [55].

Analytical studies

Etiology

Firstly, we shall attempt to summarize those coronary risk factors, for which the evidence was first reported many years ago, many but not all of which can be regarded as established, and for which we shall suggest a simple grouping system. Then we shall mention specifically four areas of etiological research which have aroused more recent interest and in which there is current activity and development, namely the fetal origins of ischemic heart disease [56, 57], the role of essential fatty acid isomers [58, 59], blood rheology [60, 61], and the more recently discovered and cloned genetic polymorphisms which have been shown to be associated with various manifestations of ischemic heart disease [62].

Established risk factors

The apparent rapid rise in IHD mortality during the first half of the twentieth century raised the question of its cause. The variation between nations in their IHD mortality generated various etiological hypotheses based upon associations between national population characteristics, e.g. diet, and the observed national IHD mortality rates. Such hypotheses led to the important early international cross-cultural studies, such as the International Atherosclerosis Project [8] and the Seven Countries Study [63], which were instrumental in providing the initial a priori evidence for some (life-style, dietary fat, and serum cholesterol) of what are now termed the established coronary risk factors.

In addition to cross-sectional cross-cultural studies, a large number of analytical within-population studies were embarked upon. Though many have been of case-referent design [e.g. 10, 64–72], the majority were prospective cohort studies, in which individuals of a geographically defined population are identified and screened, firstly for prevalent coronary disease (i.e. cases who are already clinically manifest) and secondly for their levels of hypothesized risk factors. The cohort of individuals is then followed regularly for years and their clinical cardiac outcome measured. It is such cohort studies, the first of which was Framingham [30, 73, 74], that have provided the majority of the most scientifically sound information about coronary risk factors. There have been many subsequent cohort studies addressing different populations and etiological questions, but always the outcome of interest being the incident cases. These cohort studies have included, in the United Kingdom, Whitehall I and II [31, 75], British Regional Heart Study [76, 77], Caerphilly [78–80], Renfrew and Paisley [81], and elsewhere, Seven Countries [63], US National Cooperative Pooling Project [82], Italian RIFLE Pooling Project [83], MONICA [53] and the PRC–USA Cooperative Study on Cardiovascular and Cardiopulmonary Epidemiology [84]. Some cohort studies (e.g. MRFIT [85], the WHO European Collaborative Trial [86], North Karelia Project [87, 88], and Oslo [89]), whilst set up to address questions of management strategy, have also provided valuable information about etiology.

Stamler [84] has given an excellent review of what he refers to as the four established major risk factors for coronary disease: 'rich' diet, above optimal levels of serum total cholesterol and of blood pressure, and cigarette smoking. To these could, without any controversy, be added age, gender, and the detail of the various lipoprotein subfractions.

Hyperlipidemia
The interrelationships of the lipoprotein fractions with ischemic heart disease, with each other and with other coronary risk factors are extremely complex [90, 91]. Whereas the development of coronary disease is negatively associated with high-density lipoprotein (HDL) cholesterol [92], positively associated with low-density lipoproteins (LDL) [93] and with postprandial chylomicron and very low-density lipoprotein (VLDL) remnants [94–99], but not associated with chylomicrons [90], there has been controversy about the association between the other triglyceride-rich lipoprotein, VLDL, and the development of coronary disease. The initial within-population studies demonstrated a bivariate association between plasma triglyceride and coronary disease, which disappeared on regression analyses which included the covariates total cholesterol, HDL-cholesterol, and body mass index [76, 100, 101]. This may be explained by the fact that raised VLDL levels are often associated both with reduced HDL-cholesterol levels and with an LDL fraction in which small, dense particles predominate [102]. However, subgroup analysis of the PROCAM and of the Helsinki Heart Study suggests that triglyceride levels can be used to refine coronary risk in certain subgroups defined by their LDL to HDL cholesterol ratios [103, 104]. In addition, other studies have reported not only that triglyceride level is independently associated with coronary disease, but also that in normolipidemic subjects apolipoproteins are associated with coronary disease [105].

It is possible to separate low density lipoproteins into up to 12 subfractions according to LDL particle size, which is inversely related to LDL particle density. The smaller the LDL subfraction particle size, the stronger the association with clinical manifestations of coronary disease [106–108]. This is keeping with the *in vitro* demonstration that decreasing LDL particle size and increasing LDL particle density are associated with a decreasing LDL receptor affinity, with a decreasing LDL particle antioxidant content and with an increasing susceptibility to LDL particle oxidation. These physicochemical properties are thought to provide mechanisms for the association with coronary disease; the smaller the LDL particle the more likely it is to be filtered into the arterial subendothelial space (rather than cleared from the plasma by hepatic LDL receptors), where its susceptibility to oxidation (which can only proceed once its endogenous antioxidant store has been depleted) will potentiate uptake by macrophages, cholesterol accumulation, and foam cell (and hence fatty streak) formation [109]. The susceptibility of LDL to oxidation *in vitro* is associated with extent of coronary atheroma in men [110]. In addition, small dense LDL particles have been associated with the insulin resistance syndrome, mentioned below [111–113].

High-density lipoproteins can also be subcategorized, either by their density (HDL2 vs. HDL3) or by their apolipoprotein content (apoA-I, apoA-II, or both). Attempts to use these subclasses to improve the value of HDL-cholesterol in predicting coronary disease have so far proved unsuccessful [114]. Many other apolipoproteins have been identified. Apolipoproteins apoC to apoJ are associated with HDLs [114] and LDL particles contain a single molecule of apoB [109]. For these apolipoproteins, interest is now beginning to focus upon their genotypic (rather than phenotypic) association with coronary disease.

Lipoprotein (a) (Lp(a)) is an anomalous lipoprotein that resembles an LDL particle complexed with the glycoprotein apolipoprotein (a). It has close structural homology with plasminogen and its phenotypic level is primarily under genetic control. In spite of some earlier controversy [91, 115], there has been steadily mounting evidence for the positive association of serum Lp(a) level with various manifestations both of native coronary artery disease [65, 69, 70, 116–118] and of saphenous vein aorto-coronary bypass atherosclerosis [119]. In addition, raised serum Lp(a) levels have been shown to be an independent risk factor for the development of accelerated coronary artery disease in cardiac transplant recipients [120]. Although the physiological function of Lp(a) is not established, it appears to have both thrombogenic and atherogenic properties. However, the mechanisms underlying these properties are not fully understood [121–123].

Other risk factors
As the within-population etiological analytical studies have become more advanced, the biological variables entertained as possible risk factors have expanded from basic anthropometric measures (including blood pressure), social and family history plus a relatively simple lipid profile, to include electrocardiographic and other non-invasive cardiac tests, increasingly sophisticated biochemical and hematological measures and most recently genetic markers. A wide range of other candidates for coronary risk factors has been identified, the evidence for which ranges from well-established and compelling to early and limited.

These have included lifestyle and habits in addition to smoking, such as physical fitness [124], so-called 'type A' behaviour or personality [79], socioeconomic class [27, 125], oral contraception [66, 126], hormone replacement therapy [127], obesity and dietary habit including breast feeding, alcohol [128], coffee [129], water hardness [130, 131], essential fatty acids and saturated fatty acids. They also include constitutional factors such as family history of coronary disease, ABO blood group [132], birth weight, infant growth, menopause [133, 134], reproductive history [67], glucose intolerance, forced expiratory volume in one second (FEV_1), stature [68, 135] and race [136], hematological factors such as white cell count, hematocrit, plasma viscosity, fibrinogen, factor VII coagulant activity and plasminogen activator inhibitor-1 (PAI-1) activity, and the blood levels of other measurable substances such as antioxidant vitamins [137], urate, albumin [138], chlamydial antibody [139], serum copper, ceruloplasmin, ferritin, zinc, and calcium [64, 72, 140]. In addition, the predictive value of the findings of cardiological 'screening' tests (usually a resting 12-lead electrocardiogram) performed at the recruitment stage of a cohort study have been assessed, e.g. electrocardiographic evidence of left ventricular hypertrophy was found to be an independent predictor of cardiovascular disease in the Framingham study [141].

Of the risk factor candidates listed in the previous paragraph, those for which there is reasonable evidence of at least a simple univariate association with coronary disease are listed in Table 12.1. Those in which regression analysis has revealed that the factor has a statistically significant independent association with coronary disease have been asterisked, with a typical value or range for the strength of that association (relative risk or odds ratio) placed alongside.

The risk factors can be loosely subdivided into three groups, which have been labeled intrinsic, extrinsic, and intermediate. This classification is very rough and ready and is meant to represent the spectrum from purely environmental exposure to causative agents which are eminently avoidable or correctable at one end – the extrinsic category, perhaps best exemplified by smoking – to purely inherited genetic factors about which little or nothing can be done at the other – the intrinsic category, perhaps best exemplified by gender or age. However, clearly the phenotypic severity of a large number of coronary risk factors is determined by combination of environmental and inherited influences (e.g. serum cholesterol level is determined by a combination of genetic inheritance and dietary intake), and these

Table 12.1. Reported 'risk' factors.

Intrinsic	Intermediate	Extrinsic
* Age	* Lipids (2.5)	* Smoking (3.0)
* Gender (2.5)	* Hypertension (2.0)	* Lack of physical fitness (1.4–3.2)
* Family history (1.6)	* Fibrinogen (1.7)	* Socioeconomic class (1.2–2.0)
* Diabetes (1.6)	* Factor VII (1.6)	* Contraceptive pill (0.8–2.3)
* Stature/FEV_1 (1.4)	* Albumin (0.7)	* Coffee (2.2)
* ACE gene polymorphism (1.3–3.2)		
* apoE gene polymorphism (2.0)	Impaired fibrinolysis	Essential fatty acids
Birth Weight	Alcohol	
Fibrinogen genotype	Infant growth	Chlamydial antibodies
Stromelysin gene polymorphism	Hyperuricemia	Water softness
ABO blood group	Serum ceruloplasmin	Body mass index
Personality type	Serum copper	Saturated dietary fats
Menopause	Plasma vitamin E	
Race		

*Factor has statistically significant independent association by regression analysis in at least one study. Figures in brackets represent typical values or ranges for the strength of that association (relative risk or odds ratio).

have been allocated to the intermediate category. Indeed, the situation is even more complex for not only are genes inherited, but also, to a certain extent, are environment and lifestyle (e.g. dietary habit, socioeconomic group). Furthermore, the level of one risk factor is influenced by the level of another, e.g. diabetic status and lipid level [142, 143], blood pressure, blood viscosity and body mass index [144, 145], smoking and clotting factors [146], and gender and most other factors. Hence the necessity for large scale cohort studies, analysed by regression techniques, to try and clarify which factors are independent predictors of the development of coronary disease.

The associations of obesity, hypertension, glucose intolerance, hyperinsulinemia, hypertriglyceridemia, low HDL-cholesterol, and insulin resistance have led to the postulation of the existence of an underlying metabolic disturbance, the insulin resistance syndrome, which may be present even in normoglycemic individuals and may itself be an underlying etiological factor in the development of coronary artery disease [147, 148]. Non-insulin dependent diabetes mellitus is more frequent among certain ethnic groups, many of whom have shown a recent trend to urbanization, central obesity and the development of high ischemic heart disease rates, e.g. South Asian migrants to the United Kingdom [136, 149, 150].

The aim of etiological research has been to identify, and measure the relative contribution of a range of factors to which the occurrence of coronary disease can be attributed in an entire geographically defined population (and thereby in any one individual). In any one population however, the variation in the distribution of coronary disease (particularly that occurring before the age of 55 years) could not be entirely explained by the variation in the conventional and more well-established risk factors [62]. This fueled the continued search for additional risk factors, in particular the exploration of genetic polymorphisms. However, if the components of the population's coronary disease variation due to each of the genetic polymorphisms under current investigation were simply arithmetically summated, the overall population coronary disease variation could probably be explained several times over. However this would be ignoring the interaction (in the statistical sense) between each of the polymorphisms and the other environmental risk factors.

Fetal and neonatal origins

Based on detailed records, made by English midwives and health visitors in Hertfordshire, Preston, and Sheffield between 1911 and 1930, of birth weights, placental weights, infant feeding, and growth, Professor David Barker and his group have been able to create retrospective cohorts by measuring the current clinical outcome (in terms of coronary mortality and risk factor profile) of individuals born over 50 years ago, and then relating their outcome to their neonatal and infant factors. Low birth weight or low weight at one year (or both) were associated with subsequent increased death and prevalence rates of ischemic heart disease, and with adverse coronary risk factors in adulthood – including glucose intolerance, diabetes mellitus, hypertension, central obesity, and raised clotting factors apolipoprotein B levels [151–155]. This has generated the hypothesis that adult coronary disease and its risk factors may have their origin in retarded fetal and infant growth, particularly if the retardation occurs at a critical period of fetal or infant development (or 'programming'), and that such retardation may itself be related to maternal undernutrition [56, 156, 157]. Evidence supporting extension of this hypothesis to females has recently been published [158]. However, not all the available evidence is consistent with this hypothesis [57, 159–162].

Essential fatty acids

Linoleic acid is a polyunsaturated fatty acid and is the most important of the polyenoic essential fatty acids – 'essential' because it cannot be synthesized by humans, the only source being dietary. The hypothesis that chronic dietary deficiency of linoleic acid is a cause of coronary disease was first proposed by Sinclair in 1956 [163]. Numerous subsequent cross and within-population studies have provided evidence of an inverse association between linoleic acid levels and various clinical manifestations of coronary disease [58], including male and female coronary mortality [164–166], newly diagnosed angina pectoris and incident cases of myocardial infarction [167, 168], and sudden death as the first manifestation of coronary disease [10]. This inverse association is independent of the established coronary risk factors, except for cigarette smoking, with which linoleic acid is itself inversely associated. Thus interpretation of these findings must be guarded, particularly as in dietary surveys, smokers have been shown to consume less linoleic acid than non-smokers [169], though the reason for this is not clear.

Dietary unsaturated fatty acids (including linoleic acid) from naturally occurring sources, such as vegetable or fish oils, beef fat or milk, are in their *cis*-isomer configuration. When such foodstuffs are chemically hydrogenated to produce margarine and other hardened fat products, *trans*-isomers, which have different biological properties and tend to behave as saturated fatty acids, are produced. There is some evidence to suggest that *trans*-fatty acids may be positively associated with coronary disease [170–173]. Mann has proposed that dietary exposure to *trans*-fatty acids might impair lipoprotein receptors, thereby leading to insulin resistance and coronary disease [174]. More recent evidence from two population-based case-control studies fails to support the hypothesis of a positive association between *trans*-fatty acid levels and coronary disease [175–177].

Blood rheology and coagulation

The hematological elements of leukocyte count, hematocrit, blood viscosity, hemostatic, and fibrinolytic factors, have recently (perhaps fueled by the confirmation of the thrombotic mechanism of acute coronary events [178]) received increasing recognition for their role in predisposing not only to the mechanisms of acute coronary events, but also to the development of coronary atheroma [179].

The initial reports from the Northwick Park Heart study [180, 181], that plasma fibrinogen levels and factor VII coagulant activity (VIIc) are independent predictors of the subsequent development of ischemic heart disease in middle-aged men, have since been confirmed by other studies – both prospective [182–187], measuring incidence (occurrence of new cases), and cross-sectional, measuring extent and severity of atheroma in individuals in whom coronary or other atheromatous disease was already clinically manifest, e.g. fibrinogen was shown to be associated with asymptomatic carotid intimal – medial thickness in 45–64-year-old men and women [188–193]. These latter studies support the notion that fibrin deposition (on injured intima) followed by fibrin incorporation and degradation may contribute to the growth of atheromatous plaques.

Continued follow-up of the Northwick Park Heart study cohort points to reduced fibrinolytic activity as a independent predictor of incident coronary events in 40–54-year-old males [194]. Other studies have implicated impaired fibrinolytic activity, secondary to plasminogen activator inhibitor-1 (PAI-1) activity, as a risk factor for future thrombotic ischemic events such as recurrent myocardial infarction [195–198]. It is becoming increasingly clear that evidence of activity or turnover within the hemostatic dynamic equilibrium is at least as important as the absolute plasma levels of its precursors. Evidence for this is provided by the association of an increased risk of future myocardial infarction with tissue-type plasminogen activator (t-PA) antigen level, which is thought to reflect the inhibitory effect of PAI-1 on t-PA activity [196, 199, 200]. It is also provided by the association of raised prothrombin fragment F^{1+2} and thrombin–antithrombin complex (TAT) levels with angiographically proven coronary atheroma [201]. Such increased hemostatic turnover may further contribute to atherogenesis.

Most recently, in a prospective multicenter study of 3043 patients with angina pectoris who underwent coronary angiography and were followed for two years [202], the levels of fibrinogen, von Willebrand factor antigen and t-PA antigen were independent predictors of subsequent acute coronary syndromes. The authors commented that their data were consistent with 'a pathogenic role of impaired fibrinolysis, endothelial-cell injury and inflammatory activity in the progression of coronary artery disease'. Prior studies had demonstrated that other blood constituents and elements of blood rheology, such as viscosity and leukocytes [61, 203], are important, e.g. in the Framingham Study, leukocyte count within the normal range was found to be a marker for increased risk of cardiovascular disease that is partially explained by cigarette smoking [204].

The situation is further complicated by the fact that hemostatic factors are themselves associated with other established risk factors, e.g., smoking with fibrinogen in males [205], fibrinogen with total cholesterol, triglycerides and VLDL-cholesterol in children and adolescents [206], PAI-1 activity with VLDL-triglycerides [197], blood viscosity with blood pressure, and factor VII activity with dietary fat intake [207, 208]. Taken together, these associations underline the fact that coronary risk factors can influence the subsequent development of ischemic heart disease both via a long-term atherogenic path and via an acute thrombogenic path, and emphasize the complementary roles of atherogenesis and thrombogenesis in ischemic heart disease [209].

The preceding hematological discussion has been with reference to the phenotypic levels of the factors in question. However, the gene loci that control some of these phenotypic levels have been identified, and such genetic polymorphisms either have already been, or are likely to be, added to the list of risk factors for atheroma and coronary disease [210, 211].

Genetic polymorphisms

Prior to the mid-1980s efforts to characterize the role of heritability as a risk factor for coronary disease were, with a few notable exceptions, concentrated upon studying the influence of a family history of ischemic heart disease on the risk of the future development or recurrence of the disease. There were numerous reports of the family history being an independent risk factor [212–216]. It was argued as to whether it was the risk factors for the disease or the disease itself (or both) which had been inherited. In some situations it was recognized that there was a major gene effect controlling the heritability of usually a major risk coronary factor, which had a profound effect upon the phenotype of the individual concerned, such as in familial hypercholesterolemia [217]. However, such cases were relatively rare (compared to the high prevalence of the disease) and did not explain the apparent overall heritability of the disease in the population as a whole, which was usually ascribed to multiple polygenic effects [62].

The development of genetic tools from Southern blot techniques to DNA amplification by polymerase chain reaction have enabled various mechanisms to be unveiled. Various genetic polymorphisms, which control the phenotype of some of the recognized coronary risk factors and their response to environmental influences, have been discovered, cloned and are under investigation. For lipid levels, these include those located at the apoE, apoB, apoA-I, apoC-III and apo(a) gene loci and at the apoA-I/C-III/A-IV gene cluster. For hemostatic factors, these include those located at the factor VII, PAI-1 and beta fibrinogen gene loci [211].

The genetic basis of lipoprotein disorders has recently been well reviewed [218]. About half the population variance in LDL cholesterol is thought to be genetic, only a small proportion (about 14%) of which is explained by the apoB, apoE and LDL-receptor genes (mutations or deletions of the latter of which are responsible for the autosomal dominant familial hypercholesterolemia). Elevated apoB levels are associated with up to a third of patients with premature coronary disease [219] and there is some evidence suggesting that LDL particle size in humans may be determined by a major gene effect with varying additive and polygenic effects linked to the apoA-I/C-III/A-IV gene cluster on chromosome 11 and to the cholesterol ester transfer protein gene locus on chromosome 16 [220–224]. Polymorphism of the apoE gene (specifically its E2/2 genotype) has for some time been known to be associated with Fredrickson type III hyperbetalipoproteinemia [62, 225, 226]. More recently the E4 allele of the apoE gene polymorphism has been shown to predict coronary death in males [227, 228].

Single-gene syndromes probably account for only about 1% of the population variance of HDL-cholesterol levels, however a large proportion (40–60%) appears to be due polygenic inheritance. Phenotypically, HDL-cholesterol and apoA-I levels are strongly correlated, but coronary disease due to low HDL-cholesterol levels secondary to apoA-I gene abnormalities are extremely rare (only seven families reported) and are due to homozygous single gene defects [218, 229]. Interestingly, cholesterol ester transfer protein gene mutations, which result in a phenotype with raised apoA-I and HDL-cholesterol and reduced apoB and LDL-cholesterol levels, are not uncommon in Japan (which, the reader is reminded, is firmly at the foot of the 'league table' of national certified IHD rates [230].

Hypertriglyceridemia, in Caucasians, is associated with apoC-III gene polymorphism [231, 232], which together with polymorphisms in the apoA-I/C-III/A-IV gene cluster has also been reported as being associated with coronary disease among individuals with a family history of coronary disease [224, 233]. In addition to the above human studies, work is in progress on mice genetically engineered to express human transgenes for apoA-I, apoA-II, apoA-IV, apoC-II and III, and apoE [234].

A common polymorphism for the factor VII gene has a strong influence on plasma factor VII coagulant activity and the phenotypic association between factor VII coagulant activity and triglyceride levels is confined entirely to one genotype within the polymorphism [235, 236]. Similarly, there is evidence that the phenotypic association of PAI-1 activity with VLDL triglycerides may also be confined mainly to subjects with one genotype within one of the two polymorphisms found at the PAI-1 gene locus [237, 238]. This could mean that certain genotypic-specific hypertriglyceridemic individuals might be predisposed to thrombotic complications. In a study of 121 cases and 126 controls from the Edinburgh Artery Study, an association has been found between the genotype at the beta fibrinogen locus and not only the fibrinogen phenotype but also the risk of peripheral arterial disease [210].

In addition to genetic polymorphisms which control the phenotype of recognized coronary risk factors, other polymorphisms have been discovered which control other phenotypes which are related to other aspects of the pathophysiology of ischemic heart disease, but which themselves have not previously been characterized as 'risk factors'. Their population distribution is currently being investigated and their association with different manifestations of coronary disease tested. Examples are an insertion/deletion (ID) polymorphism at the angiotensin-converting enzyme (ACE) gene [239, 240], a molecular variant thereof [241], and a common polymorphism in the stromelysin gene promoter [242].

The gene for ACE was cloned in 1988 and its ID polymorphism explains between 28% and 44% of the variability of plasma ACE, the level of which is stable in an individual but highly variable between individuals [243]. The renin–angiotensin system is an integral part of cardiovascular homeostasis and could play a role in the etiology of ischemic heart disease. A multicenter (Belfast, Lille, Strasbourg, and Toulouse) case control study of 610 cases of myocardial infarction drawn from the WHO MONICA registers and of 733 controls drawn randomly from the local general population (the ECTIM study) demonstrated that the DD genotype of the ACE polymorphism, which is associated with higher levels of plasma ACE than the ID or II genotypes, was significantly more frequent in patients with myocardial infarction than in controls, especially among subjects with low body mass index and low plasma apoB levels (i.e. those who would normally be considered at low risk according to conventional criteria) [71].

The ECTIM group have extended this work to show that the ACE polymorphism is associated both with an increased risk of fatal myocardial infarction and with a parental history of fatal myocardial infarction [244, 245]. However, in those ECTIM patients who had undergone coronary angiography, the investigators were unable to demonstrate an association between the ACE polymorphism and degree of coronary atheroma [246]. Other workers have demonstrated that the ACE polymorphism is associated with electrocardiographic left ventricular hypertrophy [247] and with a diagnosis of coronary disease defined by the Rose questionnaire and electrocardiographic Minnesota coding, in a cohort of 1226 men [80]. The molecular variant of the ACE polymorphism has been investigated in a case control study (82 cases, 160 controls) in Japan, where a significant association between the polymorphism and angiographically proven coronary disease was demonstrated [241].

Stromelysin is a metalloproteinase which may be important in the connective tissue remodeling processes involved with atherogenesis and plaque rupture. Stromelysin expression is regulated by the stromelysin gene promoter, in which a common polymorphism has been identified. An association has been demonstrated between the 6A6A genotype of this polymorphism and a greater rate of progression of angiographically proven coronary disease in men who participated in the St Thomas Atherosclerosis Regression Study [242]. The authors state that their findings support the hypothesis that connective tissue remodeling, mediated by metalloproteinases, contributes to the pathogenesis of atheroma.

The discovery of the genetic control of the renin–angiotensin system and of enzymes involved in connective tissue remodeling extends the spectrum of possible etiological factors for coronary disease, and further assists attempts to explain the variability of the occurrence of coronary disease throughout the population as a whole.

Implications

The purposes of risk factor identification are:

1. To allow a better understanding of the etiology and pathophysiology of the disease. This however, is a purely academic exercise which does not alter clinical practice, unless the hypothesis that risk factor modification improves clinical outcome can be tested.
2. The generation of the detail of the above hypotheses. However, risk factor modification is concerned with prevention (be it primary or secondary) and all that prevention implies, namely population screening and trials and implementation of intervention strategies.

References

1. Angelini P. Normal and anomalous coronary arteries: Definitions and classification. Am Heart J 1989;117:418–34.

2. Cook DG, Shaper AG, MacFarlane PW. Using the WHO (Rose) angina questionnaire in cardiovascular epidemiology. Int J Epidemiol 1989;18:607–13.
3. Cannon RO, Camici PG, Epstein SE. Pathophysiological dilemma of Syndrome X. Circulation 1992;85:883–92.
4. Romeo F, Rosano GMC, Martuscelli E, Lombardo L, Valente A. Long-term follow-up of patients initially diagnosed with Syndrome X. Am J Cardiol 1993;71:669–73.
5. Barker DJP, Hales CN, Fall CHD, Osmond C, Phipps K, Clark PMS. Type 2 (non-insulin dependent) diabetes mellitus, hypertension and hyperlipidaemia (syndrome X): Relation to reduced fetal growth. Diabetologica 1993;36:62–7.
6. Alexopoulos D, Olympios C, Psiroyiannis A et al. Hyperinsulinaemia in Syndrome X: A marker of the syndrome? J Cardiovasc Risk 1994;1:69–74.
7. Davies MJ. Unexplained death in fit young people. A category of the sudden unexpected death syndrome is needed. Br Med J 1992;305:538.
8. Geographic pathology of atherosclerosis. Lab Invest 1968;18:465–53.
9. Thomas AC, Knapman PA, Krikler DM, Davies MJ. Community study of the causes of 'natural' sudden death. Br Med J 1988;297:1453–6.
10. Roberts TL, Wood DA, Riemersma RA, Gallagher PJ, Lampe FC. Linoleic acid and risk of sudden cardiac death. Br Heart J 1993;70:524–9.
11. Bowker TJ, Burton JDK, Cary NRB, Chambers DR, Davies MJ, Wood DA. National survey of sudden adult death. J Am Coll Cardiol 1994;23:264A.
12. Fall CHD, Vijayakumar M, Barker DJP, Osmond C, Duggleby S. Weight in infancy and prevalence of coronary heart disease in adult life. Br Med J 1995;310:17–9.
13. Fazzini PF, Prati PL, Rovelli F et al. Epidemiology of silent myocardial ischaemia in asymptomatic middle-aged men (the ECCIS project). Am J Cardiol 1993;72:1383–8.
14. World Health Organisation. International Classification of Diseases, 9th revision: 1975. London: HMSO, 1977.
15. Tunstall-Pedoe H, Smith WCS, Crombie IK. Level and trends of coronary heart disease mortality in Scotland compared with other countries. Health Bulletin 1986;44:153–61.
16. Marmot MG, Booth M, Beral V. Changes in heart disease mortality in England & Wales and other countries. Health Trends 1981;13:33–8.
17. Thom TJ, Epstein FH, Feldman JS, Leaverton PE. Trends in total mortality from heart disease in 26 countries from 1950 to 1978. Int J Epidemiol 1985;14:510–20.
18. Morgan M, Heller RF, Swerdlow A. Changes in diet and coronary heart disease mortality among social classes in Great Britain. J Epidemiol Community Health 1989;43:162–7.
19. Campbell M. Death rate from diseases of the heart: 1876 to 1959. Br Med J 1963;2:528–35.
20. Campbell M. The main causes of increased death rate from diseases of the heart: 1920 to 1959. Br Med J 1963;2:712–7.
21. Office of Population Censuses and Surveys. Mortality Statistics: Cause, England & Wales (Series DH2), yearly 1979 to 1991. London: HMSO, yearly 1981 to 1993.
22. Clayton DG, Taylor D, Shaper AG. Trends in heart disease in England & Wales, 1950–73. Health Trends 1977;9:1–6.
23. Florey CduV, Melia RJW, Darby SC. Changing mortality from ischaemic heart disease in Great Britain 1968–76. Br Med J 1978;1:635–7.
24. Heller F, Hayward D, Hobbs MST. Decline in rate of death from ischaemic heart disease in the United Kingdom. Br Med J 1983;286:260–2.
25. Bowker TJ, Wilkinson P. Diagnostic transfer in ischaemic heart disease mortality trends in England, Wales and the USA. Eur Heart J 1990; 11 (Abstr Suppl): 131.
26. Tunstall-Pedoe H, Kenicer M, Iannoukos L. Decline in rate of death from ischaemic heart disease in the United Kingdom (letter). Br Med J 1983; 286:560.
27. Marmot MG, McDowall. Mortality decline and widening social inequalities. Lancet 1986;ii:274–6.
28. Bowker TJ, Wilkinson P. A comparative cohort analysis of ischaemic heart disease mortality trends in the USA and England, Wales, 1954–84. J Am Coll Cardiol 1990;15:183A.
29. Fox KM, Purcell H. Coronary heart disease: The continuing problem in the UK. Br J Cardiol 1994;1:(Suppl 2): S2–3.

30. Kannel WB, Dawber TR, Kagan A, Revotskie N, Stokes J. Factors of risk in the development of coronary heart disease – six-year follow-up experience. Ann Intern Med 1961;55:33–50.
31. Reid DD, Hamilton PJS, McCartney P, Rose G, Jarrett RJ, Keen H. Smoking and other risk factors for coronary heart disease in British civil servants. Lancet 1976;ii:979–84.
32. Durkheim E. Suicide: A study in sociology. New York: Free Press, 1951:153.
33. Kahn HA, Medallie JH, Neufeld HN et al. Serum cholesterol: Its distribution and association with dietary and other variables in a survey of 10,000 men. Isr J Med Sci 1969;5:1117–27.
34. Keys A. Diet and blood cholesterol in population surveys – lessons from analysis of the data from a major survey in Israel. Am J Clin Nutr 1988; 48:1161–5.
35. Liu K, Stamler J, Dyer A, McKeever J, McKeever P. Statistical methods to assess and minimise the role of intra-individual variability in obscuring the relationship between dietary lipids and serum cholesterol. J Chron Dis 1978;31:399–418.
36. Morgenstern H. Uses of ecologic analysis in epidemiologic research. Am J Public Health 1982;72:1336–44.
37. Elliott P. Design and analysis of multicentre epidemiological studies: The INTERSALT Study (Chapter). In: Marmot M, Elliott P (eds), Coronary heart disease epidemiology. Oxford: Oxford University Press, 1992: 166–78.
38. Bowker TJ. Covert coronary disease and non-invasive evidence of covert myocardial ischaemia – their prevalence and implications. Int J Cardiol 1994;45:1–7.
39. Langou RA, Huang EK, Kelley MJ, Cohen LS. Predictive accuracy of coronary artery calcification and abnormal exercise test for coronary artery disease in asymptomatic men. Circulation 1980;62:1196–203.
40. Erikssen J, Enge I, Forfang K, Storstein O. False positive diagnostic tests and coronary angiographic findings in 105 presumably healthy males. Circulation 1976;54:371–6.
41. Thaulow E, Erikssen J, Sandvik L, Erikssen G, Jorgensen L, Cohn PF. Initial clinical presentation of cardiac disease in asymptomatic men with silent myocardial ischaemia and angiographically documented coronary artery disease (the Oslo ischaemia study). Am J Cardiol 1993;72:629–33.
42. Froelicher VF, Thompson AJ, Walthuis R et al. Angiographic findings in asymptomatic aircrew men with electrocardiographic abnormalities. Am J Cardiol 1977;39:32–8.
43. Kohli RS, Cashman PM, Lahari A, Raftery EB. The ST segment of the ambulatory electrocardiogram in a normal population. Br Heart J 1988;60:4–16.
44. Gandhi MM, Wood DA, Lampe FC. Characteristics and clinical significance of ambulatory myocardial ischaemia in men and women in the general population presenting with angina pectoris. J Am Coll Cardiol 1994;23:74–81.
45. Family Heart Study Group: Randomised controlled trial evaluating cardiovascular screening and intervention in general practice: principal results of British family heart study. Br Med J 1994;308:313–20.
46. Shaper AG, Cook DG, Walsker M, McFarlane PW. Prevalence of ischaemic heart disease in middle aged British men. Br Heart J 1984;51:595–605.
47. Smith WCS, Kenicer MB, Tunstall-Pedoe H, Clark EC, Crombie IK. Prevalence of coronary heart disease in Scotland: Scottish Heart Health Study. Br Heart J 1990;64:295–8.
48. Gandhi MM, Lampe FC, Wood DA. Incidence, clinical characteristics and short-term prognosis of angina pectoris. Br Heart J 1995;73:193–8.
49. Armstrong A, Duncan B, Oliver MF et al. Natural history of acute coronary heart attacks. Br Heart J 1972;34:67–80.
50. Kinlen LJ. Incidence and presentation of myocardial infarction in an English community. Br Heart J 1973;35:616–22.
51. Tunstall-Pedoe H, Clayton D, Morris JN, Brigden W, McDonald L. Coronary heart attacks in East London. Lancet 1975;ii:833–8.
52. Royal College of General Practitioners, Office of Population Censuses and Surveys, Department of Health and Social Security. Morbidity Statistics from General Practice, 1981–2. London: HMSO, 1986 (Series MB5).
53. Tunstall-Pedoe H, Kuulasmaa K, Amouyei P, Arveiler D, Rajakangas, Pajak A for the WHO MONICA Project. Myocardial infarction and coronary deaths in the World Health Organisation MONICA project. Circulation 1994;90:583–612.

54. Murphy JJ, Connell PA, Hampton JR. Predictors of risk in patients with unstable angina admitted to a district general hospital. Br Heart J 1992;67:395–401.
55. Bowker TJ, Boyle RM, Fox KM, Murphy JM, Wood DA on behalf of the SAMII Study Group. Management patterns and outcome of acute myocardial ischaemia and infarction in the UK. J Am Coll Cardiol 1994;23:434A.
56. Barker DJP. Fetal origins of coronary heart disease. Br Heart J 1993;69:195–6.
57. Paneth N, Susser M. Early origin of coronary heart disease (the 'Barker hypothesis') Br Med J 1995;310:411–2.
58. Wood DA, Oliver MF. Linoleic acid, antioxidant vitamins, and coronary heart disease. In: Marmot M, Elliott P, (eds), Coronary heart disease epidemiology. Oxford: Oxford University Press, 1992:179–202.
59. McKeigue P. Trans fatty acids and coronary heart disease: Weighing the evidence against hardened fat. Lancet 1995;345:269–70.
60. Meade TW. Atheroma and thrombosis in cardiovascular disease: Separate or complementary? In: Marmot M, Elliott P, (eds), Coronary heart disease epidemiology. Oxford: Oxford University Press, 1992;287–97.
61. Lowe GDO, Fowkes FGR, Dawes J, Donnan PT, Lennie SE, Housley E. Blood viscosity, fibrinogen and activation of coagulation and leukocytes in peripheral arterial disease and the normal population in the Edinburgh Artery Study. Circulation 1993;87:1915–20.
62. Berg K. Genetics of coronary heart disease and its risk factors. In: Bock G, Collins GM, (eds) Molecular approaches to human polygenic disease (Ciba Foundation Symposium 130). Chichester, UK: John Wiley & Sons, 1987:14–33.
63. Keys A. Seven countries – a multivariate analysis of death and coronary heart disease. Cambridge, MA: Harvard University Press, 1980.
64. Kok FJ, Van Duijn CM, Hofman A et al. Serum copper and zinc and the risk of death from cancer and cardiovascular disease. Am J Epidemiol 1988;128:352–9.
65. Hoefler G, Harnoncourt F, Paschke E, Mirtl W, Pfeiffer KH, Kostner GM. Lipoprotein Lp(a): A risk factor for myocardial infarction. Atherosclerosis 1988;8:398–401.
66. Ananijevic-Pandey J, Vlajinac H. Myocardial infarction in young women with reference to oral contraceptive use. Int J Epidemiol 1989;18:585–8.
67. Talbott EO, Kuller LH, Detre K et al. Reproductive history of women dying of sudden cardiac death: A case-control study. Int J Epidemiol 1989;18:589–94.
68. Palmer JR, Rosenberg L, Shapiro S. Stature and the risk of myocardial infarction in women. Am J Epidemiol 1990;132:27–32.
69. Wiklund O, Angelin B, Olofsson S-O et al. Apolipoprotein (a) and ischaemic heart disease in familial hypercholesterolaemia. Lancet 1990;335:1360–3.
70. Rosengren A, Wilhelmsen L, Eriksson E, Risberg B, Wedel H. Lipoprotein (a) and coronary heart disease: A prospective case-control study in a general population sample of middle aged men. Br Med J 1990;301:1248–51.
71. Cambien F, Poirier O, Lecerf L et al. Deletion polymorphism in the gene for angiotensin-converting enzyme is a potent risk factor for myocardial infarction. Nature 1992;359:641–4.
72. Manttari M, Manninen V, Huttunen JK et al. Serum ferritin and ceruloplasmin as coronary risk factors. Eur Heart J 1994;15:1599–603.
73. Kannel WB. Contribution of the Framingham Heart Study to preventive cardiology. Bishop Lecture. J Am Coll Cardiol 1990;15:206–11.
74. Kannel WB. The Framingham experience. In: Marmot M, Elliott P, (eds), Coronary heart disease epidemiology. Oxford: Oxford University Press, 1992:67–82.
75. Marmot MG, Davey-Smith G, Stansfield S et al. Health inequalities among British civil servants: The Whitehall II study. Lancet 1991;337:1387–93.
76. Shaper AG, Pocock SJ, Walker M, Phillips AM, Whitehead, Macfarlane PW. Risk factors for ischaemic heart disease: The prospective phase of the British Regional Heart Study. J Epidemiol Community Health 1985;39:197–209.
77. Shaper AG, Elford J. Regional variations in coronary heart disease in Great Britain: Risk factors and changes in environment. In: Marmot M, Elliott P (eds) Coronary heart disease epidemiology. Oxford: Oxford University Press, 1992:127–39.

78. Miller NE, Bolton CH, Hayes TM et al. Associations of alcohol consumption with plasma high density lipoprotein cholesterol and its major subfractions: The Caerphilly and Speedwell Collaborative Heart Disease Studies. J Epidemiol Community Health 1988;42:220–5.
79. Gallacher JE, Yarnell JW, Butland BK. Type A behaviour and prevalent heart disease in the Caerphilly study: Increase in risk or symptom reporting? J Epidemiol Community Health 1988;42:226–31.
80. Mattu RK, Needham EWA, Galton DJ, Frangos E, Clark AJL, Caulfield M. A DNA variant at the angiotensin-converting enzyme gene locus associates with coronary artery disease in the Caerphilly Heart Study. Circulation 1995;91:270–4.
81. Isles CG, Hole DJ, Hawthorne VM, Lever AF. Relation between coronary risk and coronary mortality in women of the Renfrew and Paisley survey: Comparison with men. Lancet 1992;339:702–6.
82. Pooling Project Research Group: Relationship of blood pressure, serum cholesterol, smoking habit, relative weight and ECG abnormalities to incidence of major coronary events: Final report of the Pooling Project. J Chron Dis 1978;31:201–306.
83. Menotti A, Farchi, Seccareccia F, and the RIFLE Research Group. The prediction of coronary heart disease mortality as a function of major risk factors in over 30,000 men in the Italian RIFLE Pooling Project: A comparison with the MRFIT primary screenees. J Cardiovasc Risk 1994;1:263–70.
84. Stamler J. Established major coronary risk factors. In: Marmot M, Elliott P, (eds), Coronary heart disease epidemiology. Oxford: Oxford University Press, 1992:35–66.
85. MRFIT (Multiple Risk Factor Intervention Trial Research Group). Mortality rates after ten and a half years for participants in the Multiple Risk Factor Intervention Trial. Findings related to a priori hypotheses of the trial. Circulation 1990;82:1616–28.
86. World Health Organisation European Collaborative Group: European collaborative trial of multifactorial prevention of coronary heart disease: Final report on the 6-year results. Lancet 1986;i:869–72.
87. Puska P, Salonen JT, Tuomilehto J et al. Change in risk factors for coronary heart disease during 10 years of community intervention programme (North Karelia project). Br Med J 1983;287:1840–4.
88. Salonen JT, Tuomilehto J, Nissinen A, Kaplan GA, Puska P. Contribution of risk factor changes to the decline on coronary incidence during the North Karelia Project: A within-community analysis. Int J Epidemiol 1989;18:595–601.
89. Hjerrmann I, Valve-Byre DV, Holme I, Leren P. Effect of diet and smoking intervention on the incidence of coronary heart disease: Report from the Oslo Study Group of a randomised trial in healthy men. Lancet 1981;ii:1303–10.
90. Barter PJ. Plasma lipoproteins and coronary heart disease – overview. J Cardiovasc Risk 1994;1:193–6.
91. Assman G, Hunt BJ. Clinical chemistry and coagulation: Editorial comment. Curr Opinion Lipidol 1994;5:391–4.
92. Gordon DJ, Probsfield JL, Garrison RJ et al. High density lipoprotein cholesterol and cardiovascular disease: Four prospective American studies. Circulation 1989;79:8–15.
93. Kannel WB. High density lipoprotein: Epidemiologic profile and risks of coronary heart disease. Am J Cardiol 1983;52:93–123.
94. Groot PH, van Stiphout WA, Krauss XH et al. Postprandial lipoprotein metabolism in normolipaemic men with and without coronary artery disease. Arterioscler Thromb 1991;11:653–62.
95. Watts GF, Mandalia S, Brunt JNH, Slavin BM, Coltart DJ, Lewis B. Independent associations between plasma lipoprotein sub-fraction levels and the course of coronary artery disease in the St Thomas' Atherosclerosis Regression Study (STARS). Metabolism 1993;42:1461–7.
96. Phillips NR, Waters D, Havel RJ. Plasma lipoproteins and progression of coronary artery disease evaluated by angiography and clinical events. Circulation 1993;88:2762–70.
97. Krauss RM. Heterogeneity of plasma low-density lipoproteins and atherosclerosis risk. Curr Opin Lipidol 1994;5:339–49.
98. Karpe F, Bard JM, Steiner G, Carlson LA, Fruchart JC, Hamsten A. HDLs and alimentary lipaemia. Studies in men with previous myocardial infarction at a young age. Arterioscler Thromb 1993;13:11–22.

99. Clifton PM. Postprandial lipoproteins and coronary heart disease. J Cardiovasc Risk 1994;1:197–201.
100. Cambien F, Jacqueson A, Richard JL, Warnet J-M, Ducimetiere P, Claude JR. Is the level of serum triglyceride a significant predictor of coronary death in 'normocholesterolaemic' subjects? The Paris Prospective Study. Am J Epidemiol 1986;124:624–32.
101. Austin MA. Plasma triglyceride and coronary heart disease. Arterioscler Thromb 1991;11:1–14.
102. Austin MA, King MC, Vranizan KM, Krauss RM. Atherogenic lipoprotein phenotype: A proposed genetic marker for coronary heart disease. Circulation 1990;82:495–506.
103. Assmann G, Betteridge DJ, Gotto AM Steiner G. Management of hypertriglyceridaemic patients: Treatment classifications and goals. Am J Cardiol 1991;68 (Suppl A):30A–34A.
104. Manninen V, Tenkanen L, Koskinen P et al. Joint effects of serum triglyceride and LDL-cholesterol and HDL-cholesterol concentrations on coronary heart disease in the Helsinki Heart Study: Implications for treatment. Circulation 1992;85:37–45.
105. Barbir M, Wile D, Trayner I, Aber V, Thompson GR. High prevalence of hypertriglyceridaemia and apolipoprotein abnormalities in coronary artery disease. Br Heart J 1988;60:397–403.
106. Austin MA, Breslow JL, Hennekens CH, Buring JE, Willett WC, Kraus RM: Low-density lipoprotein subclass patterns and risk of myocardial infarction. JAMA 1988;26:1917–21.
107. Tornvall P, Bavenholm P, Landou C, deFaire U, Hamsten A. Relation of plasma levels and composition of apolipoprotein B containing lipoproteins to angiographically defined coronary artery disease in young patients with myocardial infarction. Circulation 1993;88:2180–9.
108. O'Brien R. Biological importance of low-density lipoprotein subfractions. J Cardiovasc Risk 1994;1:207–11.
109. Rajman I, Maxwell S, Cramb R, Kendall M. Particle size: The key to the atherogenic lipoprotein? J Med 1994;87:709–20.
110. Regnstrom J, Nilsson J, Tornvall P, Landou C, Hamsten A. Susceptibility to low density lipoprotein oxidation and coronary atherosclerosis in man. Lancet 1992;339:1183–6.
111. Austin MA, Hokanson JE, Brunzell JD. Characterisation of low-density lipoprotein subclasses: Approaches and clinical relevance. Curr Opin Lipidol 1994;5:395–403.
112. Selby JV, Austin MA, Newman B et al. LDL subclass phenotypes and the insulin resistance syndrome in women. Circulation 1993;88:382–7.
113. Reaven GM, Chen Y-DI, Jeppesen J, Maheux P, Kraus RM. Insulin resistance and hyperinsulinaemia in individuals with small, dense low-density lipoprotein particles. J Clin Invest 1993;92:141–6.
114. von Eckardstein A, Huang Y, Assman G. Physiological role and clinical relevance of high-density lipoprotein subclasses. Curr Opin Lipidol 1994;5:404–16.
115. Haffner SM, Moss SE, Klein BE Klein R. Lack of association between lipoprotein (a) and coronary heart disease mortality in diabetes: The Winconsin epidemiologic study of diabetic retinopathy. Metabolism 1992;41:194–7.
116. Jauhiainen M, Koskinen P, Ehnholm C et al. Lipoprotein (a) and coronary heart disease risk: A nested case control study of the Helsinki Heart Study participants. Atherosclerosis 1991;89:59–67.
117. Ridker PM, Hennekens CH, Stampfer MJ. A prospective study of lipoprotein (a) and the risk of myocardial infarction. J Am Med Assoc 1993;270:2195–9.
118. Cremer P, Nagal D, Labrot A et al. Lipoprotein (a) as a predictor of myocardial infarction in comparison to fibrinogen, LDL-cholesterol and other risk factors: Results from the Prospective Gottingen Risk Incidence and Prevalence Study (GRIPS). Eur J Clin Invest 1994;24:444–53.
119. Hoff HF, Beck GJ, Skibinski MS et al. Serum Lp(a) level as a predictor of vein graft stenosis after coronary artery by-pass surgery in patients. Circulation 1988;77:1238–44.
120. Barbir M, Kushwahi S, Hunt B et al. Lipoprotein (a) and accelerated coronary arterial disease in cardiac transplant recipients. Lancet 1992;340:1550–2.
121. Scott J. Lipoprotein (a). Be Med J 1991;303:663–4.
122. Liu AC, Lawn RM. Vascular interactions of lipoprotein (a). Curr Opin Lipidol 1994;5:269–73.
123. Sullivan DR. Lipoprotein (a). J Cardiovasc Risk 1994;1:212–6.
124. Leon AS, Connett, for the MRFIT Research Group. Physical activity and 10.5 year mortality in the Multiple Risk Factor Intervention Trial (MRFIT). Int J Epidemiol 1989;20:690–7.
125. Pocock SJ, Shaper AG, Cook DG, Phillips AN, Walker M. Social differences in ischaemic heart disease in British men. Lancet 1987;ii:197–201.

126. Stampfer MJ, Willett WC, Colditz GA, Speizer FE, Hennekens CH. A prospective study of past use of oral contraceptive agents and risk of cardiovascular diseases. N Engl J Med 1988;319:1313–7.
127. Bush TL, Barrett-Connor E. Noncontraceptive oestrogen use and cardiovascular disease. Epidemiol Rev 1985;71:80–104.
128. Ducimetiere P, Guize L, Marciniak A, Milon H, Richard J, Rufat P, for the CORALI Study Group. Arteriographically documented coronary artery disease and alcohol consumption in French men. The CORALI Study. Eur Heart J 1993;14:727–33.
129. Tverdal A, Stensvold I, Solvoll K, Foss OP, Lund-Larsen P, Bjartveit K. Coffee consumption and death from coronary heart disease in middle aged Norwegian men and women. Br Med J 1990;300:566–9.
130. Pocock SJ, Shaper AG, Cook DG et al. British Regional Heart Study: Geographic variations in cardiovascular mortality, and the role of water quality. Br Med J 1980;2(280):1243–9.
131. Lacey RF, Shaper AG. Changes in water hardness and cardiovascular death rates. Int J Epidemiol 1984;13:18–24.
132. Whincup PH, Cook DG, Phillips AN, Shaper AG. ABO blood group and ischaemic heart disease in British men. Br Med J 1990;300:1679–82.
133. Wittemann JCM, Grobbee DE, Kok FK, Hofman A, Valkenburg HA. Increased risk of atherosclerosis in women after the menopause. Br Med J 1989;298:642–4.
134. Matthews KA, Meilahn E, Kuller LH, Kelsey SF, Caggiula AW, Wing RR. Menopause and risk factors for coronary heart disease. N Engl J Med 1989;321:641–6.
135. Walker M, Shaper AG, Phillips AN, Cook DG. Short stature, lung function and risk of heart attack. Int J Epidemiol 1989;18:602–6.
136. McKeigue PM. Coronary heart disease in Indians, Pakistanis and Bangladeshis: Aetiology and possibilities for prevention. Br Heart J 1992;67:341–2.
137. Riemersma RA, Wood DA, MacIntyre CCA, Elton RA, Grey KF, Oliver MF. Risk of angina pectoris and concentrations of vitamins A, C and E and carotene. Lancet 1991;i:1–5.
138. Phillips A, Shaper AG, Whincup PH. Association between serum albumin and mortality from cardiovascular disease, cancer and other causes. Lancet 1989;ii:1434–6.
139. Saikku P, Leinonen M, Mattila K et al. Serological evidence of an association of a novel chlamydia, TWAR, with chronic coronary heart disease and acute myocardial infarction. Lancet 1988;ii:983–6.
140. Lind L, Jakobsson S, Lithell H, Wengle B, Ljunghall S. Relation of serum calcium concentration to metabolic risk factors for cardiovascular disease. Br Med J 1988;297:960–3.
141. Kannel WB, Dannenberg AL, Levy D. Population implications of electrocardiographic left ventricular hypertrophy. Am J Cardiol 1987;60:851.
142. Sacks F. Dietary fats and coronary heart disease – overview. J Cardiovasc Risk 1994;1:3–8.
143. Hannah JS, Howard BV. Dietary fats, insulin resistance and diabetes. J Cardiovasc Risk 1994;1:31–7.
144. Fowkes FGR, Lowe GDO, Rumley A, Lennie SE, Smith FB, Donnan PT. The relationship between blood viscosity and blood pressure in a random sample of the population aged 55 to 74 years. Eur Heart J 1993;14:597–601.
145. Wannmethee G, Shaper AG. The association between heart rate and blood pressure, blood lipids and other cardiovascular risk factors. J Cardiovasc Risk 1994;1:223–30.
146. Meade TW, Imeson L, Stirling Y. Effects of changes in smoking and other characteristics on clotting factors and the risk of ischaemic heart disease. Lancet 1987;ii:986–8.
147. Cambien F, Warnet J-M, Eschwege E, Jacqueson A, Richard JL, Rosselin G. Body mass, blood pressure, glucose and lipids: Does plasma insulin explain their relationships? Arteriosclerosis 1987;7:197–202.
148. McKeigue PM, Marmot MG. Mortality from coronary heart disease in Asian communities in London. Br Med J 1988;297:903.
149. McKeigue PM, Shah B, Marmot MG. Relation of central obesity and insulin resistance with high diabetes prevalence and cardiovascular risk in South Asians. Lancet 1991;337:382–6.
150. McKeigue PM, Keen H. Diabetes, insulin, ethnicity and coronary heart disease. In: Marmot M, Elliott P, (eds), Coronary heart disease epidemiology. Oxford: Oxford University Press, 1992:217–32.

151. Hales CN, Barker DJP, Clark PMS et al. Fetal and infant growth and impaired glucose tolerance at age 64. Br Med J 1991;303:1019–22.
152. Barker DJP, Bull AR, Osmond C, Simmonds SJ. Fetal and placental size and risk of hypertension in adult life. Br Med J 1990;301:259–62.
153. Law CM, Barker DJP, Osmond C, Fall CHD, Simmonds SJ. Early growth and abdominal fatness in adult life. J Epidemiol Community Health 1992;46:184–6.
154. Barker DJP, Meade TW, Fall CHD et al. Relation of fetal and infant growth to plasma fibrinogen and factor VII concentrations in adult life. Br Med J 1992;304:148–52.
155. Fall CHD, Barker DJP, Osmond C, Winter PD, Clark PMS, Hales CN. Relation of infant feeding to adult serum cholesterol concentration and death from ischaemic heart disease. Br Med J 1992;304:801–5.
156. Barker DJP, Osmond C. The maternal and infant origins of cardiovascular disease. In: Marmot M, Elliott P (eds), Coronary heart disease epidemiology. Oxford: Oxford University Press, 1992:83–90.
157. Lucas A. Programming by early nutrition in man. In: Bock GR, Whelan J (eds), 'The childhood environment and adult disease. (Ciba Foundation Symposium 156). Chichester, UK: John Wiley & Sons, 1991.
158. Fall CHD, Osmond C, Barker DJP et al. Fetal and infant growth and cardiovascular risk factors in women. Br Med J 1995;310:428–432.
159. Hasle H. Association between living conditions in childhood and myocardial infarction. Br Med J 1990;300:512–3.
160. Strachan DP, Leon DA, Dodgeon B. Mortality from cardiovascular disease among interregional migrants in England & Wales. Br Med J 1995;310:423–7.
161. Christensen K, Vaupel JW, Holm NV, Yashin AI. Mortality among twins after age 6: Fetal origins hypothesis versus twin method. Br Med J 1995;310:432–6.
162. Perry IJ, Beevers DG, Whincup PH, Beresford D. Predictors of ratio of placental weight to fetal weight in multiethnic community. Br Med J 1995;310:436–9.
163. Sinclair HM. Deficiency of essential fatty acids and atherosclerosis, ecetera (letter). Lancet 1956;i:381–3.
164. Logan RL, Riemersma RA, Thomson M et al.: Risk factors for ischaemic heart disease in normal men aged 40. Edinburgh-Stockholm study. Lancet 1978;i:949–55.
165. Riemersma RA, Wood DA, Butler S et al. Linoleic acid content in adipose tissue and coronary heart disease. Br Med J 1986;292:1423–7.
166. Tavendale R, Lee AJ, Smith WCS. Tunstall-Pedoe H. Adipose tissue fatty acids in Scottish men and women: Results from the Scottish Heart Health Study. Atherosclerosis 1992;94:161–9.
167. Wood DA, Butler S, Riemersma RA, Thomson M, Oliver MF. Adipose tissue and platelet fatty acids and coronary heart disease in Scottish men. Lancet 1984;ii:117–21.
168. Wood DA, Riemersma RA, Butler S et al. Linoleic and eicosapentaenoic acids in adipose tissue and platelets and risk of coronary heart disease. Lancet 1987;i:177–83.
169. Thomson M, Elton RA, Fulton M, Brown S, Wood CA, Oliver MF. Individual variation in the dietary intake on a group of Scottish men. J Hum Natr Dietet 1988;1:47–57.
170. Willett WC, Stampfer MJ, Manson JE et al. Intake of *trans* fatty acids and risk of coronary heart disease among women. Lancet 1993;341:581–5.
171. Ascherio A, Hennekens CH, Buring JE, Master C, Stampfer MJ, Willett WC. *Trans* fatty acids intake and risk of myocardial infarction. Circulation 1994;89:94–101.
172. Thomas LH. Ischaemic heart disease and consumption of hydrogenated marine oils in England & Wales. J Epidemiol Community Health 1992;46:78–82.
173. Siguel EN, Lerman RH. *Trans* fatty acid patterns in patients with angiographically documented coronary artery disease. Am J Cardiol 1993;71:916–20.
174. Mann GV. Metabolic consequences of dietary *trans* fatty acids. Lancet 1994;343:1268–71.
175. McKeigue P. *Trans* fatty acids and coronary heart disease: Weighing the evidence against hardened fat. Lancet 1995;345:269–70.
176. Aro A, Kardinaal AFM, Salminen I et al. Adipose tissue isomeric *trans* fatty acids and risk of myocardial infarction in nine countries: The EURAMIC study. Lancet 1995;345:273–8.
177. Roberts TL, Wood DA, Riemersma RA, Gallagher PJ, Lampe FC. *Trans* isomers of oleic and linoleic acids in adipose tissue and sudden cardiac death. Lancet 1995;345:278–82.

178. Davies MJ, Thomas A. Thrombosis and acute coronary artery lesions in sudden cardiac ischaemic death. N Engl J Med, 1984;310:897–901.
179. Hamsten A, Eriksson P, Karpe F, Silveira A. Relationships of thrombosis and fibrinolysis to atherosclerosis. Curr Opin Lipidol 1994;5:382–9.
180. Meade TW, North WRS, Chakrabarti R, Stirling Y, Haines AP, Thompson SG. Haemostatic function and cardiovascular death: Early results of a prospective study. Lancet 1980;i:1050–4.
181. Meade TW, Mellows S, Brozovic M et al.: Haemostatic function and ischaemic heart disease: Principal results of the Northwick Park Heart Study. Lancet 1986;ii:533–7.
182. Wilhelmsen L, Svardsudd K, Korsan-Bengtsen K, Welin L, Tibblin G. Fibrinogen as a risk factor for stroke and myocardial infarction. Engl J Med 1984;311:501–5.
183. Stone MC, Thorpe JM. Plasma fibrinogen – a major coronary risk factor. J R Coll Gen Pract 1985;35:565–9.
184. Kannel WB, Wolf PA, Castelli WP, A'Agostino RB. Fibrinogen and risk of cardiovascular disease. J Am Med Assoc 1987;258:1183–6.
185. Yarnell JWG, Baker IA, Sweetnam PM et al. Fibrinogen, viscosity and white blood cell count are major risk factors for ischaemic heart disease. Circulation 1991;83:836–44.
186. Ernst E, Resch KL. Fibrinogen as a cardiovascular risk factor: A meta-analysis and review of the literature. Ann Intern Med 1993;118:956–63.
187. Heinrich J, Balleisen L, Schulte H, Assman G, van de Loo J. Fibrinogen and factor VII in the prediction of coronary risk: Results from the PROCAM study in healthy males. Arterioscler Thromb 1994;14:54–9.
188. Lowe GD, Drummond MM, Lorimer AR et al. Relation between extent of coronary artery disease and blood viscosity. Br Med J 1980;280:673–4.
189. Hamsten A, Blomback M, Wiman B et al. Haemostatic function in myocardial infarction. Br Heart J 1986;55:58–66.
190. Handa K, Kono S, Saku K et al. Plasma fibrinogen levels as an independent indicator of severity of coronary atherosclerosis. Atherosclerosis 1989;77:209–13.
191. Broadhurst P, Kalleher C, Hughes L, Imeson JD, Raftery EB. Fibrinogen, factor VII clotting activity and coronary artery disease severity. Atherosclerosis 1990;85:169–73.
192. Folsom AR, Wu KK, Shahar E, Davis CE. Association of haemostatic variables with prevalent cardiovascular disease and asymptomatic carotid artery atherosclerosis. Arterioscler Thromb, 1993;13:1829–936.
193. Lassila R, Peltonen S, Lepantalo M, Saarinen O, Kauhanen P, Manninen V. Severity of peripheral atherosclerosis is associated with fibrinogen and degradation of cross-linked fibrin. Arterioscler Thromb 1993;13:1738–42.
194. Meade TW, Ruddock V, Stirling Y, Chakrabarti R, Miller GJ. Fibrinolytic activity, clotting factors and long-term incidence of ischaemic heart disease in the Northwick Park Heart Study. Lancet 1993;342:1076–9.
195. Hamsten A, de Faire U, Walldius G et al. Plasminogen activator inhibitor in plasma: Risk factor for recurrent myocardial infarction. Lancet 1987;ii:3–9.
196. Ridker PM, Vaughan DE, Stampfer MJ, Manson JE, Hennekens CH. Endogenous tissue-type plasminogen activator and risk of myocardial infarction. Lancet 1993;341:1165–8.
197. Hamsten A, Wiman B, de Faire U, Blomback M. Increased plasma levels of a rapid inhibitor of tissue plasminogen activator in young survivors of myocardial infarction. Engl J Med 1985;313:1557–63.
198. Dawson S, Henney A. The status of PAI-1 as a risk factor for arterial and thrombotic disease: A review. Atherosclerosis 1992;95:105–17.
199. Jansson J-H, Olofsson B-O, Nilsson TK. Predictive value of tissue plasminogen activator mass concentration on long-term mortality in patients with coronary artery disease: A 7-year follow-up. Circulation 1993;88:2030–4.
200. Folsom AR, Qamhieh HT, Wing RR et al. Impact of weight loss on plasminogen activator inhibitor (PAI-1), factor VII and other haemostatic factors in moderately overweight adults. Arterioscler Thromb 1993;13:162–9.
201. Kienast J, Thompson SG, Raskino C et al. Prothrombin activation fragment 1 + 2 and thrombin antithrombin III complexes in patients with angina pectoris: Relation to the presence of and severity of coronary atherosclerosis. Thromb Haemost 1994;72:550–3.

202. Thompson SG, Kienast J, Pyke SDM, Haverkate F, van de Loo JCW for the European Concerted Action on Thrombosis and Disabilities Angina Pectoris Study Group. Haemostatic factors and the risk of myocardial infarction or sudden death in patients with angina pectoris. N Engl J Med 1995;332:635–41.
203. Belch JJF. The relationship between white blood cells and arterial disease. Curr Opin Lipidol 1994;5:440–6.
204. Kannel WB, Anderson K, Wilson PWF. White blood cell count and cardiovascular disease: Insights from the Framingham Study. JAMA 1992;267:1253–6.
205. Meade TW, Imeson J, Stirling Y. Effects of changes in smoking and other characteristics on clotting factors and the risk of ischaemic heart disease. Lancet 1987;ii:986–8.
206. Sanchez-Bayle M, Cocho P, Baeza J, Vila S and the Nino Jesus Group. Fibrinogen as a cardiovascular risk factor in Spanish children and adolescents. Am Heart J, 1993;126:322–6.
207. Miller GJ, Martin JC, Webster J et al.: Association between dietary fat intake and plasma factor VII coagulant activity – a predictor of cardiovascular mortality. Atherosclerosis 1986;60:269–277.
208. Miller GJ, Cruikshank JK, Ellis LJ et al.: Fat consumption and factor VII coagulant activity in middle aged men. An association between a dietary and thrombogenic coronary risk factor. Atherosclerosis 1989;78:19–24.
209. Meade TW. Atheroma and thrombosis in cardiovascular disease: Separate or complementary? In: Marmot M, Elliott P (eds), Coronary heart disease epidemiology. Oxford: Oxford University Press, 1992:287–97.
210. Fowkes FGR, Connor JM, Smith FB, Wood J, Donnan PT, Lowe GDO. Fibrinogen genotype and risk of peripheral atherosclerosis. Lancet 1992;339:693–6.
211. Hamsten A. Haemostatic function and coronary artery disease. N Engl J Med 1995;332:677–8.
212. Nora JJ, Lortscher RH, Spangler RD, Nora AH, Kimberling WJ. Genetic-epidemiologic study of early-onset ischaemic heart disease. Circulation 1980;61:503–8.
213. ten Kate LP, Boman H, Daiger SP, Motulsky AG. Familial aggregation of coronary heart disease and its relation to known genetic risk factors. Am J Cardiol 1982;50:945–53.
214. Becker DM, Becker LC, Pearson TA, Fintel DJ, Levine DM, Kwiterovich PO. Risk factors in siblings of people with premature coronary heart disease. J Am Coll Cardiol 1988;12:1273–80.
215. Hopkins PN, Williams RR, Kuida H et al. Family history as an independent risk factor for incident coronary artery disease in a high-risk cohort in Utah. Am J Cardiol 1988;62:703–7.
216. Jorde LB, Williams RR. Relation between family history of coronary artery disease and coronary risk variables. Am J Cardiol 1988;62:708–13.
217. Moorjani S, Roy M, Gagne C et al. Homozygous familial hypercholesterolaemia among French Canadians in Quebec Province. Arteriosclerosis 1989;9:211–6.
218. Dammerman M, Breslow JL. Genetic basis of lipoprotein disorders. Circulation 1995;91:505–12.
219. Sniderman AD, Silberberg J. Is it time to measure apolipoprotein B? Arteriosclerosis 1990;10:665–7.
220. Austin MA. Genetic epidemiology of low-density lipoprotein subclass phenotypes. Ann Med 1992;24:477–81.
221. Bu X, Krauss R, Puppione D, Gray R, Rotter JI. Major gene control of atherogenic lipoprotein phenotype (ALP): A quantitative segregation analysis in 20 coronary artery disease (CAD) pedigrees (Abstract). Am J Hum Genet 1992;51:A336.
222. Austin MA, Jarvik GP, Hokanson JE, Edwards K. Complex segregation analysis of LDL peak particle diameter. Genet Epidemiol 1993;10:599–604.
223. Nishina PM, Johnson JP, Naggert JK, Krauss RM. Linkage of atherogenic lipoprotein phenotype to the low-density lipoprotein receptor locus on the short arm of chromosome 19. Proc Natl Acad Sci USA, 1992;89:708–12.
224. Rotter JI, Bu X, Cantor R et al. Multilocus genetic determination of LDL particle size in coronary artery disease families (Abstract). Clin Res 1994;42:16A.
225. Utermamm G, Pruin N, Stenmetz A. Polymorphism of apolipoprotein E III: Effect of a single polymorphic gene locus on plasma lipid levels in man. Clin Genet 1979;15:63–72.
226. Boerwinkle E, visvikis S, Welsh D, Steinmetz J, Hanash SM, Sing CF. The use of measured genotype information in the analysis of quantivive phenotypes in man. II. The role of the apolipoprotein E polymorphism in determining levels, variability and covariability of cholesterol, betalipoprotein and triglycerides in a sample of unrelated individuals. Am J Med Genet 1987;27:567–82.

227. Eichner JE, Kuller LH, Orchard TJ et al. Relation of apolipoprotein E phenotype to myocardial infarction and mortality from coronary artery disease. Am J Cardiol 1993;71:160–5.
228. Stengard JH, Zerba KE, Pekkanen J, Ehnholm C, Nissinen A, Sing CF. Apolipoprotein E polymorphism predicts death from coronary heart disease in a longitudinal study of elderly Finnish men. Circulation 1995;91:265–9.
229. Assmann G, von Eckardstein A, Funke H. High density lipoproteins, reverse transport of cholesterol and coronary artery disease. Circulation 1993;87:28–34.
230. Tall AR. Plasma cholesterol ester transfer protein. J Lipid Res 1993;34:1255–74.
231. Rees A, Shoulders CC, Stocks J, Galton DJ, Baralle FE. DNA polymorphism adjacent to the human apoprotein AI gene: Relation to hypertriglyceridaemia. Lancet 1983;i:444–6.
232. Shoulders CC, Harry PJ, Lagrost L et al. Variation at the apo AI/CIII/AIV gene complex is associated with elevated plasma levels of apo CIII. Atherosclerosis 1991;87:239–47.
233. Price WH, Kitchin AH, Burgon PRS, Morris SW, Wenham PR, Donald PM. DNA restriction fragment length polymorphisms as markers of familial coronary heart disease. Lancet 1989;i:1407–11.
234. Paigen B, Plump AS, Rubin EM. The mouse as a model for human cardiovascular disease and hyperlipidaemia. Curr Opin Lipidol 1994;5:258–64.
235. Green F, Kelleher C, Wilkes H, Temple A, Meade T, Humphries S. A common genetic polymorphism associated with lower coagulation factor VII levels in healthy individuals. Arterioscler Thromb 1991;11:540–6.
236. Humphries SE, Lane A, Green FR, Cooper J, Miller GJ. Factor VII coagulant activity and antigen levels in healthy men are determined by interaction between factor VII genotype and plasma triglyceride concentration. Arterioscler Thromb 1994;14:193–8.
237. Dawson S, Hamsten A, Wiman B, Henney A, Humphries S. Genetic variation at the plasminogen activator inhibitor-1 locus is associated with altered levels of plasma plasminogen activator inhibitor-1 activity. Arterioscler Thromb 1991;11:183–90.
238. Dawson SJ, Wiman B, Hamsten A, Green F, Humphries S, Henney AM. The allele sequences of a common polymorphism in the promoter of the plasminogen activator inhibitor-1 (PAI-1) gene respond differently to interleukin-1 in HepG2 cells. J Biol Chem 1993;268:10739–45.
239. Cambien F, Costerousse O, Tiret L et al. Plasma level and gene polymorphism of angiotensin-converting enzyme in relation to myocardial infarction. Circulation 1994;90:669–76.
240. Tiret L, Bonnardeaux A, Poirier O et al. Synergistic effects of angiotensin-converting enzyme and angiotensin II type 1 receptor gene polymorphisms on the risk of myocardial infarction. Lancet 1994;344:910–3.
241. Ishigami T, Umemura S, Iwamoto T et al. Molecular variant of angiotensinogen gene is associated with coronary atherosclerosis. Circulation 1995;91:951–4.
242. Ye S, Watts GF, Mandalia S, Humphries SE, Henney AM. Preliminary report: Genetic variation in the human stromelysin promoter is associated with progression of coronary atherosclerosis. Br Heart J 1995 (in press).
243. Tiret L, Rigat B, Visvikis S et al. Evidence, from combined segregation and linkage analysis, that a variant of the angiotensin converting enzyme (ACE) gene controls plasma ACE. Am J Hum Genet 1992;51:197–205.
244. Evans A, Poirier O, Kee F et al. Polymorphisms of the angiotensin converting enzyme gene in subjects who die from coronary heart disease. Q J Med 1994;87:211–4.
245. Tiret L, Kee F, Poirier O et al. Deletion polymorphism in angiotensin converting enzyme gene associated with parental history of myocardial infarction. Lancet 1993;341:991–2.
246. Cambien F. ACE polymorphism as a risk factor for myocardial infarction. Br J Cardiol 1995;2(Suppl 1):S4–6.
247. Schunkert H, Hense HW, Holmer SR et al. Association between a polymorphism of the angiotensin converting enzyme gene and left ventricular hypertrophy. N Engl J Med 1994;330:1634–8.

13. Symptomatology and diagnosis of coronary artery diseases

PIERS CLIFFORD and PETROS NIHOYANNOPOULOS

Coronary artery disease is most commonly caused by atherosclerosis of the epicardial arteries which supply the myocardium with oxygen and nutrients. Extension of the atherosclerotic plaque into the lumen of the artery reduces coronary blood flow and when a critical reduction in luminal diameter occurs oxygen supply can no longer meet the requirements of the myocardium, especially during exercise when oxygen consumption is increased. This results in chronic stable angina and the symptom of chest pain. If the plaque undergoes spontaneous rupture it will expose the media of the coronary artery to the luminal blood resulting in the formation of a blood clot. If, in addition to the fresh thrombus, there is increased vasomotion with vasospasm this will result in unstable angina with transient occlusion of the artery. When the vessel becomes completely and irreversibly occluded this will result in myocardial infarction. The latter two conditions most often cause chest pain at rest and constitute medical emergencies.

Clinical manifestations of coronary artery disease

Chronic stable angina

The predominant clinical manifestation of coronary artery disease is angina pectoris. This can be defined as a discomfort in the chest or adjacent areas which is caused by myocardial ischemia and is typically associated with a disturbance of myocardial function. The actual description of the pain varies between individuals, with some patients just experiencing a central dull ache whilst others describe it as a 'crushing', 'band-like' or 'vice-like' constriction in the middle of the chest. It commonly radiates to the neck, jaw or left arm. It is usually precipitated by exercise or anxiety because of the associated increase in heart rate, systolic blood pressure and myocardial oxygen demand, but it may also occur in cold weather due to coronary vasoconstriction and increased peripheral resistance resulting in a rise in arterial pressure, or after heavy meals. The pain usually lasts for seconds or minutes and is rapidly relieved by cessation of exercise, by nitrates or by the removal of the other precipitating factors. These features help distinguish pain of myocardial origin from the alternative causes of chest pain (Table 13.1).

Table 13.1. Differential diagnosis of chest pain.

Cardiovascular
    Myocardial ischemia; myocardial infarction, unstable angina, angina pectoris and aortic stenosis
    Pericarditis
    Mitral valve prolapse
    Aortic dissection

Pulmonary
    Pulmonary embolism
    Pneumonia/pleurisy

Abdominal
    Biliary disease
    Pancreatic disease
    Esophageal reflux/ulceration
    Peptic ulceration
    Subphrenic abscess

Musculoskeletal
    Intercostal neuralgia
    Myositis
    Injuries

In the majority of patients the amount of exercise required to precipitate pain is relatively constant because the myocardial oxygen consumption must reach a threshold level before the amount of blood flowing through the stenosed coronary artery becomes insufficient to meet the demand. Other individuals suffer from angina with a variable threshold and in these patients alterations in coronary vascular tone combined with a fixed stenosis are probably responsible for the decreased oxygen supply.

Because of marked inter-individual variability in the threshold for the development of angina, various grading systems have been developed. The New York Heart Association functional classification is outlined in Table 13.2. This classification is useful because it allows the comparison of different patient groups on the basis of their symptoms, but some people with coronary artery disease do not suffer from chest pain at all (silent ischemia). This is especially common in diabetics, possibly resulting from a form of sensory neuropathy. In others, the pain is rather atypical either in character, severity or position, but is associated with the usual precipitating factors. Alternatively, dyspnea on exertion may be the main pre-

Table 13.2. New York Heart Association functional classification of angina.

Class 1:	Patients with cardiac disease with no limitation of physical activity
Class 2:	Patients with cardiac disease and slight limitation of physical activity. Ordinary physical activity results in fatigue, dyspnea or anginal pain
Class 3:	Patients with cardiac disease and marked limitation of physical activity
Class 4:	Patients with cardiac disease resulting in an inability to carry out any physical activity without discomfort. Symptoms of cardiac insufficiency or of angina may be present even at rest, and these symptoms are exacerbated by exercise

senting symptom due to deterioration of left ventricular function in the presence of myocardial ischemia.

Unstable angina and myocardial infarction

Typical anginal chest pain that occurs at rest suggests coronary artery occlusion and a diagnosis of unstable angina or myocardial infarction. In unstable angina the chest discomfort is of similar quality to that of chronic stable angina but it may be more intense and can persist for up to 30 minutes. Longer episodes of pain normally signify acute myocardial infarction, especially if associated with pallor, sweating, shortness of breath or vomiting. The development of unstable angina is often heralded by a decrease in the amount of physical exercise required to provoke angina, an increase in the frequency, severity or duration of the attacks, or recent variation in the radiation of the pain.

A number of patients may also suffer myocardial infarction without the typical pains. According to the Framingham study [1] over 28% of myocardial infarctions in men and 35% in women were unrecognized. Of these, approximately half were truly silent, while in the other half some atypical symptoms were present but not sufficient for either the patient or physician to consider that myocardial infarction was occurring or had occurred.

Physical examination

General examination

In many patients with coronary artery disease the physical examination is normal or it may reveal the presence of risk factors associated with the development of atherosclerosis. In particular, the physician should look for signs of hypercholesterolemia such as corneal arcus, xanthomas or xanthelesma. Measurement of the blood pressure may reveal hypertension and retinal examination may show silver wiring, arteriovenous nipping or increased vessel tortuosity in these patients. Alternatively signs of diabetic retinopathy may be present.

Examination of the arterial system may reveal carotid or femoral bruits and in some patients there may be loss of the dorsalis pedis or posterior tibial foot pulses indicating widespread atherosclerosis.

In patients suffering from an acute myocardial infarction all these signs should be sought but additional signs may be present such as pallor, sweatiness, variability in heart rate suggestive of arrhythmias or heart block and systemic hypotension if the patient is in cardiogenic shock.

Cardiac examination

Detection of the murmurs of aortic stenosis or hypertrophic cardiomyopathy can provide evidence of non-coronary causes of cardiac chest pain and the cardiac examination also gives some indication of myocardial function. Third of fourth heart sounds in the absence of evidence of other cardiac disease suggest coronary artery disease and are indicative of the pressure and compliance of the left ventricle during diastole. Paradoxical splitting of the second heart sound may occur transiently during an ishemic attack and is associated with prolongation of ventricular contraction and delayed closure of the aortic valve. Lateral displacement of the apical impulse or the palpation of dyskinetic areas suggest left ventricular dysfunction secondary to previous myocardial infarction. Similarly, apical systolic murmurs of mitral regurgitation may result from ischemic papillary muscle dysfunction, subendocardial fibrosis or simply from stretching of the mitral annulus due to ventricular dilatation.

If the patient has suffered a myocardial infarction the detection of a pansystolic murmur may represent a flail mitral valve leaflet, ruptured papillary muscle with consequent acute mitral regurgitation, or the development of a ventricular septal defect. The latter is often associated with a precordial thrill.

Diagnosis of coronary artery disease

Prior to the performance of specific cardiac investigations it is very important to assess the patient's risk factors for the development of coronary artery disease and to exclude coexisting medical disease. Blood testing will reveal the presence of anemia, diabetes, or hypercholesterolemia and a chest X-ray is useful to assess heart size and shape, the presence of valvular calcification and to exclude pulmonary disease.

Electrocardiography

The ECG is the cheapest and most cost-effective investigation in the assessment of chest pain and in the diagnosis of coronary artery disease. The resting ECG is normal in one-third of patients with chronic stable angina and therefore does not exclude the presence of coronary artery disease. The presence of ST-segment and T wave abnormalities however are strongly suggestive of coronary artery disease. Rarely, during a routine ECG, acute ST elevation suggestive of myocardial infarction in progress is seen, in which case prompt action is required. If there is evidence of left ventricular hypertrophy this would suggest long-standing hypertension (one of the major risk factors for the development of coronary artery disease) or suggest an alternative diagnosis for the etiology of the chest pain (hypertrophic cardiomyopathy or aortic stenosis). Left bundle branch block is not a specific indicator of coronary artery disease but when it is associated with chronic ischemic heart disease it often signifies marked impairment of left ventricular function [2] and multi-vessel disease. The presence of pathological Q waves, loss of R-wave progression across the anterior chest leads or of deep symmetrical T-wave inversion gives more definite evidence of coronary artery disease and demands further assessment in the form of exercise testing.

In unstable angina and myocardial infarction the resting ECG provides greater information because the patient has ongoing ischemia when the recording is made. Active ischemia results in transient displacement of the ST-segment (depression or elevation), the distribution of which gives some indication of which coronary artery is involved. Alternatively, transient inversion of the T-waves may be seen. These changes resolve with the cessation of pain and persistence of these changes suggests myocardial necrosis has occurred. Serial ECGs will then provide information as to the stage of evolution of a myocardial infarction. In the early stages ST-segment elevation occurs in the leads representing the area of injury, which may be accompanied by ST-segment depression in other leads representing remote 'opposite' areas [3]. The T-wave may show terminal inversion whilst the ST-segment is still elevated, but normally becomes symmetrically inverted once the ST-segment has returned to baseline. Q-waves are not normally present on the initial ECG unless previous myocardial damage has occurred, but develop over the ensuing hours or days. This classic pattern of acute myocardial infarction is seen in 50–60% of patients.

Exercise electrocardiography

Performing an ECG during the course of exercise yields greater diagnostic and prognostic information than the resting ECG alone. This is because exercise induces an imbalance between the supply of oxygen to the heart in the presence of a stenosis of the coronary artery and the demands of the myocardium. The aim of the test is to provoke chest pain and/or observe ischemic changes on the ECG whilst the patient performs a graded exercise program which will induce gradual increments in the patient's heart rate and blood pressure and hence in myocardial oxygen demand. There are now numerous protocols available both for treadmill testing and, if appropriate, for bicycle exercise testing, and the one adopted depends on the clinical status of the individual to be tested and on local preferences.

The imbalance between myocardial oxygen demand and oxygen supply will be maximal when the patient achieves his or her maximal heart rate. This is calculated as 220 minus the age of the patient. The exercise test can only be considered negative if the patient achieves 85% of maximal heart rate without significant flat or down-sloping ST-segment depression (> 1 mm as compared to the isoelectric point 80 ms after the J point on the ECG). Exercise induced ST-segment depression, as opposed to ST-segment elevation, does not localize the area of myocardium at risk nor does it predict which coronary artery is involved [4]. In addition the following observations can be taken as evidence of coronary artery disease and signal the need for further invasive investigations:

(1) a drop in systolic blood pressure below pre-exercise value in the absence of known left ventricular dysfunction;
(2) exercise-induced bundle branch block;
(3) persistence of ST-segment changes into the recovery period;
(4) early onset of ST-segment depression; and
(5) exercise-induced ventricular ectopy or ventricular tachycardia.

Table 13.3. Non-coronary causes of ST-segment depression.

Severe aortic stenosis
Severe hypertension with or without left ventricular hypertrophy
Hypertrophic cardiomyopathy
Anemia
Severe hypoxia
Digitalis
Hypokalemia
Hyperventilation
Mitral valve prolapse
Tachyarrhythmias
Severe volume overload due to mitral or aortic regurgitation

The exercise test can be difficult to interpret in the presence of left ventricular hypertrophy (false positive) and there are several other non-coronary causes of ST-segment depression as outlined in Table 13.3. If the patient does not acquire target heart rate due to antianginal medication, ischemic heart disease cannot be excluded and if the diagnosis of angina is in question it may be preferable to discontinue these medications for 2 days prior to the test.

In addition, the standard exercise test can be used to assess patient prognosis. If the test is abnormal in an asymptomatic man the risk of suffering a cardiac event, usually the development of angina, is increased nine-fold compared to an individual with a negative test. However, the risk of a non-fatal myocardial infarction is not increased [5]. The risk is further increased if a strongly positive test is associated with the presence of several atherosclerotic risk factors and supportive evidence of underlying coronary disease such as coronary calcification [6]. The significance of exercise testing in patients with angiographically documented coronary artery disease was demonstrated in the CASS study [7]. Twelve percent of patients were classified as high risk with an annual mortality in excess of 5% per year when exercise workload was less than Bruce stage 1 and the exercise ECG was positive. Patients who exercised beyond Bruce stage 3 with a normal exercise ECG had an annual mortality of less than 1% per year over the four years of follow-up.

Similarly, ischemic ST-segment abnormalities seen in 30–40% of patients admitted with unstable angina on a submaximal predischarge exercise test are associated with a significantly increased risk of subsequent cardiac events. A negative test identifies a low risk subgroup with 100% 8-year survival in one study [8].

Performance of a submaximal exercise test (up to 80% of age-predicted maximum) post-myocardial infarction can be used to stratify patients into high and low risk groups and indicate the need for predischarge coronary angiography. High risk predictors include an inability to perform the test, an abnormal systolic blood pressure response, poor exercise tolerance and ST-segment depression in patients with inferior wall infarction.

Holter monitoring

Holter monitoring gives additional information to conventional electrocardiography because it provides a continuous 24-hour record of ST-segment displacement during the course of the subjects' normal daily activities and during sleep. It is of particular value in detecting silent ischemia as up to 90% of ishemic episodes detected by this technique are not associated with symptoms. It can therefore be used to assess the efficacy of antianginal medication and the possible need for revascularization, and to quantify the total ischemic load suffered by the myocardium, which may relate to prognosis. The real significance of these ST changes on Holter monitoring alone is however doubtful [9].

Some studies using continuous ECG monitoring have demonstrated that the majority of patients with chronic stable angina exhibit a mixture of painful and painless ischemic episodes with a high proportion of silent ischemic events occurring at lower heart rates than during exercise [10]. This suggests that transient ECG changes occurring during daily activities may be predominantly related to dynamic mechanisms limiting coronary arterial supply such as changes in blood pressure or coronary artery tone. When demand-driven ischemia dominates, as occurs during exercise, the chest pain appears to be more related to the magnitude of ischemia [11].

Echocardiography in the diagnosis of coronary artery disease

The presence of myocardial ischemia or infarction can account for the occurrence of chest pain, dyspnea, hypotension, new murmurs and systemic emboli. Although the clinical presentation with typical anginal pain together with the presence of characteristic electrocardiographic changes often make the diagnosis relatively straightforward without the need for further investigations, this unfortunately is not always the case.

Differential diagnosis in chest pain syndromes
Patients presenting to the accident and emergency department complaining of acute chest pain often pose a diagnostic dilemma. When a typical history of anginal pain is accompanied by ST-segment elevation, a diagnosis of evolving myocardial infarction can be made rapidly. Often however, coronary artery occlusion can be clinically and electrocardiographically non-specific. Subarachnoid hemorrhage, acute pericarditis or myocarditis, hypertrophic cardiomyopathy, and aortic dissection may all mimic acute coronary occlusion, and vice versa, with potential catastrophic results for the patient as treatment for each of these conditions may be fundamentally different. A potentially catastrophic scenario would be to give acute thrombolysis for suspected evolving myocardial infarction in a patient with aortic dissection or acute pericarditis. Conversely, not giving thrombolysis quickly in a patient with evolving myocardial infarction, because of a diagnostic uncertainty, may condemn the patient to sustain extensive myocardial damage. Echocardiography can readily recognize each of the above clinical conditions and provide the precise diagnosis, allowing for the appropriate and speedy intervention.

Detecting myocardial ischemia
The role of echocardiography in the detection of myocardial ischemia is based principally on its ability to obtain anatomical, functional and flow characteristics with

high spatial and temporal resolution. During systole, a normally functioning myocardium thickens and moves toward the centre of the left ventricular cavity. Motion impairment (asynergy) can involve one or more myocardial regions and can vary in degree from minimal (hypokinesia) through severe (akinesia), up to paradoxical systolic expansion (dyskinesia). In addition to identifying the site of infarction, echocardiography is also useful for estimating the 'functional' size of the infarction. Because the extent of myocardial injury and dysfunction can influence global left ventricular performance and long-term prognosis, these factors also have an impact on management strategies.

Complications of myocardial infarction
These are associated with increased morbidity and mortality. Congestive heart failure can be caused by severe left ventricular dysfunction involving a large myocardial segment or the presence of ventricular aneurysm which can readily be detected with two-dimensional echocardiography. Right ventricular infarction can cause hypotension, necessitating fluid administration rather than inotropic agents and this is very difficult to diagnose clinically or by ECG alone. Conversely, the right ventricle can easily be described using echocardiography and as with left ventricular dysfunction, right ventricular asynergy is a sensitive marker of myocardial infarction.

Ventricular septal rupture or papillary muscle dysfunction may easily be identified with two-dimensional and colour flow imaging in a patient who develops a heart murmur, heart failure or cardiogenic shock. Papillary muscle dysfunction and rupture can cause severe mitral regurgitation with pulmonary edema and fall in blood pressure. Echocardiography with its detailed spatial resolution can detect the underlying cardiac abnormality and assess the severity of mitral regurgitation.

Stress echocardiography
The advent of stress echocardiography has provided a useful adjunct to the exercise ECG and in patients who are unable to perform conventional exercise this may be the only method available to determine the presence of a fixed coronary stenosis. It is also of value in determining which coronary artery is responsible for the patient's symptoms.

Stress echocardiography combines cardiovascular stress with cross-sectional echocardiographic images to detect ischemia-induced wall motion abnormalities. Myocardial ischemia is accompanied by characteristic mechanical, electrical and perfusional abnormalities, each of which has been used to detect coronary artery disease and the extent of the ischemic burden. The use of transient regional asynergy as a marker for ischemia evolved after it was elegantly demonstrated that progressive coronary artery ligation in animals produced progressive regional hypokinesia of the respective myocardial segment. When total occlusion occurs then myocardial contraction ceases [12]. Subsequent studies confirmed that regional asynergy after the induction of ischemia tends to precede ECG changes and symptoms and last longer after cessation of symptoms and normalization of ECG. Stress echocardiography is appropriate where exercise ECG is unlikely to provide a satisfactory answer to the clinical question being posed and should improve the selection of patients for tertiary referral. Speed and convenience strengthen the economic argument in favor of this technique, the reliability of which was emphasized early on by results that were highly concordant if not better than gated pool imaging and single photon emission computed tomography (SPECT) perfusion imaging.

There are several types of stress that can be linked with echocardiography. The fundamental advantage of exercise echocardiography over pharmacological stress testing is that it provides excellent natural physiological cardiovascular stress, and allows ECG changes and symptoms to be analysed in combination with cross-sectional echocardiography to detect ischemia-induced wall motion abnormalities. Its diagnostic accuracy has previously been documented in atherosclerotic coronary artery disease producing regional myocardial dysfunction in patients with angina, in contrast to patients with syndrome X in whom no regional wall motion abnormalities are identified [13–15].

Dobutamine stress has now emerged as the best alternative to exercise with very similar diagnostic accuracy. Its particular use is in patients unable to exercise but it is also useful for the detection of myocardial viability.

Radionuclide imaging

In this non-invasive test, a radioactive isotope (usually thallium-201) is injected at peak exercise and an image is obtained several minutes later when the patient is at rest. Areas of reduced perfusion appear as defects on the scan and may be due to myocardial infarction or transient hypoperfusion caused by coronary artery stenosis. A repeat scan once resting heart rate has been restored will differentiate between these two possibilities. In the case of an infarct the defect will persist (a fixed defect), whereas if the area exhibits delayed reuptake then ischemia is the likely cause of the defect. If a patient cannot perform conventional exercise, maximal coronary vasodilatation can be achieved using dipyridamole or adenosine, inducing a steal syndrome from the diseased stenotic artery, the territory of which will be hypoperfused, resulting in a reversible defect on the resulting scan.

This test is expensive, requires specialized equipment, is time consuming, and involves relatively high doses of radiation, and should therefore be used with caution and rarely as a first-line investigation.

Cardiac catheterization and coronary angiography

The non-invasive tests mentioned previously are useful in establishing the diagnosis of ischemic heart disease and to some degree in assessing the prognosis, but to evaluate the actual extent of the coronary artery disease and its precise anatomical location coronary angiography is required. It is therefore essential if any revascularization procedure is being considered, for symptomatic relief or for prognostic reasons. It involves cannulation of the femoral or brachial artery and the passage of preshaped catheters over a guide wire firstly into the left ventricle and subsequently into the left and right coronary ostia. Iodinated contrast medium is then injected down these catheters to assess left ventricular function and the patency of the coronary arteries. Simultaneously pressure measurements can be obtained from the ventricle and aorta.

Left ventricular function can be assessed by estimating the end-diastolic pressure and by ventriculography. The latter demonstrates the presence of wall motion abnormalities and the presence of ventricular dilatation. It will also reveal mitral regurgitation or a ventricular septal defect. Coronary angiography demonstrates the distribution and severity of coronary artery stenoses, and in the event of a total occlusion it will reveal the extent of collateral blood flow.

Once the coronary artery anatomy has been delineated it is possible to institute appropriate therapy. If the coronary arteries appear normal the patient can be generally reassured.

Symptomatic single vessel disease, especially if there is a single discrete lesion, can be treated by coronary angioplasty. Recent studies have also provided some evidence that angioplasty has a role in the treatment of patients with stable angina and multi-vessel disease [16]. Additionally angioplasty can be used to prevent incipient myocardial infarction in patients with unstable angina, and in the treatment of early myocardial infarction where vessel patency is of great importance [17, 18].

The CASS study [19, 20] clearly demonstrated that coronary artery bypass grafting was the treatment of choice for patients with: (1) triple vessel disease and impaired left ventricular function; and (2) left main stem stenosis. These patients gain both symptomatic and prognostic benefit.

References

1. Aronow WS. Prevalence of presenting symptoms of recognised acute myocardial infarction and of unrecognised healed myocardial infarction in elderly patients. Am J Cardiol 1987;60:1182.
2. Hamby RI, Weissman RH, Prakash MN, Hoffman I. Left bundle branch block: A predictor of poor left ventricular function in coronary artery disease. Am Heart J 1983;106:471.
3. Becker RC, Alpert JS. Electrocardiographic ST-segment depression in coronary heart disease. Am Heart J 1988;115:862.
4. Froelicher VF, Yanowitz FG, Major AJT, Lancaster MC. The correlation of coronary angiography and the electrocardiographic response to maximal treadmill testing in 76 asymptomatic men. Circulation 1973;48:597.
5. Ekelund LG, Suchindran CM, McMahon LP et al. Coronary heart disease morbidity and mortality in hypercholesterolaemic men predicted from an exercise test: The Lipid Research Clinics Coronary Primary Prevention Trial. J Am Coll Cardiol 1989;14:556.
6. Sox HC, Littenberg B, Garber AM. The role of exercise testing in screening for coronary artery disease. Ann Intern Med 1989;110:456.
7. Weiner DA, Ryan TJ, McCabe CH et al. Prognostic importance of a clinical profile and exercise test in medically treated patients with coronary artery disease. J Am Coll Cardiol 1984;3:772.
8. Severi S, Orsini E, Marracini P et al. The basal electrocardiogram and the exercise stress test in assessing prognosis in patients with unstable angina. Eur Heart J 1988;9:441.
9. Klein J, Chao SY, Berman DS, Rozanski A. Is 'silent' myocardial ischaemia really as severe as symptomatic ischaemia? Circulation 1994;89:1958–66.
10. Selwyn A, Fox K, Eves M, Oakley D, Dargie H, Shillingford J. Myocardial ischaemia in patients with frequent angina pectoris. Br Med J 1978;2:1594–6.

11. Nihoyannopoulos P, Marsonis A, Joshi J, Athanassopoulos G, Oakley CM. Magnitude of silent ischaemia is greater in painful than in painless myocardial ischaemia: An exercise echocardiographic study. J Am Coll Cardiol 1995;25:1507–12.
12. Gallagher KP, Matsuzaki M, Koziol JA, Kemper WS, Ross J Jr. Regional myocardial perfusion and wall thickening during ischaemia in conscious dogs. Am J Physiol 1984;16:H727.
13. Marwick TH, Nemec JJ, Pashkow FJ, Stewart WJ, Salcedo EE. Accuracy and limitations of exercise echocardiography in a routine clinical setting. J Am Coll Cardiol 1992;19:74–81.
14. Nihoyannopoulos P, Kaski JC, Crake T, Maseri A. Absence of myocardial dysfunction during stress in patients with syndrome X. J Am Coll Cardiol 1991;18:1463–70.
15. Armstrong WF. Exercise echocardiography: Ready, willing and able. J Am Coll Cardiol 1988;11:1359–61.
16. RITA Trial participants. Coronary angioplasty versus coronary artery bypass surgery: The Randomised Intervention Treatment of Angina (RITA) trial. Lancet 1993;341:573.
17. Grines CL, Browne KF, Marco J *et al.* for the PAMI study group. A comparison of immediate angioplasty with thrombolytic therapy for acute myocardial infarction. N Engl J Med 1993;328:673.
18. Zijlstra F, Jan de Boer M, Hoorntje JCA, Reiffers S, Reiber JHC, Suryapronata H. A comparison of immediate coronary angioplasty versus intravenous streptokinase in acute myocardial infarction. N Engl J Med 1993;328:680.
19. Chaitman BP, Fisher LD, Bourassa MG. Effect of coronary bypass surgery survival patterns in subsets of patients with left main coronary artery disease. Report of the Collaborative Study in Coronary Artery Surgery (CASS). Am J Cardiol 1981;48:765.
20. Alderman EL, Bourassa MG, Cohen LS *et al.* Ten year follow-up of survival and myocardial infarction in the randomised coronary artery surgery study. Circulation 1990:82:1629.

14. Angina pectoris in patients with normal coronary arteriograms: Syndrome X

JUAN CARLOS KASKI

The definition of syndrome X

Approximately 10–30% of patients who undergo coronary arteriography for the assessment of chest pain suggestive of ischemic heart disease are found to have normal coronary arteriograms [1, 2]. Chest pain in patients who do not have obstructive coronary artery disease represents a dilemma for the treating physician.

Over 25 years ago, Likoff et al. [4] reported their findings in a group of nondiabetic women who had exertional chest pain and ischemia-like electrocardiographic (ECG) changes in the presence of normal coronary arteriograms. These patients were normotensive and had a normal hemodynamic response to exercise despite the presence of angina, ST-segment depression and metabolic evidence of myocardial ischemia during stress testing. In this [4] and other studies [5], chest pain was found to be 'severe and refractory to conventional forms of therapy' in at least some of the patients. In 1973, the term 'syndrome X' was used for the first time by Kemp [6] in an editorial comment of a paper by Arbogast and Bourassa [7] who observed that patients in a so-called 'group X' had normal left ventricular performance during pacing-induced chest pain despite ECG and metabolic changes suggestive of myocardial ischemia.

The problem of angina-like chest pain in the absence of coronary artery disease is not a 'discovery' of the angiography era. More than 100 years ago, William Osler considered that 'hysterical or pseudo-angina' (chest pain without coronary obstructions) was 'the chief difficulty' in the diagnosis of 'true' angina pectoris – that associated with coronary artery disease.

Patients with chest pain in the absence of coronary artery disease are usually considered to have 'syndrome X'. The definition of syndrome X is not uniform and although extra-cardiac causes such as esophageal dysmotility and reflux, and cardiac causes such as left ventricular hypertrophy, systemic hypertension, valvular heart disease, cardiomyopathy, and coronary artery spasm are usually excluded, different authors have different inclusion and exclusion criteria [8] The presence of 'objectively' documented myocardial ischemia is required by some investigators to define syndrome X. However, this may not be appropriate as myocardial ischemia is probably only one of the many pathogenetic mechanisms in syndrome X.

A metabolic entity characterized by hyperlipidemia, insulin resistance and hypertension, termed 'syndrome X' by Reaven [9] in 1988, defines a completely different category of patients. Although both the metabolic and cardiac syndrome X may share some pathogenetic mechanisms, the two are separate entities.

Observations by Opherk et al. [8] that coronary blood flow reserve was reduced in patients with the so-called syndrome X suggested that syndrome X was caused by myocardial ischemia. Cannon and Epstein [10] suggested that the reason for chest pain and normal coronary arteriograms was an abnormal vasodilator capacity of the coronary microcirculation located at the prearteriolar level. They coined the term 'microvascular angina' to define a condition where a microcirculatory derangement is its hallmark. The presence or absence of exercise induced ST-segment depression is of no relevance for the diagnosis of microvascular angina, neither is the presence of systemic hypertension (without left ventricular hypertrophy).

Differential diagnosis

It is accepted that chest pain in the absence of obstructive coronary artery disease is frequently non-cardiac in origin. Psychosomatic symptoms [11], including panic disorders, appear to be common in patients with chest pain and normal coronary arteries. The chest wall syndrome [12] frequently mimics cardiac pain but it may be just an innocent bystander and not the cause of the syndrome. Esophageal pain and cardiac ischemic pain may be indistinguishable in character and circumstances of occurrence and relief. It has been suggested that esophageal motor disturbances can lower the threshold for exercise-induced angina [13] and also cause ischemia-like ST-segment shifts [14]. Chest pain, however, may be cardiac in origin despite the presence of normal coronary arteriograms. Indeed, left ventricular hypertrophy of different origin and systemic hypertension are frequently associated with the syndrome of chest pain and normal coronary arteriograms. Coronary artery spasm, as seen in Prinzmetal's variant angina, is also a well-known cause of angina with normal coronary arteriograms [16] and should be carefully investigated before the diagnosis of syndrome X is made.

Clinical presentation

A female prevalence is commonly seen in syndrome X but this is not a universal finding [2]. Women with syndrome X are usually peri- or post-menopausal [17]. Chest pain is usually exertional and similar in character to that observed in patients with coronary artery disease. Angina at rest, however, is not uncommon in syndrome X patients (41%) [18]. Although usually typical, chest pain in both syndrome X and microvascular angina has atypical features. Among these are the response to sublingual nitrates which, in our experience [18, 19] are effective in less than 50% of patients, and the discrepancy between the severity and duration of chest pain and the absence of left ventricular dysfunction in the majority of patients [19, 20]. Chest pain tends to be prolonged in patients with syndrome X with 40% [18] of patients reporting episodes longer than 30 minutes.

The exercise response of patients with syndrome X is frequently indistinguishable from that of patients with coronary artery disease. Although on average, syndrome X patients tend to develop ischemia-like ST-segment changes at a higher rate – pressure product than patients with coronary artery disease [21], patterns of onset and offset of ST-segment depression are similar in syndrome X and patients with coronary artery disease, as described by Pupita *et al.* [21]. Heart rate-recovery loops are also similar in coronary artery disease and syndrome X patients [22]. Recently, we observed that a rapid increase of heart rate and blood pressure during the first stages of the exercise protocol in patients with syndrome X [23], identifies patients who may develop systemic hypertension during follow-up. We speculate that this finding may be associated with an increased sympathetic drive.

Patients with syndrome X experience ischemia-like ST-segment changes during their daily activities, as assessed by continuous ambulatory ECG monitoring [24]. The circadian distribution of the episodes of ST-segment depression is similar to that observed in coronary artery disease patients and quite opposite to that of variant angina. In patients with syndrome X, ST-segment depression occurs predominantly during waking hours. Silent ST-segment depression and angina without ST-segment shifts are also frequently found in patients with syndrome X [24]. The large majority of ischemic episodes are heart rate related although a significant proportion are not preceded by an increase of heart rate [18].

Pathogenesis

Different pathogenetic mechanisms have been proposed, which are summarized in Table 14.1.

Table 14.1. Pathogenesis of Syndrome X.

Myocardial ischemia (caused by reduced coronary flow reserve)
    Microvascular dysfunction
    Estrogen deficiency
    Endothelial dysfunction
    Coronary artery hyperreactivity
    Increased sympathetic tone
Prearteriolar constriction and 'patchy' release of adenosine
Abnormal interstitial release of potassium
Myocardial metabolic abnormality
Insulin resistance
Early cardiomyopathy
Increased pain perception

Myocardial ischemia

Anginal pain and exercise-induced ST-segment changes in patients with syndrome X are suggestive of myocardial ischemia. Myocardial ischemia has been documented in a variable proportion of syndrome X patients. Myocardial lactate production has been found in 13–100% of patients with angina and normal coronary arteriograms in different series [25] and it has been suggested that 'lactate producers' are those patients with marked ST-segment changes during atrial pacing [26]. Chest pain alone, however, does not seem to correlate with lactate production [27]. In patients with microvascular angina, evidence of lactate production has also been obtained [28–30]. The limitations of lactate measurement as an index of myocardial ischemia are well-known.

Studies of myocardial perfusion and left ventricular function using radionuclide techniques have shown ischemic responses in some patients (approximately 30%) with syndrome X and/or microvascular angina [3, 18]. However, in the majority of syndrome X patients ischemia cannot be demonstrated [19, 31–33]. A proportion of patients with microvascular angina exhibit an abnormal ejection fraction response during exercise. Cannon looked at the relationship between LV function and ST-segment shifts during exercise stress and found that 35% of patients who do not show exercise-induced ECG changes have an abnormal wall motion response, whereas 53% of those with ischemia-like ST-segment changes and 64% of those with left bundle branch block (LBBB) have a reduced ejection fraction during exercise. Contrary to findings in patients with microvascular angina, Nihoyannopoulos *et al.* [19] showed that in patients with syndrome X, LV function is normal during exercise. These observations have different possible interpretations. They may suggest that in some patients ischemia is of mild intensity, patchy or involving only thin layers of the myocardium and is therefore below the threshold of our diagnostic techniques. Another explanation is that because syndrome X is a heterogeneous syndrome, mechanisms other than myocardial ischemia are responsible for the anginal symptoms and ST-segment shifts in different patients subgroups.

Few patients with syndrome X develop heart failure over time [18]. Recent studies [34], however, suggest that a subgroup of syndrome X patients may experience deterioration of their LV function. These are patients as described by Opherk *et al.* [34] who reported that of 40 patients with syndrome X, those with LBBB (on resting or exercise ECGs) commonly demonstrated deterioration in rest and exercise LV-ejection fraction over an average follow-up of four years. Cannon *et al.* [35] studied the 4.5-year follow-up of 61 patients with microvascular angina; 25% showed significant deterioration in resting LV ejection fraction or new wall motion abnormalities. In contrast to findings by Opherk *et al.* [34], in this preliminary report, Cannon *et al.* observed that decline in LV function was not restricted to patients with LBBB. Curiously, a decline in function was actually seen more commonly in patients without ischemic appearing ECG responses to exercise stress.

Mechanisms of ischemia in patients with angina and normal coronary arteriograms

In 1983 Cannon *et al.* [28] reported limitation in great cardiac vein flow response to atrial pacing (coronary sinus thermodilution method) in patients with typical angina and normal coronary arteriograms. Repeat flow measurements during pacing stress, but after the administration of ergonovine, showed further limitation of flow reserve with increase of coronary resistance in patients with chest pain but not in those who remained symptom free. As angiography during ergonovine demonstrated no change in epicardial coronary dimensions, Cannon et al. concluded that the increase of coronary resistance was caused by constriction of the microcirculation. Lactate production was found in 10% of patients with pacing-induced chest pain. Cannon and Epstein [10] used the term 'microvascular angina' to indicate what appeared to be an increased sensitivity of the coronary microcirculation to vasconstrictor stimuli. The authors proposed that an abnormal behavior of the prearteriolar vessels was the underlying cause of the syndrome. Recently the same group [3] showed that microvascular angina patients may also show a generalized vasodilator incapacity of the microcirculation of different vascular beds, esophageal motility disorders, and abnormal bronchoconstrictor responses to metacholine inhalation. The cause of the abnormal coronary blood flow reserve is not known. Several mechanisms have been proposed: increased sympathetic drive, endothelial dysfunction affecting both epicardial and small coronary vessels, and metabolic abnormalities.

Other pathogenetic hypotheses

Adenosine release
Recently, Maseri et al. [20] suggested that the increased resistance of prearteriolar vessels, which can explain the reduced coronary vasodilative response of the coronary microcirculation in patients with syndrome X, could be associated with a local release of adenosine. Distal to the most constricted arterioles, a compensatory increase of adenosine may take place, which could cause angina even in the absence of ischemia.

Increased pain perception
The frequent finding in patients with syndrome X that chest pain is severe, long-lasting and not associated with objective signs of myocardial ischemia led investigators to consider abnormal pain perception as the underlying mechanism of the syndrome in some patients. Turiel et al. [36] showed that women with syndrome X had a reduced pain threshold for forearm ischemia and electrical skin stimulation. Shapiro et al. [37] and Cannon et al. [38] observed that catheter manipulation within the heart chambers of patients with chest pain and normal coronary arteriograms (syndrome X and microvascular angina patients, respectively) resulted in typical chest pain. The lack of an appropriate control population does not allow us to conclude whether these observations indicate that patients with syndrome X truly have an abnormal, local or generalized, sensory response or whether the findings just show the normal distribution of the phenomenon in the general population.

Ischemic cardiomyopathy
Opherk et al. [34] and Cannon et al. [23] have suggested that patients with microvascular angina may experience deterioration of left ventricular function over time. A pathogenic link between microvascular dysfunction and certain forms of cardiomyopathy has therefore been suggested. In the original paper by Opherk

et al. [8], biopsy specimens taken from left ventricular myocardium did not reveal significant morphological abnormalities or microvascular lesions. Electron microscopy however, showed swelling of mitochondria in all but one of the patients with syndrome X. These findings were interpreted by the authors as a sign of myocardial hypoxia. Other cell organelles were normal as were the arterioles, venules and capillaries. The range of analyzable vessels, however, was limited by technical difficulties. Vessels between 40 and 200 μm are not accessible to light or electron microscopy. Therefore, the results of this study do not exclude the fact that microvascular alterations could be responsible for the anginal syndrome in patients with syndrome X. Recently, Mosseri *et al.* [39] reported the presence of abnormal histological findings in the small coronary arteries of patients with angina pectoris and patent large coronary arteries. However, only six patients formed the basis of the report, and these were part of a subgroup who showed slow run-off of the contrast medium at angiography. All of the patients in Mosseri's study had left ventricular hypertrophy (four were hypertensive) and do not fall under the category of syndrome X as previously defined. Coronary microvascular dysfunction has been observed in patients with dilated [40, 41] and hypertrophic [42] cardiomyopathy.

Prognosis and treatment

With the exception of patients with LBBB, prognosis in patients with syndrome X is good in respect of survival and incidence of acute coronary events. However, management of syndrome X is difficult at present. Antianginal medications appear to be beneficial only in a relatively small proportion of patients. Antagonists of adenosine receptors (e.g. aminophylline) may be useful in those patients in whom symptoms are associated with abnormal release of adenosine [18]. Specific drugs which affect visceral neural function or central nervous system pain regulatory systems may be necessary to tackle the problem of increased pain sensitivity found in some patients with syndrome X. Recently, Cannon *et al.* [43] observed that treatment with the antidepressant agent imipramine (50 mg once a day) resulted in significant improvement of anginal symptoms. Estrogen replacement therapy may also improve symptoms in women with syndrome X who have signs of estrogen insufficiency. Treatment of insulin resistance and associated entities (obesity, hyperlipidemia and hypertension) should be also considered as this could improve angina, ST-segment changes and coronary reactivity in a subset of patients. Appropriate psychological characterization of individual patients and reassurance by the physician usually results in symptomatic improvement.

References

1. Proudfit WL, Shirley EK, Sones FM. Selective cine coronary arteriography: Correlation with clinical findings in 1000 patients. Circulation 1966;33:901–10.
2. Kemp HG, Kronmal RA, Vlietstra RE, Frye RL and the Coronary Artery Surgery Study (CASS) participants. Seven year survival of patients with normal or near normal coronary arteriograms: A CASS registry study. J Am Coll Cardiol 1986;7:479–83.

3. Cannon R, Camici P, Epstein SE. Pathophysiological dilemma of syndrome X. Circulation 1992;85:883–92.
4. Likoff W, Segal BL, Kasparian H. Paradox of normal selective coronary arteriograms in patients considered to have unmistakable coronary heart disease. N Engl J Med 1967;276:1063–6.
5. Kemp HG, Vokonas PS, Cohn PF, Gorlin R. The anginal syndrome associated with normal coronary arteriograms: Report of a six year experience. Am J Med 1973;54:735–42.
6. Kemp HG. Left ventricular function in patients with the anginal syndrome and normal coronary arteriograms. Am J Cardiol 1973;32:375–6.
7. Arbogast R, Bourassa MG. Myocardial function during atrial pacing in patients with angina pectoris and normal coronary arteriograms: Comparison with patients having significant coronary artery disease. Am J Cardiol 1973;32:257–63.
8. Opherk D, Zebe H, Wiehe E et al. Reduced coronary dilatory capacity and ultrastructural changes of the myocardium in patients with angina pectoris but normal coronary arteriograms. Circulation 1981;63:817–25.
9. Reaven G. Banting Lecture 1988: Role of insulin resistance in human diabetes. Diabetes 1988;37:1595–607.
10. Cannon RO, Epstein SE. 'Microvascular angina' as a cause of chest pain with angiographically normal coronary arteries. Am J Cardiol 1988;61:1338–43.
11. Chambers JB, Bass C. Chest pain with normal coronary anatomy: A review of natural history and possible aetiologic factors. Prog Cardiovasc Dis 1990;33:161–84.
12. Urschel HC, Razzuk MA, Hyland JW et al. Thoracic outlet syndrome masquerading as coronary artery disease (pseudoangina). Ann Thorac Surg 1973;16:239–48.
13. Schofield PM, Bennett DH, Whorwell PJ et al. Exertional gastro-oesophageal reflux: A mechanism for symptoms in patients with angina pectoris and normal coronary angiograms. Br Med J 1987;294:1459–61.
14. Dart AM, Alban-Davies H, Lowndes RH, Dalal J, Ruttley M, Henderson AH. Oesophageal spasm and angina: Diagnostic value of ergometrine (ergonovine) provocation. Eur Heart J 1980;1:91–5.
15. Richter JE, Bradley LA. Chest pain with normal coronary arteries – another perspective. Editorial. Dig Dis Sci 1989;35:1441–4.
16. Kaski JC. Mechanisms of coronary artery spasm. Trends Cardiovasc Med 1991;7:289–94.
17. Rosano G, Lindsay D, Kaski JC, Sarrel P, Poole-Wilson P. Syndrome X in women: The importance of ovarian hormones. J Am Coll Cardiol 1992;19:255A.
18. Kaski JC, Rosano GMC, Nihoyannopoulos P, Collins P, Maseri A, Poole-Wilson P. Syndrome X – Clinical characteristics and left ventricular function – A long term follow-up study (in press).
19. Nihoyannopoulos P, Kaski JC, Crake T, Maseri A. Absence of myocardial dysfunction during stress in patients with syndrome X. J Am Coll Cardiol 1991;18:1463–70.
20. Maseri A, Crea F, Kaski JC, Crake T. Mechanisms of angina pectoris in syndrome X. J Am Coll Cardiol 1991;17:499–506.
21. Pupita G, Kaski JC, Galassi AR, Gavrielides S, Crea F, Maseri A. Similar time course of ST depression during and after exercise in patients with coronary artery disease and syndrome X. Am Heart J 1990;120:848–54.
22. Gavrielides S, Kaski JC, Galassi AR et al. Recovery-phase patterns of ST-segment depression in the heart rate domain cannot distinguish between anginal patients with coronary artery disease and patients with syndrome X. Am Heart J 1991;122:1593–8.
23. Romeo F, Gaspardone A, Ciavolella M, Gioffre P, Reale A. Verapamil versus acebutolol for syndrome X. Am J Cardiol 1988;62:312–3.
24. Kaski JC, Crea F, Nihoyannopoulos P, Hackett D, Maseri A. Transient myocardial ischemia during daily life in patients with syndrome X. Am J Cardiol 1986;58:1242–7.
25. Hutchison SJ, Poole-Wilson PA, Henderson AH. Angina with normal coronary arteries: A review. Q J Med 1989;72:677–88.
26. Boudoulas H, Cobb TC, Leighton RF, Wilt SM. Myocardial lactate production in patients with angina-like chest pain and angiographically normal coronary arteries and left ventricle. Am J Cardiol 1974;84:501–5.
27. Mammohansingh P, Parker JO. Angina pectoris with normal coronary arteriograms: Hemodynamic and metabolic response to atrial pacing. Am Heart J 1975;90:555–61.

28. Greenberg MA, Grose RM, Neuburger N, Silverman R, Strain JE, Cohen MV. Impaired coronary vasodilator responsiveness as a cause of lactate production during pacing-induced ischemia in patients with angina pectoris and normal coronary arteries. J Am Coll Cardiol 1987;9:743–51.
29. Cannon RO, Bonow RO, Bacharach SL et al. Left ventricular dysfunction in patients with angina pectoris, normal epicardial coronary arteries, and abnormal vasodilator reserve. Circulation 1985;71:218–26.
30. Cannon RO, Watson RM, Rosing DR, Epstein SE. Angina caused by reduced vasodilator reserve of the small coronary arteries. J Am Coll Cardiol 1983;1:1359–73.
31. Levy RD, Shapiro LM, Wright C, Mockus L, Fox KM. Diurnal variation in left ventricular function: A study of patients with myocardial ischaemia, syndrome X, and of normal controls. Br Heart J 1987;57:148–53.
32. Crake T, Canepa-Anson R, Shapiro L, Poole-Wilson PA. Continuous recording of coronary sinus oxygen saturation during atrial pacing in patients with coronary artery disease or with syndrome X. Br Heart J 1988;59:31–8.
33. Camici PG, Marraccini P, Lorenzoni R et al. Coronary hemodynamics and myocardial metabolism in patients with syndrome X: Response to pacing stress. J Am Coll Cardiol 1991;17:1461–70.
34. Opherk D, Schuler G, Wetterauer K, Manthey J, Schwarz F, Kübler W. Four-year follow-up in patients with angina pectoris and normal coronary arteriograms ('syndrome X'). Circulation 1989;80:1610–6.
35. Cannon RO, Dilsizian V, Correa R, Epstein SE, Bonow RO. Chronic deterioration in left ventricular function in patients with microvascular angina. J Am Coll Cardiol 1991;17:28A (Abstract).
36. Turiel M, Galassi AR, Glazier JJ, Kaski JC, Maseri A. Pain threshold and tolerance in women with syndrome X and women with stable angina pectoris. Am J Cardiol 1987;60:503–7.
37. Shapiro LM, Crake T, Poole-Wilson PA. Is altered cardiac sensation responsible for chest pain in patients with normal coronary arteries? Clinical observation during catheterization. Br Med J 1988;296:170–1.
38. Cannon RO, Quyyumi AA, Schenke WH et al. Abnormal cardiac sensitivity in patients with chest pain and normal coronary arteries. J Am Coll Cardiol 1990;16:1359–66.
39. Mosseri M, Yarom R, Gotsman MS, Hasin Y. Histologic evidence for small-vessel coronary artery disease in patients with angina pectoris and patent large coronary arteries. Circulation 1986;74:964–72.
40. Cannon RO, Cunnion RE, Parrillo JE et al. Dynamic limitation of coronary vasodilator reserve in patients with dilated cardiomyopathy and chest pain. J Am Coll Cardiol 1987;10:1190–200.
41. Treasure CB, Vita JA, Cox DA et al. Endothelium-dependent dilation of the coronary microvasculature is impaired in dilated cardiomyopathy. Circulation 1990;81:772–9.
42. Cannon RO, Rosing DR, Maron BJ et al. Myocardial ischemia in patients with hypertrophic cardiomyopathy: Contribution of inadequate vasodilator reserve and elevated left ventricular filling pressures. Circulation 1985;71:234–43.
43. Cannon RO, Quyyumi AA, Mincemoyer R et al. Imipramine in patients with chest pain despite normal coronary angiograms. N Engl J Med 1994;330:1411–7.

15. Management of coronary artery disease

JOHN G.F. CLELAND

Coronary artery disease (CAD) is one of the leading causes of mortality in industrialized countries, both in the whole population and in those under the age of 65 years (Figure 15.1) and angina pectoris is one manifestation of it. As angina pectoris, by definition, is symptomatic, it is easier to identify than other manifestations of chronic CAD such as 'silent' ischemia and asymptomatic CAD. Therefore angina is an obvious target for treatment, not only to reduce symptoms but also to reduce potentially the mortality from CAD. However, the idea that by treating angina we will substantially reduce mortality from CAD may not be correct. Data from the Framingham study indicate that only about 25% of patients admitted with a myocardial infarction (MI) will have an obvious history of angina

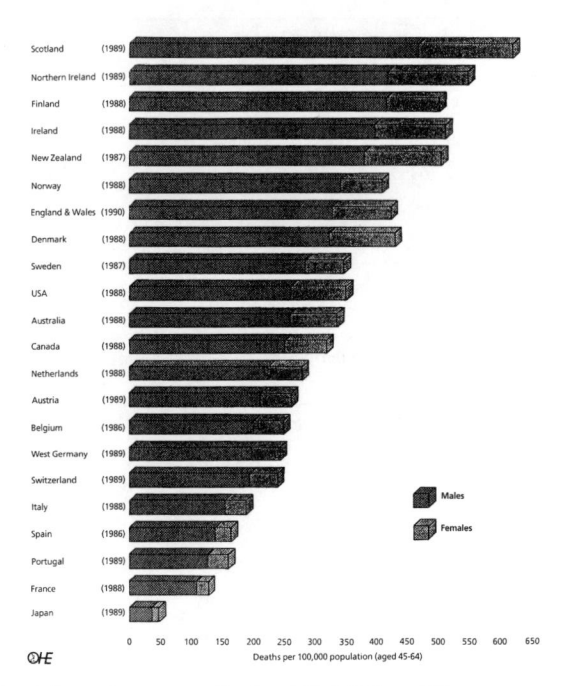

Figure 15.1. Ischemic heart disease mortality (aged 45–64) (from [1]).

A.-M. Salmasi and A. Strano (eds), *Angiology in Practice*, 187–208.
© 1996 *Kluwer Academic Publishers. Printed in Great Britain.*

prior to the event [2, 3]. Thus, 75% of patients having an infarct will be missed by any strategy that concentrates solely on the treatment of angina.

Epidemiology of angina and coronary disease

The incidence and prevalence of angina have been determined in a number of community screening programs with varying methodologies [3–11]. The most rigorous screening program was probably that of Ghandi et al. [6] and included screening of suspect cases using treadmill exercise tests. The incidence of angina appeared similar to that of previous reports in the UK and US, though not Israel [4]; methodological differences may account for this anomaly (Table 15.1 and 15.2). The prevalence of angina appears roughly similar across largely Caucasian populations, but may be higher in people from the Indian subcontinent. The overall prevalence of angina in the population over 30 years of age is 24 000 per million with about 800 per million new cases per year [6, 11].

The UK in general, and Scotland in particular, has been identified as having a high mortality from CAD. However, the quality control of death certification data is

Table 15.1. Incidence of angina pectoris

Study	n	Population	Men	Women
			(per 1000 per annum)	
HIP [3] (1969)	100 000	35–64 years	1.8	0.8
Framingham [3] (1976)	29 158	30–74 years	1.8	0.4
Medalie et al. [4] (1976)	9 764	40–65 years, men only	5.7	–
Duncan et al. [5] (1976)	28 400	35–69 years, men only	1.8	–
Ghandi [6] (1992)	191 677	Age < 70 years	1.1	0.5

Table 15.2. Prevalence of angina pectoris

Study	n	Population	Men	Women
			(per 1000 population)	
Whitehall [7] 1977	18 403	40–64 years, men only	43	
HDPP [8] 1980	UK 9734	40–59 years, men only	UK 36	
	B[a] 8509		B 50	
	I 3131		I 30	
	P 9115		P 51	
	S 1384		S 23	
RHS [8]	7735	40–59 years, men only	79	
Abernathy et al. [10] (1988)	US 473 USSR 399	50–59 years, men only	US 44 USSR 95	
Cannon et al. [11] (1988)	344 700	> 30 years	< 65 yrs: 15 > 65 yrs: 71	< 60 yrs: 6 > 60 yrs: 44

[a] B = Belgium; I = Italy; P = Poland; S = Spain.
Note that the apparently low prevalence in men 30–65 years in the study by Cannon et al. is probably because of the inclusion of patients < 40 years old who will have a low prevalence of angina.

Table 15.3. Life expectancy at birth in men and women in OECD countries; figures are for 1985–90 (reproduced from [12] with permission).

Country	Men	Women
World	61.8	65.9
Western Europe	71.9	79.0
EEC	72.1	79.5
Australia	72.9	79.5
Austria	70.6	77.8
Belgium	71.5	77.9
Canada	73.3	80.3
Denmark	72.6	78.3
Finland	71.0	78.8
France	71.9	80.0
W Germany	71.6	78.2
Greece	73.5	77.9
Iceland	74.8	80.4
Ireland	71.5	76.9
Italy	72.4	78.9
Japan	75.4	81.1
Luxembourg	71.0	77.7
Netherlands	73.5	80.2
New Zealand	71.8	77.9
Norway	73.5	80.2
Portugal	70.0	76.8
Spain	73.6	79.7
Sweden	74.2	80.1
Switzerland	73.8	80.4
Turkey	62.5	65.8
UK	72.4	78.1
USA	71.9	79.0

variable. In the context of a clinical trial we would look at total mortality in a population rather than deaths attributable to one cause. If CAD is a major killer then it should show up in variations in life expectancy between countries. When this is done the UK male population appear to live somewhat longer than people from most other industrialized nations, including Italy and France, countries generally considered to have less CAD (Table 15.3). Interestingly, the pattern is different for women, who also have much lower rates of premature CAD. National differences in mortality due to CAD may be due to over-certification of this cause of death in the UK or under-reporting in other countries.

Natural history of angina

The high prevalence compared to incidence suggests that the prognosis of patients with angina is not generally poor. The prognosis of angina pectoris treated medically is probably improving. The most recent studies suggest that, with the introduction of the widespread use of aspirin, the annual risk of MI or death are

Table 15.4. Medical prognosis of patients with angina

Study	Start year	Population	CABG	MI (p.a.)	Death (p.a.)
Framingham [13]	1958 (14 year follow-up)	119 men 110 women	?	3.1% 1.2%	2.0% 0.9%
Veterans [14]	1972–74 (18 year follow-up)	354 men	2.4%	2.3%	3.7%
ECSS [15, 16]	1973–76 (12 year follow-up)	373 men	3.0%	2.2%	2.4%
CASS [17, 18]	1979 (10 year follow-up)	780 (90% men)	3.8%	2.2%	2.1%
Italian [19]	1987 (5 year follow-up)	309 (90% men)	5.8%	2.6%	1.7%
Swedish [20]	1987 (5 year follow-up)	1009 no aspirin[a] 1026 aspirin[a]	0.7% 0.7%	1.8% 1.2%	2.1% 1.6%

[a] About 50% were women.

both less than 2% (Table 15.4). With more aggressive medical management further improvements may be expected. The procedural morbidity and mortality of percutaneous transluminal coronary angioplasty (PTCA) or coronary artery bypass graft (CABG) (see below) are similar to or exceed the annual mortality of the medically-treated condition and this must be taken into account when advising on treatment for symptoms.

Another important feature of angina is that contrary to popular belief it is not a condition in which symptoms progress inexorably. The severity of angina commonly fluctuates and 30–40% of patients will have spontaneous remission of angina for two or more years [13–21]. This is a real problem for management. The patient is usually referred to the cardiologist during an exacerbation of symptoms. It is likely that symptoms will tend to improve spontaneously. It is difficult to know if the cardiologist should act on the basis of symptoms at the time of referral or wait, and if so for how long. This is made even more difficult because the likelihood of infarction and death are greatest in the first few weeks after the symptoms appear.

Goals of treatment of angina

As with most diseases the goals of treatment involve quality of life and mortality. However, as the number of possible conditions that can be treated and treatments available increase, cost–benefit becomes an important tertiary consideration.

Quality of life is a complex issue and is easier to consider in parts rather than as a whole. However, it is an act of, sometimes mistaken faith, that by treating one aspect of the disease, the whole quality of life will be changed. Treatment to improve quality of life should be directed not only at improving symptoms and increasing mobility but also minimizing side-effects of treatment and anxiety. The anxiety, pain and complications of PTCA and CABG must be included as part of the potential morbidity related to angina. Prevention of MI and stroke are also major considerations.

There are few data on direct measurement of quality of life in angina though the appearance of CAD has a major adverse effect [22]. Opinion is divided about how well relief of symptoms and improvements in exercise testing are reflected by instruments purporting to measure quality of life.

The issue of mortality is also more complex than might appear at first sight. Everybody will die. The longer a person lives the greater the chance that something really unpleasant will happen to them before they die. A recent survey showed that sudden cardiac death was easily the most preferred way to die [23]. A selective reduction in premature death, however that is defined, and reduction in deaths other than sudden would be ideal, but probably impossible to achieve.

Lifestyle

Stopping smoking reduces the risk of reinfarction and death [24]. Smoking may negate the antianginal benefits of nifedipine [25].

Regular exercise may have an effect at least as great as treatment with a beta-blocker in those who can comply with the training programme [26]. Potentially, this is a very cost-effective treatment and, intuitively, may be considered to have the most positive effect on total quality of life. There is no evidence that exercise can reduce mortality in those with angina. Several meta-analyses of exercise rehabilitation studies after MI have suggested a favorable effect of exercise on prognosis; consideration of the studies themselves is less convincing [27]. Most of the studies compared medical neglect with medical attention and exercise. Two well-designed studies comparing the effects of light and intense exercise on outcome suggested no survival advantage to the more vigorous regime [27].

Dieting to reduce obesity is also likely to have a benefit on symptoms of angina. Reduction in dietary fat intake appear to retard progression of and possibly regress angiographic coronary atherosclerosis [28] but in post-MI patients this strategy has not reduced mortality or reinfarction [27]. Other studies have suggested a reduction in reinfarction and mortality with diets rich in vitamins antioxidants (fruit, vegetables and nuts) or fatty fish in post-infarction patients [27].

Psychological rehabilitation also has some advocates.

Other risk factors

Treating risk factors may not only reduce major morbidity and mortality but also slow, or even reverse, the tendency for angina to get worse. The most accurate 'risk factor' for the presence of coronary atheroma is identification of the atheroma itself. It is likely that patients with angina obtain much greater benefit from risk factor control than the population with less accurate risk markers. However, there are few data on the effects of risk factor control in a population who already have angina.

Studies of hypertension show that in patients over the age of 65 years, thiazide diuretics in particular are effective in reducing the rates of MI, heart failure and other manifestations of CAD. Thiazides have little adverse effect on other risk markers for CAD if used in small doses [29–31]. Their more widespread use should be encouraged. Beta-blockers have an obvious advantage in that they have been shown not only to reduce the complications of hypertension but are also very effective antianginal agents and reduce mortality in patients after MI [27]. In patients with well-preserved ventricular function, verapamil and diltiazem have been shown to improve prognosis after MI and they are also effective antianginal treatments [27]. In patients with ventricular dysfunction, ACE inhibitors have been shown to reduce the need for hospitalization for angina, recurrent MI and mortality [27].

Lipid lowering agents have been highly successful in reducing the incidence of new onset angina and other coronary events in high risk populations [32, 33]. More recently a new class of lipid lowering agent has been introduced, the HMG CoA reductase inhibitors. The benefits of these agents in reducing coronary events was startling in preliminary studies, with marked benefit after only six months of treatment [34] (Figure 15.2). Subsequently, the 4S study, that recruited patients either afer myocardial infarction or with angina only showed that simvastatin 20–40 mg/day could reduce mortality by 33% as well as recurrent myocardial infarction and the need for revascularisation by 37% [67]. Preliminary data from other studies suggest that there may not be a 'safe' level of blood cholesterol in patients with overt evidence of vascular disease.

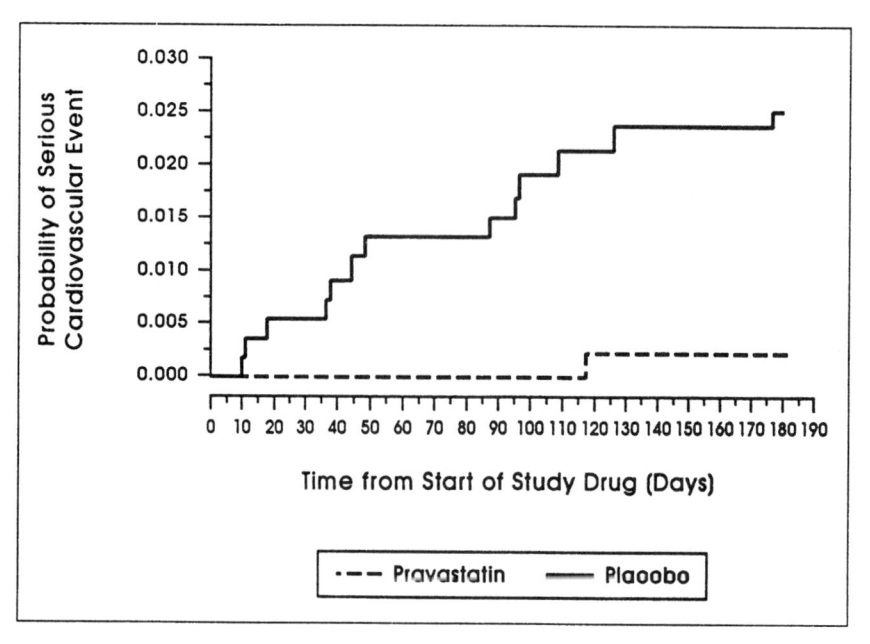

Figure 15.2. Life-table analysis of serious cardiovascular adverse events during 26 weeks of treatment with pravastatin or placebo in 1062 patients with primary hypercholesterolemia (Kaplan–Meier estimate) (reproduced from [34] with permission).

Evidence that aggressive control of diabetes *per se* has an effect on coronary events is controversial. However, treatment of hypertension and hyperlipidemia in patients with diabetes probably has an even greater impact on vascular events than in other patients with angina.

Aspirin and warfarin

The benefits of aspirin in patients after MI, at least when ventricular function is well preserved, are well publicized [27]. The SAPAT study [20] and others [35] also noted a reduction in coronary vascular events in patients treated with aspirin (Figure 15.3) and a beta-blocker (Table 15.3). In patients with heart failure and coronary disease there are sound biological reasons for believing that aspirin may be harmful and some clinical evidence to support this [68]. In addition aspirin may negate the benefits of ACE inhibition in this setting [68, 69].

The benefits of warfarin in this population may be even more striking [27, 36].

Nitrates

Nitrates dilate coronary arteries, including collateral vessels, and improve myocardial oxygen supply, but also reduce preload and afterload and thereby reduce myocardial oxygen demand [37].

Sublingual nitrates are highly effective for the relief of angina and very inexpensive. Relief of pain, even if atypical, within a minute or so, suggests that the pain is myocardial ischemia, until proven otherwise, and failure to relieve pain makes the diagnosis of angina doubtful, unless dealing with unstable angina. Short-acting nitrates may be used even more effectively by administering them before activity likely to provoke angina. Used in this fashion they will usually delay or

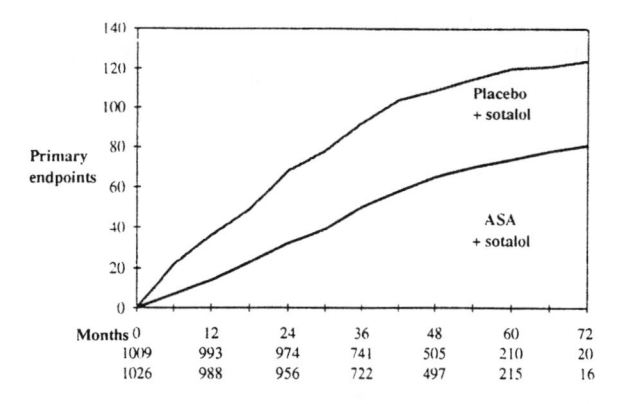

Figure 15.3. Cumulative plot of primary endpoints (ASA = aspirin). (reproduced from [20] with permission).

prevent the appearance of angina. Nitrate sprays are equally effective and preferred by some patients. The spray is generally more expensive, but as it has a longer shelf-life than sublingual nitrates, may be useful for patients with infrequent angina. Chewable isosorbide dinitrate is an alternative which also has a longer shelf-life.

There is a bewildering array of long-acting nitrate preparations. Transdermal, buccal and oral preparations are all available. Convenience, patient preference and cost should be taken into account when selecting a preparation. The most important principal is to consider the possibility of nitrate tolerance which can occur within days of initiating treatment. A nitrate-free interval of 6–8 hours is required each day to prevent tolerance from occurring.

The principal side-effect of nitrates is headache. This may be relieved by reducing the dose (or in the case of sublingual nitrates spitting the tablet out or swallowing it). Nitrates may also provoke hypotension. The low frequency of serious side-effects makes nitrates an attractive option, especially for elderly patients.

Nitrates have not been shown to reduce major events such as MI [27]. A mortality benefit was observed in patients with heart failure, many of whom had CAD, when used in combination with hydralazine [38].

Beta-blockers

Beta-blockers are one of the mainstays of treatment for angina and, having undergone a lull in the 1980s, are again fashionable [37]. Beta-blockers reduce heart rate during exertion, thereby increasing the duration of diastole during which coronary flow takes place. Other possible mechanisms of action include a reduction in myocardial contractility and afterload, thereby reducing oxygen demand. Beta-blockers should be viewed as the 'gold-standard' against which other antianginal agents should be tested.

Side-effects of beta-blockers are numerous but usually minor. Beta-blockers should not be used in asthmatics, in patients with resting limb ischemia or uncontrolled heart failure. Beta-blockers have remarkably little effect on intermittent claudication in most patients. Beta-blockers are being increasingly advocated for prevention of progression of 'controlled' heart failure. Other side-effects include impotence, cold extremities and fatigue, all reversible. Side-effects may be reduced by using highly beta-1-selective agents (atenolol, bisoprolol) or vasodilating beta-blockers (celiprolol and carvedilol). However, non-selective beta-blockers may be more effective antianginal agents and may have a greater reduction in mortality in the post-MI setting [27]. Bradycardia is a common effect of beta-blockers but should not lead to reduction in dose unless accompanied by symptoms.

There are no mortality studies of beta-blockers in angina. After MI, non-selective beta-blockers can reduce mortality by up to 36% [27].

Dihydropiridine calcium antagonists

These agents act principally by coronary vasodilatation and reducing afterload. Most studies suggests that these agents are less effective antianginal agents than beta-blockers or other classes of calcium antagonists [37]. However, the recent TIBET study indicated that nifedipine was equally effective as atenolol; the agents in combination were better than either used singly [39].

The principal side-effects are flushing, headache, swollen ankles, hypotension and, especially in elderly patients, exacerbation of angina. The latter may reflect a fall in coronary perfusion pressure and a reflex tachycardia.

There is no evidence that these agents reduce mortality in patients with angina or after MI when used alone. Indeed there is a trend to excess mortality or infarction, both in patients with minor CAD [40] and after MI [27], at least with short-acting drugs. However, when used with a beta-blocker there is some evidence, inconclusive as yet, that they exert an additional benefit in terms of reducing unstable angina and infarction [39]. Evidence that dihydropiridine antagonists can retard the progression of atheroma is very weak; the studies purporting to show such an effect are notable for the increase in coronary events in the group receiving active treatment [40–43].

Diltiazem

Diltiazem reduces exercise heart rate and myocardial contractility, and causes coronary vasodilatation. Diltiazem is as effective as a beta-blocker for controlling symptoms [37]. Diltiazem has the most favorable side-effect profile of all the calcium antagonists.

There is no evidence that diltiazem alone reduces mortality in patients with angina. A pilot study of the ACIP trial suggests that aggressive treatment with a beta-blocker and diltiazem in combination may reduce the rate of coronary events [44]. After MI, in patients with well preserved ventricular function, diltiazem probably reduces the risk of reinfarction and death [27]. This is balanced by a trend to an excess of heart failure and mortality in patients with ventricular dysfunction.

Verapamil

Verapamil reduces exercise heart rate and myocardial contractility more effectively than other calcium antagonists, but is a less potent vasodilator. Verapamil is as effective as a beta-blocker for controlling symptoms [37].

Side-effects of verapamil include constipation and an exacerbation of heart failure. Constipation often improves with time and may be less of a problem with slow-release preparations. Verapamil should be given to patients on a beta-blocker only under the most expert supervision due to the risks of inducing complete heart block or heart failure.

There is no evidence that verapamil reduces mortality in patients with angina, but the mortality of patients with angina treated with verapamil or metoprolol is very similar [70]. After MI, among patients with well preserved ventricular function, verapamil reduces the risk of reinfarction and death [27]. This is balanced by a trend to an excess of heart failure and mortality in patients with ventricular dysfunction. There is some evidence that verapamil can retard the progress of atheroma [43].

Other agents

Aminophylline is a coronary vasoconstrictor but may redirect flow from myocardial territories without disease to those served by a vessel with an epicardial coronary stenosis [45]. Aminophylline may also improve coronary collateral flow. This is the reverse of the coronary steal phenomenon induced by the coronary vasodilator, dipyridamole. Clinical experience is limited.

Evidence that ACE inhibitors, short-term, reduce or exacerbate myocardial ischemia is controversial. Any therapeutic effect is probably clinically irrelevant [46]. However, there is substantial, though not conclusive evidence that long-term ACE inhibition can reduce episodes of unstable angina and MI [27, 43].

A series of agents that may improve ischemic metabolism are being tested currently (ranolizine, trimetazidine) [47]. Sinus node modulators are also in development. As reducing heart rate not only reduces myocardial oxygen demand but also improves supply by prolonging diastole, the time when most of the coronary flow occurs, this seems logical. Amiodarone, currently used mainly as an antiarrhythmic agent, is also a very effective antianginal agent.

Transcutaneous spinal stimulation has been used for patients with intractable, inoperable angina [48].

Which agent?

The causes of (progressive) CAD must first be treated. Cholesterol lowering agents should be used extensively; it is questionable whether there is a safe level of cholesterol in the presence of angina. The aim should be to reduce total cholesterol below 5 mmol/L. It is better to treat with diet and drugs from the outset rather than prevaricate. Drugs can always be withdrawn if the diet is effective. Hypertension should be controlled, although this is often achieved by the antianginal treatment. The patient should be counseled regarding smoking, diet and exercise.

On current evidence, patients with good ventricular function should be treated with a beta-blocker, aspirin and a short-acting (sublingual) nitrate unless contraindicated. There is growing evidence that the use of a dihydropiridine calcium antagonist in addition to a beta-blocker, routinely, may further reduce coronary events [39, 44].

In patients with reversible airways obstruction or severe peripheral vascular disease, verapamil should be used instead of a beta-blocker.

In patients with poor ventricular function a beta-blocker is usually a better choice than a calcium antagonist. However, despite studies suggesting potential benefits from a beta-blocker in heart failure, some patients experience a worsening of symptoms. In these cases, reducing the dose of the beta-blocker and adding a nitrate may be effective. Newer dihydropiridine calcium antagonists may have fewer problems than the older drugs and may be used with caution. Warfarin may be a better choice than aspirin under these circumstances [687].

In patients who fail to respond adequately to a beta-blocker, adding a long-active nitrate (once daily) or a dihydropridine calcium antagonist is often effective. Adding a third agent is usually only of marginal benefit. A coronary intervention should be contemplated at this stage.

Diltiazem and nitrates are often the drugs of choice in those prone to side-effects.

PTCA

It is amazing that so much of the health budget is consumed by a procedure which is essentially untested! There is only one controlled trial of angioplasty versus

Table 15.5. Relative costs and benefits of treatment of angina.

		CABG (Million ECUs)	PTCA (Milllion ECUs)	Medical (Million ECUs)
Relative costs and benefits of treating 1000 patients for 3–6 months				
Procedure		10	4	0.1
Three months	(ACIP) [44]	10	4.3	0.5
Six months	(ACME) [21]	10	5.3	0.7
				(0.8 with lipid lowering)
Death		2%°	0	1%
Morbidity				
MI		5%°	5%	3%
(Repeat) PTCA		None°	15%	11%
(Repeat) CABG		None°	7%	0%
Total procedures		1000	1220	110
Relative costs and benefits of treating 1000 patients for 2.5 years				
Procedure		10	4	0.1
Three months	(ACIP) [44]	10	4.3	0.6
Six months	(ACME) [21]	–	5.6	1.2
2.5 years	(RITA) [50]	10.2	7.6	2.3 (approx.)
				(3.0 with lipid lowering)
Death		3.6%	3.2%	Same°
Morbidity				
MI		4.0%	6.6%	Lower°
PTCA		3.2%	18.2%	??
CABG		0.8%	18.8%	10%°
Total procedures		1040	1370	100

Van den Brand et al. [51] used to calculate interventional costs, British National Formulary 1994 used for drug costs. Costs of investigation, outpatient clinics, hospitalization other than for procedures, and drug costs in the intervention groups have not been included. Medically treated patients are costed as receiving aspirin, beta-blockers and calcium antagonists, although the patients in the trials were generally suboptimally treated by current standards. Mortality and morbidity data obtained from clinical trials [14–17, 21, 44, 50].

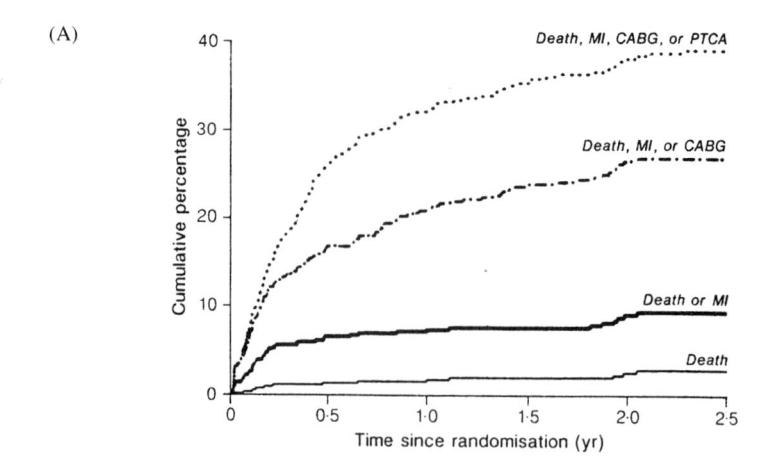

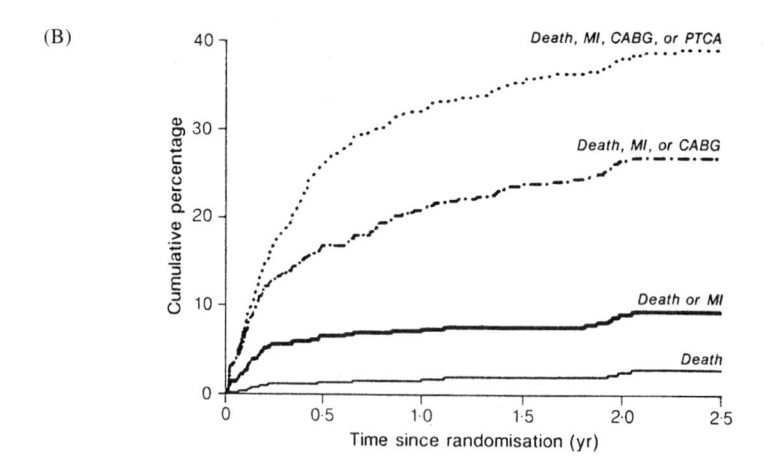

Figure 15.4. (A) Patients randomized to PTCA: cumulative risk of later PTCA, CABG, myocardial infarction, or death; (B) patients randomized to CABG: cumulative risk of later PTCA, CABG, myocardial infarction or death (reproduced from [50] with permission).

medical therapy for chronic stable angina [21]. This showed a marginal benefit in terms of relief of angina over six months of follow-up, but there was a high incidence of MI and need for CABG in the angioplasty group (Table 15.5). Thus, a small improvement in symptoms had been paid for not only in terms of cost, but also the morbidity of having the procedure itself done and the morbidity associated with the complications of the procedure [49].

Comparisons between PTCA and CABG are no more promising [50]. PTCA is associated with a greater reinfarction rate, need for repeat PTCA and need for further CABG (Figure 15.4), and similar mortality.

Data from Medicare in the United States, probably the largest interventional database, indicated that the mortality within 30 days of an angioplasty was 3.8%, and within one year was 8.2%. If the indication for angioplasty is restricted to angina, then the respective figures were 1.9% and 6.0%. Although some centers may believe that their results are better, it is likely that this large database represents the true state of affairs.

It seems doubtful whether patients are being properly informed by doctors of the risks and benefits of PTCA, otherwise patients would presumably be more reluctant to entrust themselves to the procedure [52]. It is to be hoped that PTCA will be reserved for the management of intractable symptoms, either with single vessel disease or when the patient is inoperable. There is a continuing need for ethically approved research into the possible benefits of PTCA. The role of PTCA in unstable angina and as a primary procedure after MI remains to be properly defined [27]. The routine use of angioplasty after thrombolysis is to be deplored [27].

Surgery

Six trials [14–18, 53–55] of coronary bypass surgery versus medical treatment have been conducted and only one showed a significant benefit from surgery in terms of mortality [15]. None of the trials suggested that surgery reduced the risk of MI. There is no evidence that surgery in patients without symptoms improves prognosis (Figures 15.5–15.10).

It has been argued that the reason why there was no difference between medical and surgical outcomes was that patients crossed over from medical treatment to surgery if their symptoms were too severe. This argument is flawed on at least three counts:

1. The cross-over rates were not large, in the order of 3–4% per year (Table 15.3).
2. The landmark studies with ACE inhibitors in heart failure were able to identify benefits despite cross-over rates of up to 30% [27].
3. Good medical practice is to treat those patients with intractable symptoms by surgery anyway.

Furthermore, the lack of a positive result for surgery because of inadequate study design hardly justifies the use of surgery; a more convincing positive trial result is still required. The trials thus suggest that referring patients for surgery on the basis of symptoms or inability to tolerate side-effects of medical treatment is satisfactory.

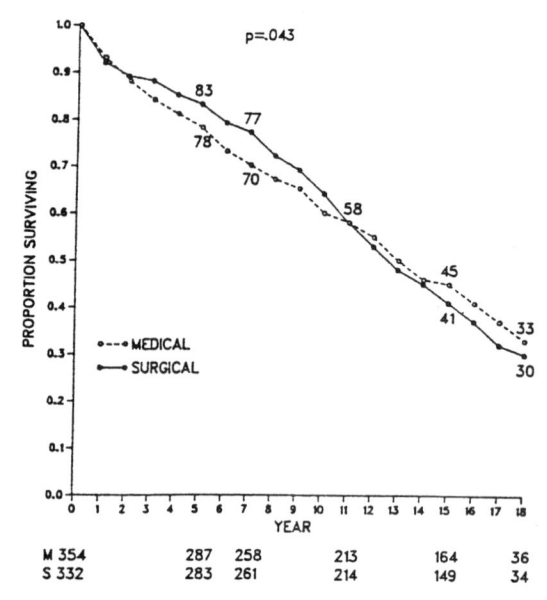

Figure 15.5. Cumulative survival rates for all patients by intent to treat. Numbers of patients at risk are given at the bottom (M, medical; S, surgical). Survival was significantly better with surgical therapy only at 7 years (reproduced from [14]).

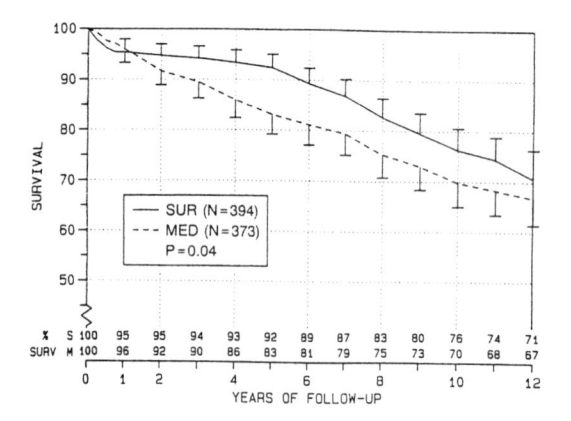

Figure 15.6. Twelve-year cumulative survival rates and 95% confidence intervals for all patients randomly assigned to eithier surgical treatment (SUR, S) or medical therapy (MED, M). N denotes number of patients, and % SURV, percentage surviving (reproduced from [15] with permission).

The mortality within 30 days of CABG according to the 1992 US Medicare system was 6.4%; within one year it was 11.8% (5.1% and 10.8% respectively, if confined to angina as the indication). These figures are no better than for the older surgical trials. It is likely that surgery on higher risk individuals accounts for much of the failure of surgical mortality to decline.

The duration of the benefits of surgery are also open to doubt. The surgical trials suggest that after five years there is little difference in the severity of symptoms or

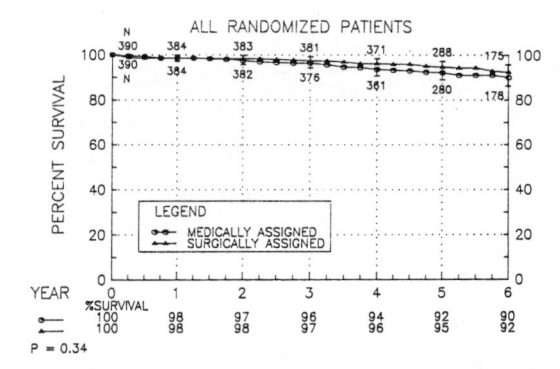

Figure 15.7. Six-year cumulative survival rates for all study patients. Numbers of patients in medical and surgical groups followed to each year appear on the curve. At time zero the number assigned to medical therapy is topmost; thereafter, the number refers to nearest data point. In these and all subsequent survival curves, the error bars represent one-half of 97.5% confidence intervals for the cumulative percent survival at each year with the use of the Greenwood standard error (reproduced from [56]).

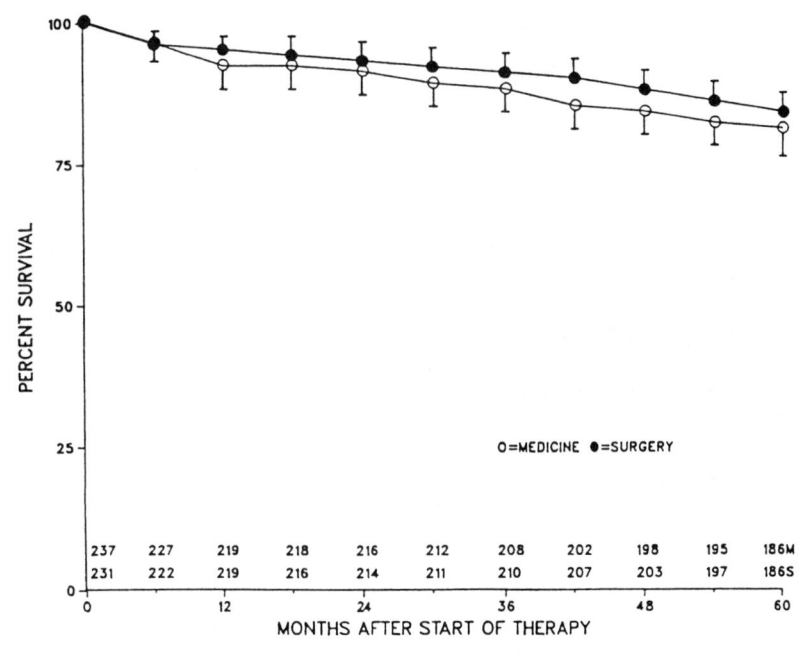

Figure 15.8. Plot of overall survival of medical and surgical patients classified by treatment assigned. Verical bars represent 1 SEM. Numbers of patients at risk in each time intervals are listed above x axis (reproduced from [57]).

the amount of medication required, whether patients are randomized to surgery or not [56, 58] (Figure 15.11). This probably reflects spontaneous improvement of symptoms in some medically managed patients and the benefits of (delayed) surgery in others. Overall the number of hospitalizations is greater in those

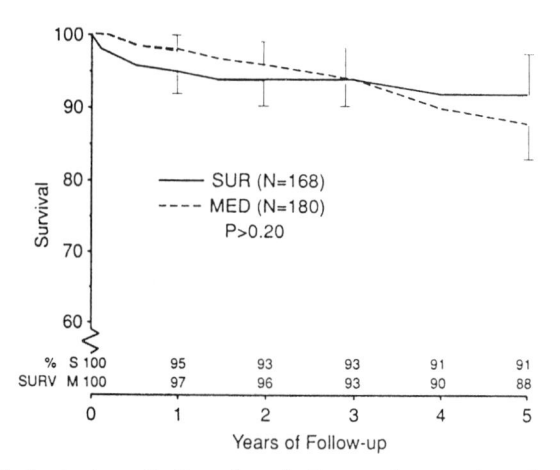

Figure 15.9. Survival rates in medically and surgically treated groups (reproduced from [54] with permission).

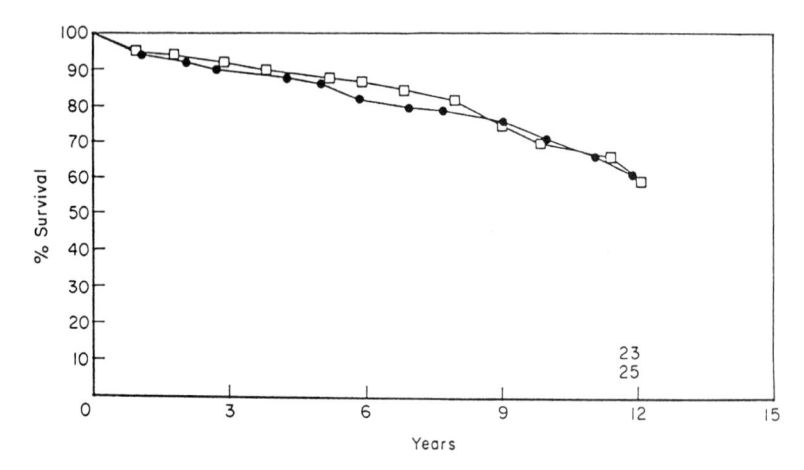

Figure 15.10. Actuarial survival curves for patients in the surgical trials analysed according to intention to treat. Surgical patients are represented by squares and non-surgical patients by circles ($N = 100$ in each group) (reproduced from [53] with permission).

randomized to surgery [56] and the rate of hospitalization, excluding initial surgery in those assigned to it, is no different between groups (Figure 15.12).

Risk stratification

There is no evidence that coronary angiography is superior to exercise testing in defining modifiable risk [59, 60] (Figure 15.13). Myocardial scintigraphy and probably more importantly measurement of ventricular function (Figure 15.14) may enhance the predictive accuracy of the exercise test. The exercise test has been crit-

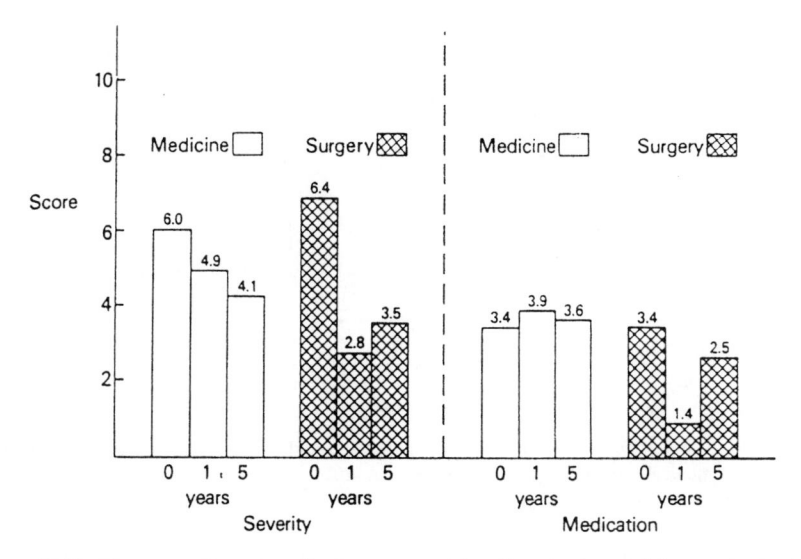

Figure 15.11. Mean severity and medication scores at baseline, 1 year, and 5 years by treatment assigned. Numbers at top of bars are mean scores (reproduced from [58] with permission).

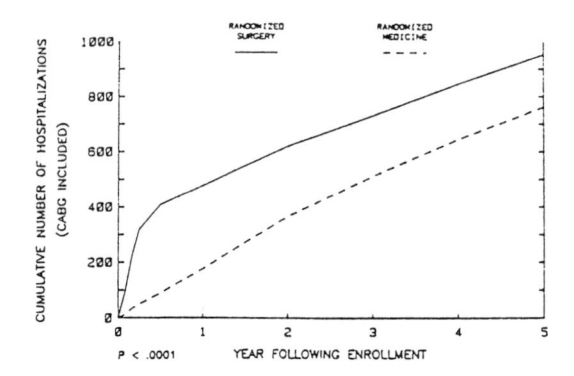

Figure 15.12. Total number of hospitalizations including those for coronary artery bypass graft surgery (CABG). Excluded are scheduled hospitalizations for coronary arteriography done on some patients at approximately 18 and 60 months after entry as part of the study protocol (reproduced from [56]).

icized in that it accurately identifies mortality but not the risk of MI [60]. As surgery and PTCA have not been shown to modify the risk of MI the argument falls down. It can also be argued that the exercise test does not reliably predict those patients with left main coronary artery stenosis. The CASS registry indicated that 7.3% of patients undergoing angiography had a left main coronary stenosis greater than 50% [61] but that only 0.3% were asymptomatic. The prognosis of left main disease is not uniformly poor [61, 62]. It is likely that the exercise test does identify those patients with left main disease who require surgery. Similarly, it would appear that exercise testing can identify those patients with three-vessel disease who do or do not need surgery.

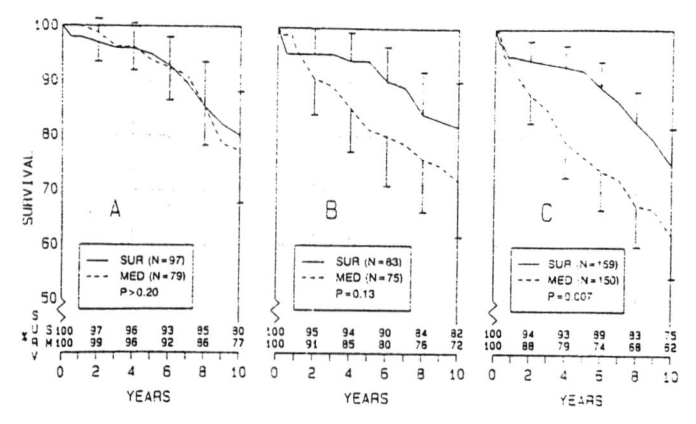

Figure 15.13. Ten-year cumulative survival rates and 95% confidence intervals for the surgically treated (SUR, S) and medically treated (MED, M) groups, stratified according to cardiovascular response to exercise graded by ST-segment depression, maximal heart rate and maximal workload. A denotes a normal or slightly positive test results, B a positive test result, and C a markedly positive test results; N denotes number of patients, and % SURV percentage surviving (reproduced from [15] with permission).

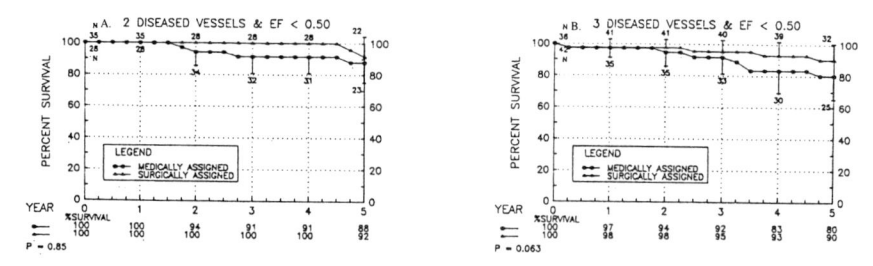

Figure 15.14. Five-year cumulative survival rates for patients with ejection fractions (EF) of less than 0.50, double (A), and triple (B) vessel disease (reproduced from [56]).

The major conceptual problem that is probably holding back modern management of CAD is the idea that lesions greater than 70% are most likely to occlude and produce an MI or death. Studies suggest exactly the opposite. Eighty percent of lesions greater than 70% that occlude do so without an acute deterioration in symptoms. Eighty percent of lesions less than 30% that occlude lead to an infarct [41, 63–65]. However, interventional cardiology is obsessed with the more benign lesion. The reason why patients with triple vessel disease do worse than patients with less affected vessels is probably not to do with the severity of the lesions but rather the surface area of the coronary arteries involved with atheroma.

There is no doubt that once an angiogram has been done it is emotionally difficult not to intervene. The obvious solution is not to do the angiogram. A critically important study is now underway in the UK which will compare the outcome in patients undergoing routine angiography for angina with those being assessed by treadmill exercise testing alone. Peer review confirms the suspicion that patients are often referred inappropriately for angiography [66] and further work in this area is required.

Conclusion

Medical management of CAD is the optimal strategy for the vast majority of patients with angina because:

1. Medical treatment is associated with the lowest morbidity, when the morbidity associated with interventional procedures is taken into account.
2. Mortality associated with medical treatment is not appreciably higher than with interventions.
3. While the real benefits of angioplasty are unknown, medical treatment has for the 'aggressive' physician improved dramatically in the last five years.
4. Medical treatment, even allowing for routine use of lipid lowering agents and two or three antianginal agents, is the least expensive short- and long-term treatment (Table 15.5).

Further trials of PTCA and surgery versus current medical therapy, and studies of the need for coronary angiography to stratify risk for patients with angina in patients selected on the basis of symptoms or exercise test result are required. Trials (RITA-2 and EMAS) which will address some of these problems are in progress, although in these trials medical treatment may be suboptimal, failing to capitalize on the recent data on beta-blocker/calcium antagonist combinations [39, 44] and trials of lipid lowering therapy [34].

References

1. Chew R. Compendium of health statistics, 8th ed. London: Office of Health Economics, 1992.
2. Cupples LA, Gagnon DR, Wong ND, Ostfeld AM, Kannel WB. Preexisting cardiovascular conditions and long-term prognosis after initial myocardial infarction: The Framingham Study. Am Heart J. 1993;125:863–72.
3. Margolis JR, Gillum RF, Feinleib M, Brasch R, Fabsitz R. Community surveillance for coronary heart disease: The Framingham Cardiovascular Disease Study. Comparisons with the Framingham Heart Study and previous short-term studies. Am J Cardiol 1976;37:61–7.
4. Medalie JH, Snyder M, Groen JJ, Neufeld HN, Goldbourt U, Riss E. Angina pectoris among 10,000 men: 5 year incidence and univariate analysis. Am J Med 1973; 55:583–94.
5. Duncan B, Fulton M, Morrison SL et al. Prognosis of new and worsening angina pectoris. Br Med J 1976;1:981–5.
6. Ghandi MM, Lampe F, Wood DA. Incidence of stable angina pectoris. Eur Heart J 1992;13:181.
7. Rose G, Reid DD, Hamilton PJS, McCartney P, Keen H, Jarret RJ. Myocardial ischaemia, risk factors and death from coronary heart disease. Lancet 1977;i:105–9.
8. WHO European Collaborative Group. Multifactorial trial in the prevention of coronary heart disease. I. Recruitment and critical findings. Eur Heart J 1980;1:73–80.
9. Shaper AG, Cook DG, Walker M, Macfarlane PW. Prevalence of ischaemic heart disease in middle aged British men. Br Heart J 1984;51:595–605.
10. Abernathy JR, Thorn MD, Trobaugh GB et al. Prevalence of ischaemic resting and stress electrocardiographic abnormalities and angina among 40–59 year old men in selected US and USSR populations. Circulation 1988;77:270–8.

11. Cannon PJ, Cannell PA, Stockley IH, Garner ST, Hampton JR. Prevalence of angina as assessed by a survey of prescriptions for nitrates. Lancet 1988;1:979–81.
12. Kannell WB, Sorlie, PD. Remission of clinical angina pectoris: The Framingham Study. Am J Cardiol 1978;42:119–23.
13. Kannel WB, Feinleib M. Natural history of angina pectoris in the Framingham study. Prognosis and survival. Am J Cardiol 1972;29:154–63.
14. Peduzzi P. Eighteen-year follow-up in the Veterans Affairs Cooperative Study of coronary artery bypass surgery for stable angina. Circulation 1992;86:121–30.
15. Varnauskas E, Olsson SB, Carlstrom E et al. Twelve-year follow-up of survival in the randomized European Coronary Surgery Study. N Engl J Med 1988;319:332–7.
16. Varnauskas E. Survival, myocardial infarction, and employment status in a prospective randomized study of coronary bypass surgery. Circulation 1985;72:V90–101.
17. Chaitman BR, Ryan TJ, Kronmal RA, Foster ED, Frommer PL, Killip T and the CASS investigators. Coronary artery surgery study (CASS): Comparability of 10 year survival in randomised and randomizable patients. JACC 1990;16:1071–8.
18. CASS principal investigators and their associates. Myocardial infarction and mortality in the coronary artery surgery study (CASS randomized trial. N Engl J Med 1984;310:750–8.
19. Romeo F, Rosano GMC, Nartuscelli E, Valente A, Reale A. Characterisation and long-term prognosis of patients with effort-induced silent myocardial ischaemia. Eur Heart J 1992;13:457–63.
20. Juul-Moller S, Edvardsson N, Jahnmatz B, Rosen A, Sorensen S, Omblus R, for the Swedish Angina Pectoris Aspirin Trial (SAPAT) group. Lancet 1992;340:1421–4.
21. Parisi AF, Folland ED, Hartigan P. A comparison of angioplasty with medical therapy in the treatment of single-vessel coronary artery disease. N Engl J Med 1992;326:10–16.
22. Pinsky JL, Jette AM, Branch LG, Kannel WB, Feinleib M. The Framingham disability study: Relationship of various coronary heart disease manifestations to disability in older persons living in the community. Am J Publ Health 1990;80:1363–8.
23. Reeves RA, Chen E. Who wants to eliminate heart disease? J Clin Epidemiol. 1994; 47:667–70.
24. Cavender JB, Rogers WJ, Fisher LD, Gersh BJ, Coggin CJ, Myers WO. Effects of smoking on survival and morbidity in patients randomized to medical or surgical therapy in the coronary artery surgery study (CASS); 10-year follow-up. J Am Coll Cardiol 1992;20:287–94.
25. Fox KM, Deanfield J, Krikler S et al. The influence of cigarette smoking on the medical management of angina. Drugs 1983;25(Suppl 2):177–80.
26. Todd IC, Ballantyne D. Effect of exercise training on the total ischaemic burden: An assessment by 24 hour ambulatory electrocardiographic monitoring. Br Heart J 1992;68:560–6.
27. Cleland JGF, MvMurray J, Ray S. Prevention strategies after myocardial infarction. Science Press, 1994.
28. Watts GF, Lewis B, Brunt JNH et al. Effects on coronary artery disease of lipid-lowering diet, or diet plus cholestyramine, in the St Thomas' Atherosclerosis Regression Study (STARS). Lancet 1992;339:563–9.
29. Dahlof B, Lindholm LH, Hansson L, Schersten B, Ekbom T, Wester PO. Morbidity and mortality in the Swedish Trial in Old Patients with Hypertension (STOP-Hypertension). Lancet 1991;338:1281–5.
30. Probstfield JL. Prevention of stroke by antihypertensive drug treatment in older persons with isolated systolic hypertension: Final results of the Systolic Hypertension in the Elderly Program (SHEP). J Am Med Assoc 1991;265:3255–64.
31. Peart S, Brennan PJ, Broughton P et al. Medical Research Council trial of treatment of hypertension in older adults: Principal results. Br Med J 1992;304:405–12.
32. The lipid research clinics coronary primary prevention trial results. I. Reduction in incidence of coronary heart disease. J Am Med Assoc 1984;251:351–64.
33. Frick MH, Elo O, Haapa K et al. Helsinki Heart Study: Primary-prevention trial with gemfibrozil in middle-aged men with dyslipidemia. Safety of treatment, changes in risk factors, and incidence of coronary heart disease. N Engl J Med 1987;317;1237–45.
34. The Pravastatin Multinational study group for cardiac risk patients. Effects of pravastatin in patients with serum total cholesterol levels from 5.2 to 7.8 mmolL (200–300 mg/dl) plus two additional atherosclerotic risk factors. Am J Cardiol 1993;72:1031–7.

35. Ridker PM, Manson JE, Gaziano JM, Buring JE, Hennekens CH. Low-dose aspirin therapy for chronic stable angina. A randomized, placebo-controlled trial. An Intern Med 1991;114:835–9.
36. Borchgrevink CF. Long-term anticoagulant therapy in angina pectoris. Lancet. 1962; 1:449–51.
37. Dollery (Ed.). Drugs and therapeutics. London: Churchill-Livingstone.
38. Cohn JN, Archibald DG, Ziesche S *et al*. Effect of vasodilator therapy on mortality in chronic congestive heart failure: Results of a Veterans Administration Cooperative Study. N Engl J Med 1986;314:1547–52.
39. Dargie HJ, Ford I, Fox KM, on behalf of the TIBET study group. Effects of ischaemia and treatment with atenolol, nifedipine SR and their combination on outcome in patients with chronic stable angina. Eur Heart J. 1996; 17:104–12.
40. Lichtlen PR, Hugenholtz PG, Rafflenbeul W, Hecker H, Jost S, Deckers JW. Retardation of angiographic progression of coronary artery disease by difedipine. Results of the International Nifedipine Trial on Antiatherosclerotic Therapy (INTACT). Lancet 1990;335:1109–13.
41. Lichtlen PR, Nikutta P, Jost S, Deckers J, Wiese B, Rafflenbeul W. Anatomical progression of coronary artery disease in humans as seen by prospective, repeated quantitated coronary angiography: Relation to clinical events and risk factors. Circulation 1992;86:828–38.
42. Waters D, Lesperance J, Francetich M *et al*. A controlled clinical trial to assess the effect of a calcium channel blocker on the progression of coronary atherosclerosis. Circulation 1990;82:1940–53.
43. Cleland JGF, Krikler DM. Modification of atherosclerosis by agents that do not lower cholesterol. Br Heart J 1993;69(Suppl.):554–62.
44. Knatterud GL *et al*. Effects of treatment strategies to suppress ischemia in patients with coronary artery disease: 12-week results of the Asymptomatic Cardiac Ischemia Pilot (ACIP) study. J Am Coll Cardiol. 1994; 24:11–20.
45. Crea F, Galassi AR, Kaski JC, Pupita G, El-Tamimi H, Davies GJ. Effect of theophylline on exercise-induced myocardial ischaemia. Lancet 1989;1:683–6.
46. Cleland JGF, Henderson E, McLenachan J, Findlay IN, Dargie HJ. Effect of captopril, an angiotensin-coverting enzyme inhibitor, in patients with angina pectoris and heart failure. J Am Coll Cardiol 1991;17:733–9.
47. Dalla-Volta S, Maraglino G, Della-Valentina P, Viena P, Desideri A. Comparison of trimetazidine with nifedipine in effort angina: A double-blind, crossover study. Cardiovasc Drugs Ther 1990;4(Suppl. 4);853–9.
48. Mannheimer C, Augustinsson L-E, Carlsoon C-A, Manhem K, Wilhelmsson C. Epidural spinal electrical stimulation in severe angina pectoris. Br Heart J 1988;59:56–61.
49. Cleland JGF, Van Den Brand M. Coronary angioplasty: Is cardiological practice in the USA really the gold standard for Europe? Eur Heart J 1993;14:1435–7.
50. Hampton JR, Henderson RA, Julian DG *et al*. Coronary angioplasty versus coronary artery bypass surgery: The Randomised Intervention Treatment of Angina (RITA) trial. Lancet 1993;341:573–80.
51. Van den Brand M, Van Halem C, Van den Brink F *et al*. Comparison of costs of percutaneous transluminal coronary angioplasty and coronary bypass surgery for patients with angina pectoris. Eur Heart J 1990;11:765–71.
52. Cleland JGF. Angioplasty versus medical therapy for single-vessel coronary artery disease. N Engl J Med 1992;326:1632–4.
53. Norris RM, White HD, Cross DB, Wild CJ, Whitlock RML. Prognosis after recovery from myocardial infarction: The relative importance of cardiac dilatation and coronary stenoses. Eur Heart J 1992;13:1611–8.
54. Lorimer AR, Karlsson T, Varnauskas E. The role of early surgery following myocardial infarction. Br J Clin Pract 1992;46:238–42.
55. Booth DC, Deupree RH, Hultgren HN, DeMaria AN, Scott SM, Luchi RJ. Quality of life after bypass surgery for unstable angina. 5-year follow-up results of a Veterans Affairs Cooperative Study. Circulation 1991;83:87–95.
56. CASS principal investigators and their associates. Coronary artery surgery study (CASS): A randomized trial of coronary artery bypass surgery. Quality of life in patients randomly assigned to treatment group. Circulation 1983;68:939–60.

57. Parisi AF, Khusi S, Deupree RH *et al*. Medical compared with surgical management of unstable angina. Circulation 1989;80:1176–89.
58. Hultgren HN, Peduzzi P, Detree K, Takaro T and the study participants. The 5 year effect of bypass surgery on relief of angina and exercise performance. Circulation 1985;72(Suppl. V):V79–83.
59. Morris CK, Ueshima K, Kawaguchi T, Hideg A, Froelicher VF. The prognostic value of exercise capacity: A review of the literature. Am Heart J 1991;122:1423–31.
60. Bogaty P, Dagenais GR, Cantin B, Alain P, Rouleau JR. Prognosis in patients with a strongly positive exercise electrocardiogram. Am J Cardiol 1989;64:1284–8.
61. Taylor HA, Deumite NJ, Chaitman BR, Davis KB, Killip T, Rogers WJ. Asymptomatic left main coronary artery disease in the Coronary Artery Surgery Study (CASS) registry. Circulation 1989;79:1171–9.
62. Hueb W, Bellotti G, Franchini-Ramires JA, Lemos da Luz P, Pileggi F. Two- to eight-year survival rates in patients who refused coronary artery bypass grafting. Am J Cardiol 1989;63:155–9, A14.
63. Fuster V, Badimon L, Badimon JJ, Chesebro JH. Mechanisms of disease: The pathogenesis of coronary artery disease and the acute coronary syndromes (first of two parts). N Engl J Med. 1991;326:242–50.
64. Fuster V, Badimon L, Badimon JJ, Chesebro JH. The pathogenesis of coronary artery disease and the acute coronary syndromes (second of two parts). N Engl J Med 1992;326:310–8.
65. Fuster V, Badimon JJ, Badimon L. Clinical-pathological correlations of coronary disease progression and regression. Circulation 1992;83(Suppl.):III 1–11.
66. Graboys TB, Biegelsen B, Lampert S, Blatt CM, Lown B. Results of a second opinion trial among patients referred for coronary angiography. J Am Med Assoc 1992;268:2537–40.
67. Pedersen TR. Randomised trial of cholesterol lowering in 4444 patients with coronary heart disease. The Scandinavian Simvastatin Survival Study (4S). Lancet. 1994; 344:1383–9.
68. Cleland JGF, Bulpitt CJ, Findlay IN *et al*. Is aspirin safe for patients with heart failure? Br Heart J 1995; 74:215–19.
69. Cleland JGF, Poole-Wilson PA. Is aspirin safe in heart failure?: more data (abstract). Heart. 1996; 75:426–7.
70. Rehnqvist N, Hjemdahl P, Billing E *et al*. Effects of metoprolol vs verapamil in patients with stable angina pectoris. The Angina Prognosis Study in Stockholm (APSIS). Eur Heart J 1996; 17:76–81.

16. Aortic aneurysm and dissection of the aorta

JACK COLLIN

Aortic aneursym

Definition

An aneurysm is an abnormal dilatation of a blood vessel. Cross-sectional dilatation is invariably accompanied by elongation of the vessel so that tortuosity is inevitable. The median diameter of the aorta is greater in men than women and increases progressively above 40 years of age in both sexes. Dilatation of part of the aorta relative to adjacent normal aorta can easily be seen to be aneurysmal but when the whole aorta dilates the diagnosis may be less obvious. Current convention classifies an infra-renal aorta as aneurysmal if the anteroposterior external diameter is 3.0 cm or greater.

Classification

Aortic aneurysms may involve any part of the thoracic or abdominal aorta and the latter are frequently continuous with aneurysms of the common iliac arteries.

Infra-renal aortic aneurysms
Seventy-five percent of all aortic aneurysms are confined to the infra-renal aorta and one in ten of them coexist with clinically significant iliac artery aneurysms. When the aortic aneurysm is continuous with common iliac aneurysms the whole is called an aorto-iliac aneurysm. Occasionally the common iliac aneurysm may be continuous with an aneurysm of the internal iliac artery. For reasons unknown aneurysms of the external iliac artery are of extreme rarity and most vascular surgeons have never seen one.

Thoracic aortic aneurysms
Historically most aneurysms of the thoracic aorta were syphilitic in origin. As syphilis has decreased in incidence and its tertiary manifestations have been prevented by effective antibiotic treatment, isolated thoracic aneurysms particularly of the ascending aorta have become less common.

The age at presentation tends to be younger than for patients with abdominal aortic aneurysms and the underlying etiologies tend to be different. Specific causes such as Marfan's syndrome, Ehlers–Danlos syndrome, Takayasu's disease and aortitis account for many cases. Some patients with chronic aortic dissection present for the first time with a thoracic aneurysm.

Thoraco-abdominal aortic aneurysms
These have attracted interest disproportionate to their incidence which is less than 2% of all aortic aneurysms. They have been subdivided into four types.

- Type I: Involves the whole of the descending thoracic aorta and the upper abdominal aorta.
- Type II: Involves the whole of the descending thoracic and abdominal aorta.
- Type III: Involves the lower half of the descending thoracic aorta and the whole of the abdominal aorta.
- Type IV: Involves the peridiaphragmatic aorta and the whole of the abdominal aorta.

The classification is arbitrary and not particularly helpful. Pragmatically the two important questions are:

(1) Is the aorta aneurysmal where the main abdominal visceral arteries arise?
(2) How much of the descending thoracic aorta is aneurysmal?

The answer to the first predicts the perioperative blood loss and to the second the expected incidence of postoperative paraplegia.

Type IV thoraco-abdominal aneurysms are by far the most common, have the lowest operative mortality (around 12%) and carry the lowest risk of postoperative paraplegia (around 5%).

Epidemiology

Aortic aneurysm is a disease of elderly men. It is rare before the age of 50 years and becomes increasingly common after 60 years of age. Its greatest relative importance as a cause of death is in men aged 70–74 years in whom it accounts for one in every 50 deaths. Much less common in women of all ages, it does not become common in the fairer sex until ten years later than in men.

As a consequence of community screening programs using ultrasonography to detect abdominal aortic aneurysms, the prevalence of the disease in the main groups at risk is now well documented. Six percent of all men aged 65–74 years have an abdominal aortic aneurysm and in a third of these it is 4.0 cm or more in diameter. Most aortic aneurysms are occult and asymptomatic so the incidence (annual rate of presentation) is substantially lower than the prevalence of the disease in the community.

Natural history

As 'giant oak trees from little acorns grow', all aortic aneurysms are initially small. The median growth rate of aneurysms less than 4.0 cm diameter is 1 to 2 mm per annum. As aneurysms become larger so their growth rates increase and when they are between 5.0 and 6.0 cm in diameter the median growth rate is 5 mm per annum.

The risk of aortic rupture increases exponentially as aneurysms grow. For aneurysms under 4.0 cm in diameter the rupture risk is less than 1% per annum. Between 4.0 and 6.0 cm in diameter the risk is less than 5% per annum. Over 6.0 cm in diameter aneurysms tend to grow rapidly and the annual risk of rupture increases progressively to almost 100% per annum. Recognition of the worsening natural history with aneurysm growth has led all vascular surgeons to recommend elective aortic replacement for patients with aneurysms of 6.0 cm or more in diameter unless their general health is so poor that the expected operative mortality or subsequent life expectancy would be prohibitive.

The place of elective aortic surgery for asymptomatic aneurysms under 6.0 cm in diameter is less certain. The natural history of the disease needs to be carefully balanced against the age and health of the patient, elective operative mortality and the individual patient's wishes and personal circumstances.

Etiology

Recognized specific causes of aortic aneurysm are Marfan's syndrome, Type IV Ehlers–Danlos syndrome and other disorders of type III collagen formation, Takayasu's disease, aortitis, tertiary syphilis and acute aortic infection (mycotic aneurysm). The etiology of the common 'degenerative aneurysm' of the elderly remains elusive.

Atherosclerosis

All middle-aged and elderly people have evidence of atherosclerotic change in the aorta and other major vessels. In most cases the association with aneurysmal dilatation is probably coincidental but in patients with symptomatic atherosclerotic occlusive disease the prevalence of aortic aneurysm is twice that in people without occlusive arterial disease. It has been suggested that ceroid, a constituent of atherosclerotic plaques, may, if released from the plaque, excite an immune response which weakens the aortic wall. This mechanism may be of particular relevance in the 10% of aortic aneurysms that are of the gross inflammatory type but a degree of inflammatory response is seen histologically in most aortic aneurysms.

Connective tissue degradation

In the normal aorta elastin limits expansion of the vessel in response to pulse pressure and controls the aortic recoil during diastole. The amount of elastin is greater in the thoracic than abdominal aorta and decreases in both with advancing age. The role of collagen appears to be to set an absolute limit to the amount of arterial expansion that can occur and its relative importance increases as the amount of elastin declines.

Both collagenase and elastase proteolytic activity have been demonstrated in ruptured and unruptured aortic aneurysms but authentic collagenase has been shown to be present only when the aneurysm has ruptured. It is uncertain whether collagenolysis is the cause or the consequence of aortic rupture. Recently a unique metalloprotease elastase has been found in aneurysm patients but its significance is uncertain.

The current state of knowledge is well summarized by the endocrinology aphorism, 'It is possible to extract a chemical from a barn door that will knock a man's hat off but it does not prove there is a hormone for politeness'.

Genetic predisposition
The occurrence of aneurysms in close relatives of patients with the disease has been noted for some years but until recently a genetic or familial predisposition to the disease has been uncertain. Ultrasound screening programs of first degree relatives of patients with aortic aneurysms have shown that in male siblings over 50 years of age the prevalence of aortic aneurysm is 25%, around five times the expected prevalence in the general population. Statistical projection of these data suggests that the life time prevalence for first degree relatives may be 50%. If such is indeed the case it points to a dominantly inherited, probably autosomal gene being responsible.

Environmental factors
As with most genetic predispositions to disease the role of environmental potentiation is to control the likelihood of developing clinically significant disease and the age of onset. It is known that aortic aneurysm is more common in:

- men;
- the elderly;
- tobacco smokers;
- hypertensives; and
- patients with chronic obstructive airways disease or occlusive arterial disease.

Tobacco smoking and hypertension are of the greatest importance since the first is preventable and the second can be controlled with appropriate medication.

As with the risk from atherosclerotic arterial disease the protective effect of female gender is progressively although incompletely lost with advancing years.

Mycotic aneurysms
Acute infective aneursyms have become increasingly common in recent years because of two perversions of the late twentieth century, namely intravenous drug abuse and the frequent consumption of white meat. In the former, microorganisms are frequently injected directly into the circulation and most of the mycotic aneurysms occur close to injection sites, particularly when venous access is exhausted and arterial injection is resorted to. The latter fad has encouraged factory farming of chickens by dealers and the users are consequently predisposed to salmonella infection. *Salmonella enteritidis* is now a common organism isolated from mycotic aneurysms.

The importance of making a diagnosis of mycotic aortic aneurysm is that the growth rate of such aneurysms is rapid and early rupture is almost inevitable. The aortic wall is rapidly destroyed by the infection and urgent aortic replacement is essential.

Clinical presentation

In current vascular surgical practice in the United Kingdom approximately one-third of patients present for the first time with a ruptured aortic aneurysm, one-third with a clinically significant but usually asymptomatic aneurysm and one-third with a small incidentally discovered clinically insignificant aneurysm.

Ruptured aneurysm
A ruptured thoracic aneurysm causes severe sudden onset chest and back pain, and a ruptured abdominal aortic aneurysm causes central abdominal and lumbar back pain. Both may be confused with myocardial infarction or aortic dissection and the latter with perforated viscus, pancreatitis or renal colic. The diagnostic factors are sudden onset associated with circulatory collapse and the intensity of back pain.

Patients are dying from the moment aortic rupture occurs. They will survive only as long as the periaortic connective tissue prevents free rupture into the peritoneal or pleural cavity. It is imperative therefore that if possible the diagnosis is made on physical examination alone. Asking for a diagnostic CT scan may be sending the patient to his death.

A small number of patients with stout retroperitoneal tissues survive chronic contained rupture for many days. Such stable patients often survive distant referral to far-away hospitals and account for the low operative mortalities reported by some tertiary referral centers. For most patients their only chance of survival is surgery within the hour at the primary referral center to arrest the hemorrhage.

Non-ruptured aneurysm
The commonest presentation is with an asymptomatic aneurysm discovered incidentally on chest or abdominal radiography, CT or MR imaging. For abdominal aneurysms, ultrasonography, the commonest abdominal examination, is now the usual means of discovery. Some patients may notice their abdominal aortic aneurysm as a visible pulsatile epigastric mass while others may experience lumbar back pain caused by pressure on the lumbar vertebrae and anterior spinal longitudinal ligament. Rare symptomatic presentations are as follows:

1. *Aortic occlusion*: The lumen of the aneurysm may obstruct by thrombosis *in situ* or if a portion of mural thrombus becomes dislodged. The onset of symptoms is usually acute with severe ischemia of both lower limbs. Because of early massive muscle infarction the outcome is usual fatal.
2. *Distal embolus*: Mural thrombus may dislodge and be propelled down one or both legs. The presentation and outcome depend on the amount of limb ischemia produced.

3. *Ureteric occlusion*: Inflammatory abdominal aortic aneurysms may draw the ureters medially and cause obstruction as they become encased in the intense, periaortitis induced, fibrosis. More commonly the ureter is obstructed by an inflammatory common iliac aneurysm as the ureter crosses the iliac artery bifurcation.
4. *Duodenal obstruction*: The third and fourth parts of the duodenum are closely adherent to the abdominal aorta. Functional but almost never mechanical high intestinal obstruction may occur as the aneurysm enlarges. The presentation is with recurrent vomiting of bile and recently ingested food.

Management

The management of patients with ruptured or symptomatic aortic aneurysms is uncontroversial.

Ruptured aortic aneurysms

Immediate surgery is required if the patient is to survive. For all practical purposes aortic rupture carries a 100% mortality and no surgeon can do worse. Hypotensive patients with an unstable circulation will not survive interhospital transfer and should be operated on by the most competent surgeon available. Patients who are not shocked and not actively bleeding can be considered for transfer to a specialist vascular surgical unit where the outcome of emergency surgery is likely to be better. It should be borne in mind that any delay can be fatal and that patient survival to operation depends on the periaortic connective tissue continuing to exert adequate tamponade. Fluid transfusion should be restricted to the minimum required to maintain tissue perfusion of vital organs. Full restoration of blood pressure and circulating volume is likely to disrupt the connective tissue tamponade and cause fatal intracoelomic rupture.

Symptomatic aortic aneurysm

Abdominal or back pain and tenderness on palpation of the aneurysm in the absence of symptoms or signs of blood loss suggest aneurysm expansion. Operation should be planned for the next available daytime operating list. Investigations should be confined to those that have an immediate bearing on the predicted operative mortality and postoperative care.

Patients who present with aortic occlusion or embolization of the lower limbs require emergency surgery to restore circulation to the ischemic tissues. Sudden aortic occlusion in patients with an aortic aneurysm is frequently fatal since there has been no opportunity for a collateral circulation to develop. Embolization of the lower limb carries a high risk of amputation.

Duodenal obstruction or ureteric occlusion from an abdominal aortic aneurysm are best treated by elective surgical replacement of the aneurysm. It is usually unnecessary to dissect free either duodenum or ureter to produce resolution of symptoms. It is advisable to catheterize an occluded ureter for 6 weeks perioperatively to maintain renal function until the obstruction resolves following aortic surgery. For duodenal obstruction the fashioning of a temporary feeding jejunostomy allows nourishment of the patient pending restoration of normal gastrointestinal transit.

Asymptomatic aortic aneurysm
The underlying principle to remember is that the sole objective of management for this group of patients is to prevent unnecessary premature death from aortic rupture. It follows that if the natural history of an aortic aneurysm is benign or the operative mortality and morbidity are high, the primary management objective is unlikely to be achieved by elective surgery. The two essential questions to be answered before rational treatment can be recommended are:

(1) What is the risk of aneurysm rupture?
(2) What is the likely operative mortality risk?

Abdominal aortic aneurysm
For abdominal aortic aneurysms under 4.0 cm in diameter there is no doubt that the natural history of the disease is benign. It is inconceivable that elective aortic resection can confer benefit even when operative mortality has been reduced to the lowest achievable level. Best management is therefore conservative medical therapy combined with annual measurement of the maximum aortic diameter by means of ultrasonography. Unless there is a specific contraindication all patients should receive prophylactic daily aspirin in order to reduce the risk of death from coexistent atherosclerotic coronary artery disease and from thromboembolic stroke. There is experimental evidence in turkeys and mice that therapy with propranolol reduces the risk of aortic aneurysm rupture. Although retrospective data in patients with aortic aneurysm lends support to the belief that propranolol reduces growth rates of small aortic aneurysms the question is as yet unanswered and a randomized controlled study is needed.

Vascular surgeons have little hesitation in recommending elective aortic replacement for patients with abdominal aortic aneurysms more than 5.5 cm in diameter. At this size aneurysms begin to grow faster and are likely soon to become of a diameter at which the annual risk of rupture greatly exceeds the operative mortality. The exceptions to this general policy occur in patients with incurable malignancy or other severe coexistent disease. Most patients are likely to prefer the option of sudden death from aortic rupture to a lingering painful death from cancer.

Best management for asymptomatic abdominal aortic aneurysms of 4.0–5.4 cm diameter is currently being studied in two randomized controlled trials of surgical or best medical treatment. In the United States Veterans Administration study patients are recruited by ultrasound screening of military veterans while in the United Kingdom study most patients have been referred in routine clinical practice. Since the trials began new evidence suggests that the natural history of such aneurysms may be more benign than was previously believed. On current evidence elective surgical treatment of asymptomatic patients with aneurysms under 5.0 cm in diameter cannot be recommended. The variable determinant of beneficial outcome is the audited operative mortality for the surgical team. Where operative mortality is known to be more than 5%, elective surgery on abdominal aortic aneurysms less than 5.5 cm in diameter should not be undertaken.

Thoracic and thoraco-abdominal aortic aneurysms
Data on the natural history of thoracic aneurysms are even less adequate than those for infra-renal abdominal aortic aneurysm. Given that the normal thoracic aorta is larger than the normal abdominal aorta, elective surgery for an asymptomatic thoracic aortic aneurysm of under 6.0 cm diameter cannot be recommended on current evidence.

The two major additional factors to be borne in mind are the operative mortality risk, particularly for thoraco-abdominal aneurysms, and the paraplegia risk.

The additional operative mortality risk associated with thoracic aneurysm surgery has two major components. Cross-clamping the thoracic aorta imposes a huge immediate afterload on the heart compared with infra-renal aortic clamping. The problem can to some extent be minimized by acute blood pressure control peroperatively but such measures require specialized anesthetic skills. For thoraco-abdominal aneurysms peroperative blood loss from the upper abdominal visceral vessels is usually considerable. The problems caused by transfusion of stored bank blood can in part be minimized by blood salvage systems to return some of the patient's lost blood by reinfusion.

The most distressing outcome of elective aortic surgery is the occurrence of post-operative paraplegia or paraparesis. The blood supply of the spinal cord is variable but embryologically is segmental. In the adult the crucial supply is derived superiorly from the vertebral arteries and inferiorly from branches of the internal iliac supplemented by thoracic and/or lumbar segmental arteries of which one or more is usually dominant. The dominant vessel generally arises at the level of the ninth thoracic vertebra but can arise higher or lower or be multiple. For infra-renal aortic surgery the paraplegia risk is around 0.5% and is increased if one or more internal iliac arteries are removed from the circulation. For the commonest thoraco-abdominal aortic aneurysm involving the whole abdominal aorta, but only the peridiaphragmatic thoracic aorta, the risk of paraplegia is around 5%. The highest risk of paraplegia occurs when the whole of the descending thoracic aorta and abdominal aorta are involved; some reports have indicated that paraplegia can be expected in one-third of patients.

Most patients regard the development of paraplegia as a fate worse than death. The patient with a large aneurysm involving the whole of the thoracic and abdominal aorta and willing to subject himself to the operative mortality and paraplegia risks of elective surgery will be encountered by few vascular surgeons.

In patients with type IV thoraco-abdominal aneurysms the decision whether to subject themselves to elective aneurysm resection or the natural history of their disease is more finely balanced. They can be advised that the combined mortality and paraplegia risk of elective surgery is not less than 15%.

Outcome after aneurysm surgery

Patients with aortic aneurysms are at risk of developing aneurysms elsewhere, particularly of the iliac, femoral and popliteal arteries. In addition after aortic surgery the adjacent aorta may eventually become aneurysmal or anastomotic arterial aneurysms can occur. Aortic aneurysm is also associated with the presence of atherosclerotic occlusive disease elsewhere; most importantly in the coronary, carotid or cerebral vasculature.

It has been claimed by some that the life expectation of patients who have had successful emergency or elective aortic aneurysm surgery is comparable to that of a normal population of the same age. For the reasons outlined above such claims are not credible. The few long-term follow-up data available point to the annual all-cause mortality after recovering from aortic aneurysm surgery being around twice that expected for the general population of the same age and gender.

Dissection of the aorta

Aortic dissection occurs when blood from the true aortic lumen enters the media of the arterial wall through an intimal breach and tracks distally creating an additional 'false' aortic lumen. Patients are usually younger than those with aortic aneurysms and specific connective tissue disorders are more common.

Classification and pathology

Earlier more complex classifications have given way to the present description of two main types of dissection.

Type A dissections account for two-thirds of cases. They begin in the ascending aorta, usually the anterior wall and may involve the aortic arch and occlude brachiocephalic, carotid or subclavian arteries. Retrograde dissection into the aortic root producing aortic valve incompetence and coronary artery occlusion or into the pericardium with cardiac tamponade are common fatal outcomes.

Type B dissections begin in the descending thoracic aorta beyond the aortic arch vessel origins, usually in the posterior wall.

The primary pathology is a degeneration of the medial layer of the aortic wall, 'cystic medial necrosis'. A breach in the intima occurs at the main shear stress points in the thoracic aorta caused by cardiac motion and directional changes in blood flow. The intimal breach is predisposed to by atheromatous plaques, subintimal hemorrhage and arterial hypertension.

Clinical presentation

The patient classically presents with sudden onset severe central chest pain which rapidly moves posteriorly into the back of the chest. The change in location of pain is an important differentiating symptom from myocardial infarction with which it is commonly confused. Pain may later migrate to the lumbar region as the dissection progresses.

Associated clinical features that more certainly point to the diagnosis are caused by partial, intermittent or complete occlusion of major arteries arising from the aorta to which the dissection has progressed. The commonest of these are acute lower limb ischemia and stroke but intestinal infarction, renal infarction, paraplegia and loss of upper limb pulses are not infrequent. Occasionally cerebral or spinal ischemic symptoms may be transient and limb pulses which were absent may return as the dissection progresses either because of distal intimal re-entry of the dissection or by the establishment of flow from the false lumen.

Management

The diagnosis can be confirmed by contrast enhanced computed tomography or in specialist units by transesophageal colour Duplex sonography. Early differentiation from myocardial infarction is essential since the administration of thrombolytic therapy, for example streptokinase, may facilitate progression of the dissection and precipitate a fatal outcome.

In all patients the systolic blood pressure should be reduced acutely to 100 mmHg or the lowest level compatible with perfusion of vital organs. For patients with type B dissections who have no arterial ischemic symptoms and for stable type A dissections presenting weeks after the onset, medical therapy may be all that is necessary.

Visceral or limb artery occlusion dictate urgent surgery to secure revascularization if death or permanent disability are to be avoided. Major stroke is generally regarded as an absolute contraindication to surgical intervention because of the risks of causing fatal hemorrhage into infarcted brain. Mesenteric ischemia has the worst prognosis for all arterial occlusions since diagnosis is often delayed until extensive intestinal infarction has occurred.

Most patients with type A dissections are now best treated by surgery to the ascending aorta. The objectives of intervention are to fix the intima in the distal ascending aorta to the other layers of the arterial wall and to prevent retrograde dissection into the aortic valve and coronary artery origins. Sometimes replacement of the aortic root with reimplantation of coronary arteries is required.

Prognosis

The outlook for patients with acute aortic dissection has been greatly improved in recent years by early diagnosis, intensive medical therapy and appropriate surgery. Long-term survival is improved by rigorous control of hypertension. Some patients will go on to develop progressive aneurysmal dilatation of the thoracic or abdominal aorta that may require elective aortic replacement.

17. Diseases of the arteries of the upper limb

MICHELE COSPITE, FILIPPO FERRARA and VALENTINA COSPITE

In 1961 Reivich et al. [1] described for the first time a syndrome caused by steno-occluding pathological processes involving the subclavian artery proximal to the emergence of the ipsilateral vertebral artery, and characterized by the activation of specific collateral pathways of the ascending aorta; that same year Fisher et al. [2] named it 'subclavian steal syndrome'. In this case the subclavian artery, stenosed or occluded at the origin, is supplied with blood from the ipsilateral vertebral artery with a reverse flow direction [3]. This allows valid compensation for hemodynamic disorders in the brachial area, at the expense, however, of the encephalic region from which blood diverted to the subclavian artery is subtracted. This phenomenon was first noted in 1886 [4], after a subclavian artery ligation for a traumatic aneurysm: the vertebral artery was ligated and the patient survived ten years. Later contributions on this subject have not only shown that subclavian steal syndrome is a reliable indicator of severe subclavian artery stenosis, though the syndrome itself is relatively benign, but have also provided a more detailed etiological framework showing that alongside arteritic, traumatic, congenital and iatrogenic forms exist others – which occur more frequently – of atherosclerotic origin [5] (Table 17.1).

Physiopathology

From a hemodynamic point of view, subclavian steal syndrome is characterized by the following physiopathological conditions [3]:

- Occlusion or stenosis of a subclavian artery before the origin of the vertebral artery. This is a condition *sine qua non*; if the occlusion involves the origin of the vertebral artery or is situated beyond this point, the perfusion of the subclavian artery by means of the vertebral artery could not occur, that is, the physiopathological fulcrum of the syndrome.
- Patency of the homolateral vertebral artery, or at least of its tract closer to the obstructed subclavian artery. In the case of high obstruction of the homolateral vertebral artery, a low recovery of the subclavian artery is in fact possible at inverted flow through the thyro-cervical trunk or anastomotic intervertebral branches.
- Subtraction of arterial blood from the cerebral circulation. The stolen blood is introduced retrogressively into the vertebral artery of the damaged side, coming

Table 17.1. Diseases leading to subclavian steal syndrome.

Intravascular pathologies
Inflammatory arteritis
Nodose polyarteritis
Thromboangitis obliterans
Horton's arteritis
Takayasu's arteritis

Infectious arteritis
Tuberculotic arteritis
Syphilitic arteritis
Rheumatoid arteritis

Embryogenetic disorders
Ascending aorta anomalies
Fibro-muscular dysplasia

Degenerative atherosclerotic arteriopathy

Extravascular pathologies
Clotting thrombogenic disorders
Cardiac embolism
Mediastinal trauma or neoplastic masses

both from the circle of Willis and, to a greater extent, directly from the contralateral vertebral artery.
– Introduction of stolen blood into the subclavian artery, below the occluded segment, in correspondence with the origin of the ipsilateral vertebral artery (Figure 17.1).

This hemodynamic situation implies several fundamental consequences:

– A possible ischemia in the territory supplied by the stenotic or obstructed subclavian artery, less than the extent of anatomical damage would imply. In other words, the functional impotence and trophic disorders of the upper limb are, in these particular patients, considerably milder than those observed in patients with obstruction – or with stenosis to the same extent – of the subclavian artery distal to or on a level with the origin of the vertebral artery. Indeed, in these latter patients, excluding the vertebral artery from the collateral circulations, the other sources of blood supply are much less efficient.
– There can be a paradoxical implication of disorders of the compromised limb. In fact, contrary to that normally observed in arteriopathics without this hemodynamic peculiarity (in whom the disorders are accentuated by exercising the limb concerned), in subclavian steal syndrome, at least in some cases, the disorders (paresthesia, cold skin, pallor of the limb) are more frequent and intense when at rest, and instead they fade or even disappear with muscular exercise. This occurs as exercising of the compromised limb activates, through a 'siphoning' mechanism, the collateral circulation. Muscular exercising, in fact, provokes local vessel dilatation with consequent reduction of district arteriole resistances; thus the 're-

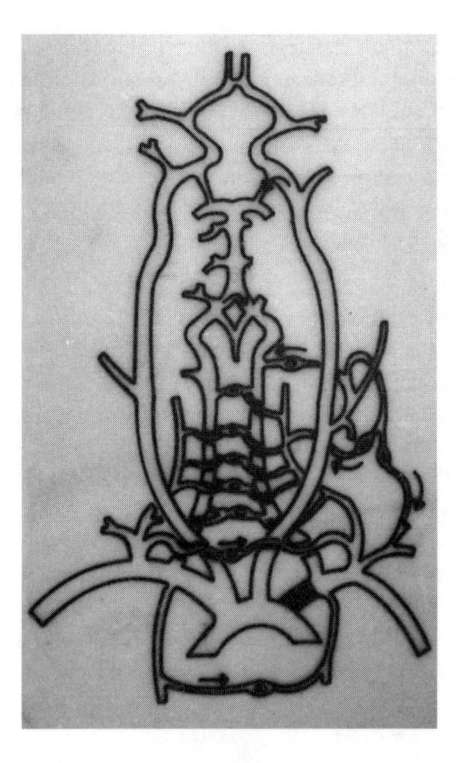

Figure 17.1. Illustration of subclavian steal syndrome.

sistance gradient' increases between the cephalic territory on one hand, and brachial territory on the other, and this induces a proportional increase in the blood flow to this latter territory.
– There are ischemic disorders of the cerebral territory, greater than the anatomical conditions of the vessels would imply. In fact, if the hemodynamic disorder in the vascular area is reduced to a lack in supply of arterial blood through the vertebral artery of the damaged side (as would happen in the case of obstruction of the subclavian artery in correspondence with the origin of the vertebral artery), the cerebral circulatory disorders would be very slight or probably absent altogether. In subclavian steal syndrome, however, the vertebral artery not only does not supply, but subtracts blood, to a considerable degree, from the basilar trunk, especially when accompanied by lesions of the carotid vessels, incapable of producing effective hemodynamic compensation. This explains therefore, how these patients show signs of cerebral circulatory disorders – dizziness, lipothymia, amaurosis fugax, etc. – even if only temporary, which are more imposing than those of the upper limb, which can become accentuated during muscular exercise of the limb itself.

It seems that the cerebral circulatory disorders are less acute than the extent of subtraction of blood could imply. This is due to a concomitant increase in flow to the brain through the other arterial trunks: the vertebral artery and contralateral carotids. It is documented by the radiological observations of an increase in diameter of the vertebral artery contralateral to the lesion, experimental research on dogs [1] and Doppler observations.

Alongside this 'paradigmatical' physiopathological situation exist others in which the stenotic or obstructive lesion affects the innominate artery. In these cases the involvment of the carotid vessels assumes the following hemodynamic variations [6]:

1. *Innominate syndrome*
   This comes about when the lesion involves the innominate artery up to the origin of the common carotid artery, which is occluded. The distinguishing hemodynamic elements are, therefore, ischemia of the carotid artery and subclavian steal syndrome. Cerebral supply is assured from the contralateral common carotid artery, that of the upper limb from activation of the vertebral–vertebral circulation (Figure 17.2).
2. *Innominate steal syndrome*
   This occurs when the lesion is limited to the proximal tract of the innominate artery, and so the common carotid artery is duly patent. Two hemodynamic variations can be seen:
   – Innominate steal syndrome with recovery of the carotid artery. In this case, the hemodynamic compensation is assured by the system of vertebral arter-

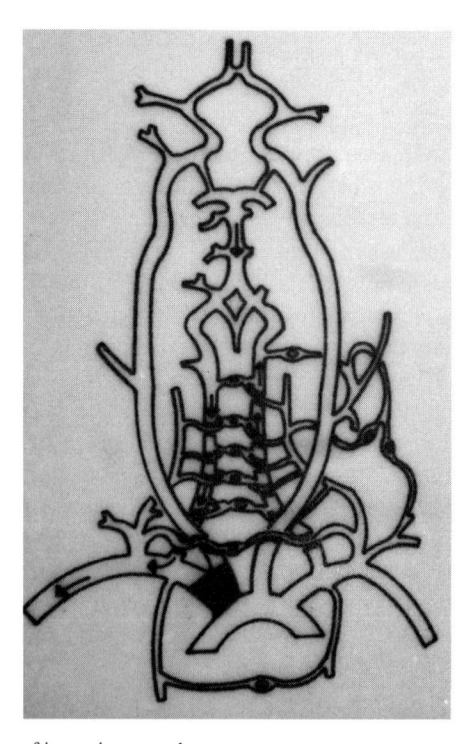

Figure 17.2. Illustration of innominate syndrome.

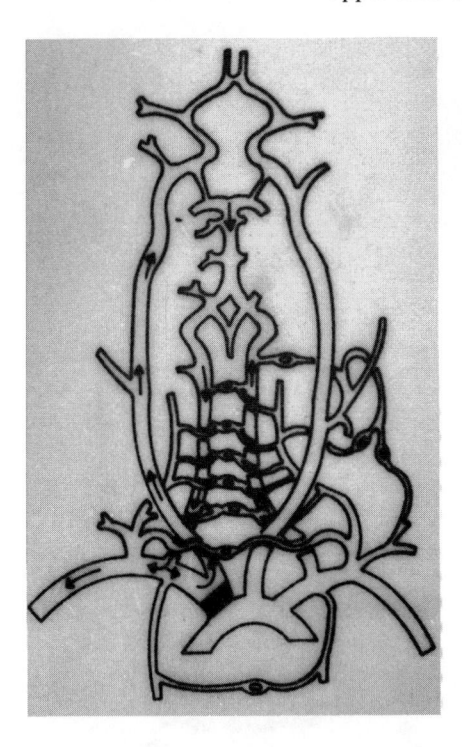

Figure 17.3. Illustration of innominate steal syndrome with recovery of the carotid artery.

ies through activation of the vertebral–vertebral circulation with antidromic flow in the ipsilateral vertebral artery to the lesion. The blood, reaching the origin of the vertebral artery, is distributed equally between the subclavian artery and the common carotid artery which is 'recovered' through the pre-vertebral subclavian artery and the patent tract of the innominate artery, where the blood flows in an antidromic manner (Figure 17.3).

– Innominate steal syndrome with flow inversion of the carotid artery. Hemodynamic compensation is assured both from the vertebrals and the carotids and is exclusively aimed at the blood supply of the upper limb. In this case, alongside the vertebral– vertebral circulation, the left common carotid–left internal carotid–anterior communicating–right internal carotid–right common carotid–right subclavian circulation is activated, with antidromic flow on the common and internal carotid homolaterals to the lesion (Figure 17.4).

In the outline of the aforementioned hemodynamic variations, the determining element is represented by the vascular resistance of the circle of Willis. In fact if these resistances are lower than those of the territory of the subclavian artery, the first variation comes about (subclavian steal syndrome with recovery of the carotid artery); if, however, they are higher, the second variation occurs (subclavian steal syndrome with flow inversion on the carotid artery).

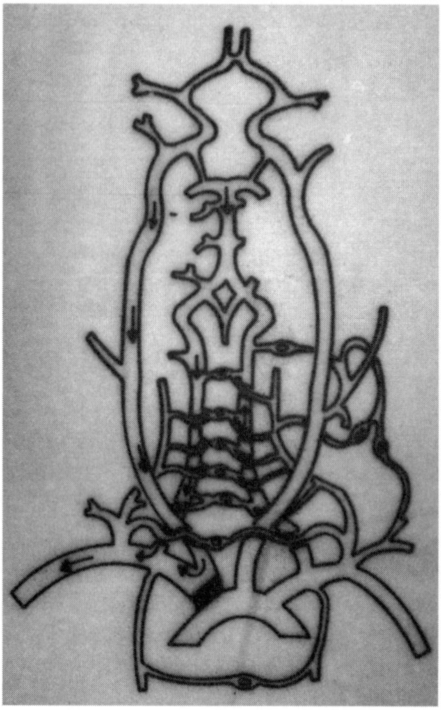

Figure 17.4. Illustration of subclavian steal phenomenon with inversion of the carotid artery.

There also exist rarer collateral circulations which intervene when the lesion of the subclavian artery or the innominate artery is accompanied by stenosis, more or less significative of the origin of the vertebral artery. In such cases:

- blood can be diverted to the subclavian artery from the external carotid artery through the upper and lower thyroid arteries;
- blood from the external carotid artery can reach the subclavian artery through the occipital artery, the deep cervical artery and the transversal artery of the neck;
- blood to the subclavian artery passes from the external carotid artery through the branches of the occipital artery and muscular branches of the vertebral artery;
- blood flows from the external iliac artery to the subclavian artery through the lower epigastric artery, the upper epigastric artery and the internal mammary artery;
- blood flows from the thoracic aorta to the subclavian artery and the axillary artery, through the intercostal branches of the internal mammary, the upper intercostal and the lateral thoracic arteries;
- blood flows from the contralateral subclavian artery through the vertebral–vertebral circulation;

- blood flows from the contralateral subclavian artery through the intervertebral branches;
- blood flows from the contralateral subclavian artery through the contralateral internal mammary artery, the intermammary branches and the homolateral internal mammary artery.

Sometimes there can be an association of collateral circulations and this mostly occurs with the vertebral–vertebral circulation, combined with the carotid–basilar, the intervertebral, the intermammary and the interthyrocervical anastomotic branches.

It is on the other hand useful to point out that in stenosis or occlusion of the innominate artery, the cerebral flow is steadily reduced, while in subclavian steal syndrome, two hemodynamic situations can form:

- subclavian steal syndrome without encephalic steal: occurs when the carotid vessels are functionally whole and therefore able to provide for, through a flow increase, the subtraction of blood from the vertebral circulation.
- subclavian steal syndrome with encephalic steal: occurs when the lesion at the level of the subclavian artery is accompanied by carotid alterations to the extent of preventing a compensatory increase in cerebral blood flow.

Finally, depending on the extent of stenosis of the subclavians and common trunk, we can also distinguish [7]:

- Intermittent steal: occurs due to severe but not full stenosis of the subclavian artery above the origin of the vertebral artery. Flow at vertebral level is directed normally toward the encephalic area during diastole and early systole. In the mid-systolic phase there is a reduction with subsequent complete flow inversion. This depends on the fact that the existing pressure difference between the vertebral artery origin reaches the level necessary for flow reversal in the vertebral artery only during systole. This type of steal is recognizable, in basal conditions, from Doppler ultrasonographic reports of subclavian artery stenosis and biphasic morphology – negative systolic and positive diastolic velocity – of vertebral artery pulse curve. Compression of the subclavian artery distal to the vertebral artery normalizes these reports due to the quantity of blood diverted to that vessel.
- Latent steal: characteristic of lesions which cause a reduction in vessel diameter of around 30% in which flow inversion is seen only after prolonged and intensive exercise of the upper limb and only in cardiac systole.

In addition, even rarer possibilities of hemodynamic compensation should be mentioned, which occur when the vertebral artery, due to embryogenetical disorders, originates directly from the aortic arch. In these cases, due to the concomitant presence of subclavian artery stenosis, activation of the vertebral–vertebral circulation is impossible; instead, a 'homolateral steal' occurs, supported by the vertebral–thyrocervical trunk circulation (Figure 17.5). The blood flows normally (forward direction) in the vertebral artery homolateral to the lesion, and through the occipital artery (branch of the same vertebral artery), is diverted in the thyrocervical trunk,

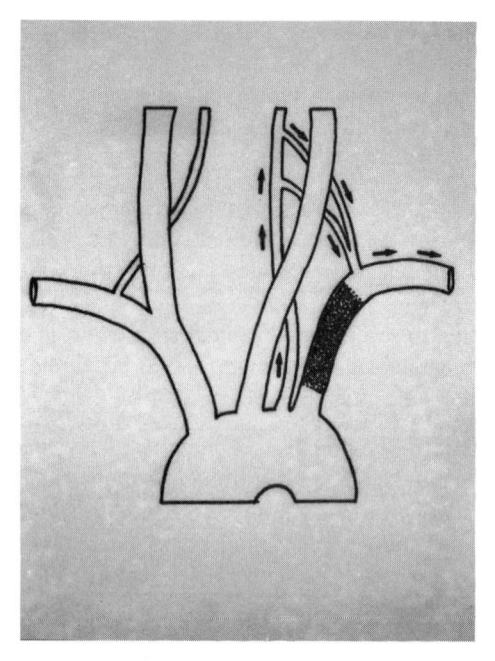

Figure 17.5. Illustration of vertebral–subclavian homolateral steal syndrome.

from which it supplies the homolateral subclavian artery in an antidromic direction (Figure 17.6).

All the above-mentioned variations have a different influence on cerebral flow and therefore a different expression on a clinical level. Indeed, while subclavian steal syndrome without encephalic steal can remain 'silent' on a clinical level for a long time, the syndromes with encephalic steal and all the syndromes involving the innominate artery cause the onset of numerous symptoms and cerebral signs, the most frequent being mental fatigue, confusion, irritability, loss of memory, equilibrium diorders, fading vision, diplopia, photopsy and scotoma.

Diagnosis

The clinical signs which can be found in a case of stenosis of a subclavian artery or innominate artery are:

- An audible systolic murmur at the level of the supraclavicular fossa, which is absent, however, in the complete occlusion of the vessel.
- A systolic blood pressure difference between the arms (equal to or greater than 20 mmHg), corresponding to a reduction in width of the sphygmic wave, noticeable also in the palpation of the radial pulse.
- In some cases it is also possible to find a murmur in the retromastoid region homolateral to the lesion or, much more rarely, in both the retromastoid regions after muscular exercise of the upper limb.

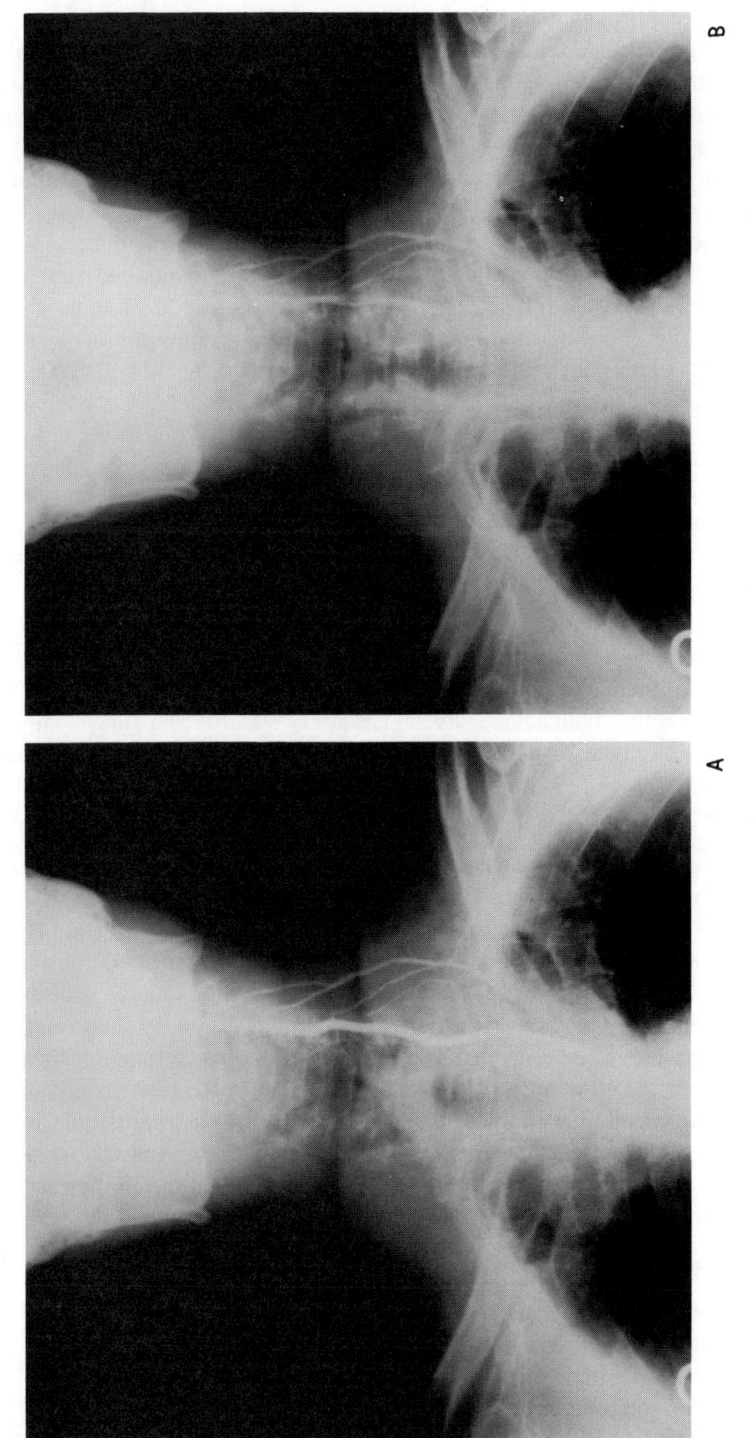

Figure 17.6. Vertebral–subclavian 'homolateral steal' syndrome. Selected photogram from selective arteriography of the left vertebral artery: (a) anomalous origin of the left vertebral artery from the aortic arch; (b) delayed supply to the left subclavian artery from a vertebral–thyrocervical trunk circulation (antidromic flow direction).

The diagnostic confirmation of subclavian steal syndrome can, however, occur only through angiographic and ultrasonographic tests. With the arteriographic technique it is possible to document both the proximal level of the lesion and reversal of flow in the homolateral vertebral artery. To this end the angiographic test should be carried out in two distinct phases: first of all with a thoracic aortography (aortic arch injection in its ascending part at pressure 4–5 atm.) to locate the obstruction; immediately afterwards with a selective arteriography (injection at manual pressure). This latter method also establishes the extent of the obstruction in cases of subclavian steal syndrome by injecting retrogressively the supplied subclavian artery as well to the distal limit of the obstruction itself (Figure 17.7). In the case of stenosis or obliteration of the innominate artery, angiography allows a correct assessment of the extent of the lesion and identification of different collateral circulations (Figures 17.8 and 17.9)

Recently, with new ultrasonographic techniques we have also gained more information on the different ways in which collateral circulations are activated [7, 8]. These tests are carried out in basal conditions – morphological criteria – and after appropriate activation maneuvers – dynamic criteria – involving the application of a blood pressure cuff to the arm homolateral to the arterial stenosis, in order to ascertain changes in resistances of the same limb: the cuff is inflated to a pressure of around 40–50 mmHg higher than humeral systolic pressure of the patient, left in place for about two minutes – the patient exercises the homolateral hand during the last minute of occlusion – and then rapidly deflated. They are reliable methods for detecting both severe subclavian artery stenosis and subclavian steal syndrome; the intermediate stages can also be detected with specificity and sensitivity of almost 100%.

The morphological criteria of subclavian steal syndrome are:

– At the level of the subclavian artery: in the case of complete occlusion, slowing down with morphological modifications of the curve above the lesion, absence of flow in the occluded tract and pressure drop below the obstruction; in the case of stenosis, turbulent flow below with morphological alterations of the curve – which appears more reduced in width the more the stenosis is occluded.
– At the level of the vertebral artery homolateral to the lesion: the sound and relative velocity curves assume characteristics similar to those found on the subclavian artery, as flow runs in retrograde direction. In the case of intermittent steal, the vertebral artery flow runs retrogressively only during systole, so the initial part of the curve will be below the baseline and the end part above. In the case of latent steal there may not be any significant alterations in the curves of the vertebrals.

The hemodynamic criteria of subclavian steal syndrome are:

– In the case of complete steal: evidence of diastolic flow on the homolateral and contralateral vertebral arteries on decompression of the cuff, the greater the extent of blood steal, the faster the speed (Figure 17.10).
– In the case of intermittent flow: variations in flow directions in the basal condition (Figure 17.11) and appearance of diastolic flow on decompression of the cuff to a lower extent than usually seen in complete steal.

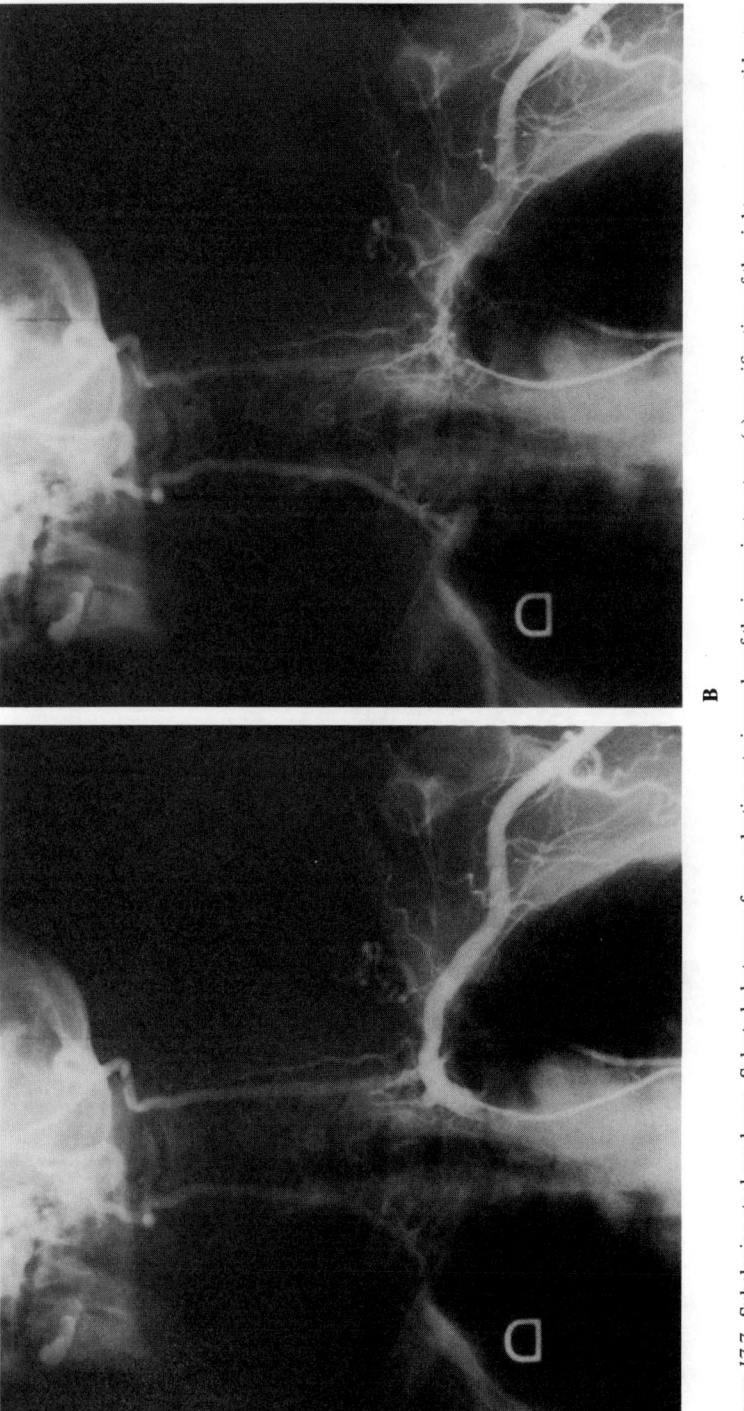

Figure 17.7. Subclavian steal syndrome. Selected photogram from selective arteriography of the innominate artery; (a) opacification of the right common carotid artery, right subclavian artery and right vertebral artery with evidence of the first segment of the contralateral vertebral artery; (b) complete opacification of the left vertebral artery which supplies, at inverted flow, the left subclavian artery.

Figure 17.8. Innominate syndrome. Selected photogram from selective arteriography of the left subclavian artery: (a) opacification of the left subclavian artery and first segment of the homolateral vertebral artery; (b) complete opacification of the vertebral artery; (c) opacification of the left vertebral artery, which supplies, at inverted flow, the subclavian artery.

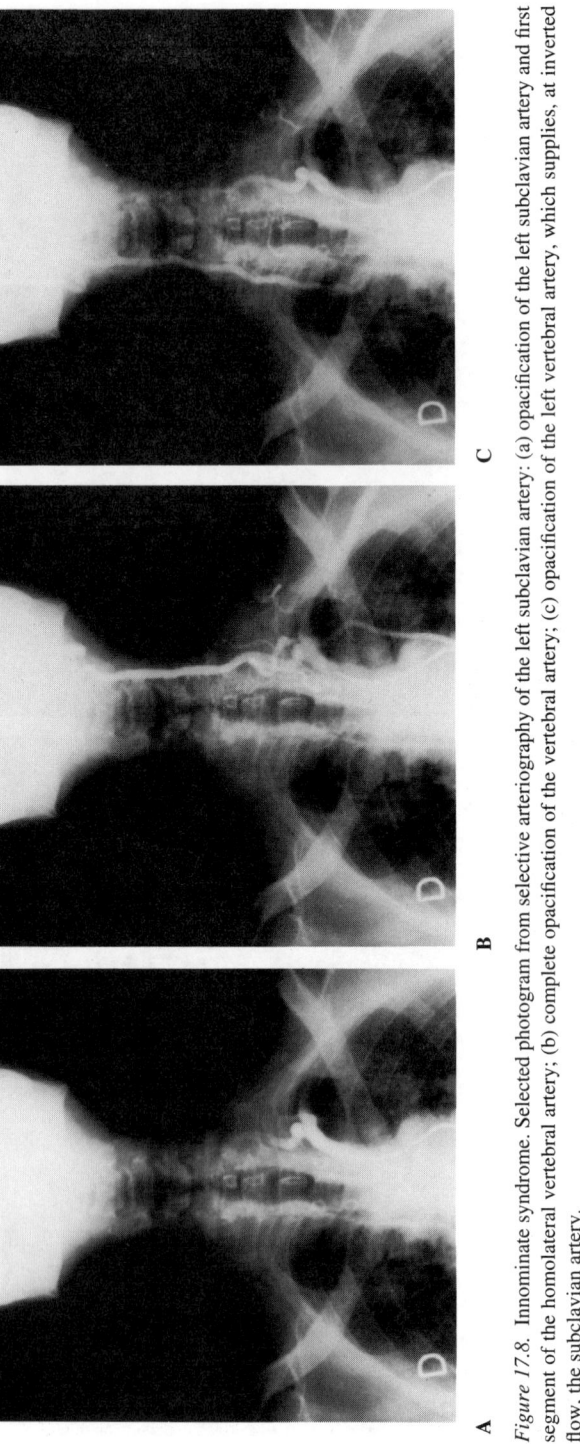

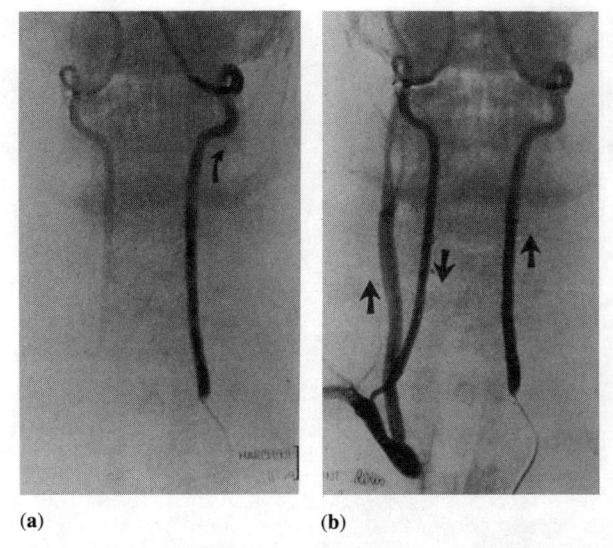

Figure 17.9. Innominate steal syndrome with recovery of the carotid artery. Selected photogram from selective arteriography of the left vertebral artery: (a) opacification of the left vertebral artery (arrow above) and first segment of the right vertebral artery; (b) opacification of the left vertebral artery, right vertebral artery, which re-channels, at inverted flow (arrow below) the subclavian artery, the innominate artery and the right common carotid artery (arrow above).

- In the case of latent steal: appearance of intermittent steal after decompression of the cuff (Figure 17.12).

These analyses are completed with the curves of the common and internal carotid arteries during the reactive hyperemia test. This allows evaluation of the efficiency of the carotid–vertebral circulation to the upper limb. In fact if we find an increase in velocity in the carotids similar to that found on the vertebrals, the quantity of blood subtracted from the brain by the latter is entirely compensated by the carotid circulation – subclavian steal syndrome without encephalic steal. If at the level of the carotids there is no increase in velocity, or if there is increase but lower than that of the vertebrals, the carotid circulation cannot assure the upkeep of a normal cerebral hematic perfusion – subclavian steal syndrome with encephalic steal.

For the innominate steal syndrome, the morphological criteria are:

- At the level of the subclavian artery homolateral to the lesion: a morphological modified curve with loss of the diastolic reflow and reduction in diastolic velocity.
- At the level of the vertebrals: the curves recorded both at the origin and at Tillaux are more or less identical to those recorded on the subclavians.
- At the level of the carotids (Figure 17.13): on the left, the curves show systolic velocity only, increased due to preferential flow; on the right, on the common and internal carotids, the curves are inverted due to retrograde flow direction – in this case, the blood, coming from the left common carotid artery through the internal carotid and the anterior communicating arteries, goes to supply the

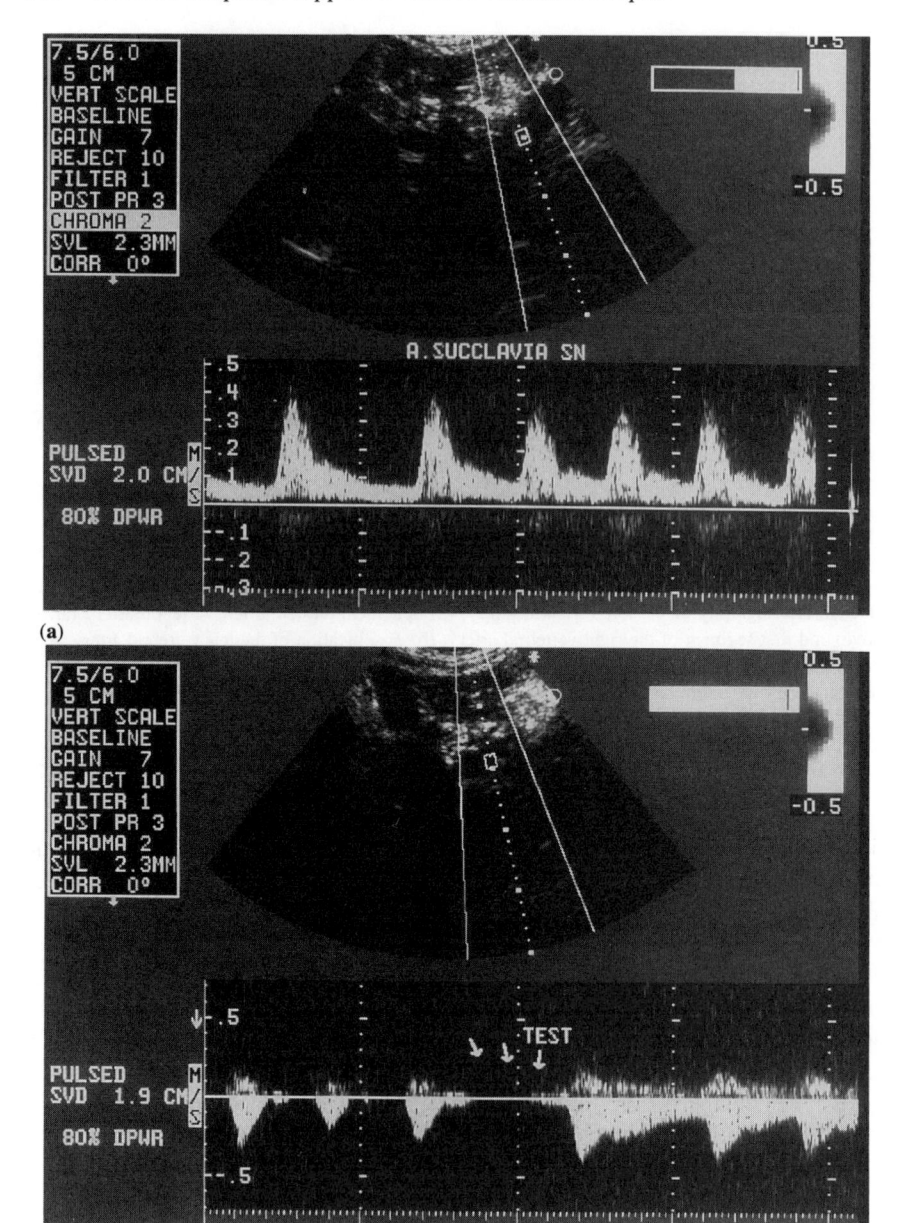

Figure 17.10. Vertebral–subclavian complete steal syndrome. Ecodoppler survey: (a) tight stenosis of left subclavian artery at the origin; (b) inverted flow on homolateral vertebral artery with marked increase in diastolic speed on decompression of the cuff (after dynamic test).

right internal carotid artery and common carotid artery, which in turn supply the prevertebral subclavian artery: this is a typical example of innominate steal syndrome with inversion of the carotid artery; on the external carotid artery and

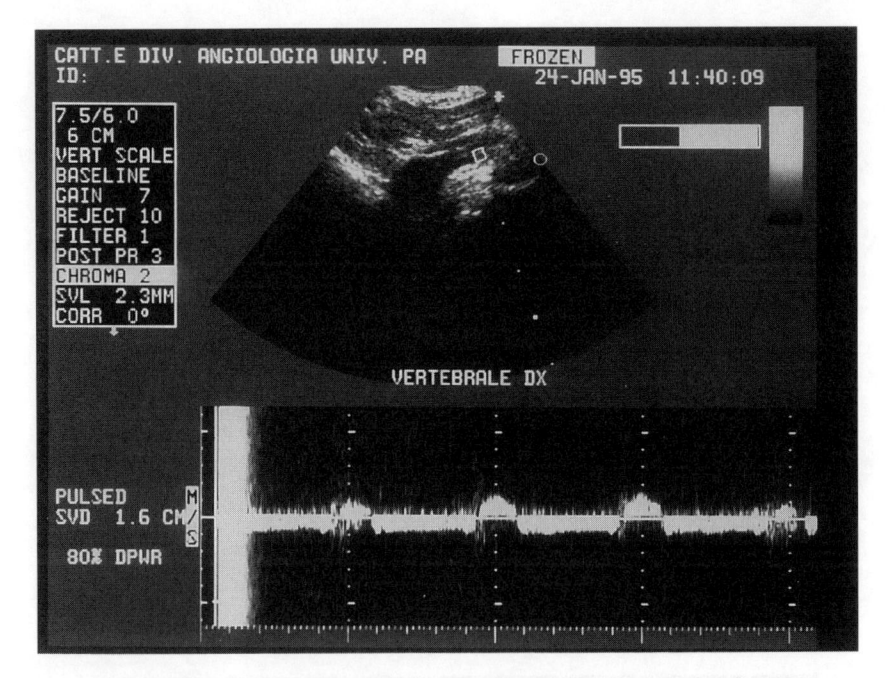

Figure 17.11. Intermittent vertebral–subclavian steal syndrome. Variations in flow direction, in the basal condition, in proportion to cardiac cycle.

ophthalmic artery, the curves show morphological modifications, but with normal flow direction (it should be remembered that the ophthalmic is rechanneled directly from the contralateral internal carotid artery through the anterior communicating artery; the external carotid artery can be rechanneled through the internal carotid artery or through vertebral–occipital circulation).

In innominate steal syndrome with recovery of the carotid artery, the trend of the Doppler curves, as regards the homolaterals subclavian artery and the vertebral artery, will be similar to that normally observed in subclavian steal syndrome, while on the homolateral common internal and external carotid arteries curves morphologically changed are obtained, decidedly reduced in width, in retrograde direction; this is an expression of the considerable slowing down in the speed of flow.

Finally, in innominate syndrome there will be no trace of flow at the level of common, internal and external carotid arteries homolateral to the lesion, while at the level of the vertebral artery and subclavian artery, Doppler behavior will be superimposable on that obtained in the case of subclavian steal syndrome.

The dynamic criteria in innominate steal syndrome with inversion of the carotid artery are:

– At the level of the subclavian artery and right vertebral artery: appearance of diastolic flow on decompression of the cuff, a sign of torrential flow in the subclavian artery below the occlusion.

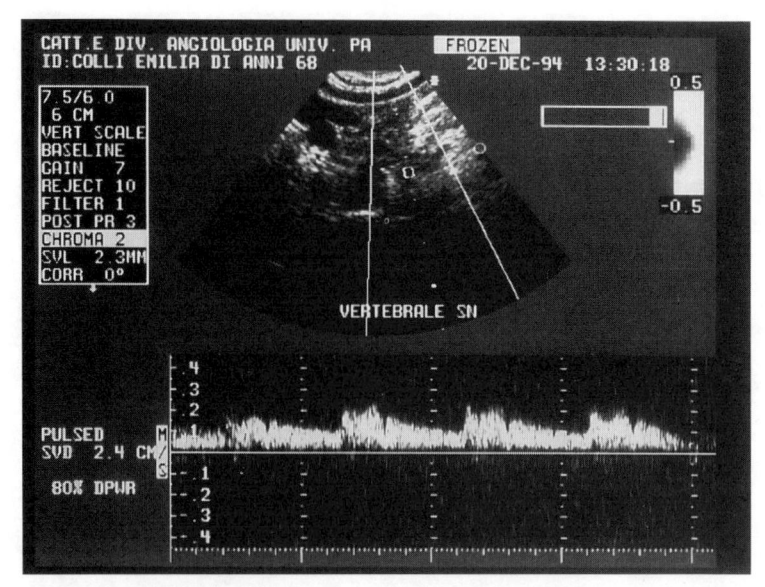

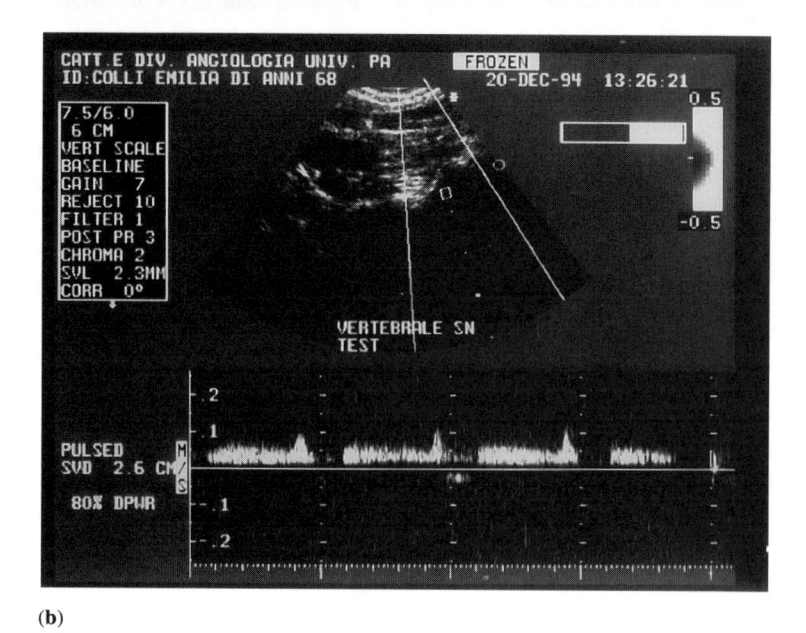

Figure 17.12. Latent vertebral–subclavian steal syndrome. (a) Anterograde flow of left vertebral artery in basal conditions. (b) After dynamic test, evidence of intermittent flow.

– At the level of the right carotid artery, on inflating the cuff, inversion of flow direction, a sign of increase in resistance abruptly induced by the cuff itself. The blood, with inverted flow in the vertebral artery, instead of flowing into the

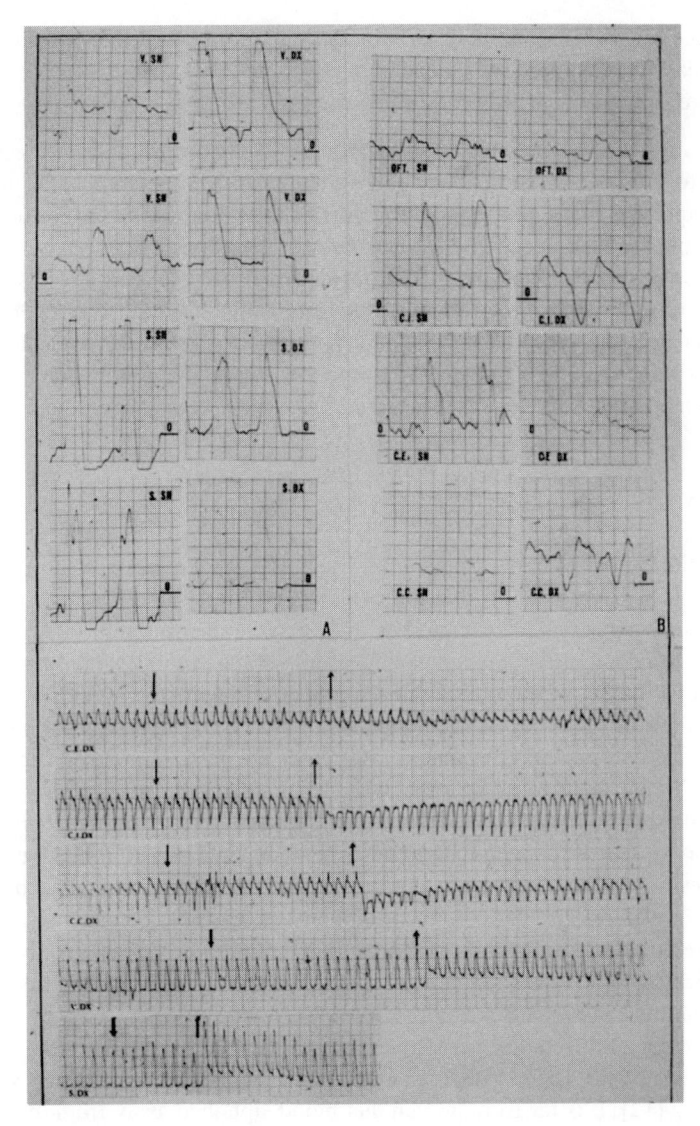

Figure 17.13. Continuous wave Doppler survey of the innominate steal syndrome with flow inversion of the carotid artery. Morphological criteria: right common carotid artery and right internal carotid artery curves; morphological alterations of the subclavian artery and vertebral artery curves. Dynamic criteria: after dynamic maneuvers of the upper limb, compression of the cuff (arrow below); decompression of the cuff (arrow above) evidence of diastolic flow in all vessels except external carotid artery.

post-vertebral subclavian artery, flows into the pre-vertebral and consequently the common carotid artery: that is the transformation of the inversion of the carotid phenomenon to recovery of the carotid; decompression revives the phenomenon of inversion of the carotid and causes an increase in diastolic flow.

- At the level of the internal carotid artery the most evident phenomenon is an increase in diastolic flow on decompression.
- There is no effect at the level of the external carotid.

In innominate steal syndrome and innominate syndrome dynamic criteria are similar to those described for vertebral–subclavian steal syndrome in that, as we have frequently mentioned, the carotid vessels are not involved in the supply of the upper limb, the task assigned exclusively to the vertebral system.

Further information can be gained through the use of Ecodoppler systems [9] which not only confirm the results of the tests with continuous wave Doppler, but also establish the morphological characteristics of the obstructing plaques and, above all, allow a more detailed study of the origin of the homolateral vertebral artery where associated lesions often occur.

Therapy

Obstruction of the proximal subclavian artery is a quite common but in most cases symptomless disease. A striking preponderance of left-sided lesions was found in several reported series of studies [10]. This may be due to the more acute angle at the point of origin of the left subclavian artery, which produces more turbulences, a well-known factor facilitating the development of atherosclerotic lesions. The rich collateral circulations around the subclavian artery and between the anterior and posterior cerebral circulations are in most cases adequate to compensate the hemodynamic impairment from the subclavian lesion, even during exercise. Symptoms of vascular insufficiency of the cerebral and brachial circulation are therefore often secondary or at least concomitant to other hemodynamically significant extracranial vessel lesions or facilitated by anatomical variations that cause a reduced efficiency of these collateral circulations [11] (as many as 20–30% of patients have an incomplete circle of Willis and consequently are able to compensate only partially). According to some recent studies examining the short and long-term results of surgical treatment in patients suffering from obstructive disease of the proximal subclavian artery of different severity, there are no correlations between the anatomical progression of the lesions, their hemodynamic consequences and the severity of symptoms [12]. It is far from proven that blood siphoned away from the brainstem by arm exercise produces ischemic symptoms, and subclavian steal syndrome may represent only a harmless hemodynamic phenomenon causing, at worst, minor vertebrobasilar transient ischemic attacks. As a result, not only the blood diversion from one territory to another but also the instability of blood perfusion-pressure, particularly in the brainstem areas, where the autoregulation system is less efficient than in the hemispheres, are responsible for vertebral blood insufficiency [13, 14].

The therapy for obstructive lesions of the subclavian artery and innominate artery consists of different surgical procedures with the aim of reproducing the complete patency of the blood flow and to avoid any worsening of the disease. A careful clinical examination and the results of invasive and non-invasive diagnostic procedures, recorded above, enable the surgeon to evaluate properly which kind of patients might obtain the best results from revascularization of the upper limb main arteries.

The etiology of subclavian steal syndrome seldom represents a fundamental factor in the choice of surgical therapy. For example, Takayasu's arteritis, due to its evolutive characteristics, has only a rare surgical indication. Aneurysms and arterial venous fistulae, on the other hand, need generally and absolutely a surgical treatment. Congenital and traumatic lesions of the upper limb arteries, should be managed surgically only if symptomatic and therefore hemodynamically significant.

Several of the most employed surgical techniques for the treatment of subclavian steal syndrome can be divided according to type of access (Table 17.2).

Table 17.2. Surgical management of subclavian steal syndrome.

Transthoracic access
Subclavian thromboendarterectomy
Subclavian thromboendarterectomy with patch
Aorto–subclavian bypass

Extrathoracic access
Carotid–subclavian bypass
Subclavian–carotid transposition
Axillo–axillary bypass
Subclavian–subclavian bypass

Subclavian percutaneous transluminal angioplasty

There has been an evolution in the surgical approach to subclavian insufficiency, beginning with transthoracic procedures, such as thrombo-endarterectomy (TEA) of the innominate artery occlusion, described by Davis et al. [15] in 1956 and the use of a graft to bypass an occluded innominate artery and right common carotid artery in 1957 by DeBakey et al. [16].

At present, various therapeutic approaches are available, including transthoracic *in situ* repairs, extrathoracic procedures and the most recent method of percutaneous transluminal angioplast (PTA).

Nearly all vascular surgeons only operate on patients with symptoms of arm ischemia or disabling cerebral symptoms; doubts remain about which procedure should be performed [17]. When only limb symptoms are present, revascularization of the subclavian artery is the correct treatment. However, when cerebral symptoms are dominant and there is concomitant carotid artery disease, it is not well-established if the restoration of anterograde vertebral artery blood flow on its own improves vertebral symptoms or, on the other hand, if carotid TEA, without subclavian revascularization, is sufficient to eliminate transient ischemic attacks [18]. According to the literature, many surgeons focus their attention on only one vascular system, often disregarding the other [19–22]. The results of this approach have not always been encouraging, whereas a combined subclavian and carotid approach is to be preferred in patients whose brachial and cerebral circulations are compromised.

Extrathoracic approach has now widely replaced transthoracic access, which became unpopular as a result of the high morbidity and mortality rates reported in several follow-up studies [23, 24]. Procedures that avoid any kind of transthoracic approach are quicker, safer and as effective. Two similar and frequently used procedures are carotid–subclavian bypass and subclavian–carotid transposition. Both methods employ a supraclavicular approach to the proximal subclavian artery and the cross-clamping of the ipsilateral common carotid artery [25]. It could lead to potential risks of central neurological deficits; as a consequence, alternative forms of bypass grafting, such as axillo–axillary bypass, first reported by Myers *et al.* [26] in 1971, have been advocated. This offers distinct advantages [27] over the alternative procedures, already described, avoiding sternotomy, clavicular section and the 'carotid steal phenomenon' [28], a possible consequence of carotid–subclavian bypass, and is a simple, well-tolerated, effective and durable technique. Disadvantages of the axillo–axillary bypass include the potential for kinking across the pectoralis major muscle and the necessity to rearrange the graft in case of a subsequent sternotomy [27].

Subclavian PTA is a well-established treatment for patients with subclavian artery stenosis and brachial or cerebral symptoms [29]. The increasing use of PTA is reducing the number of candidates for surgery. Nevertheless, its efficacy for recanalizing a complete subclavian obstruction is not yet determined because of the too small number of treated patients and their relatively short mean follow-up period, and surgery remains mandatory in such cases. According to several authors [30], the improving technology over the last few years (digital subtraction angiography, more sophisticated guidewire, thinner diagnostic and dilatation catheters and stents) favored a more successful recanalization rate. In particular, stent placement is of considerable help in patients with residual stenosis of thrombotic material as it theoretically might diminish embolic debris by trapping it against the arterial wall [31]. Indications for subclavian PTA in asymptomatic patients should be carefully weighed, according to the presence or absence of other localizations of atherosclerotic disease; for example the treatment of asymptomatic subclavian stenosis in the case of axillary–femoral bypass or internal mammary bypass grafts is generally recommended, even if prognosis is worsened when combined lesions impair the carotid as well as the vertebral circulations. In the case of isolated subclavian artery stenosis with subclavian steal syndrome, the management remains controversial: the lack of absolute safety of PTA in such patients should emphasize that indications have to be very selective; on the other hand, in view of the higher surgical risk, if treatment is decided upon, angioplasty should be preferred to surgery [32].

Medical therapy has in general only few indications in subclavian steal syndrome, especially if an obstructive lesion has already formed. It is beneficial, however, in the treatment of aspecific inflammatory diseases involving the upper limb vessels, particularly during the initial period. When the subclavian artery lesion is caused by syphilis or TB the use of antibiotics is necessary. Vasodilator drugs are inefficacious and in some circumstances harmful, due to 'steal phenomena' secondary to their use and to the fact that the hypotension provoked by them could compromise the cerebral vascular circulation, already damaged. Antiplatelet drugs are widely used in secondary prevention, in order to avoid complication of obstructive vascular lesions and the spreading of the thrombotic process to other vascular districts (please refer to chapter 22 for more details).

References

1. Reivich M, Holling HE, Roberts B, Tode JF. Reversal of blood flow through the vertebral artery and its effect on cerebral circulation. N Engl J Med 1961;265:878–85.
2. Fisher CM. A new vascular syndrome 'the subclavian steal'. N Engl J Med 1961;265:912–3.
3. Cospite M, Palazzolo F, Geraci E. Considerazioni sulla fisiopatologia e sulla diagnostica della cosidetta 'subclavian steal'. Diag Ter 1965;7:225–38.
4. Smyth AW. Successful operation in a case of subclavian aneurysm. New Orleans Med Rec 1866;1:4–7.
5. Botta GC. Ricordi di eziologia ed anatomia patologica delle lesioni dei tronchisopraaortici. Atti Soc Ital Chir 1969;1:58–75.
6. Battezzati M, Belardi P, Becchi G, Cianfanelli G. Fisiopatologia del circolo brachiale dipendente. Atti Soc Ital Chir 1969;I:91–123.
7. Antignani PL, Amato B, De Fabritiis A, Laglia P, Poli L. Il doppler ad onda continua. GIUV (ed.). Torino: Centro Scientifico Torinese, 1985;46–57.
8. Pourcelot L, Ribadeau-Dumas JL, Fagret D, Planiol TH. Apport de l'examen doppler dans le diagnostic du vol sous-clavier. Rev Neurol 1977;133:309–23.
9. Erickson SJ, Mewissen MW, Foley WD et al. Color Doppler evaluation of arterial stenosis and occlusion involving the neck and thoracic inlet. Radiographics 1989;9(3):389–406.
10. Fields WS, Lemak NA. Joint study of extracranial arterial occlusion, VII. Subclavian steal – a review of 168 cases. J Am Med Assoc 1972;272:1139–43.
11. Bornstein N, Norris J. Subclavian steal: A harmless hemodynamic phenomenon? Lancet 1986;11:303–5.
12. Branchereau A, Magnan P, Espinoza H, Bartoli J. Subclavian artery stenosis: hemodynamic aspects. J Cardiovasc Surg 1991;32:604–12.
13. Yonas H, Steed DL, Latchaw RE, Gur D, Peitzman AB, Webster EW. Relief of nonhemispheric symptoms in low flow states by anterior circulation revascularization; a physiological approach. J Vasc Surg 1987;5:289–97.
14. Naritomi H, Sakay F, Meyer JS. Pathogenesis of transient ischemic attacks within the vertebrobasilar arterial system. Arch Neurol 1979;36:121–8.
15. Davis J, Grove W, Jiulian OC. Thrombic occlusion of the branches of the aortic arch, Martorell's syndrome. Ann Surg 1956;144:124–6.
16. De Bakey M, Morris G, Jordan G et al. Segmental thrombo-obliterative disease of branches of aortic arch. J Am Med Assoc 1958;166:988–96.
17. Criado FJ. Extrathoracic management of aortic arch syndrome. Br J Surg 1982;69(suppl): S45–51.
18. Mingoli A, Feldhaus R, Farina C, Naspetti R, Schultz R, Cavallaro A. Concomitant subclavian and carotid artery disease: The need for a combined surgical correction. J Cardiovasc Surg 1992;33:593–8.
19. Beebe H, Stark R, Johnon M, Jolly P, Hill L. Choices of operation for subclavian vertebral arterial disease. Am J Surg 1980;139:618–24.
20. Rosenthal D, Cossman D, Ledig CB, Collow AD. Results of carotid endarterectomy for vertebrobasilar insufficiency: An evaluation over ten years. Arch Surg 1978;113:1361–4.
21. Sandman W, Kniemeyer HW, Jaeschock R, Hnnerici M, Aulich A. The role of subclavian–carotid transposition in surgery for supra-aortic occlusive disease. J Vasc Surg 1987;5:53–8.
22. McNamara JO, Heyman A, Silver D et al. The value of carotid endarterectomy in treating transient cerebral ischemia of the posterior circulation. Neurology 1977;22:682–4.

23. Mannik JA. Extrathoracic operations for lesions of the vessels arising from the aortic arch. In: Greenhalgh RM (ed), Indications in vascular surgery. London: Saunders, 1988:63–9.
24. Crawford ES, Stowe CL, Powers RW Jr. Occlusion of the innominate, common carotid and subclavian arteries: Long term results of surgical treatment. Surgery 1983;94:781–91.
25. Kretschmer G, Teleky B, Marosi L et al. Obliterations of the proximal subclavian artery: To bypass or to anastomose? J Cardiovasc Surg 1991;32:334–9.
26. Myers WO, Lawton BR, Sautter RD. Axillo–axillary bypass graft. J Am Med Assoc 1971;217:826.
27. Weiner R, Deterling R, Sentissi J, O'Donnel T. Subclavian artery insufficiency. Arch Surg 1987;122:876–80.
28. Otis L, Rush M, Thomas M et al. Carotid steal syndrome following carotid subclavian bypass. J Vasc Surg 1984;1:649–52.
29. Duber C, Klose KJ, Kopp H, Schild H, Hake V. Angioplastie der arteria subclavia. Technik, fruh und spartergebuisse. Dtsch Med Wochenschr 1989;114:496–502.
30. Mathias K, Luth I, Haarmann P. Percutaneous transluminal angioplasty of proximal subclavian artery obclusion. Cardiovasc Intervent Radiol 1993;16:214–8.
31. Iannone L, Toom R, Le Master Rayl K, Percutaneous transluminal angioplasty of the innominate artery combined with carotid endarterectomy. Am Heart J 1993;126:1466–9.
32. Millaire A, Trinca M, Marache P, De Groote P, Jabnet JL, Duclan G. Subclavian angioplasty: Immediate and late results in 50 patients. Cathet Cardiovasc Diagn 1993;29:8–17.

18. Raynaud's syndrome

SHERRYL A. WAGSTAFF and MICHAEL J. GRIGG

Raynaud's syndrome presents a number of difficulties and confusions for primary care physicians. At least some of the 'mystique' of the condition is due to the changing nomenclature. In 1862, the year he received his medical degree in Paris, Maurice Raynaud published his inaugural thesis, 'Sur l'asphyyxia locale et la gangrene' [1], and henceforth the widely recognized clinical entity of extremity vasospasm became known as *Raynaud's disease*. Raynaud's original 25 patients exhibited digital gangrene despite the presence of palpable wrist pulses and Raynaud himself proposed that the underlying abnormality producing such severe vasospasm was sympathetic nerve overactivity. This theory held sway for almost a century but is incorrect. Not only do these patients not have systemic sympathetic overactivity but vasospasm alone does not result in digital gangrene.

In 1901, Hutchinson [2] recognized that a number of diverse conditions may manifest as digital ischemia e.g. atherosclerosis, scleroderma etc., and redefined the disease as a phenomenon. This was further clarified by Allen and Brown [3] who defined Raynaud's disease as idiopathic and *Raynaud's phenomenon* as being a manifestation of a more serious and potentially more progressive underlying disease process. Allen and Brown were attempting to distinguish between those patients who followed a benign course and those patients who progressed to develop tissue loss of the digits. However, with increasingly sophisticated immunologic testing, an increasing proportion of patients are recognized to have, or eventually to develop evidence of, an underlying autoimmune disorder. Thus, the misleading primary Raynaud's disease and secondary Raynaud's phenomenon are now replaced with the more encompassing term of *Raynaud's syndrome*.

Clinical presentation

Raynaud's syndrome is episodic vasospasm of the digits, usually of the upper limb but occasionally of the lower limb as well. The digits between attacks are generally normal in terms of color, temperature and sensation. The attacks typically begin in adolescence and are initiated by exposure to cold and emotional stimuli and are usually completed 15 to 60 minutes after cessation of the stimulus. The classical triad of color changes of pallor, cyanosis and rubor may be evident but often one of the latter two color changes is less obvious. The vasospasm of Raynaud's syndrome is symmetrical and about 90% of those who seek medical advice are female. Paresthesia and mild discomfort, especially during the rubor phase are common but overt pain is rare in the absence of ischemic ulceration. Digital tissue loss does not occur with vasospasm alone but indicates structural change and anatomical obstruction of digital and palmar arteries is present with a correspondingly worse prognosis.

Pathophysiology

Lewis [4, 5] proposed that vascular wall hyperresponsiveness to cold was due to a 'local fault' in the vessel. His experiments involved local anesthetic blocks of both somatic and autonomic nerves. These blocks did not prevent vasospasm in response to cold stimuli. Maurice Raynaud's theory of a hyperactive sympathetic nervous system appeared to be disproved yet cervical sympathectomy continued to be used because of the beneficial results observed. Although an initial hyperemia is observed, vasospasm can still be precipitated albeit with a more severe cold stress. The overall results however are disappointing, particularly in the longer term.

If the adrenergic system is involved in the production of vasospasm, then either there is an excessive abundance of the stimulating agent or there is an excessive response to stimulation. From the time of Lewis in the 1930s, the pendulum has swung toward the concept of excessive response. Coffman and Cohen [6] emphasized that digital blood flow either perfused the nutrient capillary bed or was shunted through arteriovenous communications. Cold stress applied to normal fingers resulted in decreased arteriovenous shunt flow but unaltered nutrient capillary blood flow, whereas in patients with Raynaud's syndrome there was a reduction in both. More importantly, they showed that pretreatment with reserpine, a sympathetic blocking agent, resulted in increased nutrient capillary flow. This was amongst the first evidence suggesting that enhanced adrenergic neuroeffector activity had a role in the pathophysiology of Raynaud's syndrome.

More recently attention has focused on α-adrenergic receptors in vascular smooth muscle, specifically α_2-adrenergic receptors. In 1983, Keenan and Porter [7] reported significantly elevated levels of α_2-receptors in circulating platelets in patients with vasospasm compared to controls and suggested a correlation may occur with vascular smooth muscle. The possibility of an increased receptor population provides a mechanism for a 'final common pathway' for a variety of stimuli. The concept of altered receptor population may have implications for other clinical entities involving vasospasm e.g., migraine, variant angina. Experimental work with regard to α-adrenergic receptors in general is continuing but of particular interest is the possibility that the population of receptors is not fixed but may be modulated by activity in response to stimuli.

From a practical point of view it is tempting to divide Raynaud's syndrome into vasospasm and vaso-obstruction. However, patients, particularly if observed over a long period, tend to demonstrate features of both. It is likely that vasospasm and vaso-obstruction are merely opposite ends of the same spectrum and thus such separation is artificial. Certainly the two processes are not mutually exclusive.

Vasospasm is the reversible cessation of blood flow. Patients with Raynaud's syndrome which is primarily vasospastic do not have demonstrable anatomical abnormalities of their palmar or digital arteries. During an attack, blood flow ceases as the constrictive force in the vessel wall exceeds the distending intraluminal pressure; but in between attacks, there is normal digital artery pressure and blood flow. The normal systolic brachial to digital pressure gradient in normal patients is 15 mmHg. In patients who have significant anatomical vaso-obstruction the gradient is greater than 15 mmHg [8]. To achieve such a gradient however a patient has to have developed obstruction of both digital arteries of the one digit. Thus, a declining resting pressure is a comparatively late manifestation of a pathological structural change occurring in the wall of the digital artery.

Whilst vasospasm and vaso-obstruction may be considered as different ends of the same disease spectrum, it may not be correct to consider them to be on the same temporal spectrum, i.e. vasospasm may not always be the initial manifestation leading to vaso-obstruction. There is evidence to suggest that the presence of vaso-obstruction sufficient to cause a significant resting systolic pressure gradient will in itself precipitate a vasospastic response in response to a cold stimulus [9], i.e. anyone with digital artery obstruction resulting in a fall in resting perfusion pressure will experience Raynaud's syndrome.

Much of the interest in the pathophysiology of Raynaud's syndrome has centered on the so-called critical closing point of the microcirculation in response to a cold stimulus. Digital skin temperature, which has a linear type relationship to digital blood flow, has been a convenient and thus favored research and investigative modality. In normal patients exposure to a cold stimulus results in decreasing digital temperature and a linearly decreasing digital artery perfusion. The same is true of patients with Raynaud's syndrome until digital skin temperature reaches a 'critical' temperature, often around 28°C when there is sudden constriction of the wall of the vessel and cessation of blood flow [10]. Grigg et al. [11] were interested in the recovery of vessels after cessation of the cold stimulus and repeated observations on digital rewarming reported by Porter et al. in 1975 [12]. They observed in normal patients that digital skin temperature, and thus digital blood flow, began increasing immediately the cold stimulus was withdrawn. The rate of increase was as much as 1–2°C per minute. In patients with vasospastic Raynaud's syndrome but with normal resting digital pressures, rewarming did not occur with withdrawal of the cold stimulus. Instead, a variable latent period of some minutes was observed. When rewarming did occur, it did so at the same rate of increase as observed in normal patients. In contrast, those patients with evidence of vaso-obstruction i.e., reduced resting digital pressures, often began with colder digital temperatures, and experienced similar latent periods after cessation of the cold stimulus, but once rewarming began were unable to achieve the same rate of increase of digital temperature. It was postulated that this pattern signified a structural as well as a physiological defect in the digital arteries.

The classical clinical triad of color changes is explained in terms of changes in the microcirculation – pallor being arteriolar constriction, cyanosis when the capillary bed is suffused by deoxygenated blood, possibly due to persistence of venule constriction after arteriolar relaxation, and rubor in response to a relative reactive hyperemia.

Epidemiology

The prevalence of Raynaud's syndrome is unknown and will vary according to geographical area and to whether or not the general population has been surveyed or whether only patients presenting for medical advice are reviewed. Certainly the condition is more common in cold, damp climates. Porter *et al.* [13] have reported that as many as 30% of the population living in such areas questioned at random have at one time experienced symptoms suggestive of a diagnosis of Raynaud's syndrome, with the vast majority being female.

Of medicolegal interest is the association of Raynaud's syndrome with certain types of employment – specifically those who work in chronically cold environments, for example, workers in the food processing industry and those who work with vibrating tools. A number of studies have demonstrated that sustained exposure to vibrating tools results in a significant increase in the incidence of Raynaud's syndrome [14, 15]. The development of subintimal fibrosis has been implicated with evidence of palmar and digital vessel obstruction [16].

Diagnostic evaluation

The diagnosis of Raynaud's syndrome is based upon the clinical history. No special diagnostic tests are required to establish the diagnosis and these should be reserved for the identification of underlying disorders and for quantitating the severity of ischemia. The clinical features required for diagnosis are well recognized – episodic digital ischemia in response to cold or emotional stimuli. It is worth noting that bilateral, symmetrical digital involvement is usual. The recent onset of unilateral involvement should focus the clinician's attention on the proximal arterial tree (Figure 18.1). Clinical features suggestive of an underlying connective tissue disorder should be sought, e.g., arthralgia, dry mouth or eyes, dysphagia, etc. A history of smoking and medication may also have management implications. The list of disorders reported to be associated with Raynaud's syndrome is extensive (Table 18.1).

Despite the importance of clinical diagnosis, the vascular laboratory can be of assistance in providing objective evidence for Raynaud's syndrome, evidence of severity of disease, deterioration over time and in determining the efficacy of treatment. The most commonly employed tests in our vascular laboratory are digital plethysmography and digital blood pressure measurements, together with cold water immersion testing and recording skin temperature recovery time [11]. Neilsen and Lassen have described an 'occlusive digital hypothermic challenge test' [17] which has been reported to be both highly specific and sensitive. A double inlet digital cuff is positioned over the proximal phalanx of the finger.

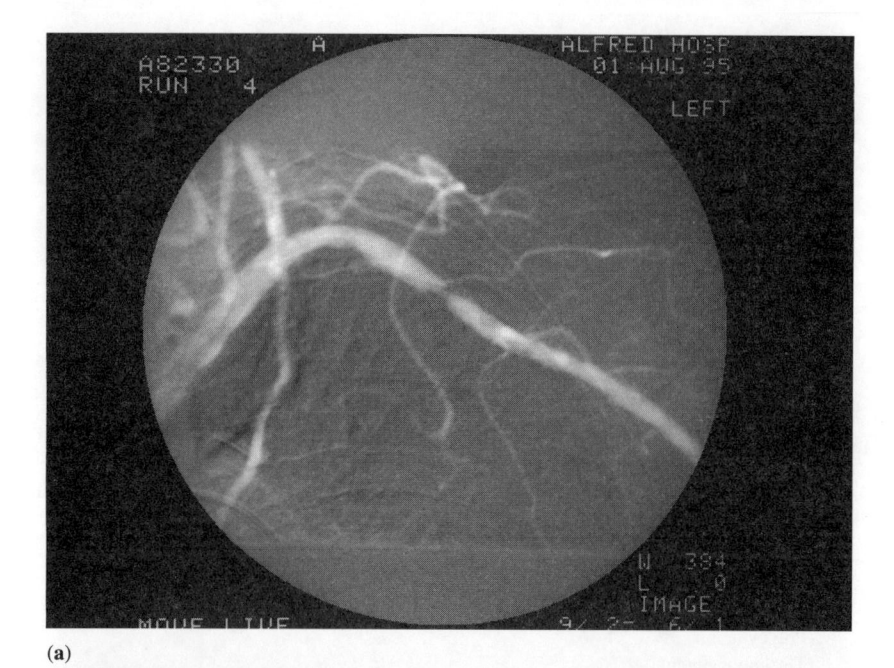

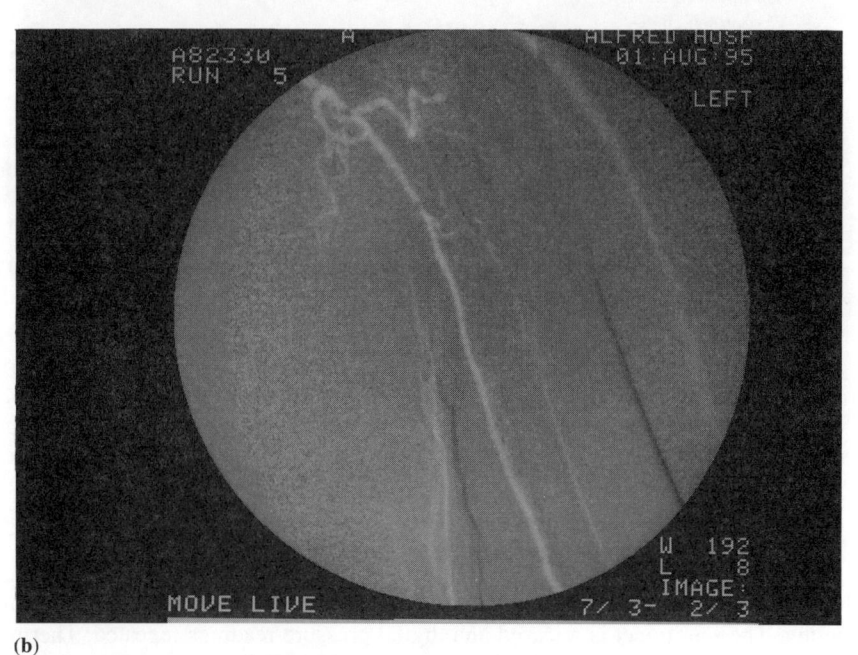

Figure 18.1. Angiogram of a 70-year-old lady who presented with sudden onset of severe Raynaud's syndrome affecting her left hand only. Brachial and radial pulses were absent to palpation and a systolic bruit was audible in the left supraclavicular fossa. She had a past history of bilateral lower limb arterial bypasses indicating the presence of significant atherosclerosis. The stenoses in the subclavian (a) and axillary (b) arteries were successfully dilated with balloon angioplasty.

Table 18.1. Conditions associated with the development of Raynaud's syndrome

Connective tissue diseases
Scleroderma
Systemic lupus erythematosus
Rheumatoid arthritis
Dermatomyositis
Polyarteritis nodosa
Sjögren's syndrome
Reiter's syndrome

Neurovascular compression syndromes
Thoracic outlet syndromes
Carpal tunnel syndrome

Arterial diseases
Thromboembolic syndromes
Buerger's disease
Arteritis
Atherosclerosis

Hematological disorders
Leukemia
Polycythemia
Thrombocythemia
Cryoproteinemia
Paraproteinemia

Drugs and poisons
Ergot-based agents
Methysergide
Beta blockers
Arsenic
Heavy metals

Miscellaneous
Neoplasms
Pheochromocytoma
Hypothyroidism
Pulmonary hypertension
Reflex sympathetic dystrophy
Frostbite
Chronic renal failure
Hepatitis

Baseline digital pressure measurements are made followed by 5 minutes of ischemic cooling. The tourniquet is released and digital pressure readings repeated. Thermal entrainment, first described by Lafferty *et al.* in 1983 [18] may be the most sensitive test available but its complexity has not encouraged widespread application.

Laser Doppler flowmetry has been used to detect blood cell flux in the skin of the fingertip and has been suggested to be helpful in diagnosis and grading of vasospastic disorders [19] but the technique remains experimental due to difficulties with interpretation. Nailfold capillaroscopy has similar difficulties but has been suggested as a means of determining those patients with Raynaud's syndrome who are likely to develop problems beyond vasospasm. The number and length of capillary loops per millimeter of the nailfold surface can be assessed [20].

Arteriography of the hand and digital vessels has largely been replaced by noninvasive testing but remains the definitive method of assessment of the proximal arterial tree.

The extent of hematological and biochemical testing that should be undertaken on individual patients can be difficult to determine. Certainly clinical history and examination can be helpful as can response to simple management measures. Possible baseline tests are listed in Table 18.2 but the possibilities for more extensive testing are virtually unlimited, particularly with the likely introduction of increasingly sophisticated immunological tests.

Table 18.2. 'Screening' investigations which may be considered for patients presenting with Raynaud's syndrome.

Full blood examination, ESR, Urea, Creatinine, Electrolytes, Liver function tests
Urinalysis
Anti-nuclear antibodies, Rheumatoid factor, Cold agglutinins, Anti-cardiolipin antibodies, Lupus inhibitor
Serum protein electrophoresis, Complement levels, Immunoglobulin electrophoresis

Treatment

The majority of patients with Raynaud's syndrome are young women who are concerned that the symptoms which they are experiencing are indicative of 'poor circulation' with future implications for cardiovascular and cerebrovascular problems. Reassurance and explanation can be of considerable benefit. General advice with regard to avoidance of cold and other detrimental stimuli, particularly cessation of smoking, is also helpful. Encouragement to wear warm gloves and preferably mittens is appropriate. For more severely affected patients who are required to spend time outside for their employment, battery-powered heated gloves are commercially available. The so-called swinging arms maneuver has been suggested as a simple means of overcoming a vasospastic episode [21].

There are no medications which will 'cure' Raynaud's syndrome *per se*; many have undesirable side-effects and this should be explained to patients. Nitroglycerin, both topically and sublingually has been tried with some success [21] but the calcium channel blocking agents, initially nifedipine but more recently felodipine, have been the mainstay of drug treatment for a number of years. These drugs have largely replaced sympathetic blocking agents such as reserpine, methyldopa and prazosin primarily due to problems with side-effects, even though the calcium channel blocking agents themselves can produce unacceptable symptoms such as headache, flushing and peripheral edema in some patients. Serotonin antagonists such as ketanserin were reported to have a beneficial effect but are now rarely used. Thymoxamine with α-adrenergic inhibition properties has also been shown to be of value in a double-blind placebo controlled trial in patients with primarily vasospasm problems and was comparatively benign in terms of production of side-effects (22). Pentoxifylline has not been of benefit in our experience in patients with Raynaud's syndrome whose problems are primarily vasospastic in nature, but at least on theoretical grounds may be of assistance to those patients with digital artery obstruction.

In cases of severe digital ischemia, intravenous guanethidine delivered as for a Bier's block technique can be of value. Low molecular weight dextran (Dextran 40) and even therapeutic defibrination using ancrod (Arvin) have also been tried. Plasmapheresis may be appropriate in some patients particularly if there is evidence of cryoglobulinemia or increased blood viscosity.

Intravenous prostaglandin E1 has been reported to be beneficial [23]. Central venous infusion over 72 hours has been used on those patients with more extreme problems of digit tissue necrosis with early gratifying effects of improved perfusion as evidenced by relief of pain and increased digital temperature. Although the benefits are short-lived (days to weeks) this agent can be useful in overcoming a particularly severe exacerbation.

In those patients with digital ulceration, careful cleansing and dressings are required together with systemic antibiotics if secondary infection as evidenced by cellulitis develops. Local topical antibiotic agents are of little value either as treatment or as prophylaxis. Debridement during washing or even limited surgical debridement can be beneficial.

Cervical sympathectomy has been widely employed in the past but anecdotal reports of short-term and limited benefit have not been sufficient to prevent the demise of this technique from the armamentarium of most clinicians involved with the treatment of patients with Raynaud's syndrome, particularly those with digital ulceration due to underlying vascular obstruction. The innovations of microsurgical techniques have been applied to the problem by way of digital artery sympathectomy, which involves stripping of the adventitia from the digital arteries, and by way of microsurgical bypass procedures. Despite being described more than a decade ago [24], convincing evidence of efficacy is still awaited. It may be that the only value of surgery in dealing with Raynaud's syndrome is minor digital amputation of those fortunately rare patients in whom tissue destruction is extreme.

Summary

Raynaud's syndrome involves episodic digital pallor and/or cyanosis in response to cold and occasionally emotional stimuli. It is very common in colder climates affecting as many as 20–30% of the female population. Often beginning in adolescence, it fortunately follows a benign course in the majority of patients who require only reassurance and symptomatic treatment. The development of arterial obstruction can result in more severe symptoms of tissue loss, i.e. digital ulceration, and is usually associated with an underlying autoimmune connective tissue disorder.

References

1. Raynaud, M. On local asphyxia and symmetrical gangrene of the extremities. In: Selected monographs. London: New Syndenham Society, 1888.
2. Hutchinson J. Raynaud's phenomena. Med Press Circ 1901;123:403–10.
3. Allen EV, Brown GE. Raynaud's disease; a critical review of minimal prerequisites for diagnosis. Ann Intern Med 1928;1:535–42.
4. Lewis T. Experiments relating to the peripheral mechanism involved in spastic arrest of the circulation in the fingers, a variety of Raynaud's disease. Heart 1929;15:7–13.
5. Lewis T, Pickering G.W. Observations upon maladies in which the blood supply to the digits ceases intermittently or permanently and upon bilateral gangrene of the digits; observations relevant to so-called Raynaud's disease. Clin Scin 1933;1:327–35.
6. Coffman P, Cohen AS. Total and capillary fingertip blood flow in Raynaud's phenomenon. N Engl J Med 1971;285:259–63.
7. Keenan E, Porter JM. Alpha 2 adrenergic receptors in platelets in patients with Raynaud's syndrome. Surgery 1983;94:204–9.
8. Downs AR, Gaskell P, Morrow I et al. Assessment of arterial obstruction in vessels supplying the fingers by measurement of local blood pressures and skin temperature response test – correlation with angiographic evidence. Surgery 1975;77:530–6.
9. Hiraii M. Cold sensitivity of the hand in arterial occlusive disease.Surgery 1979;85:140–4.
10. Porter JM. Raynaud's syndrome in: Sabiston DC, (ed.), Textbook of surgery. Philadelphia: Saunders, 1986:1930.
11. Grigg MJ, Nicolaides AN, Papadakis K, Wolfe JHN. The efficacy of thymoxamine in primary Raynaud's phenomenon. Eur J Vasc Surg 1989;3:309–13.
12. Porter JM, Suiden RL, Bardenen EJ. et al. The diagnosis and treatment of Raynaud's phenomenon. Surgery 1975;11–23.
13. Porter JM, Friedman EJ, Mills JL, Taylor LM. Occlusive and vasospastic disease involving distal upper extremity arteries – Raynaud's syndrome. In: Rutherford (ed.), Vascular surgery, 3rd edn. Philadelphia: Saunders; 1989; 844–57.
14. Chatteyee DS, Petrie A, Taylor W. Prevalence of vibration induced white finger. Br J Ind Med 1978;35:208–13.
15. Taylor W, Pelman PL. Raynaud's phenomenon of occupational origin. Acta Chir Scand 1976;465(Suppl. 27).
16. James PB, Galloway RW. Arteriography of the hand in men exposed to vibration. In: Taylor W, Pelmean PL, (eds), Vibration white finger in industry. London: Academic Press, 1975:31.
17. Neilsen SL, Lassen NA. Measurement of digital blood pressure after local cooling. J Appl Physiol 1977;43:907–10.
18. Lafferty K, de Trafford JC, Roberts VC et al. Raynaud's phenomenon and thermal entrainment: An objective test. Br Med J 1983;286:90–2.
19. Allen JA, Devlin MA, McGrann S, Doherty CC. An objective test for the diagnosis and grading of vasospasm in patients with Raynaud's syndrome. Clin Sci 1992;82:529–34.
20. Mannarino E, Pasqualini L, Fedeli F et al. Nailfold capillaroscopy in the screening and diagnosis of Raynaud's syndrome. Angiology 1994;45:37–42.
21. Peterson LL, Vorhies C. Raynaud's syndrome. Treatment with sublingual administration of nitroglycerine, swinging arms manoeuvre and biofeedback training. Arch Dermatol 1983;119:396–9.
22. Nicolaides AN, Grigg MJ. New concepts in the evaluation and treatment of patients with Raynaud's phenomenon. In: Veith FJ (ed.), Current critical problems in vascular surgery. Veith FJ, St Louis: Quality Medical Publishing, 1989:246–53.
23. Pardy B, Hoare M, Eastcott HHG. Prostaglandin El in severe Raynaud's phenomenon. Surgery 1982;92:953–65.
24. Flatt AE. Digital artery sympathectomy. J Hand Surg 1980;5:550–6.

19. Flow dynamics and pathophysiological mechanisms of diseases of lower limb arteries

GIUSEPPE MARIA ANDREOZZI

The arterial diseases of the lower limbs are a clinical syndrome sustained by the reduction of the districtual blood flow in one or both limbs. In 80% atherosclerosis is the most important inducing factor, but in the remaining 15–20%, it is due to other diseases, such as diabetes or inflammatory arteritis. For all etiologies, a common pathophysiological understanding is valid. The disease starts when, from the anatomic phase of the atherosclerotic process, it transforms into atherosclerotic illness with a reduction of arterial diameter (stenosis) [1–4].

The arterial network of the lower limbs is a system with high resistances which makes it possible to maintain a good perfusion both at rest and during muscular work. Different factors regulate the cutaneous and muscular perfusion of the lower limbs: cardiac output, arterial blood pressure, blood velocity, the microcirculation and the un-Newtonian characteristics of blood.

The appearance of stenosis induces pathophysiological changes, involving all the determinants of flow dynamics, from the macrocirculation to the microcirculatory and metabolic patterns, that determine the compensation or decompensation of the illness [5].

Velocity

Blood velocity through the stenosis is related to its degree. For a single and small stenosis the blood velocity will be reduced downstream just after the lesion and the flux laminarity does not change; for severe (> 50%) or large stenosis the blood velocity decreases significantly, missing producing turbulences and missing the flux laminarity (Figure 19.1).

The author wishes to thank Drs Signorelli, Martini, Di Pino, Barresi, Busacca, Leone and Pennisi for working in the vascular laboratory and for the bibliographic review, and Mr Paul Dennis, teacher at the Regency School of English (Ramsgate, Kent, UK) for the text revision.

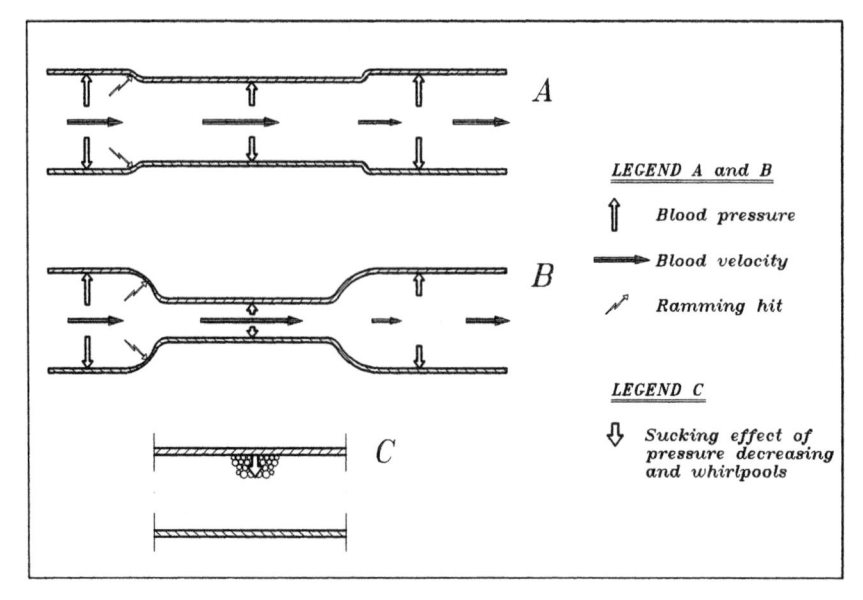

Figure 19.1. Velocity and pressure changes through the stenosis, under and over 50%. The reduction of the lateral pressure causes a *sucking effect* on the arterial wall, increasing the endothelial damage.

Pressure

The blood pressure upstream from the stenosis is equivalent to the systemic pressure; near the stenosis it is sometimes higher (*ramming hit*), downstream it is lower. The pressure also decreases within the stenosis (Bernouilli theorem), increasing the whirlpools. This causes a sucking effect on the arterial wall that takes part in the evolution of the endothelial damage, and in the growth of the atherosclerotic lesions (Figure 19.1). The drop in pressure, in the case of the isolated stenosis, diminishes proportionally leaving the lesion. This hemodynamic advantage is less important than the hydrodynamic one, due to several factors such as the post-stenotic wall conditions, the closeness of a bifurcation, and the un-Newtonian property of the blood fluid.

Flow

With reference to the variations of flow, it is necessary to take into account some peculiarities of the arterial system in the limbs. It has the capacity to work in two totally different ways: at rest and during muscular activity. The flow is determined by the Hagen–Poiseuille law ($Q = \Delta P \pi r 4/8 \eta l$), and is therefore reduced proportionally with the drop in pressure induced by the stenosis. When the flux is low (at rest), however, the important decrease of the pressure does not show significant change in the districtual flow, because of the high resistances downstream. During muscular activity, when the flux is high due to arteriolar vasodilation, the lowering

Pathophysiology of lower limb arterial diseases

of arteriolar peripheral resistance without increase of pressure (stenosis), causes a significant reduction of the flow.

In the advanced stages of the illness the most important organic damage is the obstruction; the blood flow is stopped along the principal arteries and the perfusion of the lower areas of the limbs is sustained by the collateral circulation and depends directly on the microcirculation [6].

Microcirculation

The teleology of the circulatory system is tissue nutrition, with exchanges between intra- and extravascular districts. The exchanges from blood to the tissues, and vice versa, require the blood flow to have a low velocity and pressure, to be proportional to the tissue requirements.

Downstream the hemodynamic features of the resistance vessels are widely varied. The Reynolds number is lower than 1.00, so the flux from inertial becomes viscous, and the denominator of the Hagen–Poiseuille law influences the flow more than does the numerator. The microhemodynamics are controlled by the central nervous system, hormones and local substances [6].

Microhemodynamics

The effectors of microcirculatory homeostasis are the arterioles. In healthy subjects they are submitted to rhythmic vasoconstriction and dilation (*vasomotion*), with consequent periodic perfusion of the tissue (*flowmotion*) (Figure 19.2). The rhythmic perfusion also induces rhythmic changes of the microhematocrit within the capillaries. This mechanism appears to control the release and reabsorption from and toward the tissue [7–9]. Local control is sustained by the homeostatic balance of several substance produced by the endothelial cells, as *prostacyclin* (PGI_2), *nitric oxide* (NO), *endothelin-1* (ET-1), *tissue plasminogen activator* (tPA) and its inhibitor (PAI-1), *heparin-like substances, heparin cofactor 2, and S-protein*.

PGI_2, derived from arachidonic acid (by the action of phospholipase A_2) and synthesized by cyclooxygenase), has a typical vasodilating and antiplatelet aggregation activity [10, 11]. NO, synthesized from L-arginine by NO synthetase, also has a vasodilating and antiaggregant activity; it is inhibited by M-mono-methyl-L-arginine [12, 13]. A specific NO agonist is acetylcholine, which induces NO release by the M_2 muscarinic receptor. The action of PGI_2 is mediated by cAMP, while NO increases cGMP, with a feedback control on PGI_2 and NO. This reaction induces dephosphorylation of the light chain of myosin with decontraction of smooth muscle cells. NO and PGI_2 are synergistic in inhibition of platelet aggregation, but it is PGI_2 which usually controls the regulation of vascular tone [14]. ET-1 contracts the smooth muscle cells in two phases. The fast phase quickly moves Ca^{++} storage, activating phospholipase C, which stimulates hydrolysis of phosphatidylinositol biphosphate and production of inositol triphosphate and diaglycerol. The slow

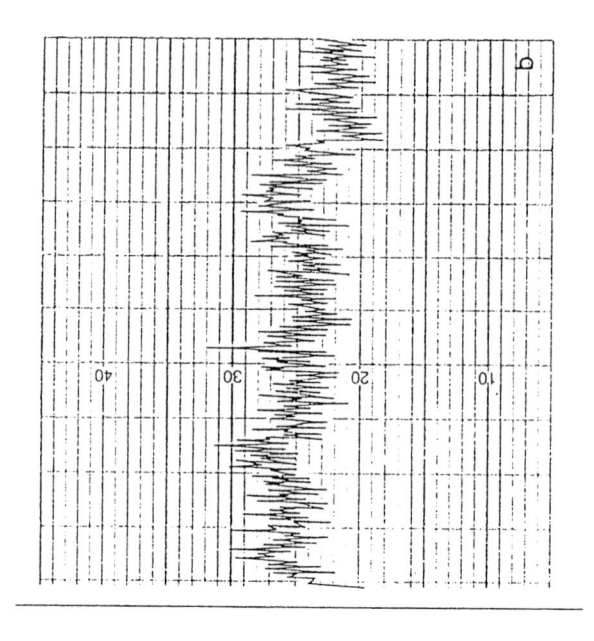

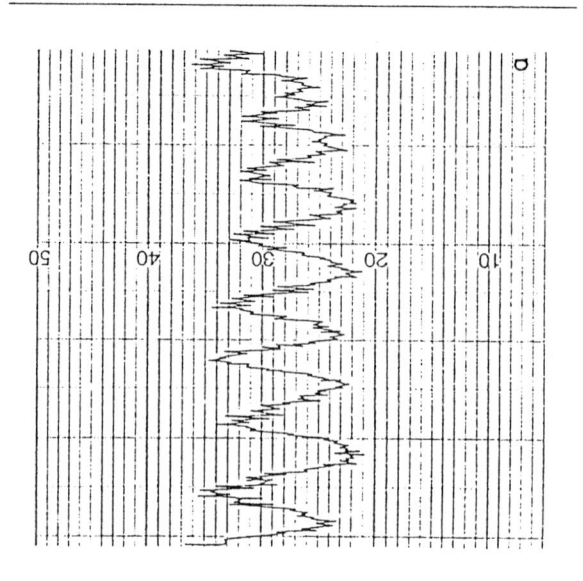

Figure 19.2. Laser Doppler output signal. Waves with different amplitude and frequency; low frequency waves (4–10 cycles/min, LFW), and high frequency waves (15–30 cycles/min, HFW). (a) Prevalence of LFW on normal skin with microcirculatory autoregulation; (b) better evidence of HFW in patient with critical limb ischemia (lost autoregulation).

phase is sustained by activation of Ca^{++} voltage dependent and independent channels. The endothelium also releases ET-1 after stimulation by angiotensin II, thrombin and adrenaline [15]; it also improves during production of superoxide anions, but the vasoconstriction from superoxide anions seems to be related to a direct action on the endothelium, to inhibition of NO and to a block of PGI_2, rather than to ET-1 release [16, 17]. Other endothelial vasocontracting factors are the cyclic endoperoxide PGH_2, thromboxane A_2 and the isoprostanes, derived from cyclooxygenation or lipoperoxidantion, which have high aggregation and constricting activity [18, 19].

All these activities of endothelial cells are continously stimulated according to the tissue metabolic requirements. At rest there is a balance between activators and inhibitors. Physiological or pathological events are characterized by the loss of this balance, with prevalence of one system. Together these systems, are part of the *microvascular flow regulating system* (MFRS) which is the basis of the local autoregulation of the microcirculation (Figure 19.2) [20].

Moreover the microcirculatory perfusion does not only depend on vasomotion and flowmotion, but is also influenced by the rheological determinants from the geometry of the vascular bed to the characteristics of the perfusion fluid and the role of the circulating cells [6].

Geometry of microvessels

The progressive reduction of vessel diameter increases the apparent blood viscosity, increasing the shear stress. Under 150 μm this apparent hyperviscosity is balanced by the *plasma skimming* (Fahraeus–Lindqvist effect) maintaining a good perfusion in the smaller vessels [21]. If the real viscosity increases over 4.5–5.0 cps, as in peripheral arterial diseases, the threshold of capillary diameter of the Fahraeus–Lindqvist effect becomes lower with subsequent perfusion reduction.

Red cells

The red cells play a very important role with reference to *hematocrit* and also *membrane deformability* [22]. The physiological stimulus to red cell deformability is the residual pressure gradient between arterioles and capillaries; in pathological conditions the residual pressure is very low and the deformability decreases significantly, proportionally to the degree of disease. In peripheral arterial disease this low deformability is secondary to the low perfusion pressure; in diabetic patients it can be primarily sustained by metabolic damage to the membrane [23–26].

Platelets

The platelet is very important for the production of vasoactive and cell stimulating substances, such as *platelet derived growth factor* (PDGF), *ADP, thromboxane A_2, serotonin,* and for the stimulation of *platelet activating factor* (PAF) release from leukocytes [27, 28].

Leukocytes

The role of the leukocyte is very important in microvascular perfusion; leukocytes have been indicated as being responsible for flowmotion, because they take a very long time to pass through microvessels, and also because of several particular interactions with the endothelial cells. The leukocyte–endothelium interaction is regulated by two mechanisms, the receptor system and the soluble substances system. The most important receptor molecules are the *integrins, selectins* and *immunoglobulins*, located on the cellular surfaces of leukocytes and endothelium; they regulate contact, rolling and adhesion of the leukocytes. To the latter group belong the *interleukins, tumor necrosis factor alpha*, PAF, leukotrienes and some fractions of the *complement system* (C4a, C5a); all these cytokines are released from endothelium and leukocytes [29]. They particularly activate recruitment, chemotaxis and migration of white cells, and other cell activities [30, 31].

Integrins, selectins and immunoglobulins do not appear on the cellular surface at the same time; GMP 140 (rolling selectin) is a molecule which appears rapidly, and ICAM and ECAM (adhesion immunoglobulin and selectin) appear 1 hour after stimulation. After stimulation the leukocyte activates these molecular systems and changes its status from *resting leukocyte* to *primed leukocyte*. If the stimulation continues it will change again into an *activated leukocyte* and will perform all the cellular reactions (chemotaxis, phagocytosis, cytolysis) [32] (Figure 19.3). This control system is defined as the *microvascular defense system* (MDS) [20]; it is activated whenever necessary (trauma, phlogosis, immunology, neoplasm). Also, recent studies involving this leukocyte mechanism in non-phlogistic diseases, such as *atherosclerosis* [3], *ischemia* [33], *shock* [34], *reperfusion syndrome* [35–37], *diabetic microangiopathy*, have shown an increase in chemotaxis and leukocyte adhesion in damaged tissue [37–39], and a correlation between tissue damage and leukocyte activation [40, 41], endothelium toxic substance and superoxide production [42–46].

To summarize, the physiology of the arterial perfusion of the lower limbs is sustained by a dynamic balance between the MFRS and MDS, with the activators and inhibitors continously being released and removed or deactivated, guaranteeing a prompt response when needed, physiologically or pathologically [6].

The presence of arterial disease with consequent changes in the pressure velocity and blood flow disturbs this dynamic balance leading to MDS prevalence. This induces a deregulation of the MFRS, with maldistribution of the local flux, free radical production and tissue toxicity [6, 47].

Pathophysiology and clinical features

Clinical evidence of peripheral arterial disease begins with a symptomatology related to all the mechanisms mentioned above. The natural history has a very slow evolution (15–20 years), due to the time needed for the anatomic damage to affect the hemodynamics, and to the efficiency of the compensation mechanism. Peripheral arterial disease has been classified into four stages (*Leriche and Fontaine classification*).

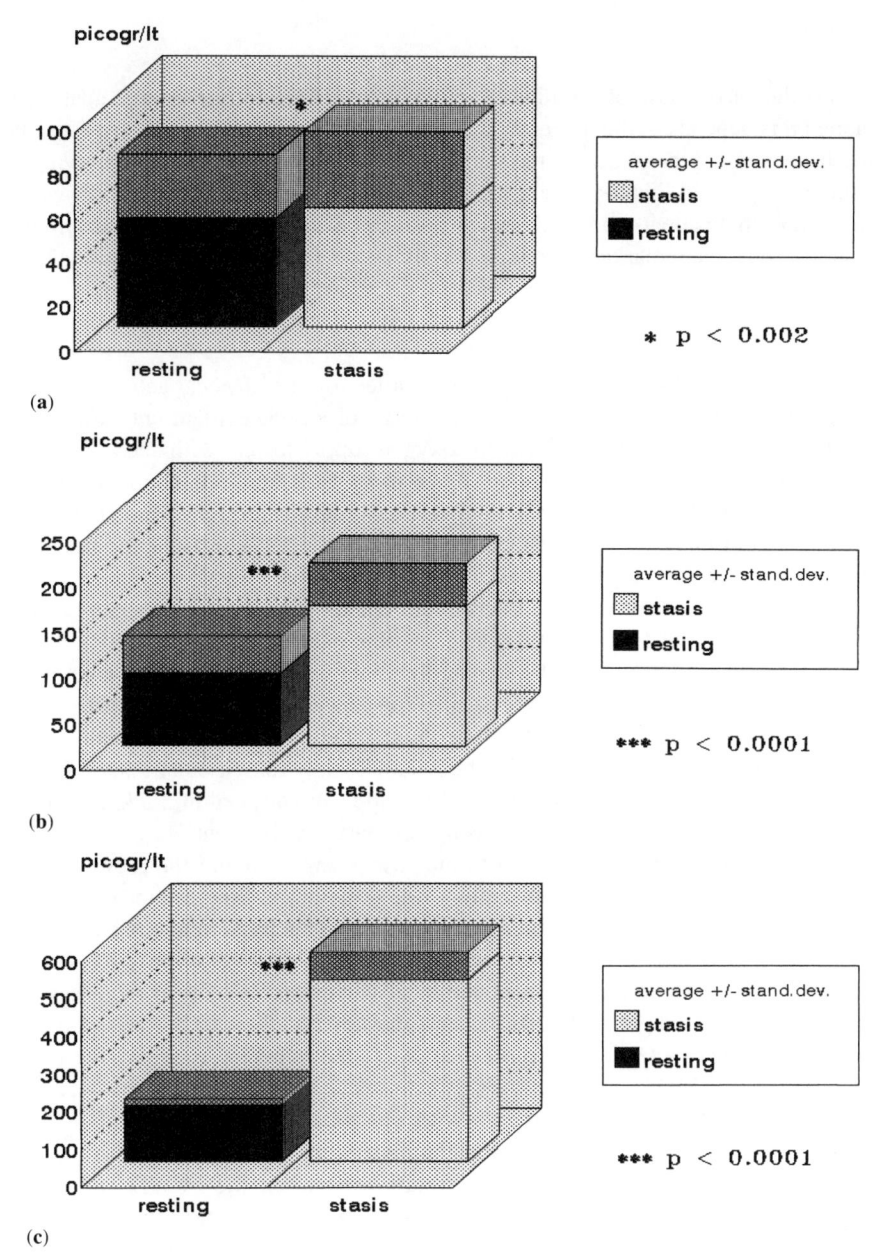

Figure 19.3. Production of interleukin-6: (a) in healthy control subjects, low level at rest (50 ± 28.87 pg/L) and small increase after 10 min of venous stasis (54.67 ± 34.64 pg/L); (b) in chronic venous insufficiency, higher resting level at rest (78.57 ± 40.62 pg/L) than in healthy controls; significant increase after 10 min of venous stasis (152.86 ± 46.38 pg/L); (c) in peripheral arterial disease, Fontaine's stage 2nd B: highest resting value of our experiment (150 ± 19.05 pg/L), and very significant increase during treadmill test (4 km/h, slope 7%) (484.16 ± 72.02 pg/L). The chronic hemodynamic damage (arterial stenosis and obstruction or venous hypertension) stimulates the leukocytes from the *resting* to the *primed* condition; every new stimulation changes the *primed leukocyte* into an *activated leukocyte*.

Stage I

This is the early phase of the illness, and is often believed to be asymptomatic, although this depends on the patient's way of life. A sedentary life rarely overlaps the mechanism of compensation. If the subject is more active, the illness will be symptomatic with pain. In this last case the patient could be classified as stage II. However we believe that patients can be classified as stage I if affected by an evident symptomatology due to a remarkable stress, e.g. walking for 1–2 km or a long climb [47].

Stage II

In this stage the illness is clinically evident after routine physical activity. At rest the patient is completely asymptomatic. Arterial disease is evident only after muscular stress because during walking the oxygen supply lowers with need. A typical symptom is *intermittent claudication*. It is a paroxystic pain, related to the level of arterial stenosis. It affects the calf, thigh, gluteus muscle and foot. Patients refer to it as a cramp (muscular acidosis) or hypostenia of the muscle (ischemic neuritis); stoping exercise without sitting makes this symptomatology disappear.

Clinical features to assess the intermittent claudication are measurement of the pain free walking distance (PFWD) and the time needed for recovery (tR). These measurements can be achieved by standardizing muscular stress with an ergometer. The treadmill test is the most useful, using constant walk and slope. Usually a 7% slope is utilized with a speed of 4 km per hour. The test must be used with care to avoid coronary problems. A study by the Italian Society for Vascular Pathology has shown that an ergometric charge with a 15% slope and a speed of 2.5 km per hour is a sensible equivalent without increasing coronary involvement [48].

At this stage MFRS deregulation to the vasoconstriction and the prevalence of MDS only occurs during muscular effort, when the blood flow cannot increase in relation to the oxygen requirement from the muscle. This leads to hypoxia and acidosis with appearance of effort pain (*claudication*). If stress is stopped the MFRS prevails, restoring autoregulation of the local perfusion. Initially it increases vasodilation and disaggregant activity, and washes out the catabolites produced during the ischemia (*reactive hyperemia*). After the hyperemia it resets in a new balance with the MDS.

In stage II, therefore, all patients with claudication can be classified, with 600–700 m or 100 m PFWD, but the pathophysiology of these two groups is very different. The first shows a direct correlation between the PFWD and transcutaneous pO_2, whilst the latter shows a decrease in this correlation and an increase of the inverse correlation with transcutaneous pCO_2 (Figure 19.4). This behavior suggests that patients with PFWD over 150 m are characterized by ischemia related to muscular work, while patients with PFWD under 150 m are characterized by a worsening of the aerobic conditions of cellular metabolism. For a better classification a stage IIA and a stage IIB have been established [47, 49].

The pathophysiology of stage IIB is sustained by blood flow reduction, permanent hypoxia, prevalence of the MDS, and low activity of the MFRS, which will always be unable to restore the autoregulation. The perfusion will decrease both in the muscle (reduction of the PFWD) and in the skin (pallor and cyanosis).

Other symptoms frequently present in subjects suffering from peripheral arterial disease are disturbances of sexual function, particularly impotence, due to a total or partial defect of penis erection, sustained by internal iliac artery or common iliac artery occlusion or stenosis. The pudendal artery can also be affected. There may also be an inability to maintain an erection, due to hypoperfusion of the spinal cord at L5 S1, induced by stenosis of the medullar arteries coming from the aorta.

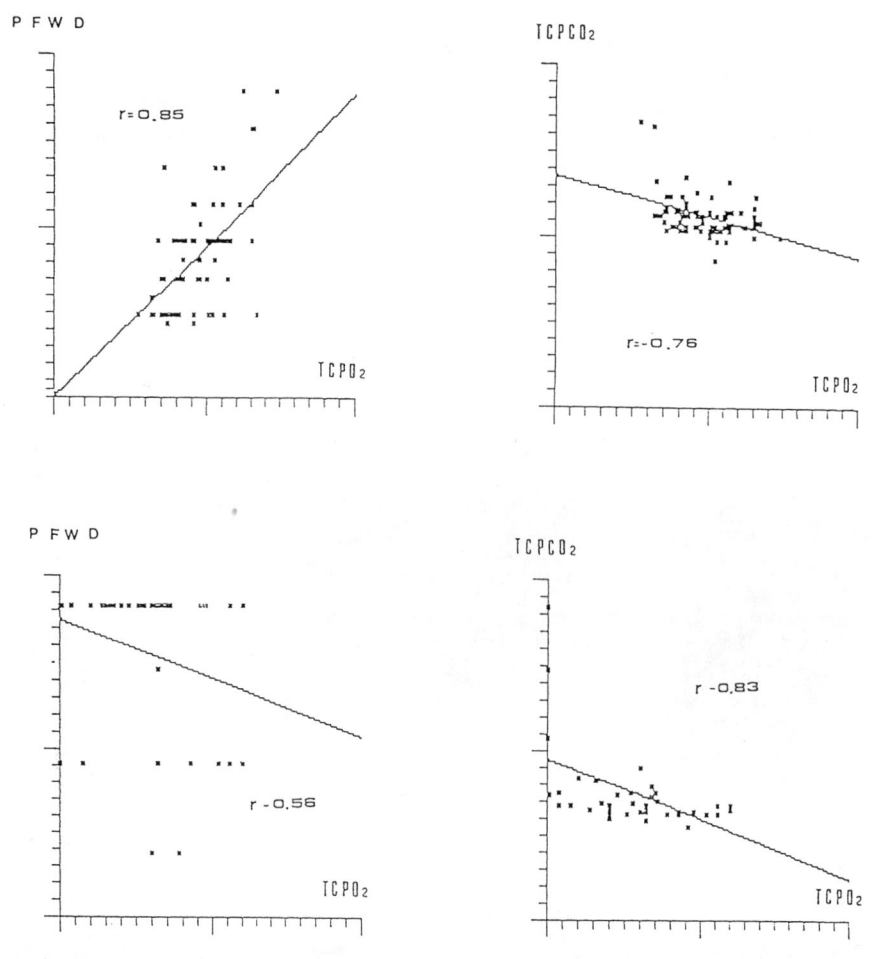

Figure 19.4. Analysis of the variance between the pain free walking distance, transcutaneous pO_2 and transcutaneous pCO_2. (a) Fontaine's stage IIA: high significant correlation between PFWD and transcutaneous pO_2 ($r = 0.85$); significant inverse correlation between transcutaneous pO_2 and transcutaneous pCO_2 ($r = -0.76$); (b) Fontaine's stage IIB: inverse and low significant correlation between PFWD and transcutaneous pO_2 ($r = -0.56$), and increase of the inverse correlation between transcutaneous pO_2 and transcutaneous pCO_2 ($r = 0.83$). This behavior indicates a worsening of the cellular metabolism, sustained by the decrease of the arterial and arteriolar inflow.

Stage III

The third stage is characterized by *rest pain* due to severe cutaneous hypoxia and ischemic neuritis. It is a continuous pain, which occurs particularly during the night, as it increases in the supine position. The patient spontaneously seeks the orthostatic position, to decrease the pain, making the leg bend out of the bed. Moreover the pain is made worse by cold and improves by heating the foot. The skin color changes gradually at this stage and often the patient does not report this symptom to the doctor. When the arteriopathy affects only one limb it is possible to note a *pale color* of the skin. In the advanced phase the pale color is always present, often with *cyanosis*. The cyanosis indicates a pathophysiological deterioration in the history of the arteriopathy. It indicates stasis and precedes gangrene [47] (Figure 19.5).

The third stage is the stage of absolute arterial insufficiency; there is no correlation between PFWD and transcutaneous pO_2 and there is a significant increase in transcutaneous pCO_2. This stage is characterized by the prevalence of the MDS with a reduction in the ability of the MFRS to restore a good perfusion. Microcirculatory reactivity disappears and stasis increases with worsening of the hypoxia and acidosis. Leukocyte activation is very strong, with great endothelial damage, and production of endothelial toxic substances and free radicals [6].

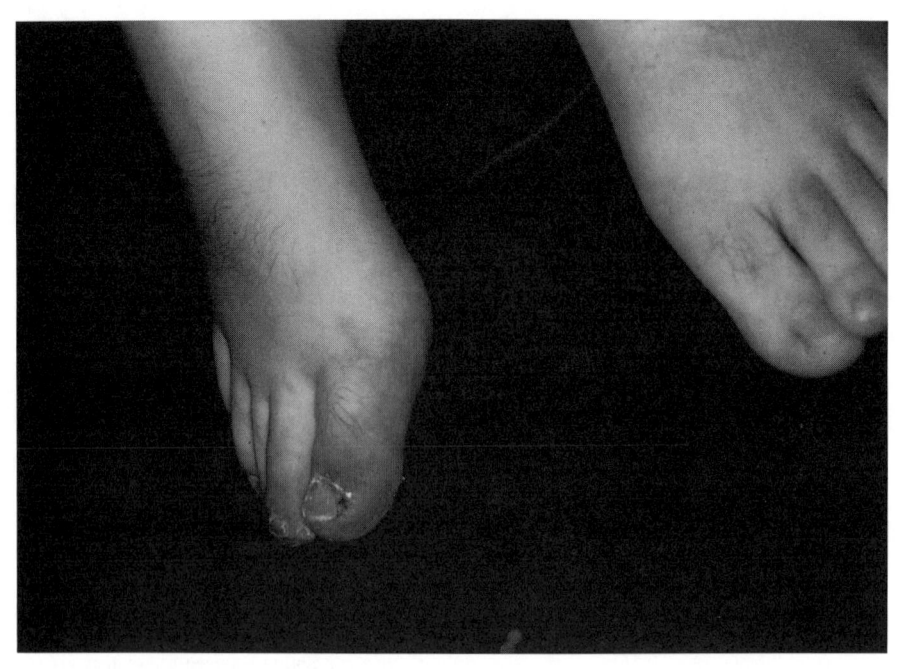

Figure 19.5. Cyanosis of the big toe, with intermittent rest pain, a prelude of critical limb ischemia (*unstable arteriopathy*).

Stage IV

This stage is characterized by *trophic injuries* sustained by hypoxia and acidosis, which hardly stress the compensation mechanisms. The trophic damage appears as different kinds of lesion, from *alopecia* to *skin lesions around the nail*, from *ulcers between fingers* to *necrosis* and *gangrene* (Figure 19.6). The gangrene can be dry or humid. Dry gangrene is sustained by a sudden death of tissues that are well demarcated from healthy areas. This can be tolerated by patients, particularly when the area is small; pain often disappears. Humid gangrene begins when the worsening of ischemia is very rapid; it is always preceded by cyanosis followed by edema and gangrene. Humid gangrene occurs even at the focus of infection in a dry necrosis. The main factor which induces the start of the trophic damage is the passage from ischemia to hypoxia and acidosis. In this stage tissue damage and free radical production is very high; the necrosis passes through a prolonged phase of necrobiosis during which reabsorption of catabolites occurs. This causes the clinical features such as fever, leukocytosis and increased erythrocyte sedimentation rate.

Critical limb ischemia

In the 40 years since the Leriche and Fontaine classification, there has been great progress in the pathological and clinical features of peripheral arteriopathies. The possibility of microcirculatory assessment, the discovery of thrombolytic drugs and prostanoids, the opening of new frontiers in surgery and angioradiology have

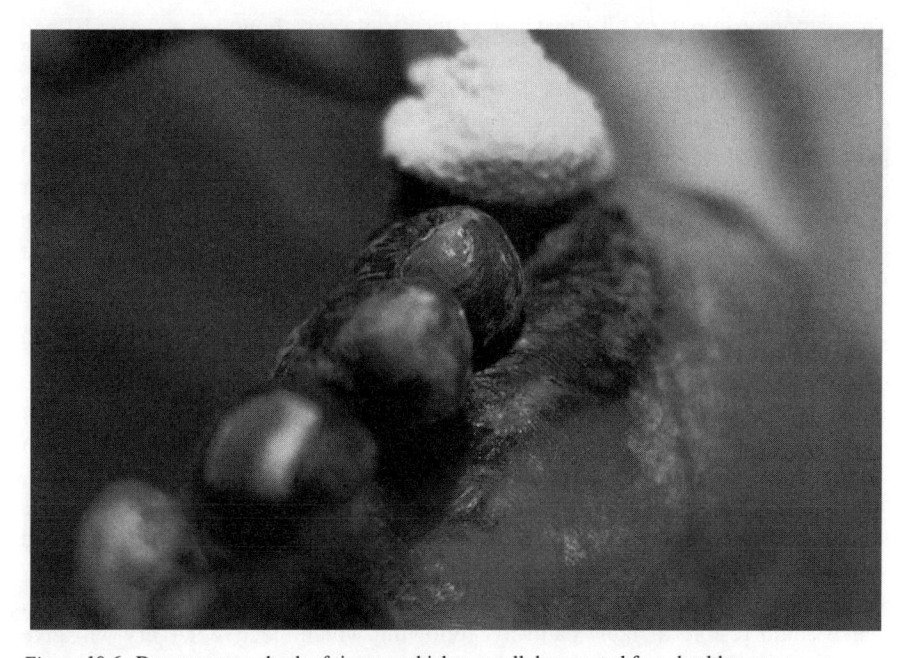

Figure 19.6. Dry gangrene; death of tissues, which are well demarcated from healthy areas.

radically changed the approach to the disease. Evolution through the four stages, from claudication to amputation can be prevented; a patient in stage III may recover to stage IIB, and even to stage IIA.

This has necessitated a revision of the Leriche and Fontaine classification. In 1989 the *European Consensus Conference* proposed the term *critical limb ischemia* (CLI), underlining the risk of the third and fourth stages leading to amputation. CLI has been defined by the following criteria:

- persistently recurring rest pain, requiring regular analgesia for more than two weeks;
- ulceration or gangrene of the foot or toes;
- ankle systolic blood pressure < 50 mmHg;
- toe systolic blood pressure < 30 mmHg (if ankle blood pressure is unreliable because of artery calcification as in diabetes; measurement with strain gauge plethysmography) [50].

This definition has been subsequently clarified, using some parameters, the most important of which are:

- transcutaneous oxygen pressure of the ischemic area ≤ 10 mmHg, which does not increase with inhalation of 100% oxygen;
- absence of arterial pulsations of the big toe (strain gauge plethysmography) after vasodilation;
- marked structural or functional changes of skin capillaries in the affected are [51].

The pathophysiology of CLI matches in the strict sense Fontaine's stages III and IV. More recently some authors have included in this risk phase the worsening of stable arteriopathy, the stage IIB. This stage, in fact, is characterized by an inverse and low significant correlation ($r = -0.56$) between PFWD and transcutaneous pO_2, while stage IIA shows a direct and very significant correlation ($r = 0.85$) (Figure 19.4). This signifies deterioration of the aerobic condition of the cellular metabolism, a prelude to CLI [47, 52]. This deterioration occurs concurrently with *cyanosis*, which can also appear without rest pain, and which is an expression of *microcirculatory stasis*.

We have suggested for this pathophysiological condition the name *unstable arteriopathy*, sustained mainly by microcirculatory decompensation, without macrocirculatory deterioration [47].

There are therefore two pathways which can lead to CLI, the micro- and the macrocirculatory pathways. The first is sustained by a lost of balance between MFRS and MDS, and increase of vasoconstrictor, aggregant and coagulative factors, with leukocyte activation. The second, while usually following the first, involves the macrocirculation with decrease of ankle systolic blood pressure, rest pain and skin necrosis. This theory suggests a possible pharmacological treatment of the unstable arteriopathy, with calcium heparin [53], prostanoids [54] or thrombolysis [55], which could restore a stable pathway, following which elective surgery will give better results than emergency surgical intervention, as in salvage surgery.

Instrumental examinations

The first diagnostic approach after anamnesis and clinical examination is measurement of systolic blood pressure along all the arteries of the lower limbs. The normal ratio between ankle and brachial blood presure is over 1.00; a ratio under 0.85 signifies a significant arterial stenosis. A decrease of more than 20–25 mmHg between two near sections (femoral and popliteal arteries) also indicates significant stenosis.

The next step is recording of the analogical signal of the Doppler continuous wave which is able to locate the stenosis and its hemodynamics (Figure 19.7). From the anatomic point of view the next examination is angiography, used for preoperative study.

Functional assessment is by measurement of district flow. The best technique is strain gauge plethysmography with venous occlusion, which can measure rest flow, peak flow after ischemia, time to peak flow and the half time of the post-ischemia hyperemia. The rest flow is not different between healthy subjects and patients because of the high peripheral resistances of the arteries of the limbs. For this reason, in clinical practice, resting flow measurement cannot distinguish patients from the controls; this can be done by assessment of blood flow after ischemic or muscular stress. After 3 min of ischemia (performed with a cuff inflated over the systolic blood pressure), is increased 3 or 4 times in healthy subjects. This ability is reduced in proportion to the degree of illness in arteriopathic patients (Figure 19.8).

The microcirculatory pathway can be investigated using the most recent techniques, laser-Doppler and transcutaneous measurement of O_2 ($tcpO_2$) and pCO_2 ($tcpCO_2$). The first is useful for investigation of microhemodynamics at rest and after ischemia, assessment of vasomotion and flowmotion, the presence of the veno-arteriolar reflex and restoration of autoregulation after ischemic stress (Figure 19.9). The latter is very helpful in assessment of some pathophysiological features. It can indicate arteriolar perfusion (*resting $tcpO_2$*), tissue damage (*resting tcp CO_2*) [49, 52], ability of the microcirculation to improve arteriolar perfusion (*$tcpO_2$ during oxygen breathing*) [56], microcirculatory hyperemia and tissue reperfusion (*oxygen recovery time* and *oxygen recovery index after ischemia*) [57, 58], tissue ability to regain a normal metabolic function (*half $tcpO_2$ recovery time after ischemia*) [49, 59], tissue resistance to ischemia, and the prognosis of patients with CLI (*$tcpCO_2$ production during ischemia and $tcpCO_2$ during postural tests*) [60–62] (Figure 19.10).

Addendum

Up to now, we have relied on these concepts, especially the $tcpCO_2$, for assessment of the skin necrosis risk, because this parameter measures the *tissue acidosis degree*, at rest and during ischemia. Nevertheless, in our investigation we went on to better define, in microcirculatory and tissue keys, the reactive hyperemia phenomenon.

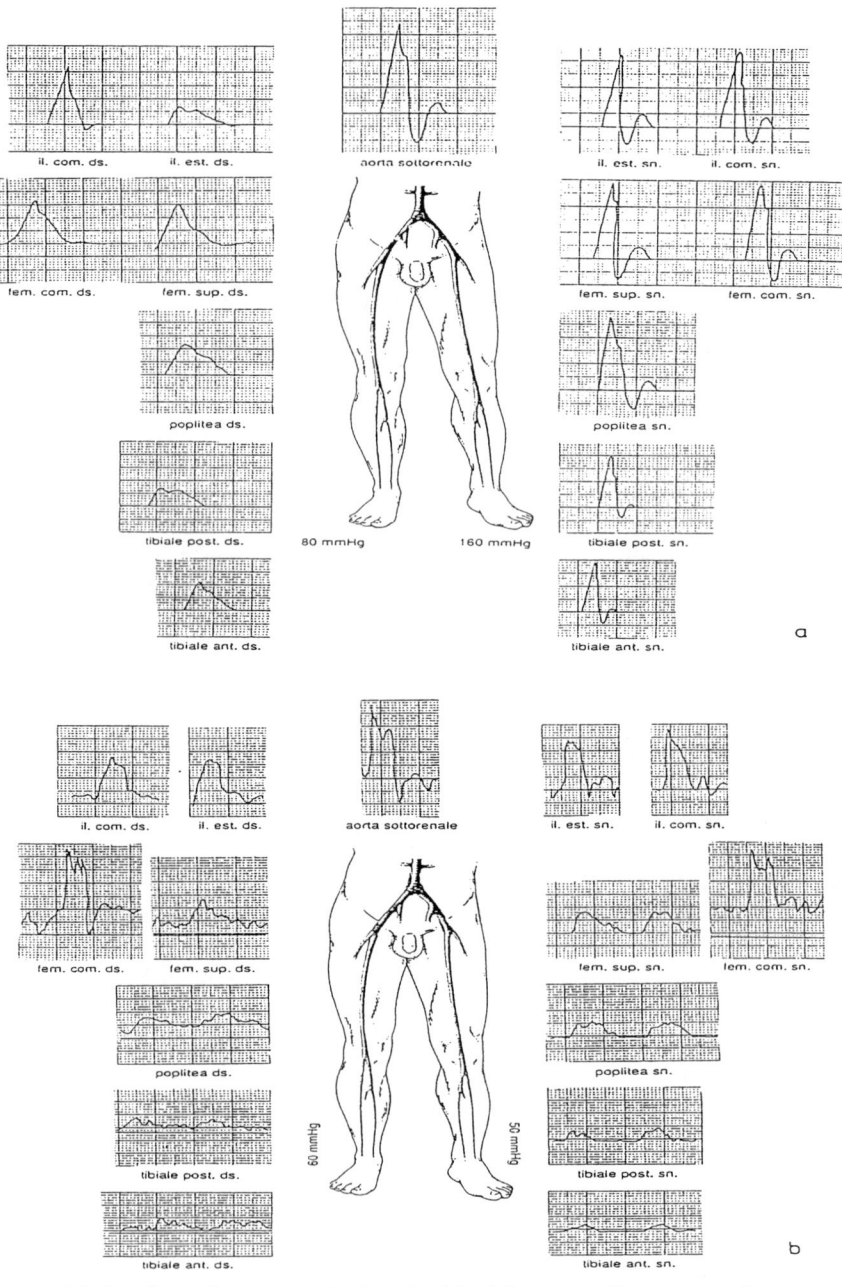

Figure 19.7. Doppler continuous wave. (a) Stenosis of the right common iliac artery, good spontaneous (collateral vessels) revascularization. Significant decrease of right ankle systolic blood pressure; demodulation of all waves on the right side; presence of continuous flow velocity in the femoral arteries, which disappears in the downstream measurements. (b) Multiple stenosis and obstruction of the right and left arterial axis. Very important reduction of the ankle systolic blood pressure; severe demodulation of all waves from the under kidney aorta to the tibial arteries.

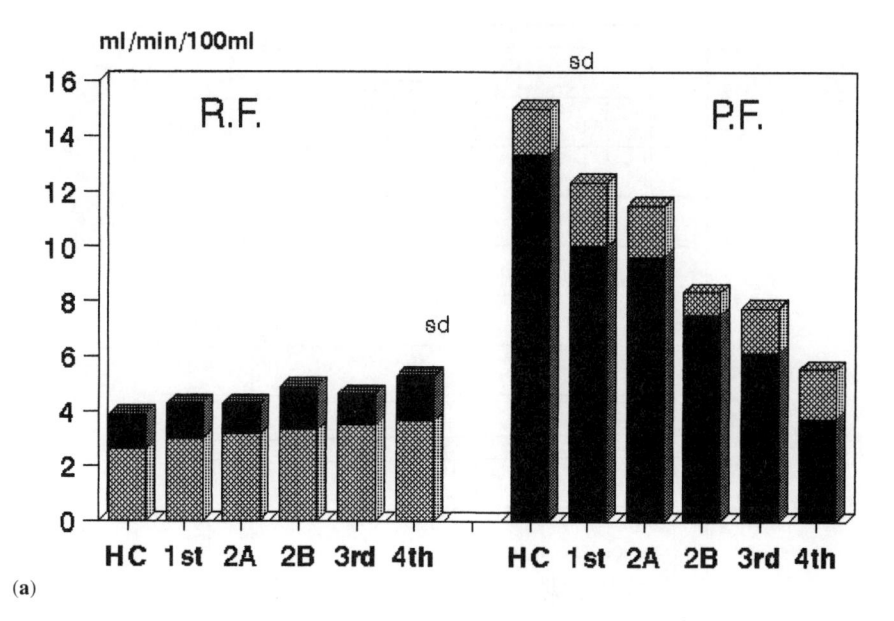

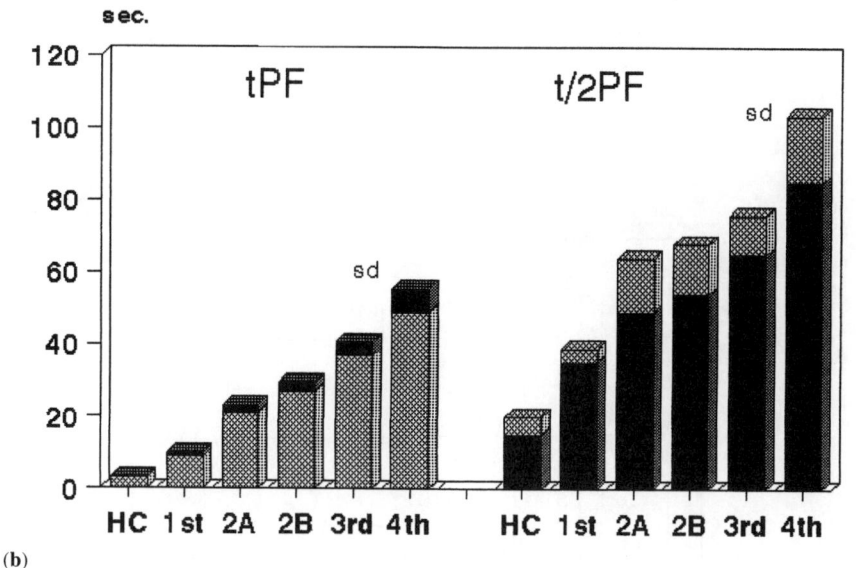

Figure 19.8. Strain gauge plethysmography. (a) Rest flow with no difference between healthy controls and patients. Peak flow (maximal reactive hyperemia after ischemic stress) with proportional decrease to the degree of disease. Note that the rest and the peak flow at the fourth stage have the same value; this is due to the permanent exciting vasodilating status of the patients, because of the high hypoxia. (b) The time parameters show an increase in the time of appearance of hyperemia after ischemia (tPF), related to the stenosis or obstruction; the duration of the hyperemia (t/2PF) is increased, related to the microcirculatory capability of washing out the ischemic catabolites.

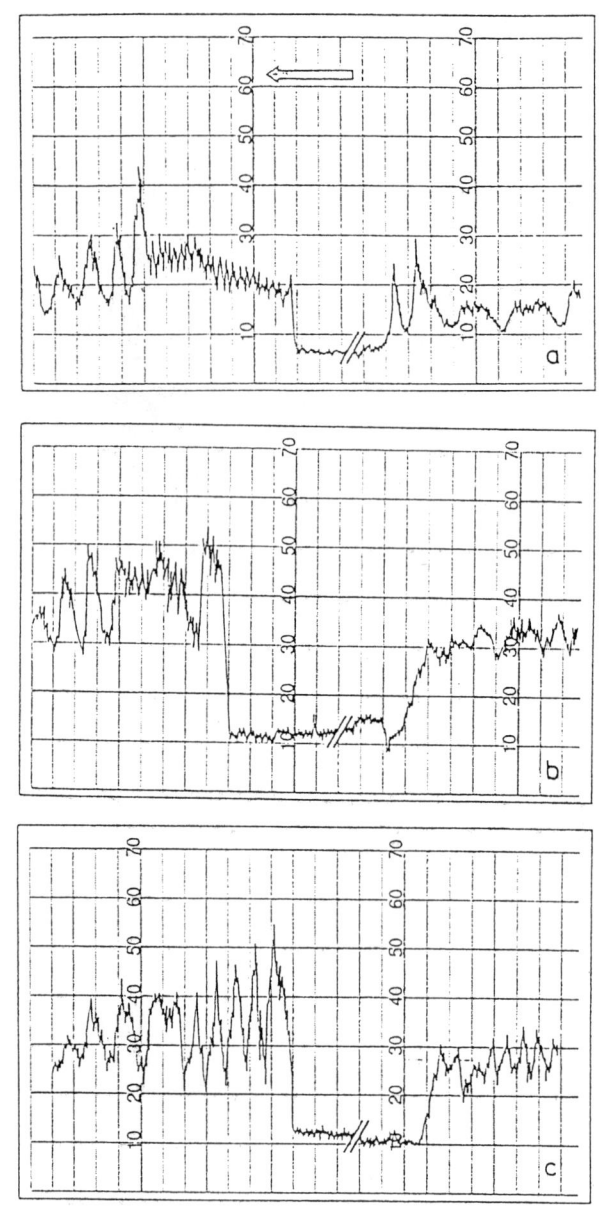

Figure 19.9. Big toe laser-Doppler output signal, in a patient with critical limb ischemia, during iloprost infusion (2.5 ng/kg/min). (a) t0, resting flow with low-frequency waves (LFW, 1.5–2.0 cycles/min) and evidence of high-frequency waves (HFW); post-ischemic flow with only HFW; restoration of autoregulation (LFW) after 80 sec. (b) t 60 min, resting flow with LFW 5 cycles/min; HFW less evidence; post ischemic flow with restoration of autoregulation after 15 sec; HFW still evident for 60 sec. (c) t 120 min, resting flow with marked increased of LFW (7 cycles/min); HFW not clearly visible; post-ischemic flow with poor evidence of HFW and restoration of autoregulation after 10 sec.

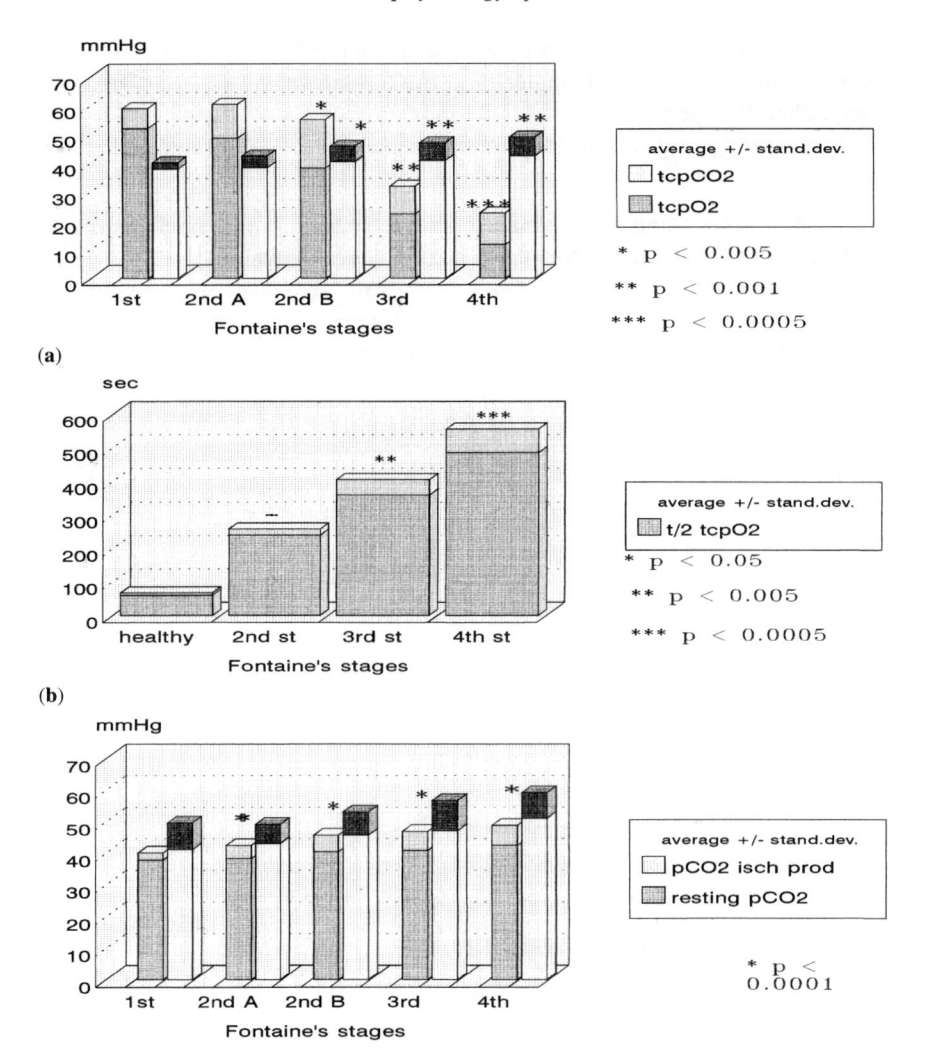

Figure 19.10. (a) Resting metatarsal transcutaneous pO_2 ($tcpO_2$) and pCO_2 ($tcpCO_2$) in patients with peripheral arterial disease. Progressive reduction of $tcpO_2$, related to the reduction of arterial and arteriolar inflow. Progressive increase of $tcpCO_2$ at Fontaine's stages IIB, III and IV, related to severe tissue damage assessing the deterioration of the cellular metabolism, sustained by reduced responsiveness of the oxidative enzymes, with lactate production. (b) Half recovery time of $tcpO_2$, after 3 min of ischemia in patients with peripheral arterial disease. During the ischemic test (calf cuff inflated over systolic blood pressure), $tcpO_2$ falls to zero-level, concomitant with the cessation of arterial inflow. After removing ischemia, in healthy controls the half value of the rest-level is restored in 60 sec. This time becomes gradually longer with different stages of peripheral arterial disease. It indicates the tissue ability to regain a normal metabolic function. (c) Metatarsal $tcpCO_2$ at rest and during ischemia in patients with peripheral arterial disease. During the ischemic test, when $tcpO_2$ falls to zero-level, $tcpCO_2$ increases. By measuring the resting value and value at 3 min, and subtracting the first from the second, $tcpCO_2$ production can be calculated. It increases proportionally with the degree of disease, and is a measure of tissue resistance to ischemia, an important prognostic value.

We are investigating this aspect by long-term continous recording of the microhemodynamic events (laser Doppler) and the tissue events ($tcpO_2$ and $tcpCO_2$) during ischemia–reperfusion.

The following points are the most important suggestions from our preliminary results:

(i) the 3 minutes standard ischemia is able to induce an ischemia (with laser Doppler at biological ZERO), but it hardly induces a hypoxia;
(ii) prolonging the stress until the $tcpO_2$ reaches the zero level, we noted that the time of hypoxia is longer in healthy controls than in patients;
(iii) after the reperfusion the LD reaches the peak flux immediately in healthy controls and later in patients;
(iv) during the hemodynamic reperfusion $tcpCO_2$ continues to increase and always reaches its plateau after the laser Doppler peak flux;
(v) the duration of the $tcpCO_2$ plateau is longer in patients than in healthy controls.

This behavior means that, in spite of the increasing oxygen, the cells only slowly recover their breathing capacity, proportionately to the tissue injury. If the $tcpCO_2$ production during 3 minutes of ischemia is already a reliable parameter, a higher reliability could probably be given by measuring the time of hypoxia, the $tcpCO_2$ plateau, and the recovery slope of $tcpCO_2$ [63].

References

1. Ross R, Glomset JA. Atherosclerosis and the arterial smooth muscle cell. Science 1973;180:1332–9.
2. Ross R, Glonset JA. The pathogenesis of atherosclerosis. N Engl J Med 1976;295:369–77.
3. Ross R. The pathogenesis of atherogenesis – an update. N Eng J Med 1986;314:488.
4. Di Perri T. Le arteriopatie ostruttive degli arti. Fisiopatologia e clinica. Rel 87° Congr Soc It Medicina Interna, Pozzi ed, Roma 1986.
5. Andreozzi GM. Manuale di Semeiotica Strumentale Angiologica. Editoriale Grasso ed, Bologna, 1992.
6. Andreozzi GM, Martini R, Di Pino L, Signorelli S. Clinical physiology of the microcirculation In: Borgatti E, & De Fabritiis A (eds), New trends in vascular exploration. Turin: Minerva Medica, 1994:25–36.
7. Intaglietta M. Vasomotion as a normal microvascular activity and a reaction to impaired homeostasis. In: Vasomotion and flowmotion in the microcirculation. Progr Appl Microcirc, Karger ed, Basel, 1989, XVI–9.
8. Colantuoni A, Bertuglia A, Intaglietta M. Microvessels diameter changes during hemorrhagic shock in unanesthetized hamster. Microvasc Res, 1983;30:133–42.
9. Colantuoni A, Bertuglia A, Intaglietta M. Variations of rhythmical diameter changes at the arterial microvascular bifurcation. Pflugers Arch 1985;403:280–95.
10. Needelman P, Marshall GR, Sobel BE. Hormone interactions in the isolated rabbit heart: Synthesis and coronary vasomotor effects of prostaglandins, angiotensin and bradykinin. Cir Res 1975;37:802–8.
11. Dusting GJ, Vane JR. Some cardiovascular properties of prostacyclin (PGI_2) which are not shared by PGE_2. Circ Res 1980;46(Suppl):183–7.
12. Palmer RMJ, Ferrige AG, Moncada S. Nitric oxide release accounts for the biological activity of endothelium-derived relaxing factor. Nature 1987;327:524–6.

13. Ignarro LJ, Harbison RG, Wood SK, Kadowitz PJ. Activation of purified soluble guanylate cyclase by endothelium-derived relaxing factor from intrapulmonary artery and vein: Stimulation of acetylcholine, bradykinin and arachidonic acid. J Pharmacol Exp Ther 1986;237:893–900.
14. Vane JR, Anggard EE, Botting RM. Regulatory functions of the vascular endothelium. N Engl J Med 1990;323:27–36.
15. Yanagisawa M, Masaki T. Molecular biology and biochemestry of the endothelins. Trends Pharmacol Sci 1989;10:374–9.
16. Katusic ZS, Vanhoutte PM. Superoxide anion is an endothelium-derived contracting factor. Am J Physiol 1989;257:H33–H7.
17. Rubanyi GM, Vanhoutte PM. Superoxide anions and hyperoxia inactivate endothelium-derived relaxing factor. Am J Physiol 1986 250:H822–H927.
18. Shephered JT, Katusic' ZS. Endothelium-derived vasoactive factors I. Endothelium-dependent relaxation. Hypertension 1991;18:III-76–III-85.
19. Katusic' ZS, Shephered JT. Endothelium-derived vasoactive factors II. Endothelium-dependent contraction. Hypertension 1991;18.III-86–III-92.
20. Lowe G. Pathophysiology of critical leg ischaemia: In: Dormandy JA, Stock, G (eds), Critical leg ischaemia, its pathophysiology and management. Berlin–Heidelberg: Springer-Verlag, 1990:33.
21. Dintenfass L. Blood microrheology. Viscosity factors in blood, ischaemia and thrombosis. London: Butterworths, 1971.
22. Di Perri T. Rheological factors in circulatory disorders. Angiology 1979;30:480–6.
23. Forconi S, Pieragalli D, Gerrini M et al. Hemorheology and peripheral arterial disease. Clin Haemorheol 1987;7:146–58.
24. Andreozzi GM, Signorelli S, Magnano V, Tornetta D, Ferrara M, Interlandi S. Profilo emoreologico del vasculopatico diabetico. Giorn It Diabet 1986;6:113–5.
25. Caimi G, Catania A, D'Asaro S et al. Red cell phospholipids and membrane microviscosity in diabetics. Clin Hemorheol 1988;8:939–44.
26. Caimi G, Serra A, Lo Presti R, Sarno A. Red cell membrane protein lateral mobility in diabetes mellitus. Horm Metab Res 1992;24:409–11.
27. Moritz MW, Reimers RC, Kendall-Baker R et al. Role of cytoplasmic and releasable ADP in platelet aggregation induced by laminar shear stress. J Clin Lab Med 1983;101:537–44.
28. Braquet P, Touqui L, Shen TY et al. Perspectives in platelet-activating factor research. Pharmacol Rev 1987;39:97–145.
29. Mantovani A, Dejana E. Cytokines as communication signals between leukocytes and endothelial cells. Immunol Today 1989;10:370.
30. Niedbala MJ. Cytokine regulation of endothelial cells extracellular proteolysis. Agents Act 1993;42(Suppl):179–93.
31. Burke Gaffhey A, Kenan AK. Modulation of human cell permeability of the cytokines interleukin-1 alpha/beta, tumor necrosis factor and interferon gamma. Immunopharmacology 1993;25:1–9.
32. Tajana G, Peluso G. Macrophage and aging. In: Davidson (ed.), cutaneous development aging and repair, Springer Verlag, 1988:273–8.
33. Ernst E, Hammerschmidt DE, Bagge U, Matrai S, Dormandy JA. Leukocytes and the risk of ischaemic disease. J Am Med Assoc 1987;2318:257.
34. Bagge U. Leukocytes and capillary perfusion in shock. In: Meiselman HJ, Lichtyman MA (eds), White cells mechanism: Basic science and clinical aspects. Alan R Liss, 285 La Celle PL, 1984.
35. Lefer AM, Araki H, Okamatsu S. Beneficial action of free radical scavenger in traumatic shock and myocardial ischaemia. Circ Shock 1981;8:273.
36. Das DK, Engelman RM. Mechanism of free radicals generation during reperfusion of ischaemic myocardium. In: Oxygen radicals. Karger Publ, 1990:97.
37. Powell WJ Jr, DiBona DR, Flores J, Leaf A. The protective effect of hyperosmotic mannitol in myocardial ischemia and necrosis. Circulation 1976;54:603.
38. Lucchesi BR, Werns SW, Fantone JC. The role of the neutrophils and radicals in ischemic myocardial injury. J Mol Cell Cardiol 1989;21:1241.

39. Davies SW, Ranyaldalayan K, Wickens DJ, Dormandy TL, Timmins AD. Lipids peroxidation associated with successful thrombolysis. Lancet 1990;339:741–3.
40. Gey KF, Brubacher GB, Stahelin HB. Plasma levels of antioxidant vitamins in relation to ischemic heart disease and cancer. Am J Clin Nutr 1987;45:1368–77.
41. Guarneri C, Flamigni F, Caldarera CM. Role of oxygen in the cellular damage induced by reoxygenation of hypoxic heart. J Ned Cell Cardiol 1980;12:797–808.
42. Warren JS, Ward PA. Oxidative injury to the vascular endothelium. Am J Med Sci 1986;292:97–103.
43. Yagi K. Assay for serum lipid peroxide level and its clinical significance. In: Lipid peroxides in biology and medicine. New York: Academic Press, 1982:231–41.
44. Andreozzi GM, Signorelli S, Martini R *et al.* Leukocytic chemotaxis and malonyldialdehyde in stasis and ischaemia in experimental human models '*in vivo*'. Proceedings Eur Congr Intern Union Phlebology, Budapest September 6–10, 1993. Brentwood, Essex: MultiScience Publication, 1993:28–32.
45. Andreozzi GM, Signorelli S, Martini R, Di Pino L. Hemodynamic and cellular effects in ischaemia and stasis: Clinical and experimental models (Invited lecture 18th Europ Conf Microcirculation). Int J Microcirc Clin Exper 1994;s1 14:247 (abstract 451).
46. Sironi M, Breviario F, Proserpio P *et al.* IL-1 stimulates IL-6 production in endothelial cells. J Immunol 1989;15,142:549–53.
47. Andreozzi GM. L'ischemia critica. La Presse Médicale (ed it) 1993:3s 3–40.
48. Signorelli S, Antignani PL, De Fabritiis A *et al.* Il test da sforzo al tappeto ruotante. Confronto di quattro differenti protocolli. Min Angiol 1991;16:sl, 84.
49. Andreozzi GM, Signorelli S, Butto G *et al.* Oxygen transcutaneous tensiometry ($tcpO_2$) for microcirculatory evaluation of peripheral arterial disease. Cardiovascular World Report 1990;3:37–9.
50. Dormandy JA, Stock G, (eds), Critical leg ischaemia, its pathophysiology and management. Berlin–Heidelberg: Springer-Verlag, 1990.
51. European Working Group on Critical Leg Ischemia. Second European Consensus Document on Critical Leg Ischemia. Circulation 1991;84(4):1–26.
52. Andreozzi GM. Dynamic measurement and functional balance of $tcpO_2$ and $tcpCO_2$, in peripheral arterial disease. J Cardiovasc Diagn Proc 1995;13:155–63.
53. Andreozzi GM, Signorelli S, Cacciaguerra G *et al.* Three-month therapy with calcium-heparin in comparison with ticlopidine in patients with peripheral arterial occlusive disease at Leriche–Fontaine IIb class. Angiology 1993;44(4):307–13.
54. Andreozzi GM, Di Pino L, Li Pira M, Butto G, Martini R, Signorelli S: Iloprost, stable analogue of prostacyclin, is able to improve the tissue resistance to ischaemia? Int J Angiol 1994;13:68–9.
55. Andreozzi GM, Signorelli S, Di Pino L, Martini R, Pharmacological treatment of critical limb ischaemia: Experience of urokinase and iloprost. Intern Angiol 1994;13(S1):8.
56. Bongard O, Krahenbuhl B. Predicting amputation in severe ischaemia: The value of transcutaneous pO_2 measurement. Bone Joint Surg 1988;70N:465–67.
57. Caspary L, Creutzig A, Alexander K. Variability of $tcpO_2$ measurement at 37 degrees C and 44 degrees C in patients with claudication in consideration of provocating tests. Vasa 1993;22(2):129–36.
58. Slagsvold CE, Kvernebo K, Stranden E *et al.* Postischemic transcutaneous oxygen tension response in assessment of peripheral atherosclerosis. Vasc Surg 1988;22:101–9.
59. Slagsvold CE, Stranden E, Rosén L, Kroese AJ. Role of blood perfusion and tissue oxygenation in the postischemic transcutaneous pO_2 response. Angiology 1992;43:155–62.
60. Signorelli S, Butto G, Martini R, Di Pino L, Andreozzi GM. Dynamic parameters of transcutaneous gas analysis in peripheral arterial disease. Int J Microcirc Clin Exp 1994;14(1):178.
61. Andreozzi GM, Riggio F, Butto G *et al.* Transcutaneous pCO_2 level as an index of tissue resistance to the ischaemia. Angiology 1995;46:1097–102.
62. Palermo G, Allegra C. $TcpO_2$ $tcpCO_2$ in critical limb ischaemia. Int J Microcirc Clin Exp 1994;14(1):177.
63. Andreozzi GM, Martini R, Di Pino L, Signorelli S. Prognostic value of $tcpO_2$–$tcpCO_2$ and assessment of the skin necrosis risk (abstract). Int J Microcirculation Clin Exp 1996; 16(S1):41.

20. Epidemiology and risk factors of diseases of lower limb arteries

GILLIAN C. LENG and F. GERRY R. FOWKES

Epidemiology

The first large scale cardiovascular survey to include peripheral arterial disease began in 1949 in the town of Framingham, USA, where a cohort of 5209 men and women was selected from the general population for examination and subsequent follow-up [1]. Since then major population studies have also been conducted in other countries, including Switzerland [2], Finland [3], Denmark [4] and the United States [5]. In 1989, a longitudinal study was established in Edinburgh to examine a wide range of risk factors in a cohort of over 1500 subjects [6]. This is probably the largest survey specifically designed to study peripheral atherosclerosis, and the results should provide important insights into the etiology of the disease.

Incidence and prevalence of lower limb atherosclerosis

Most epidemiological surveys have concentrated on identifying the prevalence of intermittent claudication. This is the most common symptom of lower limb atherosclerosis, and its prevalence is therefore a good indicator of the degree of morbidity in the general population. In 1962, Professor G. Rose at the London School of Hygiene devised a questionnaire to diagnose intermittent claudication in epidemiological surveys [7], and this was subsequently adopted by the World Health Organization (WHO) and used throughout the world. Unfortunately, although this questionnaire is known to be very specific, it is only moderately sensitive [8, 9], but until a more accurate alternative is adopted [9] it remains the most valid way of making international comparisons.

The prevalence of more severe symptoms of limb ischemia, such as rest pain, have generally not been determined in population surveys. This is primarily because the symptoms are uncharacteristic and therefore easily confused with other causes of leg pain such as arthritis and venous disease, making them difficult to diagnose by questionnaire. However, as the majority of patients with critical ischemia are referred to hospital for treatment, fairly complete data can be obtained from hospital records.

To detect less severe peripheral atherosclerosis that might not be symptomatic, several population surveys have also included noninvasive physiological tests of blood flow. The most widely used test has been the measurement of ankle systolic pressures [4, 6, 10], but a few studies have also included more sophisticated tests including analysis of pulse wave forms on oscillography [10, 11], a reactive hyperemia test [6, 10], and B-mode ultrasound scanning of the popliteal artery [5]. In the five-year follow-up of the Edinburgh Artery Study, duplex scanning was included to allow both the site of atheroma and the velocity of blood flow to be determined. Autopsy studies also provide accurate documentation of the extent of lower limb atherosclerosis in selected groups, but these data may not be representative of the general population.

Symptomatic disease
The prevalence of intermittent claudication determined throughout the world using the WHO questionnaire shows much variation, ranging from 0.6% in North American women [12] to 6.9% in men in Moscow [13] (Table 20.1). Some of this variation reflects true international differences, but unfortunately none of these studies are strictly comparable because of different age structures in the populations, possible errors of translation and healthy worker effects. In those studies which include women, the prevalence is generally found to be higher in men of equivalent age [4, 6, 12, 16], but in both women and men the prevalence of intermittent claudication increases with age [6, 10, 16] (Figure 20.1). A similar pattern is seen in the incidence of disease, which lags behind in women by about ten years and also increases with age [19].

The incidence of critical limb ischemia, estimated from the number of major amputations, ranges from 500 to 1000 per million population per year. This takes into account the fact that a considerable number of patients die prior to amputation, and that the majority of patients benefit from reconstructive surgery [20]. There are approximately 50 000 admissions each year in England and Wales with a diagnosis of

Table 20.1. International prevalences of intermittent claudication determined using the WHO questionnaire in subjects aged 40–60 years selected from the general population.

Authors	Study location	Prevalence (%)	
		Males	Females
Isaacson, 1972 [14]	Malmo, Sweden	2.8	NI[a]
Bothig et al., 1976 [13]	Berlin, Germany	3.4	NI
	Moscow, Russia	6.9	NI
De Backer et al., 1979 [15]	Belgium	1.4	NI
Schroll and Munck, 1981 [4]	Glostrup, Denmark	5.8	1.3
Reunanen et al., 1982 [16]	Finland	3.0	2.0
Pomrehn et al., 1986 [12]	North America	0.9	0.6
Gofin et al., 1987 [10]	Jerusalem, Israel	1.3	1.9
Dagenais et al., 1991 [17]	Quebec, Canada	4.2	NI
Fowkes et al., 1991 [6]	Edinburgh, Scotland	2.4	2.2

[a] NI – Female subjects not included.

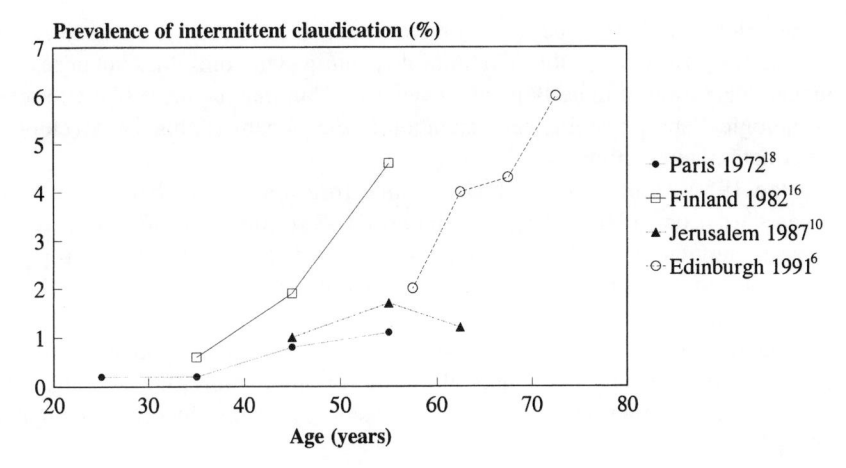

Figure 20.1. Prevalence of intermittent claudication in men by age in community-based studies.

peripheral arterial disease, and of these over 15 000 have major surgery including amputation [21].

Asymptomatic disease
In general the prevalence of peripheral arterial disease detected by noninvasive procedures is about three times greater than the prevalence of intermittent claudication [4, 6, 22], with a similar distribution by age and sex [23]. Unfortunately, because there is a lack of standardization between different surveys, it is impossible to form true comparisons. An autopsy study of 293 unselected cases carried out in Oxford in the 1960s, found that 15% of men and 5% of women had disease severe enough to produce more than 50% stenosis of at least one artery [24]. More surprisingly, none of the men and only one of the women were completely free of atherosclerotic plaques in their common iliac arteries [24]. Similar results have also been found in autopsy studies in Pittsburgh [25] and Malmo, Sweden [26].

Natural history

The natural history of peripheral arterial disease has been examined in population studies in Framingham [19, 27], Basle [11], London, Whitehall [28], Denmark [29], and Finland [16]. The degree of morbidity has been determined by amputation rates and, more subjectively, by assessing the degree of symptoms. However, the increasing availability of bypass surgery, angioplasty and thrombolytic therapy means that measuring the degree of morbidity may no longer be a true reflection of the natural progression of the disease.

Morbidity
Studies in which claudicants have been asked to assess changes in the severity of their symptoms with time suggest that at least half will improve, less than one-third

will deteriorate [30–35], and that improvement will be greater if the subject stops smoking [36]. However, subjective improvement in symptoms does not necessarily indicate regression of underlying atherosclerosis, but may be more likely to reflect psychological and physiological adaptation to the ischemia, plus the development of a collateral circulation.

In the 1950s, almost 10% of claudicants followed up for between two and 15 years went on to require leg amputation [30–35]. More recently, however, the five-year cumulative incidence of amputations was as low as 1% [27], a drop probably produced by increasing therapeutic intervention. Patients are more likely to proceed to amputation if they are heavy smokers when diagnosed [37] and if they continue to smoke [38]. Diabetes is probably also an exacerbating factor [39], and a raised systolic pressure may reduce the need for amputation [35], although some evidence suggests that diabetes and hypertension have no influence on the natural history [37].

Mortality

The five-year cumulative mortality rates for males with intermittent claudication range from 4.8% [28] to 17% [27]. Mortality rates are invariably higher in men than in women [16, 40, 41], but the relative risks of death are similar [40]. Mortality rates also increase with age, although the relative risks fall with age [32, 39–41]. Similar patterns have also been found in subjects followed up for ten years [27, 32, 34, 40].

The increased mortality rate is undoubtedly associated with smoking: smokers have relative risks of between 1.5 and 3.0 compared with non-smokers, and there is improved survival among subjects who stop smoking [16, 30, 38, 39]. Some studies have also shown increased risks associated with raised blood pressure [16, 34, 41], serum cholesterol [16] and diabetes mellitus [30].

Patients with intermittent claudication are therefore likely to die sooner than their healthy counterparts, but peripheral arterial disease itself is very rarely the cause of death [34]. Most patients die from ischemic heart disease, which accounts for 33–60% of deaths, followed by cerebrovascular disease and other vascular diseases [29, 32, 34, 36, 40, 41]. Follow-up studies have shown that subjects with intermittent claudication have three times the risk of dying from ischemic heart disease, and twice the risk of dying from stroke as the general population [16, 28, 42].

Risk factors

The most well established risk factors for the development of peripheral arterial disease are cigarette smoking and raised blood lipids, but hypertension, diabetes, elevated hemostatic factors and many others are probably also important. Conclusive evidence for the role of individual risk factors requires long-term follow-up studies of large cohorts of the general population, but unfortunately relatively few studies have been performed to date.

Smoking

Cigarette smoking is probably the single most powerful risk factor for peripheral vascular disease [43]. Cross-sectional surveys of the general population suggest that smokers may have more than seven times the risk of developing peripheral arterial disease than non-smokers, although some studies show a much smaller risk (Table 20.2). This variation can be accounted for partly by differences in age, sex and nationality of the study population, the presence of arterial disease, and also by the criteria used to define a smoker and the fact that under-reporting of smoking undoubtedly occurs. Current smoking appears to contribute to 14–53% of disease [23], and if ex-smokers are also included the figures become even higher [3, 15, 16, 44–46]. In the Framingham study, 16 years of follow-up suggested that 78% of cases of intermittent claudication could be attributable to smoking [1]. Multivariate analyses suggest that smoking has an independent effect greater than other risk factors [1, 4, 47].

Smoking appears to be a more important risk factor for the development of peripheral arterial disease than for ischemic heart disease [48], although it is not clear why this should be. It has been suggested that the increased hydrostatic pressure in the leg arteries may result in damaged endothelial cell junctions, thus permitting a greater influx of nicotine into the subendothelial space [49]. Alternatively, it may be simply a dose–response effect in which more smoking produces more severe disease, and as claudicants tend to be older [23] they presumably have more advanced atherosclerosis.

Lipids

Numerous clinical and epidemiological studies have examined the role of serum cholesterol, triglyceride and lipoproteins in the etiology of peripheral arterial disease, and more recently essential fatty acids and antioxidants have also been studied as potential risk factors.

Table 20.2. Risk of developing peripheral arterial disease in male smokers selected from the general population.

Author	Age of population (years)	Definition of a smoker	Relative risk
Higgins and Kjelsberg, 1967 [44]	20–79	Current smoker	1.9
Bothig et al., 1976 [13]	50–54	≥ 10 cigarettes/day	1.4
Heliovaara et al., 1978 [3]	55–74	≥ 1 cigarette/day	7.4
De Backer et al., 1979 [15]	40–55	Current smoker	1.4
Reunanen et al., 1982 [16]	30–59	Current smoker	1.7
Gofin et al., 1987 [10]	40–60	Current smoker	1.1
Dagenais et al., 1991 [17]	35–64	Cigar and/or pipe	2.8
		1–20 cigarettes/day	3.8
		≥ 21 cigarettes/day	4.0

Triglycerides

Elevated levels of serum triglycerides have been identified in patients with peripheral arterial disease in numerous case control studies [50–57]. Similarly, the majority of cross-sectional surveys carried out in the general population have also shown a univariate association with triglyceride levels [4, 6, 12, 45, 58], but others have shown no significant relationship [10, 16, 29, 59]. However, when multivariate analyses are performed to adjust for the influence of other risk factors, including other lipids, no independent relationship can be found between triglycerides and the occurrence of peripheral arterial disease (Table 20.3). The longitudinal relationship between serum triglyceride and the future development of peripheral arterial disease has been examined in the Basle Study [61] and in the Glostrup Study [4]. Of 2759 men in the Basle Study, 174 developed disease during a five-year period, and of these 59% had elevated baseline levels of triglyceride. In the Glostrup Study, the fasting serum triglyceride level at 50 years of age was correlated with the ankle brachial pressure index ten years later. However, again this relationship disappeared on multivariate analysis adjusting for smoking, blood pressure and serum cholesterol. Recent evidence from the Edinburgh Artery Study suggests that the strong univariate relationship between triglyceride and arterial disease can mostly be explained by the correlation between triglyceride levels and non-HDL cholesterol [6]. Current evidence therefore indicates that the association between triglycerides and peripheral arterial disease is comparable to that with ischemic heart disease: a strong univariate association disappearing on multivariate analysis.

Table 20.3. Association between serum triglycerides and peripheral arterial disease in community-based cross-sectional studies.

Author	Age of population (years)	Definition of peripheral arterial disease	Association of triglycerides with disease	
			Univariate	Multivariate
Hughson et al., 1978 [45]	50–69	Claudication	Positive*	
De Backer et al., 1979 [15]	40–55	ABPI[a]	No association	
Schroll and Munck, 1981 [4]	50	ABPI	Positive*	No association
		Claudication + ABPI	Positive*	
Reunanen et al., 1982 [16]	30–59	Claudication	No association	
Pomrehn et al., 1986 [12]	≥ 20	Claudication	Positive‡	
		ABPI	No association	
		Exercise test	Positive*	No association
Gofin et al., 1987 [10]	≥ 25	ABPI	No association	
		Claudication + ABPI	No association	No association
Hale et al., 1988 [58]	≥ 65	Claudication	Positive***	
Fowkes et al., 1992 [60]	55–74	Claudication	Positive***	No association
		ABPI	Positive***	No association

[a] Ankle brachial pressure index.
Statistical significance: * = $p < 0.05$; *** = $p < 0.001$; ‡ = not known.

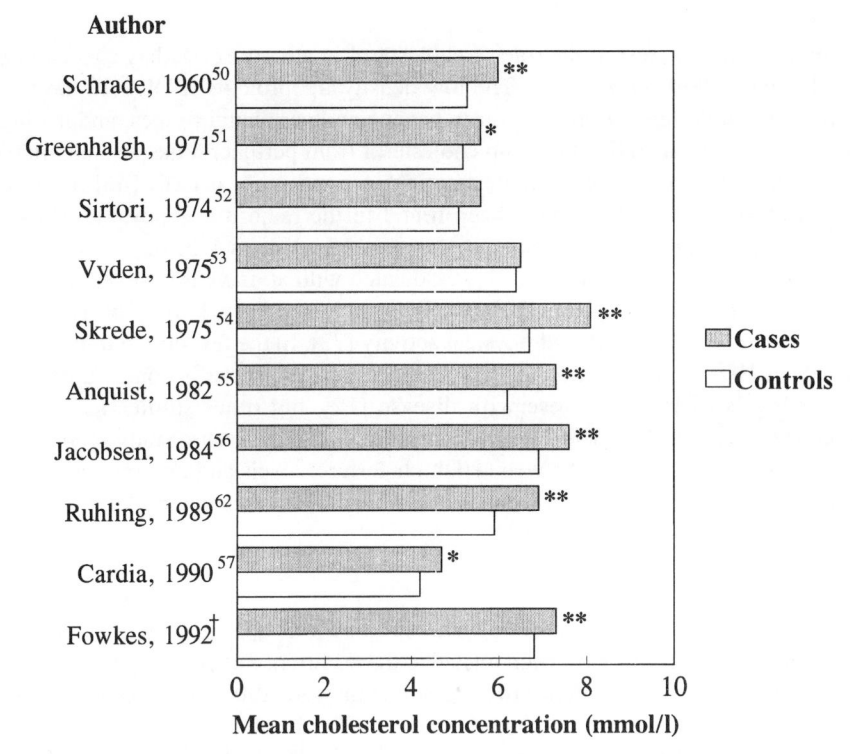

Figure 20.2. Serum cholesterol levels in clinical cases and controls in studies of peripheral arterial disease. Control subjects were all matched by age and sex. † Unpublished data from the Edinburgh Artery Study. * = $p < 0.05$; ** = $p < 0.01$.

Cholesterol
Elevated levels of serum cholesterol in patients with peripheral arterial disease have also been identified in the majority of hospital-based case-control studies (Figure 20.2), but significantly elevated levels have not been found in all studies, particularly in those where the age–sex matching was poor [63, 64]. Similarly, although most cross-sectional studies in the community show elevated cholesterol levels in diseased subjects [4, 6, 10, 16, 65], a few have shown no relationship [12, 15, 45]. In the Edinburgh [6] and Dunedin [58] cross-sectional studies, the relationship with serum cholesterol persisted after adjustment for other risk factors, but this was not the case in the Israeli study [10]. However, positive associations between serum cholesterol and the development of peripheral arterial disease have been found in two longitudinal studies: after 26 years of follow-up in the Framingham Study, serum cholesterol was found to be a significant, but weak risk factor for intermittent claudication [19]; and after ten years follow-up in the Danish Study, serum cholesterol was found to correlate with ankle brachial pressure indices, independent of other risk factors [4]. Therefore, on balance, there is sufficient evidence to indicate that elevated cholesterol levels are an independent risk factor for the development of peripheral arterial disease.

Lipoproteins

In recent years interest in the role of cholesterol in atherogenesis has concentrated on the lipoprotein subfractions. The low density lipoproteins (LDL) are the main carriers of cholesterol from the liver to hepatic and peripheral tissues, and the high density lipoproteins (HDL) pick up cholesterol from peripheral tissues and arterial walls and return it to the liver, thus acting in opposition to LDL [66]. Reduced levels of HDL cholesterol have been found in the majority of hospital cases of peripheral arterial disease compared with control subjects [55, 62, 67–69], with only one exception [70], and are also associated with an increased severity of peripheral arterial disease [56, 71]. Low HDL cholesterol levels may be related to cigarette smoking and reduced physical activity [72]. In the few community studies in which HDL cholesterol levels have been examined, there is some support for lower levels of HDL in those with disease [12], but other studies showed no significant relationship [10]. However, in the Edinburgh Artery Study there was a strong inverse relationship between HDL cholesterol levels and intermittent claudication, which persisted on adjustment for other lipids, obesity, smoking, diabetes and alcohol consumption [6].

Apolipoproteins

Each LDL particle contains a large protein known as apolipoprotein B (apo B). Apolipoprotein B levels have been related to the occurrence of coronary heart disease [73], and there is some evidence to suggest that they are also associated with peripheral arterial disease. In a case-control study of 88 male subjects, Pilger *et al.* found that those with peripheral atherosclerosis had significantly higher levels of apo B than the controls [70], and in a larger study of 205 patients there were significant differences in the apo B gene locus in patients compared to the healthy population [74].

A small proportion of LDL particles also include another large protein, apolipoprotein(a). This subfraction of LDL is known as lipoprotein(a), and has been identified in much larger concentrations in those with a family history of early onset coronary heart disease, and it is also an independent risk factor for myocardial infarction or coronary death [75]. It has been suggested that apolipoproteins may discriminate between cases of peripheral arterial disease and normal subjects better than either lipid or lipoprotein levels [70], although recent research has shown that lipoprotein(a) levels were not significantly raised in men with asymptomatic femoral atheroma, although they were independently related to the presence of carotid plaques [76].

Essential fatty acids and antioxidants

Essential fatty acids are derived from two parent molecules, linoleic acid (n-6 series) and alpha-linolenic acid (n-3 series). Deficiencies of linoleic acid were first noted in plasma cholesterol esters of patients with coronary, aortic and peripheral vascular disease in 1969 by Kingsbury *et al.* [77]. Subsequent studies have shown that low levels of linoleic acid are associated with an increased risk of developing coronary heart disease [78–80], and throughout Europe low levels of linoleic acid are known to be inversely related to the gradient of coronary heart disease [81]. In

Scotland, men with coronary heart disease have lower than expected levels of adipose linoleic acid [80], which represents a risk independent of the classical factors associated with disease [82]. There is some evidence that arachidonic acid (n-6) and eicosapentaenoic acid (n-3) levels are also lower in those with coronary heart disease [79, 82]. Few studies have examined the role of essential fatty acids in peripheral arterial disease, but in the Edinburgh Artery Study diseased cases were found to have lower levels of n-3 fatty acids, particularly docosapentaenoic acid, than matched controls [83].

Recently, naturally-occurring antioxidants, particularly vitamins E and A, have also been shown to be deficient in patients with coronary and peripheral vascular disease [84, 85]. The presence of antioxidants protects polyunsaturated fatty acids from peroxidation, and lipid peroxides have been known for many years to be correlated with the severity of aortic atherosclerosis [86]. In one recent study, plasma lipid peroxide levels were found to be significantly higher in both cases of peripheral arterial disease and ischemic heart disease than in control patients [87]. Therefore a deficiency of antioxidants may promote the development of atherosclerosis both by reducing the levels of essential fatty acids, and by promoting the formation of lipid peroxides.

Hypertension

Elevated blood pressure has been associated with the development of peripheral arterial disease in many studies. Most case-control studies and cross-sectional surveys show associations with only systolic pressure [4, 10, 14, 15, 56, 58, 88], although a few implicate both systolic and diastolic pressure [45, 89], have conflicting results [13] or show no association [16]. However, as blood pressure may be elevated secondary to arterial disease, its role in the etiology of peripheral atherosclerosis can only be clearly seen in follow-up studies. Unfortunately, the results from the cohort studies are not consistent: the Framingham study reported a three-fold increased risk of intermittent claudication at 26 years follow-up, primarily associated with a raised systolic pressure [19]; the Danish study found both initial systolic and diastolic pressures were correlated with the ankle pressure index after ten years [4]; whereas the Basle study did not find any independent association between blood pressure and the development of intermittent claudication [47]. Therefore the importance of elevated blood pressure as a risk factor for arterial disease has not been clearly established in epidemiological studies. However, the presence of hypertension might be expected to exacerbate movement of nicotine across endothelial cell membranes, thus providing a mechanism whereby raised blood pressure would act as a risk factor for peripheral arterial disease.

Hemostatic factors

Recent studies have examined the association between various hemostatic factors and the presence of peripheral arterial disease. Fibrinogen concentration in the blood is believed to be a particularly important factor in the development of atherosclerosis, as high plasma levels have been identified in subjects with intermittent claudication in numerous case-control studies [68, 90–97]. In population surveys, cigarette smoking has been related to elevated fibrinogen concentrations [98–103], and after smoking cessation the concentration falls [16]. Other factors that may influence fibrinogen levels include age, obesity, social class, serum cholesterol, diabetes mellitus, intake of cereal fiber, alcohol consumption, use of oral contraceptives and the menopause [98, 99, 101–106]. Recent evidence from the Edinburgh Artery Study also shows an increased risk of peripheral atherosclerosis due to variation at the β fibrinogen locus [107].

Blood viscosity has also been found to be higher in cases of intermittent claudication than in control subjects [63, 91–93, 108], and some studies have identified a similar association with elevated hematocrit [10, 90–92, 109], although after 26 years follow-up in the Framingham study a raised hematocrit was not associated with a greater risk of intermittent claudication [19]. Diseased subjects also have an increased fibrinogen lysis time [110], decreased fibrinolytic activity [68], raised levels of Factor VIII [90, 96], Factor XIII [111], plasminogen [90] and antiplasmin [96]. Alterations in platelet function have been identified in patients with peripheral arterial disease, including low platelet counts [91], increased platelet aggregability [112] and decreased platelet survival time [113], although others have not identified any significant changes [90, 93]. Beta-thromboglobulin, a marker of platelet release, is also elevated [113]. Serum uric acid, which may increase platelet aggregability [114], has been identified at higher levels in cases of peripheral arterial disease than in controls [20, 52, 115], but this was not confirmed in the Danish longitudinal study [4]. These results all suggest that patients with peripheral atherosclerosis have an increased thrombotic tendency, but the mechanism through which the various hemostatic factors may contribute to chronic vessel wall pathology is unclear.

Glucose metabolism

Diabetes mellitus
Peripheral arterial disease is a well-known complication of diabetes mellitus [116]. In a general population-based Finnish study of subjects aged 30 to 59 years, the age-adjusted prevalence of intermittent claudication was 3.4 times higher in diabetic men, and 5.7 times higher in diabetic women [16]. Another Finnish study found the age-adjusted incidence of intermittent claudication was significantly higher in diabetics than in non-diabetics after a five-year follow-up period [117], and similarly after five years follow-up of male civil servants in the Israeli Ischaemic Heart Study the incidence rates of claudication doubled in those with previously diagnosed diabetes [118]. After 20 years follow-up in the Framingham Study, the age-adjusted incidence rates for men were 12.6 per 1000 person years for diabetics, and 3.3 for non-diabetics [19].

Glucose intolerance
Glucose intolerance has not been clearly implicated as a risk factor for peripheral arterial disease in the general population. Community studies in Oxford [45],

Finland [16] and Jerusalem [10] found that the prevalence of intermittent claudication was not related either to a high fasting blood glucose, or to blood glucose following an 'oral glucose load', and the Basle study actually found an inverse association between the degree of glucose tolerance and the occurrence of disease [47]. Both the Basle [47] and Danish [4] longitudinal studies have also produced conflicting results. However, the Aachen study [90] and a cross-sectional study in Moscow and Berlin [46] did find glucose tolerance to be impaired more commonly in individuals with intermittent claudication.

Hyperinsulinemia and insulin resistance
Recent interest has focused on the possible role of insulin in the development of atherosclerosis. Hyperinsulinemia results when pancreatic hypersecretion occurs in response to peripheral insensitivity to insulin-stimulated glucose uptake (insulin resistance). Both insulin resistance and hyperinsulinemia are thought to play an important role in the etiology and clinical course of non-insulin dependent diabetes, hypertension and ischemic heart disease [119, 120]. Associations have also been demonstrated between hyperinsulinemia and abnormalities of lipid metabolism and coagulation [121]. Elevated fasting levels of insulin have been shown to be an independent risk factor for the development of ischemic heart disease [122], and might therefore also be expected to be a risk factor for peripheral arterial disease. In small cohort studies, an association between high insulin levels and peripheral arterial disease was shown to be independent of other risk factors [123, 124], but the role of insulin resistance as an independent risk factor for peripheral arterial disease needs further evaluation.

Personality

The association between personality and risk of developing coronary heart disease has been the subject of much research, but relatively little work has been carried out into its relation with peripheral arterial disease. In one small study of 26 claudicants and 13 control subjects there were no significant differences between Type A personality scores, although those with claudication had more Type A characteristics, and the responses to anger-related questions suggested that patients with intermittent claudication were poor at controlling expressions of anger [125]. In the Edinburgh Artery Study, a hostile personality was found to be related to both asymptomatic and symptomatic disease, suggesting that hostility may be a risk factor for atherogenesis rather than simply a response to atherogenesis [126]. A recent review of personality type in relation to disease concluded that those with type A personality were more at risk of developing both cerebrovascular and peripheral vascular disease, but did not have an increased risk of incurring other illnesses [127].

Alcohol

Cases of peripheral arterial disease in the Edinburgh Artery Study had higher intakes of alcohol than matched controls, and this difference remained statistically significant after adjusting for age, sex and the levels of nutrients [128]. However, there is some evidence that drinking alcohol in small quantities is a negative risk factor for peripheral arterial disease, although when intake exceeds two units per day it becomes detrimental, an effect which may be mediated by alterations in blood pressure, lipid levels and the coagulation system [129].

Physical activity

The relationship between physical activity and ischemic heart disease has been widely investigated, with most studies showing that exercise is associated with a lower rate of heart disease in later life [130–136]. Fewer studies have examined the relationship between exercise and peripheral arterial disease. In the Framingham Study, an association was found between low levels of physical activity and the development of intermittent claudication, but the association was not significant after adjustment for age [137]. In the Finnish cohort of the Seven Countries Study, however, 'claudication was clearly associated with sedentary habits' at the ten year follow-up [138]. In the Edinburgh Artery Study, the risk of peripheral arterial disease was inversely related to previous physical activity in early middle age, particularly amongst male smokers [139]. Exercise is also known to improve symptoms of intermittent claudication, possibly by normalizing certain rheological variables [108].

Conclusions

Atherosclerotic disease of the arteries of the lower limb is a major cause of morbidity in many Western countries, particularly in the elderly, and is associated with an increased mortality risk. The distribution of peripheral arterial disease throughout the population is similar to that of coronary and cerebrovascular disease, and it therefore represents an important marker of generalized atherosclerosis. Patients with intermittent claudication are two to three times more likely to die than the general population, primarily from coronary heart disease. Further longitudinal studies are required to study the associated coronary and cerebrovascular risks in more detail, particularly in order to identify high-risk groups.

General conclusions about the etiology of peripheral vascular disease may be drawn from cross-sectional surveys, but more conclusive results are required from longitudinal studies. The most important risk factor is probably smoking, and this may also be responsible for the abnormalities in hematocrit, blood viscosity and serum fibrinogen seen in patients with peripheral arterial disease. High blood pressure, especially systolic pressure, may have a significant independent effect, and similarly total and HDL cholesterol both appear to be independent risk factors. Future results from follow-up studies in Denmark, the United States and Scotland should enable the important risk factors, and their interrelationships, to be clearly established. The development of more sophisticated methods of assessing peripheral arterial disease noninvasively should open up opportunities for further epidemiological research, and enable accurate estimates of the prevalence of both symptomatic and asymptomatic disease to be obtained.

References

1. Kannel WB, Shurtleff D. The Framingham study. Cigarettes and the development of intermittent claudication. Geriatrics 1973;28:61-8.
2. Widmer LK, Greensher A, Kannel WB. Occlusion of peripheral arteries: A study of 6400 working subjects. Circulation 1964;30:836-42.
3. Heliovaara M, Karvonen WJ, Vilhunden R, Punsar S. Smoking, carbon monoxide and atherosclerotic diseases. Br Med J 1978;1:268-70.
4. Schroll M, Munck O. Estimation of peripheral arteriosclerotic disease by ankle blood pressure measurements in a population study of 60 year-old men and women. J Chron Dis 1981;34:261-9.
5. The ARIC Investigators. The atherosclerosis risk in communities (ARIC) study: Design and objectives. Am J Epidemiol 1989;129:687-702.
6. Fowkes FGR, Housley E, Cawood EHH et al. Edinburgh Artery Study: Prevalence of asymptomatic and symptomatic peripheral vascular disease in the general population. Int J Epidemiol 1991;20:384-92.
7. Rose GA. The diagnosis of ischaemic heart pain and intermittent claudication in field surveys. Bull WHO 1962;27:645-58.
8. Fowkes FGR. The measurement of atherosclerotic peripheral arterial disease in epidemiological surveys. Int J Epidemiol 1988;17:248-54.
9. Leng GC, Fowkes FGR. The Edinburgh Claudication Questionnaire: An improved version of the WHO/Rose questionnaire for use in epidemiological surveys. J Clin Epidemiol 1992;45:1101-9.
10. Gofin R, Karic JD, Friedlander Y et al. Peripheral vascular disease in a middle-aged population sample. The Jerusalem Lipid Research Clinic Prevalence Study. Int J Med Sci 1987;23:157-67.
11. Da Silva A, Widmer LK. Arterienprojekt. Peripher arterielle Verschusskrankheit. In: Widmer LK, (ed.), Venen-, Arterien-, Krankheiten, Koronare Herzkrankheit bei Berufstatigen. Bern: Verlag, 1981:137-237.
12. Pomrehn P, Duncan B, Weissfeld L et al. The association of dyslipoproteinaemia with symptoms and signs of peripheral arterial disease. The Lipid Research Clinic Prevalence Study. Circulation 1986;73(Suppl 1):100-7.
13. Bothig S, Metelisa VI, Barth W et al. Prevalence of ischaemic heart disease, arterial hypertension and intermittent claudication, and distribution of risk factors among middle-aged men in Moscow and Berlin. Cor Vasa 1976;18:104-18.
14. Isacsson S. Venous occlusion plethysmography in 55 year-old men: A population study in Malmo, Sweden. Acta Med Scand 1972;537(Suppl):1-62.
15. De Backer IC, Kornitizer M, Sobolski J, Denolin H. Intermittent claudication – epidemiology and natural history. Acta Cardiol 1979;34:115-24.
16. Reunanen A, Takkunen H, Aromaa A. Prevalence of intermittent claudication and its effect on mortality. Acta Med Scand 1982;211:249-56.
17. Dagenais GR, Maurice S, Robitaille NM, Gingras S, Lupein PJ. Intermittent claudication in Quebec men from 1974–1986: The Quebec Cardiovascular Study. Clin Invest Med 1991;14:93-100.
18. Richard JL, Ducimetiere P, Elgrishi I et al. Depistage par questionnaire de l'insuffisance coronarienne et de la claudication intermittente. Rev Epidemiol Med Soc Sante Publ 1972;20:735-55.
19. Kannel WB, McGhee DL. Update on some epidemiological features of intermittent claudication: The Framingham Study. J Am Ger Soc 1985;33:13-8.
20. Norgren L. Definition, incidence and epidemiology. In: Dormandy J, Stock G, (eds), Critical leg ischaemia – its pathophysiology and management. Heidelberg: Springer-Verlag, 1990:7-13.
21. Department of Health and Social Security. Office of Population Censuses and Surveys. Hospital Inpatient Enquiry. London: HMSO, 1986.

22. Criqui MH, Fronek A, Klauber MR et al. The sensitivity, specificity and predictive value of traditional clinical evaluation of peripheral arterial disease: Results from non-invasive testing in a defined population. Circulation 1985;82:516–31.
23. Fowkes FGR. Epidemiology of atherosclerotic arterial disease in the lower limbs. Eur J Vasc Surg 1988;2:283–91.
24. Mitchell JRA, Schwartz CJ. Arterial disease. Oxford: Blackwell, 1965.
25. Roberts JC, Moses C, Wilkins RH. Autopsy studies in atherosclerosis. Circulation 1959;20:511–9.
26. Sternby NH. Atherosclerosis in a defined population. An autopsy study in Malmo, Sweden. Acta Pathol Microbiol Scand 1968;(Suppl):194.
27. Kannel WB, Shurtleff D. The natural history of arteriosclerosis obliterans. Cardiovasc Clin 1971;3:37–52.
28. Rose G, McCartney P, Reid DD. Self-administration of a questionnaire on chest pain and intermittent claudication. Br J Prev Soc Med 1977;31:42–8.
29. Agner E. Natural history of angina pectoris, possible previous myocardial infarction and intermittent claudication during the eighth decade. Acta Med Scand 1981;210:271–6.
30. Silbert S, Zazeela H. Prognosis in arteriosclerotic peripheral vascular disease. J Am Med Assoc 1958;166:1816–21.
31. Singer A, Rob C. The fate of the claudicator. Br Med J 1960;2:633–6.
32. Bloor K. Natural history of arteriosclerosis of the lower extremities. Ann R Coll Surg Eng 1961;28:36–52.
33. Schadt DC, Hines EA, Juergens JL, Barker NW. Chronic atherosclerotic occlusion of the femoral artery. J Am Med Assoc 1961;175:937–40.
34. Begg TB, Richards RL. The prognosis of intermittent claudication. Scott Med J 1962;7:341–52.
35. Taylor GW, Calo AR. Atherosclerosis of arteries of lower limbs. Br Med J 1962;1:507–10.
36. Mathieson FR, Larsen EE, Wulff M. Some factors influencing the spontaneous course of arterial vascular insufficiency. Acta Chir Scand 1970;136:303–8.
37. Cronenwett JL, Warner KG, Zelenock GB et al. Intermittent claudication. Current results of non-operative management. Arch Surg 1984;119:430–5.
38. Juergens JL, Barker NW, Hines EA. Arteriosclerosis obliterans: Review of 520 cases with special reference to pathogenic and prognostic factors. Circulation 1960;21:188–95.
39. Hughson WG, Mann JI, Tibbs DJ et al. Intermittent claudication: Factors determining outcome. Br Med J 1978;1:1377–9.
40. Kallero KS. Mortality and morbidity in patients with intermittent claudication as defined by venous occlusion plethysmography. A ten year follow-up study. J Chron Dis 1981;34:455–62.
41. Jelnes R, Gaardsting O, Hougard Jensen K et al. Fate in intermittent claudication: Outcome and risk factors. Br Med J 1986;293:1137–40.
42. Kannel WB, Skinner JJ, Schwartz MJ, Shurtleff D. Intermittent claudication: Incidence in the Framingham study. Circulation 1970;41:875–83.
43. Levy LA. Smoking and peripheral vascular disease. Epidemiology and podiatric perspective. J Am Podiatr Med Assoc 1989;79:398–402.
44. Higgins MW, Kjelsberg M. Characteristics of smokers and non-smokers in Tecumseh, Michigan. Am J Epidemiol 1967;86:60–77.
45. Hughson WG, Mann JI, Garrod A. Intermittent claudication: Prevalence and risk factors. Br Med J 1978;1:1379–81.
46. Gyntelberg F. Physical fitness and coronary heart disease in male residents in Copenhagen aged 40–59. Dan Med Bull 1973;20:1–4.
47. Da Silva A, Widmer LK, Ziegler HW et al. The Basle longitudinal study: Report on the relation of initial glucose level to baseline ECG abnormalities, peripheral arterial disease and subsequent mortality. J Chron Dis 1979;32:797–803.
48. Gordon T, Kannel WB. Predisposition to atherosclerosis in the head, heart and legs. J Am Med Assoc 1972;221:661–6.
49. Powell JT. Smoking. In: Fowkes FGR (ed.), Epidemiology of peripheral vascular disease. London: Springer-Verlag, 1991:141–54.

50. Schrade W, Boehle E, Biefler R. Humoral changes in arteriosclerosis. Investigations on lipids, fatty acids, ketone bodies, pyruvic acid, lactic acid, and glucose in the blood. Lancet 1960;ii:1409–16.
51. Greenhalgh RM, Rosengarten DS, Mervart I et al. Serum lipids and lipoproteins in peripheral vascular disease. Lancet 1971;ii:947–50.
52. Sirtori CR, Biasi G, Vercellio G et al. Diet lipids and lipoproteins in patients with peripheral vascular disease. Am J Med Sci 1974;268:325–32.
53. Vyden JK, Thorner JK, Nagasawa K et al. Metabolic and cardiovascular abnormalities in patients with peripheral arterial disease. Am Heart J 1975;90:703–8.
54. Skrede S, Kvarstein B. Hyperlipidaemia in peripheral atherosclerotic arterial disease. Acta Clin Scand 1975;141:333–40.
55. Anquist KA, Johnson O, Ericsson M, Tollin C. Serum lipoproteins and apolipoproteins A1 and A11 in male patients with peripheral arterial insufficiency. Acta Chir Scand 1982;148:675–8.
56. Jacobson UK, Dige-Pedersen H, Gyntelberg F, Svendsen UG. 'Risk factors' and manifestations of arteriosclerosis in patients with intermittent claudication compared to normal persons. Dan Med Bull 1984;31:145–8.
57. Cardia G, Grisorio D, Impedovo G et al. Plasma lipids as a risk factor in peripheral vascular disease. Angiology 1990;41:19–22.
58. Hale WE, Marks RG, May FE et al. Epidemiology of intermittent claudication: Evaluation of risk factors. Age and Ageing 1988;17:57–60.
59. Muller-Buhl U, Schettler G. Common prevalence of coronary and peripheral vascular disease. Bol Assoc Med P R 1988;80:289–90.
60. Fowkes FGR, Housley E, Riemersma RA et al. Smoking, lipids, glucose intolerance and blood pressure as risk factors for peripheral atherosclerosis compared to ischaemic heart disease in the Edinburgh Artery Study. Am J Epidemiol 1992;135:331–340.
61. Da Silva A, Widmer LK. Occlusive peripheral arterial disease. Early diagnosis, incidence, course, significance. Berne: Hans Huber, 1980.
62. Ruhling K, Zabel-Langhenning R, Till U, Thielmenn K. Enhanced net mass transfer of HDL cholesteryl esters to Apo B-containing lipoproteins in patients with peripheral vascular disease. Clin Chim Acta 1989;184:289–96.
63. Dormandy JA, Hoare E, Colley J et al. Clinical, haemodynamic, rheological and biochemical findings in 126 patients with intermittent claudication. Br Med J 1973;4:576–81.
64. Bradby GV, Valente AJ, Walton KW. Serum high density lipoproteins in peripheral vascular disease. Lancet 1990;ii:1271–4.
65. Davey Smith G, Shipley MJ, Rose G. Intermittent claudication, heart disease risk factors, and mortality. The Whitehall Study. Circulation 1990;82:1925–31.
66. Gotto AM. Interrelationship of triglycerides with lipoproteins and high-density lipoproteins. Am J Cardiol 1990;66:20A–23A
67. Kirstein P, Olsson AG. HDL cholesterol is low in young and increases with age in male claudicators. Atherosclerosis 1979;33:145–8.
68. Lipinska I, Lipinski B, Gurewich V. Lipoproteins, fibrinolytic activity and fibrinogen in patients with occlusive vascular disease and in healthy subjects with a family history of heart attacks. Artery 1979;6:254–64.
69. Trayner IM, Mannarino E, Clyne CAC, Thompson GR. Serum lipids and high density lipoproteins in peripheral vascular disease. Br J Surg 1980;67:497–9.
70. Pilger E, Pristautz H, Pfeiffer KH, Kostner GM. Retrospective evaluation of risk factors for peripheral atherosclerosis by stepwise discriminant analysis. Arteriosclerosis 1988;3:57–63.
71. Beach KW. The correlation of arteriosclerosis obliterans with lipoproteins in insulin dependent and non-insulin dependent diabetes. Diabetes 1979;28:836–40.
72. Bihari-Varga M, Szekely J, Gruber E. Plasma high density lipoproteins in coronary, cerebral and peripheral vascular diseases. The influence of various risk factors. Atherosclerosis 1981;40:337–45.
73. Editorial. Apolipoprotein-B and atherogenesis. Lancet 1988;i:1141–2.

74. Monsalve MV, Young R, Wiseman SA et al. DNA polymorphism of the gene for apolipoprotein B in patients with peripheral arterial disease. Atherosclerosis 1988;70:123–9.
75. Rosengren A, Wilhelmsen L, Eriksson E, Risberg B, Wedel H. Lipoprotein (a) and coronary heart disease: A prospective case-control study in a general population sample of middle-aged men. Br Med J 1990;301:1248–51.
76. Cambillau M, Simon A, Amar J et al. Serum Lp(a) as a discriminant marker of early atherosclerotic plaque at three extracoronary sites in hypercholesterolemic men. Arterioscler Thromb 1992;12:1346–52.
77. Kingsbury KJ, Morgan DM, Stovold R, Brett CG. The relationship between plasma cholesteryl polyunsaturated fatty acids, age and atherosclerosis. Postgrad Med J 1969;45:591–601.
78. The Pooling Research Group. Relationship of blood pressure, serum cholesterol, smoking habit, relative weight and ECG abnormalities to incidence of major coronary events. Final report of the pooling project. J Chron Dis 1978;31:201–306.
79. Miettenen TA, Naukkarinen V, Huttunen JK, Mattila S, Kumlin T. Fatty acid composition of serum lipids predicts myocardial infarction. Br Med J 1982;282:993–6.
80. Wood DA, Butler S, Riemersma RA et al. Adipose tissue and platelet fatty acids and coronary heart disease in Scottish men. Lancet 1984;2:117–21.
81. Logan RL, Riemersma RA, Thomson M et al. Risk factors for ischaemic heart disease in normal men aged 40. Edinburgh–Stockholm Study. Lancet 1978;1:949–54.
82. Wood DA, Riemersma RA, Butler S et al. Linoleic and eicosapentaenoic acids in adipose tissue and platelets and risk of coronary heart disease. Lancet 1987;1:177–82.
83. Leng GC, Horrobin DF, Fowkes FGR et al. Plasma essential fatty acids, cigarette smoking, and dietary antioxidants in peripheral arterial disease. Arterioscler Thromb 1994;14:471–8.
84. Riemersma RA, Wood DA, MacIntyre CCA et al. Risk of angina pectoris and plasma concentrations of vitamins A, C and E and carotene. Lancet 1991;337:1–5.
85. MacRury SM, Muir M, Hume R. Seasonal and climatic variation in cholesterol and vitamin C: Effect of vitamin C supplementation. Scot Med J 1992;37:49–52.
86. Harland WA, Gilbert JD, Steel G, Brooks CJW. Lipids of human atheroma, Part 5. The occurrence of a new group of polar sterol esters in various stages of human atherosclerosis. Atherosclerosis 1971;13:239–46.
87. Stringer MD, Gorog PG, Freeman A, Kakkar VV. Lipid peroxides and atherosclerosis. Br Med J 1989;298:281–4.
88. Skalkidis Y, Katsouyanni K, Petridou E et al. Risk factors for peripheral arterial occlusive disease: A case-control study in Greece. Int J Epidemiol 1989;18:614–8.
89. Reid DD, Holland WW, Hummerfelt S, Rose G. A cardiovascular survey of British postal workers. Lancet 1966;1:614–8.
90. Kiesewetter H, Jung F, Kotitschke G et al. Prevalence, risk factors and rheological profile of arterial vascular disease; first results of the Aachen study. Folia Haematol (Leipz) 1988;115:587–93.
91. Stormer B, Horsch R, Kleinschmidt F et al. Blood viscosity in patients with peripheral vascular disease in the areas of low shear rates. J Cardiovasc Surg 1974;15:577–84.
92. Lowe GDO, Saniabadi A, Turner A et al. Studies on haematocrit in peripheral arterial disease. Klin Wochenschr 1986;64:969–74.
93. Hell KM, Balzereit A, Diebold U, Bruhn HD. Importance of blood viscoelasticity in arteriosclerosis. Angiology 1989;40:539–46.
94. Baxter K, Wiseman S, Powell S, Greenhalgh R. Pilot study of a screening test for peripheral arterial disease in middle-aged men: Fibrinogen as a possible risk factor. Cardiovasc Res 1988;22:300–2.
95. Christe M, Frischi J, Lammle B et al. Filter coagulation and fibrinolysis parameters in diabetes mellitus and in patients with vasculopathy. Thromb Haemostat 1984;52:138–43.
96. Christe M, Delley A, Marbet GA et al. Fibrinogen, Factor VIII related antigen, anti-thrombin III and alpha 2-antiplasmin in peripheral arterial disease. Thromb Haemostat 1984;52:240–2.
97. Ciuffetti G, Mannarino E, Pasqualini L et al. The haemorheological role of cellular factors in peripheral vascular disease. VASA 1988;17:168–70.

98. Meade TW, North WRS, Chakrabarti R, Naines AP, Stirling Y. Population-based distribution of haemostatic variables. Br Med Bull 1977;33:283–8.
99. Markowe HLJ, Marmot MG, Shipley MJ et al. Fibrinogen: A possible link between social class and coronary heart disease. Br Med J 1985;291:1312–4.
100. Kannel WB, D'Agostino RB, Belanger AJ. Fibrinogen, cigarette smoking, and risk of cardiovascular disease: Insights from Framingham Study. Am Heart J 1987;113:1006–10.
101. Rosengren A, Wilhelmsen L, Welin L et al. Social influences and cardiovascular risk factors as determinants of plasma fibrinogen concentration in a general population sample of middle-aged men. Br Med J 1990;300:634–8.
102. Lee AJ, Smith WCS, Lowe GDO, Tuunstall-Pedoe H. Plasma fibrinogen and coronary risk factors: The Scottish Heart Health Study. J Clin Epidemiol 1990;43:913–9.
103. Yarnell JWG, Fehily AM, Milbank J, Rubiki AJ, Eastham R, Hayes TRM. Determinants of plasma lipoproteins and coagulation factors in men from Caerphilly, South Wales. J Epidemiol Commun Health 1983;37:137–40.
104. Meade TW, Imeson J, Stirling Y. Effects of changes in smoking and other characteristics on clotting factors and the risk of ischaemic heart disease. Lancet 1987;ii:986–8.
105. Kannel WB, Wolf PA, Castelli WP, D'Agostino RB. Fibrinogen and risk of cardiovascular disease: The Framingham Study. J Am Med Assoc 1987;258:1183–6.
106. Fuller JH, Keen H, Jarrett RJ et al. Haemostatic variables associated with diabetes and its complications. Br Med J 1979;ii:964–6.
107. Fowkes FGR, Connor JM, Smith FB et al. Fibrinogen genotype and risk of peripheral atherosclerosis. Lancet 1992;339:693–6.
108. Ernst EE, Matrai A. Intermittent claudication, exercise and blood rheology. Circulation 1987;76:1110–4.
109. Kallero KS; Bergentz SE, Lindell SE, Janzon L. Elevated haematocrit in patients with intermittent claudication with special regard to men below the age of 60. Biblthca Haematol 1981;47:173–84.
110. Nestel PJ. Fibrinolytic activity of the blood in intermittent claudication. Lancet 1959;2:373–4.
111. Kloczko J, Wojtukiewicz M, Bielawiec M, Zuch A. Alterations of haemostasis parameters with special reference to fibrin stabilisation, factor XIII and fibronectin in patients with obliterative atherosclerosis. Thromb Res 1988;51:575–81.
112. Lowe GDO, Renney MM, Johnston RV et al. Increased platelet aggregation in vascular and nonvascular illness: Correlation with plasma fibrinogen and effect of ancrod. Thromb Res 1979;14:377–8.
113. Zahavi J, Zahavi M. Enhanced platelet release action, shortened platelet survival time and increased platelet aggregation and plasma thromboxane B2 in chronic obstructive arterial disease. Thromb Haemostat 1985;53:105–9.
114. Winocour PD, Turner MR, Taylor TG, Munday KA. Gout and cardiovascular disease (letter). Lancet 1977;1:959–60.
115. Greenhalgh RM, Laing SP, Cole PV, Taylor GW. Smoking and arterial reconstruction. Br J Surg 1981;68:605–7.
116. Laakso M, Ronnemaa T, Pyorala K et al. Atherosclerotic vascular disease and its risk factors in non-insulin dependent diabetics and non-diabetic subjects in Finland. Diabetes Care 1988;11:449–63.
117. Siitonen O, Uusitupa M, Pyorala K, Voutilainene E, Lansimies E. Peripheral arterial disease and its relationship to cardiovascular risk factors and coronary heart disease in newly diagnosed non-insulin dependent diabetics. Acta Med Scand 1986;220:205–12.
118. Herman JB, Medalie JH, Goldbourt U. Differences in cardiovascular morbidity and mortality between previously known and newly diagnosed adult diabetics. Diabetologica 1977;13:229–34.
119. Reaven GM. Insulin resistance and compensatory hyperinsulinaemia: Role of hypertension, dyslipidemia, and coronary heart disease. Am Heart J 1991;121:1283–8.
120. Reaven GM. Banting lecture 1988. Role of insulin resistance in human disease. Diabetes 1988;37:1595–607.
121. Zavaroni I, Bonora E, Pagliara M et al. Risk factors for coronary artery disease in healthy persons with hyperinsulinaemia and normal glucose tolerance. New Engl J Med 1989;320:702–6.

122. Ducimetiere P, Eshcwege E, Papoz L et al. Relationship of plasma insulin levels to the incidence of myocardial infarction and coronary heart disease mortality in a middle-aged population. Diabetologica 1980;19:205–10.
123. Uusitupa MIJ, Niskanen LK, Siitonen O, Voutilainen E, Pyorala K. Five-year incidence of atherosclerotic vascular disease in relation to general risk factors, insulin level, and abnormalities in lipoprotein composition in non-insulin-dependent diabetic and nondiabetic subjects. Circulation 1990;82:27–36.
124. Sorge F, Schwartzkopff W, Neuhaus GA. Insulin response to oral glucose in patients with a previous myocardial infarction and in patients with periphral vascular disease. Diabetes 1976;25:586–94.
125. Cottier C, Addler R, Vorkauf H et al. Pressurised pattern or Type A behaviour in patients with peripheral arteriovascular disease: Controlled retrospective exploratory study. Psychosom Med 1983;45:187–93.
126. Deary IJ, Fowkes FGR, Donnan PT, Housley E. Hostile personality and risks of peripheral arterial disease in the general population. Psychosom Med 1994;56:197–202.
127. Suls J, Sanders GS. Type A behaviour as a general risk factor for physical disorder. J Behav Med 1988;11:201–26.
128. Donnan PT, Thomson M. Diet and alcohol. In: Fowkes FGR, (ed.), Epidemiology of peripheral vascular disease. London: Springer-Verlag, 1991:207–16.
129. Criqui MH. The roles of alcohol in the epidemiology of cardiovascular diseases. Acta Med Scand 1987;717(Suppl):73–85.
130. Morris JN, Heady JA, Raffle PAB, Roberts CG, Parks JW. Coronary heart disease and physical activity at work. Lancet 1953;ii:1111–20.
131. Kahn HA. The relationship of reported coronary heart disease mortality to physical activity at work. Am J Public Health 1963;53:1058–67.
132. Paffenbarger RS, Laughlin ME, Gima AS, Black RA. Work activity of longshoremen as related to death from coronary heart disease and stroke. N Engl J Med 1970;282:1109–14.
133. Morris JN, Chave SPW, Adam C, Sirey C, Apstein L. Vigorous exercise in leisure-time and the incidence of coronary heart disease. Lancet 1973;i:333–9.
134. Leren P, Askevold EM, Foss OP et al. The Oslo Study. Cardiovascular diseases in middle-aged and young Oslo men. Acta Med Scand 1975;588(Suppl):1–38.
135. Powell KE, Thompson PD, Casperen CJ, Kendrick JS. Physical activity and the incidence of coronary heart disease. Ann Rev Public Health 1987;8:253–87.
136. Zimmet PZ, Collins VR, Dowse GK et al. The relation of physical activity to cardiovascular disease risk factors in Mauritians. Am J Epidemiol 1991;134:862–75.
137. Kannel WB, Sorlie P. Some health benefits of physical activity. The Framingham Study. Arch Intern Med 1979;139:857–61.
138. Keys A, Aravanis C, Blackburn HW et al. Epidemiological studies related to coronary heart disease: Characteristics of men aged 40–59 in the seven countries. Acta Med Scand 1966;460(Suppl):169–90.
139. Housley E, Leng GC, Donnan PT, Fowkes FGR. Physical activity and risk of peripheral arterial disease in the general population: Edinburgh Artery Study. J Epidemiol Comm Health 1993;47:475–80.

21. Clinical assessment of diseases of lower limb arteries

KENNETH A. MYERS and WINSTON CHONG

Occlusive or aneurysmal disease in arteries to the lower limbs usually can be recognized by characteristic symptoms and signs. This may suffice if future management is to be conservative but it is necessary to know the nature, site and extent of the pathology if intervention is contemplated and this then requires further investigation. Noninvasive vascular laboratory assessment is now centered around duplex ultrasound scanning leading to arteriography which can be more selective than in the past. The preferred method for assessment depends on the patient's presentation, the surgeon's preference, the degree of genuine interaction between the surgeon and radiologist and the expertise of the radiologist and ultrasonographer. This chapter explores how we assess disease according to its manifestations, based upon an unusual degree of collaboration between surgeons and radiologists in our unit.

What techniques do we use?

We now confine our evaluation to the history and examination, continuous-wave Doppler ultrasound with ankle/brachial pressure indices, toe pressures measured by strain gauge plethysmography, colour-Doppler duplex ultrasonography and intraarterial digital subtraction angiography. We no longer use any other form of plethysmography, measurement of tissue oxygen tensions, segmental pressures, conventional or intravenous digital subtraction angiography or intraarterial pressure measurements. We have little experience with laser-Doppler flowmetry in clinical practice and we look forward to further experience to evaluate the value of magnetic resonance angiography and spiral computed tomographic angiography.

In our experience, mistakes most often result from a poor history and examination. Clinical assessment determines whether disability is sufficient to proceed to investigation. If so, this can commence with a duplex ultrasound scan which indicates what forms of intervention are likely to succeed. It is now our general policy to recommend the least invasive treatment option for the initial intervention in most patients. If the surgeon and patient agree that intervention is warranted then an arteriogram is performed, either prior to open surgery or frequently at the same time as endovascular intervention. We find that the duplex scan and the arteriogram complement each other – one cannot replace the other and either alone no longer provides sufficient information in many patients.

Continuous-wave Doppler ultrasound and pressure indices

The hand-held pocket continuous-wave Doppler ultrasound device is the 'vascular surgeon's stethoscope' and is used as part of the routine clinical assessment. This examination can highlight stenoses detected by a change in the pitch of the Doppler signal, and areas of occlusion with drop-out of the expected signal in the artery.

The continuous-wave Doppler unit is used to measure the systolic pressure at the ankle and the arm, recording the higher pressure from signals in the posterior tibial and dorsalis pedis arteries – the test cannot be performed if both are occluded in the leg and foot. The normal systolic pressure measured at the ankle is higher than that measured in the arm so that the ratio of the two should be greater than 1.00. An ankle/brachial pressure index (ABI) < 0.95 at rest or after exercise shows that stenotic or occlusive disease is present [1]. False results can be due to inability to compress rigid calf arteries on the one hand or unrecognized stenotic disease in the subclavian arteries on the other. A change in the ABI > 0.15 is usually considered significant [2] but the variance in routine clinical practice may be > 0.20 [3]. Toe pressures measured by strain-gauge plethysmography are useful if there is an obvious artefact due to inability to compress calf arteries or if no signal is obtained from the distal arteries; the normal toe/brachial pressure index is 0.80–0.90 [4].

We routinely also measure post-exercise pressures at one minute after walking the patient on a treadmill at 3 km/h with an incline of 7° for two minutes or until claudication prevents walking. The distances travelled to onset of claudication and inability to continue are recorded, and the site of pain or other reasons for restriction are noted. It is valuable to know whether the post-exercise pressure falls if the resting pressure was normal, but it must be admitted that there is no evidence that the post-exercise measurement further helps clinical assessment if the resting index was already reduced, nor evidence that the time to recovery relates to any clinical parameters. We do not use post-reactive hyperemia pressure measurements although we appreciate that they could be helpful in subjects who cannot walk [5]. We have found that there is a poor correlation between measured walking distance and blood flow in the legs [6] or ABIs [7]. Threshold levels of ABIs have been used to define the presence of critical ischemia [8] but we do not believe that these are reliable.

The continuous-wave Doppler unit can record the common femoral and ankle pulse wave-forms. These have been used to detect proximal aortoiliac disease by the pulsatility index [9], principal component analysis [10], Laplace transform [11] or power frequency spectrum analysis [12]. However, we concluded that visual assessment of the common femoral artery wave-form after exercise was as accurate [13]. In fact, we no longer rely on any form of common femoral wave-form analysis to diagnose aortoiliac disease, for the wave-form can normalize within a short distance beyond a localized stenosis, while it does not distinguish a tight stenosis from an occlusion, detect minimal or moderate disease, or determine whether disease affects one or multiple segments.

Color-Doppler duplex ultrasound scanning

It is our practice to limit the area to be examined – if post-exercise ABIs are normal then there is little point in scanning that limb. However, if ABIs confirm that disease is present on one or both sides then it is our practice to scan the entire length from the aorta to the distal crural arteries. Although it is occasionally difficult to view all of the iliac arteries, particularly if the patient has not been adequately fasted, lateral and inferior windows as well as the anterior view usually demonstrate the vessels. An experienced vascular ultrasonographer will view all infrainguinal vessels in all patients.

For stenotic or occlusive disease, we measure both the maximum peak systolic velocity and the ratio of the velocity at a stenosis to the velocity in the *proximal* artery (V2/V1) to determine the degree of stenosis. Several studies have evaluated the relation between degrees of stenosis evaluated by duplex scanning and arteriography [14–17] – the criteria that we use are shown in Table 21.1. A probable occlusion is diagnosed if it is seen that a collateral leaves above and reenters below the occlusion and that there is a high resistance signal in the proximal artery and a damped signal in the distal artery. However, due to the high-pass filter in all colour-Doppler duplex ultrasound machines, it may not be possible to distinguish a trickle of flow through a tight stenosis from an occlusion. For aneurysmal disease, duplex scanning is used to measure the true diameters and to assess inflow and outflow disease.

Past studies have shown excellent agreement between the findings from duplex scanning and intraarterial digital subtraction angiography though neither show as good agreement with intraarterial pressure measurements [18]. Duplex scanning can provide just as reliable information for making clinical decisions as the arteriogram [19] provided that the investigation is performed in a highly experienced unit. However, we find that there is a tendency to underestimate the extent of disease, for the most proximal lesion will usually be clearly identified but multiple

Table 21.1. Criteria for evaluation of degree of stenosis.

Percent stenosis	Peak systolic velocity	Velocity ratio[a]	Doppler signal
1–29%	< 150 cm/s	< 1.5:1	Triphasic Clear window
30–49%	150–200 cm/s	< 2:1	Triphasic Filling in under systolic peak
50–75%	205–400 cm/s	< 4:1	Monophasic Spectral broadening
> 75%	> 400 cm/s	> 4:1	Monophasic Window filled

[a] The velocity ratio is a product of the velocity at the stenosis to that in the artery *above* the stenosis.

stenoses or occlusions may not be apparent due to progressive damping of the flow signal and consequent loss of information. The B-mode image provides appreciable additional information to the Doppler signal.

Intraarterial digital subtraction angiography

The principle of digital subtraction angiography is to digitize and store the images on a computer and then convert them back to images on a screen, masking the stationary background signals from bones and soft tissues. Post-processing improves the signal's quality by frame integration, edge enhancement and noise smoothing, but these can lead to misrepresentation or loss of information unless performed with care. Artefacts can result from patient movement resulting in inadequate subtraction leading to a false 'stenosis' or 'occlusion', but this can be corrected by mask reregistration and pixel shifting. The largest field of view available with most recently available commercial units is 14–16 cm so that a full study from the renal arteries to the feet may require up to ten runs to cover the region depending on the number of oblique projections, selective external iliac injections, field size and height of the patient. Road-mapping is an invaluable feature for it allows live manipulation of a guide wire or catheter in the opacified vessel which greatly helps to negotiate a tortuous or tightly stenosed artery.

Defining the distal arteries is enhanced if the catheter tip is selectively placed into each external iliac artery. The femoral artery can be punctured on the side with the worst symptoms so that the catheter can be withdrawn into the ipsilateral side. Alternatively, the catheter can be passed over the aortic bifurcation to the contralateral side and this is preferred if it is anticipated that the patient will proceed to a bypass graft so as not to contaminate the groin. Distal definition is even better if antegrade femoral puncture is used. The brachial approach is chosen if the femoral route is difficult or impossible due to common femoral or aortoiliac disease but we no longer favour axillary puncture because it is difficult to avoid a hematoma which can cause a nerve palsy. We have no experience with access via the subclavian or popliteal arteries. We have had no need to use adjuvant techniques such as balloon occlusion above the injection site, peripheral arterial vasodilatation by drugs or reactive hyperemia. Fluoroscopy and digital subtraction angiography with a high-quality image intensifier are invaluable for assessing the options, progress and outcome during open surgery.

Most arteriograms are performed as outpatient procedures, but patients who are diabetic, who are being treated with anticoagulant drugs or who live alone require admission for preliminary medical management and postoperative care. We routinely provide an information sheet to increase patient acceptance and for medicolegal protection (Appendix). A small dose of oral diazepam is usually adequate for sedation, intravenous fluids are required only for patients who are diabetic or have impaired renal function, and all are monitored through the procedure by electrocardiography and pulse oximetry. They rest lying flat for 4 hours after the procedure and are then discharged if there are no apparent complications provided that there are adults to care for them overnight.

Assessment for atherosclerotic stenotic or occlusive disease

What is the distribution of disease?

Arteriograms in non-diabetic patients were analysed by Aston et al. [20]. There was aortoiliac disease in 11%, superficial femoral artery disease in 42%, combined disease at both sites in 16% and predominant infrapopliteal disease in 31%. At least one calf artery was occluded in 51%, usually affecting the anterior tibial artery and most often sparing the peroneal artery, and only 16% had a complete pedal arch. The distribution was much the same irrespective of whether the presentation was with intermittent claudication or critical ischemia. A community study by Widmer et al. [21] found predominant disease in the aorta in 2%, the iliac arteries in 14%, superficial femoral arteries in 49%, crural arteries in 23%, and arteries to the upper limbs in 12%.

How do we diagnose whether disease is present?

This is a clinical diagnosis. A rigorous history should lead to a classical description of intermittent claudication and any variation from the typical story should raise concerns as to an alternative diagnosis of musculoskeletal, arthritic, chronic venous or neurological disorders. The history of rest pain should also be predictable with either a deep pain or burning sensation in the feet which develops an hour or so after sleeping as the systemic blood pressure falls and is relieved by hanging the legs or walking. It can be difficult to distinguish whether ulceration is due to ischemia or chronic venous disease and the two are often associated in elderly patients so that the relative contribution from each can be difficult to assess – the severity of pain is as good a guide as any. The problem is particularly marked in diabetics where the contribution of ischemia and neuropathy can be difficult to assess since neuropathy frequently results in the ulceration being relatively painless.

Palpation for pulses and auscultation for bruits down the full length of the arteries to the lower limbs is essential. Abnormal findings may only become manifest after exercising the patient and this should be a routine part of the examination. However, assessment of whether a pulse is normal, reduced or absent can be difficult. Patients attending our clinic were examined blindly by several surgeons who were asked to record the nature of the femoral and popliteal pulses – there was moderately good agreement as to whether the femoral and popliteal pulses were present or absent but no agreement beyond that expected from chance as to whether pulses were normal or diminished [22].

ABIs can be helpful to confirm or exclude the presence of disease; an ABI < 0.95 at rest or following exercise indicates that there is disease. ABIs have been used to distinguish whether an ulcer is caused by arterial or venous disease and whether an ulcer or conservative amputation is likely to heal or not [23] but we are reluctant to rely on these in clinical practice. Duplex scanning is only rarely required and arteriography should never be required to diagnose whether disease is present.

How is the site of disease determined?

The site and severity of symptoms helps to localize the site and extent of disease. However, appreciable aortoiliac stenosis with a superficial femoral artery occlusion frequently causes calf claudication alone with no thigh or buttock claudication [24]. Rarely, isolated buttock, thigh or foot claudication can result from localized internal iliac, profunda femoris or crural artery disease. A femoral bruit can result from proximal aortoiliac disease or from a stenosis in the profunda femoris or proximal superficial femoral arteries [25]. Considerable disease may be present without symptoms in the less affected side. The history and examination give little if any information about the extent of outflow disease beyond the major site of occlusion.

Techniques which relate common femoral or thigh pressures to the ankle pressures to distinguish the relative contributions from proximal and distal disease [26, 27] are theoretically attractive, for it is most frustrating to perform intervention for proximal disease only to have no clinical improvement, but we have not felt that the accuracy from these is sufficient for clinical decision-making.

The duplex scan is invaluable for mapping out the site and extent of disease. The level of the proximal end of the stenosis or occlusion is measured relative to the major artery bifurcation above the lesion (the aortic, common iliac, common femoral or popliteal bifurcations) and the length of the lesion is recorded. We consider that arteriography is the method that currently most precisely defines the distribution of disease.

How do we decide whether intervention is required?

The options for patient management range from conservative expectant treatment through endovascular intervention to open surgical reconstruction. Which is chosen depends on the severity of ischemia and the resultant disability. In spite of many attempts to measure severity by objective physiological parameters, the patient's perception of disability, particularly for intermittent claudication, remains the most helpful guide.

Many patients with intermittent claudication will seek intervention provided that it is minimally invasive but will avoid treatment if the only option is an extensive bypass graft. It is here that the duplex ultrasound scan is most helpful to show whether disease is limited and in a site accessible for endovascular intervention or whether it is extensive or relatively inaccessible so as to require open surgical reconstruction. If the presentation is with critical ischemia, then time may not allow preliminary assessment by duplex scanning and the patient may go straight to arteriography, but many patients can be successfully managed by endovascular intervention so that we prefer to perform the duplex scan first if possible. Various options for management according to the severity of symptoms are shown in Figures 21.1–21.3.

Clinical assessment of lower limb arterial diseases 295

```
                    Clinical Assessment
                            |
               Advise Conservative Treatment
                            |
                  No Further Investigations
                            |
                      Regular Review
```

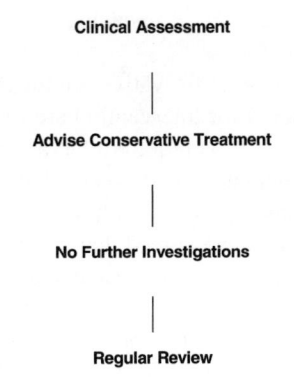

Figure 21.1. Management of mild claudication.

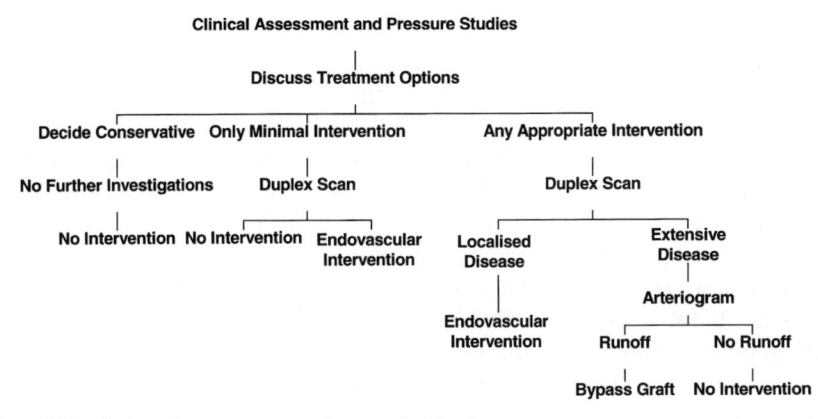

```
              Clinical Assessment and Pressure Studies
                            |
                    Discuss Treatment Options
   _____|_____
   |                       |                        |
Decide Conservative   Only Minimal Intervention   Any Appropriate Intervention
   |                       |                        |
No Further Investigations  Duplex Scan            Duplex Scan
   |                 _____|_____           _____|_____
No Intervention   No Intervention  Endovascular   Localised       Extensive
                                   Intervention   Disease         Disease
                                                     |               |
                                                 Endovascular     Arteriogram
                                                 Intervention   ____|____
                                                                |        |
                                                              Runoff   No Runoff
                                                                |        |
                                                           Bypass Graft  No Intervention
```

Figure 21.2. Options for management of severe claudication.

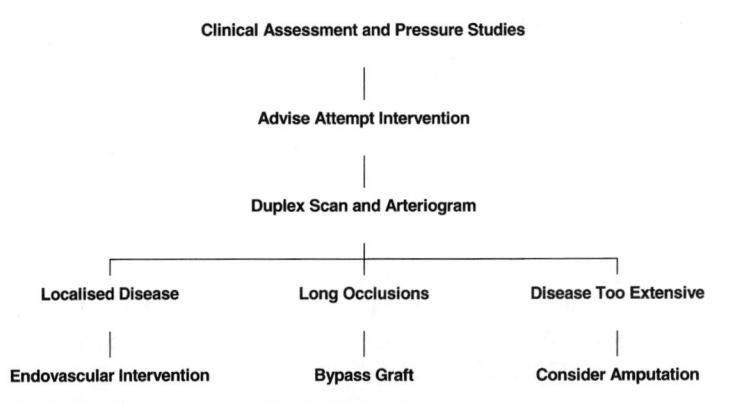

```
              Clinical Assessment and Pressure Studies
                            |
                    Advise Attempt Intervention
                            |
                    Duplex Scan and Arteriogram
       _____|_____
       |                    |                     |
  Localised Disease    Long Occlusions      Disease Too Extensive
       |                    |                     |
Endovascular Intervention  Bypass Graft     Consider Amputation
```

Figure 21.3. Options for management of critical ischemia.

How do we proceed if intervention is recommended?

As management options include conservative, endovascular or open surgical approaches, all patients considered for intervention are jointly discussed by surgeons and radiologists. In our hospital, it is required that a consultant surgeon be present for every open operation. Experience led us to conclude that endovascular intervention has at least as great a potential for difficult decision making and complications as open surgery. Because of this, we agreed that it would be appropriate for a vascular surgeon to be present at every endovascular procedure if possible. In time, this resulted in the surgeons becoming highly competent for endovascular procedures and the surgeons and radiologists became more involved in complex advanced endovascular techniques. Because both the radiologists and surgeons are personally involved, there is a strong tendency for minimally invasive endovascular intervention to be sought as the first option.

The conventional approach has been to proceed directly to arteriography after clinical examination and measurement of ABIs. Retrograde femoral puncture is performed on the side of the lesion and arteriography involves viewing the full length of the arteries. The radiologist can immediately proceed to endovascular treatment if this is shown to be feasible, but this then carries some problems. Most arteriograms are preformed as outpatient procedures whereas it is still our policy to admit patients overnight after endovascular intervention. Further, this approach places great responsibility on the radiologist working in isolation to choose the appropriate treatment, given that the radiologist is usually not familiar with the patient's precise general and local condition. At the very least, it must be certain that the treating vascular surgeon is immediately available to deal with any complications. If the lesions are complex and management is uncertain, then the arteriogram is usually completed and subsequently reviewed with the surgeon to determine whether subsequent endovascular intervention or open surgery is appropriate.

It is for this reason that an alternative approach has been developed. The site of disease can be accurately defined by adequate clinical assessment followed by non-invasive duplex ultrasound scanning in most patients, and this then allows an arteriogram which focuses on the likely site of disease. We now increasingly combine the diagnostic arteriogram with endovascular intervention and the preliminary information from the duplex scan allows us to organize the procedure accordingly. Duplex scanning is used to detect and localize disease and preliminary arteriography is only warranted if the duplex scan is inadequate. The preliminary duplex scan assesses the inflow and outflow, the site and length of the lesion and whether there is significant common femoral disease at the potential puncture site. This gives advance warning as to whether there is unilateral or bilateral disease, whether unilateral or bilateral punctures will be required for endovascular intervention and which side or site should be punctured. The duplex scan does tend to underestimate disease and the extent of treatment required is often greater than anticipated. This approach is shown in Figures 21.4–21.6.

Clinical assessment of lower limb arterial diseases 297

Clinical Assessment and Duplex Scanning
|
Aortic or Bifurcation Disease
|
Select Site Arteriogram Puncture
├── **Stenoses** → **Bilateral Retrograde Femoral Puncture**
└── **Occlusion** → **Brachial Puncture**

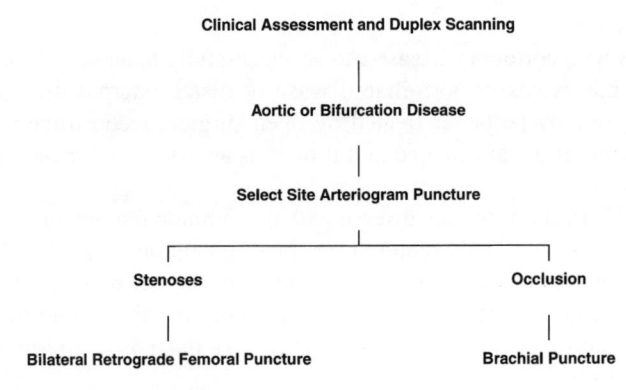

Figure 21.4. A policy for arteriography – I.

Clinical Assessment and Duplex Scanning
|
Iliac Artery Stenoses or Occlusions
|
Select Site Arteriogram Puncture
├── **Unilateral**
│   ├── **Common Femoral Normal** → **Retrograde Ipsilateral Femoral**
│   ├── **Ipsilateral Common Femoral Stenosed** → **Retrograde Contralateral Femoral with Crossover**
│   └── **Both Common Femorals Stenosed** → **Brachial Puncture**
└── **Bilateral** → **Retrograde from Worse Side with Crossover**

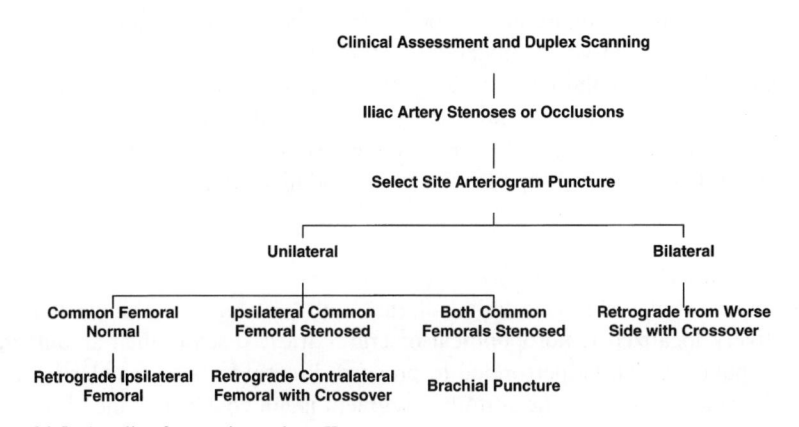

Figure 21.5. A policy for arteriography – II.

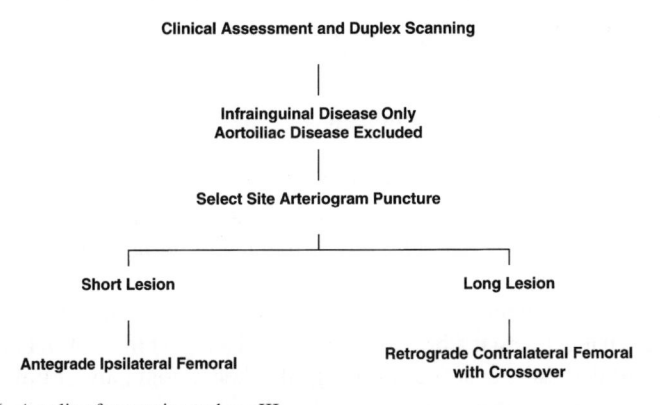

Clinical Assessment and Duplex Scanning
|
**Infrainguinal Disease Only
Aortoiliac Disease Excluded**
|
Select Site Arteriogram Puncture
├── **Short Lesion** → **Antegrade Ipsilateral Femoral**
└── **Long Lesion** → **Retrograde Contralateral Femoral with Crossover**

Figure 21.6. A policy for arteriography – III.

Aortoiliac disease

Most patients with aortoiliac disease can be successfully managed by endovascular intervention but extensive aortoiliac disease or distal external iliac or common femoral disease may be better treated by open surgical reconstruction. Proximal aortoiliac disease is always treated first if there is an associated superficial femoral artery occlusion.

For aortic bifurcation stenotic disease with no common femoral disease, bilateral femoral punctures are usually required for 'kissing balloon' dilatation. If there is a common femoral stenosis, then a diagnostic contralateral puncture may be performed to determine whether endovascular intervention is feasible by a brachial approach. An aortic occlusion requires preliminary diagnostic arteriography by a brachial approach.

More distal unilateral iliac artery disease is best confirmed and treated by ipsilateral puncture if the common femoral artery is widely patent, or by contralateral puncture with crossover if there is unilateral common femoral stenosis or a brachial approach if there are bilateral common femoral stenoses. Bilateral iliac artery disease can be treated with unilateral puncture and a crossover to dilate the contralateral side then withdrawal to dilate the ipsilateral side. The more distal the disease, the more easy it is to deal with by contralateral puncture and crossover for an ipsilateral puncture may be too close to the lesion. The crossover technique can be used to dilate combined superficial femoral and iliac artery stenoses on the same side.

Femoropopliteal disease

If the duplex scan excludes aortoiliac disease with confidence and shows that there is relatively localized femoropopliteal or crural artery disease, then an antegrade femoral puncture can be performed to proceed directly to endovascular intervention. If the duplex scan of the aortoiliac segment is not conclusive, then it is better to perform contralateral retrograde femoral puncture for a routine arteriogram. If the duplex scan shows that the lesion is long and commences at or close to the origin of the superficial femoral artery, then a contralateral retrograde femoral arteriogram with crossover to the external iliac artery is performed to define the runoff to assess how best to plan a bypass graft.

Assessment for acute thromboembolism

It is increasingly difficult to diagnose whether acute ischemia is due to embolism or thrombosis. To some degree, this is not important since subsequent treatment is much the same, be it by regional fibrinolytic therapy or thromboembolectomy with possible bypass grafting.

Assessment should include searching for a site for a thrombus in the heart, particularly in the patient who is fibrillating or has had a recent myocardial infarct, and this is now best determined by transesophageal echocardiography. If time allows, a duplex ultrasound scan can detect the site of occlusion and whether the clot is fresh, and in particular whether there is preexisting atherosclerotic disease in the affected artery, all of which can influence choice as to the most appropriate treatment.

If there is a circulation into the leg, then preliminary arteriography is worthwhile to assess further the site of occlusion and perhaps determine the likelihood of an embolus by seeing a sharp cut-off at the upper end of the occlusion. However, if there is no circulation into the leg then there is no point in preoperative arteriography for if blood cannot get to the distal vessels then contrast will not either. In this situation, we prefer to perform the diagnostic arteriogram during the course of fibrinolysis or on-table following thromboembolectomy.

Assessment for aneurysms

There is an increasing desire in the vascular community to screen communities by ultrasound to detect asymptomatic abdominal aortic aneurysms (AAAs) in an attempt to reduce the number of patients presenting with rupture. The yield, for example in males over 50 years old is approximately 2–8% [28]. This is considerably increased by focusing on high-risk groups such as first-degree male relatives and patients with hypertension or symptomatic coronary, cerebrovascular or peripheral arterial disease [28–30]. The cost–benefit from ultrasound screening for AAAs probably warrants the effort [31] but this requires evaluation in larger trials.

Abdominal palpation to detect an AAA is to be encouraged but is unreliable, for many large aneurysms are not detected in obese patients while a tortuous aorta is frequently misdiagnosed as an AAA in a thin patient. Calcification will demonstrate an AAA on a plain X-ray, but this is seen in the minority of cases. B-mode ultrasound is the most reliable technique to detect an AAA and gives a good measure of the diameter, though is not as good as computerized tomography (CT). The CT scan is required in every patient with an AAA large enough for intervention to be considered (usually more than 4.5–5 cm diameter) and it should extend from the aortic arch to the pelvis. There have been attempts to relate the absolute diameter to the size of the patient, for example to the adjacent vertebral body [32], but this does not appear to have been widely accepted. The CT scan will also show relevant abnormalities such as a horseshoe kidney, double inferior vena cava or retroaortic left renal vein.

There are divergent opinions as to the value of digital subtraction angiography in patients being considered for conventional open repair of an AAA. One view argues that it is essential to show associated stenoses or anomalous origins of the renal arteries and aneurysmal or occlusive disease of the iliac arteries which influence the technique of the operation. The alternate opinion is that these can all be diagnosed and dealt with (or ignored) at operation.

Our unit has embarked on a program of bifurcated endoluminal grafts using the Mialhe stentor (Mintec Pty Ltd) which is inserted through a femoral arteriotomy. Presently this is only used in technically suitable patients with an AAA > 5 cm diameter and either a general contraindication to open surgery or a hostile abdomen. This requires precise measurements of the length and diameter of the neck which must be able to grip the device above the AAA, the outflow artery diameters to ensure that the common iliac arteries can grip the distal ends and that the external iliacs are large enough for the sheath to pass, and the length of the aorta and each common iliac to allow the device to be manufactured to size. The diameter of the neck and the AAA are assessed from the CT scan, the diameters of the common iliacs and the lengths are obtained from a digital subtraction angiography using a pigtail catheter with multiple 1-cm graduations, and the diameters of the external iliacs are measured from duplex ultrasound scans.

Approximately 30% of patients with AAAs also have popliteal aneurysms (and vice versa) and these are either asymptomatic or present with acute occlusion. A popliteal aneurysm can usually be diagnosed by palpation, and if there is doubt then it is readily confirmed by a duplex ultrasound scan. An arteriogram is usually required to define precisely occlusions in the runoff crural arteries.

Assessment of non-atherosclerotic diseases

Buerger's disease

This disease was first documented by Von Winiwarter in 1879 [33] and fully described by Buerger in 1908 [34]. It affects young patients who are predominantly male and always smokers. Inflammatory changes affect distal arteries and veins leading to a chronic phase of fibrosis and recanalization. The presentation is usually with critical ischemia; the experience is that there are lower limb symptoms only in 60%, upper limb symptoms only in 30%, and both in 10%, but that arteriography reveals changes in all lower limb arteries and most upper limb vessels [35, 36] There are characteristic arteriographic appearances with marked bilateral symmetry showing apparently normal vessels above abrupt occlusions, corkscrew collaterals and tortuous recanalized distal vessels. In the lower limbs, this most often affects crural arteries but can extend up to the femoral or even to the iliac arteries.

Takayashu's disease

This condition was first identified by Morgagni in 1761 and clearly described by Takayashu in 1908 [37]. It affects children and young adults with a female preponderance. Inflammatory changes in the arterial wall lead to intimal proliferation and stenosis or occlusion, or weakening of the arterial wall leading to aneurysms. This predominantly affects the aorta at any site from the arch to its distal end. In the early acute phase, there is a nonspecific illness with skin lesions, fever, arthralgia, anemia and a raised erythrocyte sedimentation rate, but these may not be recognized. Some years later, sequelae of aortic disease become manifest and in the lower limbs this may lead to peripheral bruits or absent pulses with or without symptoms. There is no specific test to confirm the diagnosis. Arteriographic changes are characteristic with diffuse irregular involvement of the aorta and stenoses or occlusions in one or more of its major branches.

Cystic adventitial arterial disease

This condition results from degeneration in the wall analogous to a ganglion, and usually affects the popliteal artery. Most patients are male and the onset is usually with rapidly progressive claudication. The typical arteriographic finding is a smooth narrowing of the arterial lumen with normal proximal and distal vessels – the 'scimitar sign'.

The popliteal entrapment syndrome

There are several variants associated with entrapment of the popliteal artery, usually by the medial head of the gastrocnemius and rarely by the deeper popliteus muscle. While the artery is patent, flow is restricted only with vigorous exercise and this can be confirmed by loss of pedal pulses, particularly if the ankle is actively or passively dorsiflexed with the knee extended. This can also be demonstrated by a duplex scan although many normal subjects block their popliteal arteries with active plantar-flexion [38]. Arteriography shows a characteristic appearance usually with medial deviation of the proximal popliteal artery and either post-stenotic dilatation or segmental occlusion of the mid-popliteal artery.

Fibromuscular dysplasia

Rarely, this affects the external iliac artery and the patient may present with claudication, embolism causing the 'blue toe syndrome' or acute ischemia from dissection. The arteriographic appearance is characteristic with focal stenoses and intervening mural dilatations.

Conclusions

As new techniques for intervention become established, so do techniques for diagnosis evolve. In the era when open surgical bypass operations prevailed, clinical assessment followed by arteriography to demonstrate the entire circulation below the renal arteries was the standard management. We are now able to choose between surgical bypass and an array of endovascular procedures. Accordingly, we are now obliged to focus more on the diseased segment. Spectacular advances in non invasive techniques for investigation, particularly by color-Doppler ultrasound scanning, allow an approach which provides more information and causes less trauma to the patient.

Appendix

The arteriogram – instructions for patients

An appointment has been made for you to have an arteriogram as a day patient at .... Hospital on .... at .... You will need to be in the department by .... Please follow these instructions.

Preparation

- As you will need to rest for *four (4) hours* after the test, you may wish to bring a book or magazine or a small radio or tape deck with personal headphones.
- No solid food is to be taken for *three (3) hours* prior to the examination.
- Drink plenty of clear fluids (not milk) until you come into the hospital.
- If you have diabetes please have your normal breakfast and your usual medication. If you are an insulin-dependant diabetic you may require an intravenous line to be inserted before the procedure.
- Continue your usual medications except for Lasix (frusemide) which should not be taken on the morning of the procedure.
- If you are taking aspirin or cardiprin, stop them 24 hours prior to the procedure.
- If you are taking anticoagulants such as warfarin, please follow your treating doctor's instructions regarding stopping these before the procedure.
- Please ensure that you bring all of your usual medications with you.

The procedure

A nurse will help you change into a gown and will prepare you for the examination. A radiologist (doctor) will explain to you what will be done and answer your questions. You will then be taken to the procedure room where a medical imaging technologist will position you on the X-ray table. A nurse will prepare you by washing your groin with antiseptic and covering you with sterile drapes.

The doctor will inject local anesthetic into the groin area, after which you should experience very little discomfort. A very thin catheter (tube) is placed into your artery and a special radiographic solution is injected. You may experience a sensation like a warm flush, which is a normal response to the injection. At the same time the technologist will be taking X-rays and it is very important that you do not move at this time. The doctor, nurse and technologist will be with you all the time and will answer any questions you may have. Occasionally, the doctor may use an artery in your arm instead of an artery in the groin.

After the procedure

- You will remain resting in the Diagnostic Imaging waiting area for observation for at least *four (4) hours* after the procedure.
- You must not drive yourself or take public transport home. Please arrange in advance for someone to drive you home and stay overnight with you.
- It is advisable to wear loose fitting clothing.
- Bed rest is advised for the remainder of the day and you should avoid strenuous exercise for the next two days.
- Drink plenty of fluids but no alcohol for 24 hours.
- If bleeding from the puncture site should occur, you should apply firm direct pressure to the site and call for assistance.
- If you are concerned or experience any of the side effects listed below, ring the Radiology Department or Accident and Emergency Center through .... Hospital Phone ....

Complications

It is necessary to warn patients of occasional complications from this procedure. It is not possible to anticipate every recorded rare complication. If you have any questions concerning possible complications please discuss them with your treating doctor *before* the procedure.

- Uncommon side effects include allergic reaction to radiographic contrast material, severe bruising to the puncture site, or swelling or oozing at the puncture site.
- Rarely, dislodgment of a thrombus (clot) from within a blood vessel can interrupt blood flow resulting in tingling or numbness and change in color or temperature of a leg or arm.
- Extremely rarely, there is a risk of very severe complications as with any procedure in medicine.

References

1. Yao JST, Hobbs JT, Irvine WT. Ankle systolic pressure measurements in arterial diseases affecting the lower extremities. Br J Surg 1969;56:676–9.
2. Baker JD, Dix D. Variability of Doppler ankle pressures with arterial occlusive disease: An evaluation of ankle index and brachial–ankle pressure gradient. Surgery 1981;89:134–7.
3. Fisher CM, Burnett A, Makeham V, Kidd J, Glasson M, Harris JP. Variation in measurement of ankle brachial pressure index in routine clinical practice. Cardiovasc Surg. Accepted for publication.
4. Carter SA, Lezack JD. Digital systolic pressures in the lower limbs in arterial disease. Circulation 1971;43:905–14.
5. Hummel BW, Hummel BA, Mowbry A *et al.* Reactive hyperemia vs treadmill exercise testing in arterial disease. Arch Surg 1978;113:95–8.

6. Myers KA. Haemodynamic studies in peripheral vascular disease. Master of Surgery Thesis, University of Melbourne, 1968.
7. Myers KA. Preoperative assessment of lower limb ischaemia. In: Greenhalgh RM (ed.), Diagnostic techniques and assessment procedures in vascular surgery. Grune and Statton: London, 1985:217–39.
8. Tyrrell MR, Wolfe JHN. Critical leg ischaemia: An appraisal of clinical definitions. Br J Surg 1993;80:177–80.
9. McPherson DS, Evans DH, Bell PRF. Common femoral artery Doppler waveforms: A comparison of three methods of objective analysis with direct pressure measurements. Br J Surg 1984;71:46–9.
10. Sheriff S, Barber DC. Principal component factor analysis. In: Salmasi A-M, Nicolaides AN (eds), Cardiovascular applications of Doppler ultrasound. Churchill Livingstone: Edinburgh, 1989:71–84.
11. Skidmore R, Woodcock JP. Physiological interpretation of Doppler-shift waveforms – I Theoretical considerations. Ultrasound Med Biol 1980;6:7–10.
12. Harward TRS, Bernstein EF, Fronek A. The value of power frequency spectrum analysis in the identification of aortoiliac artery disease. J Vasc Surg 1987;5:803–13.
13. Myers KA, Williams MA, Nicolaides AN. The use of Doppler ultrasound to assess disease in arteries to the lower limbs. In: Salmasi A-M, Nicolaides AN (eds), Cardiovascular applications of Doppler ultrasound. Churchill Livingstone: Edinburgh, 1989:289–314.
14. Cossman DV, Ellison JE, Wagner WW et al. Comparison of contrast arteriography to arterial mapping with color-flow duplex imaging in the lower extremities. J Vasc Surg 1989;10:522–8.
15. Fletcher JP, Kershaw JP, Chan LZ et al. Noninvasive imaging of the superficial femoral artery using ultrasound duplex scanning. J Cardiovasc Surg 1990;31:364–7.
16. Polak JF, Karmel MI, Mannick JA et al. Determination of the extent of lower-extremity peripheral arterial disease with color-assisted duplex sonography: Comparison with angiography. Am J Radiol 1990;155:1085–9.
17. de Smet AAEA, Visser K, Kitslaar PJEHM. Duplex scanning for grading aortoiliac obstructive disease and guiding treatment. Eur J Vasc Surg 1994;8:711–5.
18. Legermate DA, Teeuwen C, Hoeneveld H et al. Value of duplex scanning compared with angiography and pressure measurement in the assessment of aortoiliac arterial lesions. Br J Surg 1991;78:1003–8.
19. Kohler TR, Andros G, Porter JM et al. Can duplex scanning replace arteriography for lower extremity arterial disease. Ann Vasc Surg 1990;4:280–7.
20. Aston NO, Lea Thomas M, Burnand KG. The distribution of atherosclerosis in the lower limbs. Eur J Vasc Surg 1992;6:73–7.
21. Widmer LK, Greensher A, Kannel WB. Occlusion of peripheral arteries – a study of 6400 working subjects. Circulation 1964;30:834–52.
22. Myers KA, Scott DF, Devine TJ et al. Palpation of the femoral and popliteal pulses: A study of the accuracy as assessed by agreement between multiple observers. Eur J Vasc Surg 1987;1:245–9.
23. Ramsey DE, Manke DA, Sumner DS. Toe blood pressure – a valuable adjunct to ankle pressure measurement for assessing peripheral arterial disease. J Cardiovasc Surg 1983;24:43.
24. Brewster DC, Perler BA, Robinson JG, Darling RC. Aortofemoral graft for multilevel occlusive disease: Predictors of success and need for distal bypass. Arch Surg 1982;117:1593–600.
25. Carter SA. Arterial auscultation in peripheral vascular disease. J Am Med Assoc 1981;246:1682–6.
26. Faris I, Tonnesen KH, Agerskov K et al. Femoral artery pressure measurement to predict the outcome of arterial surgery in patients with multilevel disease. Surgery 1982;92:10–5.
27. Rutherford RB, Jones DN, Martin MS et al. Serial hemodynamic assessment of aortobifemoral bypass. J Vasc Surg 1986;4:428–35.
28. Pleumakers HJCM, Hoes AN, van der Does E et al. Epidemiology of abdominal aortic aneurysms. Eur J Vasc Surg 1994;8:119–28.
29. McSweeney STR, O'Meara M, Alexander C et al. High prevalence of unsuspected abdominal aortic aneurysms in patients with confirmed symptomatic peripheral or cerebral arterial disease. Br J Surg 1993;80:582–4.
30. Bengtsson H, Nilsson P, Bergqvist D. Natural history of abdominal aortic aneurysm detected by screening. Br J Surg 1993;80:718–20.

31. Nichols EA, Norman PE, Lawrence-Brown MMD et al. Screening for abdominal aortic aneurysms in Western Australia. Aust NZ J Surg 1992;62:858–61.
32. Russell JGB. Is screening for abdominal aortic aneurysm worthwhile? Clin Radiol 1990;41:182–4.
33. von Winiwater F. Ueber eine eigenthumliche form von endarteritis und endophlebitis mit gangren des fusses. Arch Klin Chir 1879;23:202.
34. Buerger L. Thrombo-angiitis obliterans: A study of the vascular lesions leading to presenile spontaneous gangrene. Am J Med Sci 1908;136:567.
35. Ohta T, Shionoya S. Fate of the ischaemic limb in Buerger's disease. Br J Surg 1988;75:259–62.
36. Shionoya S. Buerger's disease: Diagnosis and management. Cardiovasc Surg 1993;1:207–14.
37. Hall S, Buchbinder R. Takayasu's arteritis. Rheum Dis Clin N Am 1990;16:411–22.
38. Akkersdijk WL, de Ruyter JW, Lapham R, Mali W, Eikelboom BC. Colour duplex ultrasonographic imaging and provocation of popliteal artery compression. Eur J Vasc Endovasc Surg 1995;10:342–5.

22. Management of peripheral obstructive arterial disease of the lower limbs

SALVATORE NOVO

Peripheral obstructive arterial disease of the lower limbs is determined by a single or multiple stenosis and/or occlusion of the iliac–femoral–popliteal arterial axis determining a reduction of the perfusion of the muscles and the skin of the lower limbs and thus a progressive tissue ischemia [1].

The disease may be considered the third most important complication of atherosclerotic disease, after coronary artery disease and cerebrovascular disease [2–4].

Cigarette smoking, diabetes and hypertension may be considered the most important risk factors for the start and evolution of the disease, while hypercholesterolemia and hypertriglyceridemia seem to play a less important role [5, 6].

From the pathophysiological point of view, some alterations of macrocirculation and microcirculation may be considered as factors involved in the evolution of the disease from the asymptomatic stage until the appearance of rest pain and gangrene [7–21].

Table 22.1 summarizes some factors modulating the hemodynamic value of the stenosis at the macrocirculatory level [7–10], thus influencing the progression of peripheral arterial disease (PAD) to critical leg ischemia (CLI). Table 22.2 lists other factors that may worsen the microcirculation and thus PAD [11–14].

The evolution of PAD into gangrene may be particularly frequent in diabetic patients [15–21], due to the alterations reported in Table 22.3.

The goal of therapy of PAD is to slow the evolution of the atherosclerotic plaque worsening the stenosis, to improve macro- and microcirculation, to prevent or reduce pain of the legs and to prevent or treat trophic lesions [22].

Table 22.1. Factors that may worsen macrocirculation in PAD.

Number and entity of atherosclerotic stenoses
Entity of the collateral circulation
Progression of the atherosclerotic plaque
– Rapid growth, breaking of the plaque with thrombosis, intraplaque hemorrhage
– Thrombophilic syndrome
Influence of systemic hemodynamics
– Cardiac output
– Systemic arterial blood pressure

A.-M. Salmasi and A. Strano (eds), Angiology in Practice, 307–321.
© 1996 Kluwer Academic Publishers. Printed in Great Britain.

Table 22.2. Factors worsening microcirculation and tissue metabolism in PAD.

Hemorheological alterations
- Reduced red cell deformability
- Increased fibrinogen and plasmatic viscosity
- Increased viscosity of the whole blood
- Platelets and coagulation activation
- Inhibition of fibrinolysis
- Leukocyte activation

Metabolic alterations
- Decreased peripheral supply of O_2
- Anerobic metabolism
- Decreased mitochondrial synthesis of ATP
- Activation of glycolysis with reduction of glycogen storage
- Dysfunction of the Na^+/K^+ pump, with K^+ loss and increase of intracellular Na^+
- Cellular reinflation
- Breaking of lysosomes with release of hydrolase and cellular lysis
- Local metabolic acidosis

Storage of metabolic products
- PGE_1 and histamine (increasing vasopermeability)
- 5-HT (determining vein contraction)
- Bradykinin (inducing arteriole dilatation)

Table 22.3. Alterations induced by diabetes mellitus and worsening PAD

Increased glycosylation of membrane proteins with increased rigidity of erythrocytes and increased viscosity
Increased adhesion and aggregation of platelets
Increased production of TXB_2
Decreased endothelial synthesis of PGI_2 and NO
Increased levels of von-Willebrand factor and fibrinogen
Increased PAI-1 and decreased tPA
Increased adhesion of activated leukocytes to endothelium
Increased release of free radicals from the activated leukocytes
Increased oxidized LDL
Increased thickness of basal membrane of capillaries and alterations of endothelial function of exchange
Increased vasopermeability and peripheral edema
Increased infection caused by alterations of immune system

The treatment must take into consideration: correction of risk factors, physical training, hygienic–dietetic measures and specific medical treatments [22].

Correction of risk factors

The correction of risk factors is very important for prevention of the progression of atherosclerotic lesions responsible for the start and evolution of the disease [22, 23].

Smoking

Patients must be informed of the increased risk induced by smoking and must be persuaded to stop [23]. Stopping smoking typically produces a two to three times increase in walking distance and an evident improvement of symptoms and slows the progression of PAD from the initial stages to CLI. Patients who continue smoking present a worsening of symptoms and in most cases an evolution into gangrene [22, 23].

Diabetes mellitus

Diabetes mellitus is one of the most important risk factors for PAD and increases more than ten times the evolution into gangrene [7, 8, 15, 22]. In diabetic patients it is very important to obtain a good metabolic compensation to prevent CLI and gangrene and to avoid the evolution of dry gangrene into humid gangrene because of infections [22, 23]. Blood sugar should be normalized as soon as possible and insulin should be administered in patients with CLI [23].

Dyslipidemias

The importance of high levels of total cholesterol, LDL-C, Apo-B lipoproteins and triglycerides as risk factors for PAD is continuously increasing as well as the role of low levels of HDL-C and of Apo AI lipoproteins. There is increasing evidence that the correction of hyperlipoproteinemias can be beneficial in slowing disease progression or sustaining a partial regression of atheroslerotic lesions and thus an improvement of PAD [22, 24].

Hypertension

Arterial hypertension determines deep alterations of the hemodynamics (increased shear stress) inducing endothelial damage and favors the start and the growth of atherosclerotic plaques and thus the formation of arterial stenoses. When PAD is established hypertension may contribute to determine a transtenotic gradient of pressure useful for maintaining a good peripheral perfusion. In such a situation the treatment of arterial hypertension must be slow and gradual [23]. In fact, a sudden decrease of blood pressure could induce a worsening of clinical symptoms, through the reduction of the transtenotic gradient of pressure [22, 23]. ACE-inhibitors and calcium-antagonists are the first choice drugs to treat hypertension in patients with PAD, while beta-blockers should be avoided especially in patients with CLI. Beta-blockers may in fact reduce peripheral perfusion through a diminution of cardiac output and a reflex skin vasoconstriction mediated by an alpha-adrenergic hypertonicity.

Hygienic–dietetic measures

Diet

A diet with a caloric intake sufficient to maintain a normal body weight and well balanced in the supply of carbohydrates, saturated and unsaturated fatty acids, vegetable and animal proteins, may be useful to correct some deleterious risk factors such as diabetes, hyperlipoproteinemias and arterial hypertension [22].

A regular intake of vegetables can supply antioxidizing nutrients such as vitamins E, A and C whose role as antiatherogenic substances has been frequently demonstrated [25].

Physical activity and training

Physical activity is of great importance in patients with intermittent claudication. The main effects of regular training [26–28] are summarized in Table 22.4. Because of these effects, physical activity is indicated in patients with PAD stages I and II, in whom walking distance can be increased. Individuals who perform a daily exercise program can expect a doubling or tripling of walking distance within three months [29–31]. In more advanced stages of the disease, physical activity may be performed in rehabilitation centers.

Table 22.4. Effects of physical training on the clinical evolution of PAD.

Improvement of walking technique and particularly coordination and flexibility of skeletal muscles
Development of the collateral circulation and optimization of collateral blood flow distribution
Enhancement of capillary perfusion and capillarization of skeletal muscle
Improved distribution of blood between muscles and skin
Better extraction and utilization of O_2 from the ischemic muscle
Increased activity of the antioxidant enzymes
Decreased total cholesterol and triglycerides and increased HDL cholesterol
Increased transtenotic gradient of pressure through increased blood pressure and decreased peripheral vascular resistance
Positive influence on blood fluidity

Posture maneuvers

In arteriopathies of stage III and IV, beneficial effects can be obtained by the downward tilting of the foot from the bed for brief periods, in the lowest possible position without inducing edema [22, 23]. This maneuver favors an increase in hydrostatic pressure which causes a transient increase of perfusion through the stenosis in the ischemic leg and often results a decrease in rest pain. The maneuver must be of only a short duration to avoid the increase of venous pressure and the lack of reabsorption of fluid from the interstitium to the venous bed with formation of edema. In fact, edema may exert compression on the capillary bed and thus may worsen the evolution of CLI [22, 23].

Foot hygiene

Hygiene of the extremities is of great importance in patients with PAD since mild cutaneous trauma may favor the appearance of trophic lesions evolving into gangrene. Patients with PAD must wear wide and sensible shoes, to ensure that pressure by footwear is avoided; avoid any trauma when performing pedicure; pare nails with extreme attention; always maintain clean and dry skin; avoid skin contact with chemical substances; wash feet in water less than 25°C; avoid cold or warm stimuli; and apply lotion to feet after drying. Patient with advanced PAD should also not step into the bath without checking the water temperature; not use hot water bottles or heating pads; not use chemical agents to treat calluses or corns; not walk barefoot; and not wear tight stockings [22, 23].

Pharmacological therapy

There are several possible benefits of vasoactive drugs in PAD [28] as reported in Table 22.5.

Hemodilution

Hemodilution has been used in the therapy of peripheral arterial disease for several years [22, 23, 28, 31]. The main effects of this therapy are listed in Table 22.6.

Table 22.5. The benefits of vasoactive drugs in patients with PAD.

Improvement of blood fluidity through reducing plasma viscosity and increasing red cell deformability
Inhibition of pathologically increased thrombocyte aggregation
Inhibition of leukocyte activation and reduced release of activated free radicals of oxygen
Increased capillary circulation
Neutralization of endothelial damage caused by the vasoconstrictive effect of systemic vasoactive substances such as serotonin, catecholamines, angiotensin II, etc.

Table 22.6. Main effects of hemodilution in patients with PAD.

Decreased hematocrit
Decreased erythrocyte aggregation
Improvement of cutaneous microcirculation
Increased intramuscular PO_2
Increased pain-free walking distance

The effect of twice a week hemodilution, both with or without venesection, seems to be better than physical activity twice a week, obtaining an increase in pain-free walking distance of 30.4%, 36.7% and 20.1% respectively [32]. The improvement of walking distance induced by hemodilution is better in patients with a high hematocrit [31].

Drugs acting on muscular metabolism

Propionyl-L-carnitine (PLC) is a drug which has been recently studied in a patient with PAD. PLC supplementation is indicated in the treatment of patients with PAD to correct the alterations in carnitine homeostasis which occur in ischemic skeletal muscles.

PLC reduces the lactate concentration in venous blood, restores carnitine – a very important substrate in fat metabolism – to normal, and improves enzyme activities and transcutaneous pO_2 in the ischemic muscle [33]. The superiority of PLC over L-carnitine in improving walking capacity in patients with peripheral vascular disease has been demonstrated [34]. In a double-blind, crossover study comparing L-carnitine versus placebo [35], the absolute walking distance increased from 174 ± 63 meters under placebo to 306 ± 122 meters on active drug ($p < 0.01$). A favorable action of PLC on hemocoagulative and hemorheological parameters has also been shown [36].

Drugs improving hemorheology

The amelioration of hemorheology is of crucial importance in patients with PAD because the improvement of the microcirculation in the capillary bed can have significant effects on the clinical symptoms of patients.

Pentoxifylline is the most studied drug in this field. In six controlled studies [37–42] the dose of the drug ranged from 600 to 1200 mg and the duration of the treatment from 1 to 6 months. In all the studies there was a significant increase of pain-free walking distance ranging from 45 to 470 meters [37–42]. In the study performed by Ciuffetti *et al.*, pentoxifylline inhibited free radicals production and granulocyte expression adhesion receptors [41].

In a controlled study performed by our group [42], we demonstrated a significant increase of walking distance in comparison with placebo and a significant improvement of some coagulative (decreased fibrinogen) and hemorheological parameters (decrease of whole blood and plasmatic viscosity).

Another drug which improves hemorheology is buflomedil (43). A recent meta-analysis showed a significant increase of absolute walking distance and pain-free walking distance in actively treated patients with PAD stage II in comparison with patients treated with placebo [44].

Antiserotoninergic drugs

Ketanserin is an antagonist of S2 receptors for serotonin tested in several placebo-controlled studies [45]. It was extensively evaluated in the PACK study (Prevention of Atherosclerotic Complications using ketanserin). Ketanserin increased walking distance similarly to placebo while the ankle/arm pressure ratio was increased only by the active drug [46]. The number of nonfatal and fatal cardiovascular events was not significantly different in the active group in comparison with the placebo group. Excluding patients treated contemporaneously with ketanserin and potassium-losing diuretics from the analysis, ketanserin obtained a 23% reduction of fatal and nonfatal cardiovascular events [47]. Ketanserin prolongs the QT interval, however, and thus the combined use of ketanserin and potassium-losing diuretics can be harmful [47].

Naftidrofuryl is an old drug that recently was demonstrated to act mainly as an inhibitor of serotoninergic receptors. A meta-analysis [48] of five double-blind, placebo-controlled studies performed in patients with stage II PAD in which naftidrofuryl was used at 600 mg/day and including 888 patients according to the intention to treat analysis (447 on naftidrofuryl and 411 on placebo), showed a significant increase of pain-free walking distance in patients on active treatment ($p < 0.002$). Moreover, this analysis demonstrated a clear and significant decrease of cardiovascular critical events (CLI, vascular surgery, cerebral or cardiac events – 32 versus 50, 7.7% versus 12.3%, $p < 0.02$) and thus a better outcome in patients on active treatment [48].

Antiplatelet drugs

Several antiplatelet drugs have been employed in the treatment of PAD on the basis of the involvement of platelets in the genesis and progression of atherosclerosis.

There is evidence that aspirin, alone or in combination with dipyridamole, may delay the progression of atherosclerosis in peripheral arteries of patients with PAD [49].

In a recent double-blind, placebo-controlled, multicenter study in which 154 patients were on placebo and 148 on active treatment with indobufen 200 mg twice a day, the intention to treat analysis showed an increase of pain-free walking distance from 125.1/63.4 to 153.1/86.8 meters with placebo, and from 127.6/66.5 to 227.9/174.4 meters with indobufen ($p < 0.01$). Also the absolute walking distance increased significantly ($p < 0.01$) [50].

Several studies have taken into consideration the efficacy of ticlopidine in the therapy of patients with intermittent claudication. In a double-blind, placebo-controlled, clinical trial [51] in patients with stage II PAD, the drug was employed at the dosage of 250 mg twice a day for six months. The pain-free walking distance doubled in 73% of patients on active treatment in comparison with 39% of patients on placebo ($p < 0.001$).

In our experience ticlopidine, alone or in combination with captopril, significantly increases pain-free and absolute walking distances in patients with intermittent claudication and mild to moderate arterial hypertension [52]. In another double-blind, placebo-controlled, multicenter study [53], in which were enrolled 151 patients with intermittent claudication, in a mean follow-up of 21 months, ticlopidine 250 mg twice a day, the intention to treat analysis showed a significant increase of the ankle – arm pressure ratio after exercise and a significant increase of the absolute walking distance [53].

Finally, ticlopidine 500 mg daily was used for six months in a double-blind, placebo-controlled study, in 192 patients with CLI and ulcers. The percentage of ulcers healing was higher (24% vs. 14%, $p < 0.01$) and the percentage of amputations lower (2% vs. 4%, $p < 0.01$) in patients on active treatment [54].

Defibrotide

Defibrotide is a drug with antithrombotic and hemorheological properties. A met-analysis [55] was recently performed on ten placebo-controlled trials including patients with stage II PAD (406 on defibrotide and 337 on placebo). The drug was employed at a dose regimen of 400 to 800 mg daily, the duration of the treatment ranging from 60 to 180 days. These was a significant increase of absolute walking distance [55].

Calcium-heparin

A recent randomized study comparing ASA 300 mg twice a day and calcium heparin 12500 IU twice a day in 60 patients with stage IIb PAD [56], treated for three months and then followed for six months, showed a significant increase of pain-free and absolute walking distances with both drugs. Moreover, the benefit was more evident on calcium heparin and the results were maintained in the follow-up [56].

In another randomized study calcium heparin increased significantly pain-free and ambulatory walking distances as well as did ticlopidine. Transcutaneous pO_2 was also improved [57].

Future perspective

Future perspectives include the use of drugs restoring the integrity of vascular function, inhibitors of thrombus formation, and inhibitors of cellular migration and myointimal proliferation [58].

Treatment of patients with CLI

A meta-analysis of randomized, placebo-controlled trials in patients with PAD in Fontaine stage III and IV was recently published by Loosemore *et al.* [59]. Randomized, placebo-controlled trials in patients with CLI have been performed using the drugs listed in Table 22.7. These drugs have potential useful action on the microcirculation, reducing rest pain and accelerating the healing of trophic ulcers [1]. The meta-analytic evaluation of all trials showed significant benefit over placebo for the cumulative endpoint, death plus major amputation, only in patients treated actively with Iloprost [59].

Table 22.7. Randomized placebo-controlled trials in patients with CLI.

Drugs employed	Number of trials
Ancrod	2
Naftidrofuryl	2
PGE_1	4
PGI_2	3
Iloprost	6

Fatal and nonfatal endpoints in patients with PAD

One of the main goals of treatment of PAD [60] is not only the control of claudication but also the prevention of cardiovascular events that frequently complicate the course of the disease (50% myocardial infarction, 15% stroke, 10% vascular disease of the abdomen). Since the majority of these events are of thrombotic origin, antiplatelet agents are being increasingly evaluated in clinical trials.

In the STIMS study [61], performed by administering ticlopidine 500 mg/day in comparison with placebo, the intention to treat analysis showed a 29% decrease of total mortality. Even better results were obtained in the EMATAP study [62].

Twenty-two trials were considered for meta-analysis in patients with PAD treated with different antiplatelet drugs [63]; cardiovascular events were 195/1649 on placebo and 160/1646 on antiplatelet drugs (9.72% vs. 11.82%), with a significant reduction of all events ($-21.6\%, p < 0.01$).

Interventional therapy

Patients with localized disease, for example stenoses or short occlusions, may be treated with angioplasty; the results are not as good in more extensive disease. If feasible, angioplasty should be considered as the first option because of a low complication rate and it does not preclude future surgery [23, 64]. Relatively localized stenosis, single or multiple, is the ideal indication for balloon angioplasty [64].

In selected occlusions of the femoral/popliteal segments it is also possible to obtain good primary results [65, 66], but occlusions longer than 3 cm are prone to reocclusion [67]. Also some total iliac occlusions can be recanalized if less than 5 cm [23, 64]. Devices for atherectomy can have a role in such occlusions, using wire catheter techniques or with the aid of thrombolytic therapy [23, 64]. Diabetic patients have an higher percentage of occlusion after angioplasty of the femoral artery [68]. Long iliac occlusions, superficial femoral occlusions that start at the vessel origin, extensive calf vessel occlusions and heavily calcified lesions are often regarded as contraindications [64]. Absolute contraindications to angioplasty are aortic occlusions, thrombosed popliteal aneurysms and severe hemorrhagic disorders [23, 64]. The disadvantages of angioplasty are possible acute rethrombosis and recurrences increasing with occlusions > 10 cm with poor runoff. In up to 3% of cases, complications require local or bypass surgery [69]. The approximate primary technical success is 70–95% for stenosis/occlusions of iliac arteries and from 75–95% for femoral/popliteal stenosis/occlusions. The patency rate of vessels at two years is 85% for iliac localizations and 50% for femoral/popliteal [23]. In general the percentage of successful angioplasty is higher for proximal and recent stenosis [23, 64]. Locally catheter-delivered infiltration of a thrombolytic agent into the thrombus is probably safer than systemic therapy, although hemorrhagic complications may also occur [70–72].

Thrombolysis may be useful to treat acute thrombosis after angioplasty, but some workers prefer to use fibrinolytic therapy before balloon dilatation, especially in the iliac artery, where even one-year old occlusions often contain lysable material [73]. Balloon dilatation is usually needed after lysis to dilate an underlying stenosis [23, 64]. The catheter suction embolectomy may be particularly effective for removing emboli that have resulted from angioplasty or locally catheter-delivered thrombolytic therapy [74].

In recent years new devices such as laser atherectomy or rotational atherectomy are being used as recanalizing tools and may be used in some total occlusions too chronic for fibrinolytic therapy and too resistant for conventional guide wire passage (75–78).

Atherectomy may be useful to remove, rather than displace and split the material, while stents are useful to maintain the artery open and to avoid reocclusions [79–80].

Surgical procedures

Endarterectomy and often bypass grafting is usually the treatment of choice for patients with CLI because they have often long obstructions that are less effectively treated by other means [81–82]. Bypass grafting may be obtained by veins or by synthetic materials and the percentage of one-year patency decreases from 90% of aorto–iliac to 50% of femoro–tibial [23]. Autologous vein graft gives the best results below the knee [83–84].

Early graft failure is rare and may result from incorrect choice of operation [85]. Late graft failure is usually caused by thrombosis, intimal hyperplasia and progressive atherosclerosis and is more frequent in current smokers and in patients with higher levels of fibrinogen [86]. Vein graft stenosis may be treated by angioplasty or surgery [87].

Graft occlusion may require a secondary surgical procedure, surgical thrombectomy, thrombolysis of the occluded graft and amputation [23].

Amputation

The primary amputation should be performed only if the possibility of a revascularization procedure has been excluded at a vascular center [23]. About 70% of below-knee amputations heal primarily, about 15% by secondary intervention and 15% need an above knee amputation [88]. In some cases primary amputation may be better than subjecting the patient to repeated bypass or reopening procedures with little chance of success and increasing mortality and morbidity [23].

Conclusions

Medical therapy of peripheral vascular disease may be performed in the following steps:

1. Correct risk factors, in particular smoking and diabetes.
2. Physical activity is very useful from stage I to IIb.
3. In stage IIb, angioplasty or vascular surgery may be performed according to the above recommendations, especially in patients in which intermittent claudication prevents usual activities.
4. Metabolic drugs such as PLC may be useful in the precocious stage of the disease.
5. Hemodilution plus vasoactive drugs are more useful from stages II to III, and with hemorheological alterations.
6. Prostanoids are useful in patients with CLI unsuitable for interventional therapy or vascular surgery.
7. Antiplatelet drugs may be useful to slow the progression of atherosclerotic lesions and to prevent fatal and nonfatal atherothrombotic complications of target organs (acute myocardial infarction, transient ischemic attacks, stroke, acute peripheral occlusion).

References

1. Novo S. The patient with intermittent claudication. In: Bloch Thomsen, PE, Clement, DL (eds), Everyday problems in clinical cardiology. Amsterdam, The Netherlands: Excerpta Medica Vol. 5, 6, 1995:3–10.
2. Criqui MH, Fronek A, Barrett-Connor E et al. The prevalence of peripheral arterial disease in a defined population. Circulation 1985;71:510–15.
3. Kannel WB, Skinner JJ, Schwartz MJ, Shurtleff D. Intermittent claudication: Incidence in the Framingham Study. Circulation 1970;XLI:875–83.
4. Balkau B, Vray M, Eschwege E. Epidemiology of peripheral arterial disease. J Cardiovasc Pharmacol 1994;23(Suppl.3):S8–16.
5. Rosenbloom MS, Flanigan DP, Schuler JJ. Risk factors affecting the natural hystory of intermittent claudication. Arch Surg 1988;123:867–70.
6. Novo S, Avellone G, DI Garbo V et al. Prevalence of risk factors in patients with peripheral arterial disease: A clinical and epidemiological evaluation. Int Angiol 1992;11:218–29.
7. Scheffler A. Pathophysiological aspects of leg ischemia. In: Strano A, Novo S (eds), Advances in vascular pathology. Amsterdam: Elsevier, 1990:749–55.
8. Lowe GDO. Pathophysiology of critical limb ischemia. In: Dormandy J, Stok G (eds), Critical leg ischemia: Its pathophysiology and management. Berlin: Springer-Verlag, 1990:17–38.
9. Strano A, Novo S, Davi' G, Avellone G, Pinto A. Haemostatic alterations in peripheral arteriopathies. In: Cajozzo A, Perricone R, Di Marco P, Palazzolo P (eds), Advances in haemostasis and thrombosis London: Plenum Publishing Corporation, 1985:213–22.
10. Novo S, Avellone G, Pinto A, Davi' G. Blood fibrinolysis in atherosclerosis and high risk metabolic disorders. In: Strano A, (ed.) Advances in coagulation, fibrinolysis, platelet aggregation and atherosclerosis. Rome: CEPI, 1976:249–55.
11. Di Perri T. Haemorheological aspects of leg ischemia. In: Strano, Novo S (eds). Advances in vascular pathology. Amsterdam: Elsevier, 1990:757–70.
12. Vane JR. Regulatory functions of the vascular endothelium. N Engl J Med 1990;323:27–36.

13. Hichman P, McCollum PT, Belch JF. Neutrophils may contribute to the morbidity and mortality in claudicants. Br J Surg 1994;81:790–8.
14. Strano A, Pinto A, Novo S, Clemenza F. Metabolic and haemorheological aspects in ischemia of the lower limbs. In: Lenzi S, Descovich GC (eds). Atherosclerosis, clinical evaluation and therapy. Lancaster: MTP Press Limited, 1982:445–52.
15. Edmonds ME. The diabetic foot: Pathophysiology and treatment. Clin Endocrinol Metab 1986;15:889–916.
16. Brownlee M, Cerami A, Vlassara H. Advanced glycosylation and products in tissue and the biochemical basis of diabetic complications. N Engl J Med 1988;20:1315–21.
17. Mac Rury SM, Lowe GDO. Blood rheology in diabetes mellitus. Diabetic Med 1990;7:285–91.
18. Ernst E, Dale E, Hammerschmidt MD, Bagge U, Matrai A, Dormandy J. Leukocytes and the risk of ischemic diseases. J Am Med Assoc 1987;257:2318–24.
19. Ostermann H, Van De Loo J. Factors of the haemostatic system in diabetic patients. Haemostasis 1986;16:386–416.
20. Davi' G, Catalano I, Averna M et al. Thromboxane biosynthesis and platelet function in diabetes mellitus. N. Engl J Med 1990;322:1769–74.
21. Kluft C, Potter Van Loon BJ, De Maat MPM. Insulin resistance and changes of haemostatic variables. Fibrinolysis 1992;6(Suppl.3):11–6.
22. Strano A, Novo S. Possibilities and limits of medical therapy in vascular atherosclerotic disease of the limbs. In: Carlson LA, Paoletti R, (eds), Proceedings of the International Conference on Atherosclerosis. New York: Raven Press, 1978:423–7.
23. Andreani D, Bell P, Bollinger A et al. (European Working Group on Critical Leg Ischemia). Second European Consensus Document on chronic critical leg ischemia. Circulation 1991;84:4(Suppl.):1–26.
24. Olsson AG, Ruhn G, Erikson U. The effect of serum lipid regulation and the development of femoral atherosclerosis in hyperlipidaemia: A non randomized controlled study. J Intern Med 1990;227:381–91.
25. Gaziano MJ, Hennekens H. Vitamin antioxidants and cardiovascular disease. Curr Op Lipidol 1992;3:291–4.
26. Zetterquist S. The effect of active training on the nutritive blood flow in exercising ischemic legs. Scand J Clin Lab Invest 1970;25:101–11.
27. Dahlhof AG, Holm J, Schersten T, Sivertssen R. Peripheral arterial insufficiency; effect of physical training on walking tolerance, calf blood flow and blood flow resistance. Scand J Rehab Med 1976;8:19–26.
28. Spitzer S, Bach R, Schieffer H. Walk training and drug treatment in patients with peripheral arterial occlusive disease stage II. A review. Inter Angio 1992;11:204–10.
29. Clifford PC, Davies PW, Hayne JA, Baird RN. Intermittent claudication: Is a supervised class worthwhile? Br Med J 1980;6:1505–6.
30. Maas U. Naftidrofuryl bei arterieller Verschlusskrankeit. Dtsch Med Wschr 1984;109:745–8.
31. Kiesewetter H, Jung F, Erdlenbruch W, Wenzel E. Haemodilution in patients with peripheral arterial occlusive disease. Int Angiol 1992;11:169–75.
32. Kiesewetter H, Jung F, Birk A, Spitzer S. Hypervolemic haemodilution with or without venesection in peripheral arterial occlusive disease stage II. Int Angiol 1994;13:1–4.
33. Brevetti G, Angelini C, Rosa M et al. Muscle carnitine deficiency in patients with severe peripheral vascular disease. Circulation 1991;84:1490–5.
34. Brevetti G, Perna S, Saba' C et al. Superiority of L-propionyl-carnitine versus L-carnitine in improving walking capacity in patients with peripheral arterial disease: An acute intravenous, double-blind, study. Eur Heart J 1992;13:251–5.
35. Brevetti G, Chiariello M, Furlano G et al. Increase in walking distance in patients with peripheral vascular disease treated with L-carnitine. Circulation 1988;77:767–73.
36. Pola P, Flore R, Tondi P, Nolfe G. Rheological activity of propionyl-L-carnitine Drugs. Exp Clin Res 1991;XVII:191–6.
37. Tonak J, Knecht H, Groitl H. Zur Behandlung von Durchblutungsstorungen mit Pentoxifillin. Med Wschr 1977;31:467–2.

38. Lindgard F, Jeines R, Bjorkman H. Conservative drug treatment in patients with moderately severe chronic occlusive peripheral arterial disease. Circulation 1989;80:1549–56.
39. Porter JM, Cutler BC, Lee BY. Pentoxifylline efficacy in the treatment of intermittent claudication: Multicenter controlled double-blind trial with objective assessment of chronic occlusive arterial disease patients. Am Heart J 1982;104:66–72.
40. Di Perri T, Carandente O, Vittoria A, Guerrini M, Messa GL. Studies on the clinical pharmacology and therapeutic efficacy of pentoxifylline in peripheral obstructive arterial disease of the lower limbs. Angiology 1984;35:427–35.
41. Ciuffetti G, Paltriccia R, Lombardini R, Lupattelli G, Pasqualini L, Mannarino M. Treating peripheral arterial occlusive disease: Pentoxifylline vs exercise. Int Angiol 1994;13:33–9.
42. Strano A, Davi' G, Avellone G, Novo S, Pinto A. Double-blind, cross-over study of the clinical efficacy and the haemorheological effects of pentoxiphylline in patients with occlusive arterial disease of the lower limbs. Angiology 1984;35:459–66.
43. Trubestein G. Buflomedil bei arterieller verschlubkrankheit. Ergebnisse einer kontrollierten studie. Dtsch Med Wschr 1982;107:1957–64.
44. Bissanti A. Blufomedil: Meta-analysis of clinical controlled trials. Basi Raz Ter 1993;XXIII(Suppl.4):1–6.
45. Clement D, Duprez D. Effects of ketanserin in the treatment of patients with intermittent claudication: Results from 13 placebo-controlled parallel group studies. J Cardiovasc Pharmacol 1987;10(Suppl.3):S89–95.
46. PACK Claudication Substudy Investigators. Randomized placebo-controlled, double-blind trial of ketanserin in claudicants: Changes in claudication distance and ankle systolic pressure. Circulation 1989;80:1544–8.
47. PACK Group. Prevention of atherosclerotic complications: Controlled trial of ketanserin. Br Med J 1989;298:424–30.
48. Lehert P, Comte S, Gamand S, Brown TM. Naftidrofuryl in intermittent claudication: A retrospective analysis. J Cardiovasc Pharmacol 1994;23(Suppl.3):S48–52.
49. Hessvh, Mietaschk A, Deichsel G. Drug-induced inhibition of platelet function delays progression of peripheral occlusive arterial disease. A prospective double-blind arteriography controlled trial. Lancet 1985;1:415–9.
50. Tonnesen KH, Albuquerque P, Baitsch G et al. Double-blind controlled multicenter study of indobufen versus placebo in patients with intermittent claudication. Int Angiol 1993;12:371–7.
51. Cloarec M, Caillard Ph, Mouren X. Double-blind clinical trial of ticlopidine versus placebo in peripheral atherosclerotic disease of the leg. Thromb Res 1986;160:316.
52. Novo S, Abrignani MG, Pavone G, Zamueli M, Pernice C, Geraci AM, Longo B, Caruso R, Strano A. Effects of captopril and ticlopidine, alone or in combination, in hypertensive patients with intermittent claudication. Int Angiol 1996; 15:169–74.
53. Balsano F, Coccheri S, Libretti A et al. Ticlopidine in the treatment of intermittent claudication: A 21-month double-blind trial J Lab Clin Med 1989;114:84–91.
54. Katsumura T, Mishima Y, Kamiya K, Sakaguchi S, Tanabe T, Sakuma A. Therapeutic effects of ticlopidine, a new inhibitor of platelet aggregation, on chronic arterial occlusive diseases, a double-blind study versus placebo. Angiology 1982;33:357–67.
55. Ferrari PA, Clerici G, Gussoni G, Nazzari M. Defibrotide versus placebo in the treatment of intermittent claudication. A meta-analysis. Drugs Invest 1994;7(3):157–60.
56. Allegra C, Carlizza A, Sardina M. Long-term effects of low dose calcium-heparin versus ASA in patients with peripheral arterial occlusive disease at IIb Leriche–Fontaine stage. Thromb Haemostasis 1993;69:401.
57. Andreozzi GM, Signorelli SS, Cacciaguerra G et al. Three-month therapy with calcium-heparin in comparison with ticlopidine in patients with peripheral arterial occlusive disease at Leriche–Fontaine IIb class. Angiology 1993;44:307–13.
58. Shepherd JT, Bergan JJ, Cohen RA et al. Report of the task force on vascular medicine. Circulation 1994;89:532–5.
59. Loosemore TM, Chalmers TC, Dormandy JA. A meta-analysis of randomized placebo controlled trials in Fontaine stages III and IV peripheral occlusive arterial disease. Int Angiol 1994;13:133–42.

60. Dormandy J, Mahir M, Ascadj G et al. Fate of the patient with chronic leg ischemia. J Cardiovasc Surg 1989;30(1):50–7.
61. Janzon L, Bergqvist D, Boberg J et al. Prevention of myocardial infarction and stroke in patients with intermittent claudication; effects of ticlopidine. Results from STIMS, the Swedish Ticlopidine Multicentre Study. J Intern Med 1990;227:301–8.
62. Blanchard J, Carreras LO, Kinderman M and the EMATAP Group. Results of EMATAP: A double-blind placebo-controlled multicentre trial of ticlopidine in patients with peripheral arterial disease. Nouv Rev Fr Hematol 1993;35:523–8.
63. Antiplatelet Trialist's Collaboration. Collaborative overview of randomized trials of antiplatelet therapy – I: Prevention of death, myocardial infarction and stroke by prolonged antiplatelet therapy in various categories of patients. Br Med J 1994;308:81–106.
64. Pentecost MJ, Criqui MH, Dorros G et al. Guidelines for peripheral percutaneous transluminal angioplasty of the abdominal aorta and lower extremity vessels. A statement for health professionals from a special writing group of the Council on Cardiovascular Radiology, Arteriosclerosis, Cardiothoracic and Vascular Surgery, Clinical Cardiology and Epidemiology and Prevention, the American Heart Association. Circulation 1994;89:511–5.
65. Morgenstern HR, Getrajdman GI, Laffey KJ, Bixon A, Martin EC. Total occlusion of the femoral popliteal artery: High technical success rate of conventional balloon angioplasty. Radiology 1989;172:937–40.
66. Krepel VM, van Andel GJ, van Erp WFM, Breslau PJ. Percutaneous transluminal angioplasty of the femoropopliteal artery: initial and long term results. Radiology 1985;156:325–8.
67. Gallino A, Mahler F, Probst P, Nacgbur B. Percutaneous transluminal angioplasty of the lower limbs – 5 years follow up. Circulation 1984;70:619–23.
68. Spence RK, Freiman DB, Gatenby R et al. Long term results of transluminal angioplasty of the iliac and femoral arteries. Arch Surg 1981;116:1377–86.
69. Belli AM, Knox AM, Procter AE, Welsh CL. The complication rate of percutaneous peripheral balloon angioplasty. Clin Radiol 1990;41:380–3.
70. Motarjeme A. Thrombolytic therapy in arterial occlusion and graft thrombosis. Semin Vasc Surg 1989;2:155–78.
71. Van Breda A, Katzen BT. Thrombolytic therapy of peripheral arterial disease. Semin Intervent Radiol 1985;2:354–66.
72. Beridge DC, Makin GS, Hopkinson BR. Local low dose intra-arterial thrombolytic therapy: The risk of stroke and major haemorrhage. Br J Surg 1989;76:1230–3.
73. Auster M, Kadir S, Mitchell SE et al. Iliac artery occlusion: Management with intrathrombus streptokinase infusion and angioplasty. Radiology 1984;153:385–8.
74. Moody P, Gould DA, Harris PL. Venous graft surveillance improves patency in femoro-popliteal bypass. Eur J Vasc Surg 1990;4:117–21.
75. Cumberland DC, Taylor DI, Welsh CL et al. Percutaneous laser thermal angioplasty: Initial clinical results with a laser probe in total peripheral arterial occlusions. Lancet 1986;1:1457–9.
76. Valbracht C, Liermann DD, Prignitz I et al. Low speed rotational angioplasty in chronic peripheral occlusions: Experience in 83 patients. Radiology 1989;172:327–30.
77. Michaels JA. Percutaneous arterial recanalization. Br J Surg 1990;77:373–9.
78. Wright JG, Belkin M, Greenfield AJ, Guben JK, Sanborn TA, Menzoian JO. Laser angioplasty for limb salvage: Observations on early results. J Vasc Surg 1989;10:29–38.
79. Hofling B, Backa D, Lauterjung L et al. Percutaneous removal of atheromatous plaques in peripheral arteries. Lancet 1988;1:384–6.
80. Rousseau HP, Raillat CR, Joffre FG, Knight CJ, Ginestet MC. Treatment of femoro-popliteal stenosis by means of self-expandable endoprostheses: Mid-term results. Radiology 1989;172:961–4.
81. Adar R, Critchfield GC, Eddy DM. A confidence profile analysis of the results of femoro-popliteal percutaneous transluminal angioplasty in the treatment of lower leg ischaemia. J Vasc Surg 1989;10:57–67.
82. Bell PFR. Indications for aortoiliac and aortofemoral bypass grafts for lower limb ischaemia. In: Greenhalg RM, (ed.), Indications in vascular surgery, Philadelphia: Saunders, 1988:189–213.
83. Rutherford RB, Jones DN, Bergentz SE et al. Factors affecting the patency of infrainguinal bypass. J Vasc Surg 1988;8:236–46.

84. Brewster DC, LaSalle AJ, Darling C. Comparison of above knee and belove knee anastomosis in femoropopliteal bypass grafts. Arch Surg 1981;116:1013–8.
85. Patel KC, Semel L, Clauss RH. Extended reconstruction rate for limb salvage with intraoperative pre-construction angiography. J Vasc Surg 1988;7:531–8.
86. Wiseman S, Kenchington F, Dain R et al. Influence of smoking and plasma factors on patency of femoro-popliteal vein graft. Br Med J 1989;299:643–7.
87. Wolfe JHN, Thomas ML, Jamieson CW, Browse NL, Brunald KG, Rutt DL. Early diagnosis of femorodistal graft stenoses. Br J Surg 187;74:268–70.
88. Cederberg PA, Pritchard DJ, Joyce JW. Doppler-determined segmental pressure and wound healing in amputations for vascular disease. J Bone Joint Surg 1983;65A:363–5.

23. Pathophysiology and clinical manifestations of diseases of the renal, celiac and mesenteric arteries

PAOLO FIORANI, FRANCESCO SPEZIALE, MARCO MASSUCCI, ENRICO SBARIGIA and MAURIZIO TAURINO

Renovascular occlusive disease

Renovascular occlusive disease is defined by Maxwell et al. [1] as 'the presence of one or more occlusive lesions in the main renal artery or in one or more of its main branches' and has two important clinical manifestations:

- renovascular hypertension, i.e. hypertension caused by renal artery disease, which can potentially be cured or improved with renal revascularization or nephrectomy; and
- renovascular renal insufficiency which can be defined as a renal insufficiency caused by a reduction of renal blood flow.

Incidence

In an autoptic study [2] of normotensive patients, renal artery occlusive disease was found in 49% of 256 patients. Other studies in which the patients were evaluated by angiography for different reasons (overall for concomitant aortic occlusive and aneurysmal disease) show a frequency rate of renal artery stenosis varying from 19 to 59% [3–10].

The main etiology of renovascular disease is atherosclerosis, accounting for 60–70% of cases, while fibromuscular dysplasia is responsible in 25–30% of cases [2, 11–14]. Many studies have confirmed how stenotic lesions of the renal artery follow a different course depending on whether they are atherosclerotic or dysplastic [11, 15–17].

Atherosclerosis in the renal arteries usually involves ostium and extends 1–2 cm into the renal artery with a typical tapering in the distal direction, and often with maximal narrowing within 1 cm from the aortic inner wall or atherosclerotic plaque overlay [2].

The natural history of these lesions has been well defined: Wollenweber et al. [11], reporting 30 patients followed for an average of 28 months, found that there was progression in 63% of cases; Meany et al. [15] reported progression of renal arterial stenosis in 36% of patients in a follow-up of 6 months to 10 years.

In a recent analysis by Tollefson and Ernst [16], 194 sequential aortograms were performed in 48 patients: the study shows a progression of disease in 44% of cases with a high risk of occlusion (22%) in stenoses of 75–99%.

In dysplastic-type stenoses, the evolution of lesions is less frequent, compared to atherosclerotic disease. The percentage of evolutive dysplastic stenoses is reported in literature as 16–33% [15, 17–18]. The evolution of stenosis into full obstruction is rare and is prevalently seen in subadventitial fibroplasty forms [19].

On the other hand the natural history of patients with atherosclerotic renal artery disease shows that progressive arterial obstruction occurs in patients treated medically, and renal function continues to deteriorate in approximately 40% of cases [20]. This occurs as result of the efficacy of the therapy in lowering the blood pressure [11, 15–16]. It is also well-known that drugs which inhibit the renin–angiotensin system cause a deterioration of renal function when there is a reduced renal perfusion in patients with bilateral lesions or renal artery stenosis in a solitary kidney [21].

Blood flow in a stenotic renal artery depends on systemic blood pressure, the degree of stenosis, poststenotic intrarenal perfusion pressure and vascular resistance. Clinical and experimental investigations have shown that the area of the renal artery must be reduced by 85% to result in a significant reduction of pressure and flow distal to the stenosis [22, 23].

Clinical manifestations

Renovascular occlusive disease may be found as an incidental anatomic lesion without functional significance. It may produce renovascular hypertension by activation of the renin–angiotensin–aldosterone system, and may lead to the progressive loss of excretory function, culminating in end-stage renal disease.

Renovascular hypertension

Renovascular hypertension is an uncommon but important cause of hypertension. Its prevalence is a source of debate because there has never been a suitable, simple screening test to document its presence. It is estimated that it may involve 5–10% of the hypertensive population [1, 12, 24–26].

Pathophysiology

Demonstration of the relationship between renal artery disease and blood pressure elevation, and the pathogenesis of renovascular hypertension is still source of debate. The kidney is an important site of blood pressure regulation because of its influence on circulating plasma volume as well as its activity in modulation of vasomotor tone. The pathophysiological process is complex but it has been demonstrated that renovascular hypertension is induced by the renin–angiotensin–aldosterone system. It is a complex feedback mechanism which participates in a wide variety of homeostatic processes and, under varying conditions, is able to maintain either a stable blood pressure or blood volume [27, 28].

Specialized smooth-muscle cells, richly innervated, located in the distal end of the afferent arterioles in juxtaposition to the renal glomerulus, are sensitive monitors of perfusion pressure. The reduction in intraarteriolar pressure stimulates the cells of the juxtaglomerular apparatus to release renin, a proteolytic enzyme, that has no physiological activity by itself. It acts as the starter of the renin–angiotensin sequence, interacts with angiotensinogen, an alpha-2 globulin manufactured in the liver, to produce angiotensin I, an inactive decapeptide, that is converted to the potent vasoconstrictor, angiotensin II, by a converting enzyme. Angiotensin II is an octapeptide, has a very short plasma half-life, and is rapidly inactivated by multiple enzymes in blood and tissues. Angiotensin II also increases blood pressure, in addition to its vasoconstrictor properties, through stimulation of aldosterone release from the zona glomerulosa of the adrenal cortex. This, in turn, increases plasma volume by increasing sodium and water resorption in the renal tubules. Blood pressure, plasma volume and plasma sodium content are therefore increased.

Another specialized group of cells located in the kidney, adjacent to the juxtaglomerular apparatus, the macula densa, acts as a sensor of sodium concentration in the distal tubules and thereby exerts a positive feedback mechanism on renin release. These mechanisms increase perfusion pressure to the juxtaglomerular cells; renin production and release is suppressed and blood pressure is modulated within a narrow range.

Goldblatt et al. [29] showed in 1934 that constriction of a renal artery in the dog produced a blood pressure increase. He postulated that this was due to production of renin by the ischemic kidney. After a few days, however, the renin level may return to normal despite persistence of the hypertension. Although the mechanism of the acute phase of hypertension following constriction of a renal artery is renin dependent, the mechanism of the continuing hypertension differs depending on the presence or absence of the contralateral kidney [30–31].

Two models of hypertension were described by Goldblatt et al. in the experimental animal [29].

The first is the 'two-kidney-one-clip model' in which one renal artery is constricted in the presence of a normal contralateral kidney; in this model there is an increased secretion of renin by the poststenotic kidney and a suppression of renin secretion from the opposite kidney. Sodium retention is minimal and so hypertension is essentially renin-dependent.

The second model is the 'one-kidney-one-clip model' in which renin secretion falls to normal but sodium is retained with consequent volume expansion. Therefore the hypertension is essentially volume-dependent.

Characteristics of renovascular hypertension

The most frequently quoted discriminating factors which suggest the presence of renovascular hypertension are: recent onset of hypertension; severity of hypertension, which is mainly diastolic; young age; lack of a family history of hypertension; and the presence of an abdominal bruit.

Renovascular renal insufficiency

The other pathological condition secondary to renovascular occlusive disease is renal insufficiency, ischemic renal dysfunction or ischemic nephropathy which usually occurs with severe hypertension.

Renovascular renal insufficiency is usually a progressive condition that may be symptom-free for a considerable time. The presence of stenosis of the renal artery is not predictable from either the existence of hypertension or from abdominal renal function [7].

The pathophysiology of the renal insufficiency is not well defined: in purely ishemic injuries the decreased supply of oxygen may result in impairment of the energy-dependent function of the cells. In metabolically active cells, such as tubular cells, energy sources are quickly depleted. As a result, the structural integrity of the cells may be broken [32]; this is however only one part of a complex pathophysiological process where, besides ischemia, hypertensive injuries, nephrosclerosis, microembolization etc. may play a very important role.

The incidence of renovascular disease as a cause of terminal renal insufficiency is reported to be around 16.5% [33]. The clinical presentation of patients with ischemic nephropathy can be classified, according to Weibull [33], as follows:

1. Acute renal failure precipitated by reduction in blood pressure, usually due to treatment with ACE-inhibitors in addition to antihypertensive therapy.
2. Progressive azotemia in patients with known renovascular hypertension which is pharmacologically controlled.
3. Progressive azotemia in elderly patients with refractory hypertension.
4. Unexplained progressive azotemia in elderly patients.
5. Repeated pulmonary edema, often more difficult to treat than usual, in elderly patients [34, 35].
6. history of flank-pain with or without hematuria in the presence of abdominal bruit in combination with hypertension and azotemia.

Clinical signs and symptoms which should lead to the suspicion of renovascular insufficiency are similar to those of renovascular hypertension in combination with impaired renal function. To prevent renovascular renal insufficiency it is important to take into consideration the progressive nature of atherosclerotic disease which causes total occlusion in a considerable percentage of cases.

The natural history of patients with atherosclerotic renal artery disease shows that progressive arterial obstruction occurs in patients treated medically and renal function continues to deteriorate in approximately 40% of cases. This occurs as a result of the efficacy of the therapy in lowering the blood pressure [20]. As previously mentioned, drugs which inhibit the renin–angiotensin system cause a deterioration of renal function when there is a reduced renal perfusion in patients with bilateral lesions or renal artery stenosis in a solitary kidney [21].

These observations have reinforced the importance of correction of the renal artery lesions to secure normal renal perfusion and preserve renal function. Therefore the indications for intervention in hypertensive patients have changed in recent years and the aim of surgical treatment is to provide a long-lasting normal kidney perfusion in order to preserve a renal function.

Mesenteric and celiac occlusive disease

Anatomical considerations

The blood supply to the intestine is provided by the celiac axis, superior mesenteric artery and inferior mesenteric artery; in the physiological state, over 90% of the splanchnic blood flow is provided by the celiac axis and the superior mesenteric artery.

The superior mesenteric artery provides blood to the small bowel and right half of the colon. The small bowel may derive a significant amount of its blood supply from the inferior mesenteric artery by way of the meandering mesenteric artery when there is complete or partial superior mesenteric arterial occlusion [36].

The meandering mesenteric artery is a large continuous communicating link between the left branch of the middle colic and the left colic arteries. The inferior mesenteric artery and its branches are connecting links between the superior mesenteric arterial and hypogastic arterial circulation.

This system is capable of great flexibility; in fact it is possible for the gut to survive without two and occasionally three of these vessels. This is possible because of the extensive collateral circulation that exists between them and because the other vessels that participate in the blood supply of the gut are capable of considerable increase when necessary.

Terminal branches of the gastroduodenal and superior pancreaticoduodenal arteries anastomose with branches of the inferior pancreaticoduodenal artery to provide the collateral pathway between the celiac axis and SMA.

Pathophysiology
The bowel is usually not affected by ischemic injury because of its abundant collateral circulation. Collateral pathways around occlusions of smaller mesenteric arterial branches are provided by the primary, secondary and tertiary arcades in the mesenters of the small bowel and the marginal arterial complex of Drummond in the mesocolon.

Inside the bowel wall itself, there is a network of communicating submucosal vessels which can maintain the viability of segments of the intestine in which the extramural arterial supply has been lost.

There is good clinical evidence that when gradual occlusions of the major mesenteric arteries occur, and in acute occlusions when mesenteric vasocostriction does not supervene, the collateral blood supply is normally adequate to maintain intestinal viability.

Occlusion of a major vessel results in the opening of collateral pathways in response to the fall in pressure distal to the obstruction. Increased blood flow through this collateral circulation continues as long as the pressure in the vascular bed distal to an obstruction remains below the systemic arterial pressure. When vasoconstriction develops in the distal bed, arterial pressure rises, which causes a narrowing of differential pressure, and a decrease in flow; if normal blood flow is reconstituted, flow through collateral channels ceases.

Low flow produces, initially, mesenteric vascular responses that try to maintain an adequate intestinal flow. If the reduced flow is prolonged, active vasoconstriction develops and may persist even after the correction of the primary cause of mesenteric ischemia. Therefore mesenteric vasoconstriction has an important role during an acute occlusive episode and for varying periods after correction of its cause.

The pathophysiology of the postprandial pain of mesenteric vascular origin is not yet well understood. Experimental evidence does suggest that mesenteric blood flow increases following food ingestion.

Acute intestinal ischemia

Reduction in visceral blood flow by one of several pathologic processes may produce the clinical syndrome of acute or chronic intestinal ischemia.

During the last years there has been increasing recognition of the importance and frequency of intestinal ischemia. Acute ischemia occurs in approximately 1 per 1000 admissions to major medical centers.

A generalized poor perfusion, as in shock or with a failing heart, or as a result of either local morphologic or functional changes can cause a reduction in blood flow to the intestine. Narrowing of the major mesenteric vessels, emboli of atheromatous material or blood clot, thromboses, vasculitis as part of a systemic disease, or mesenteric vasoconstriction can all lead to inadequate circulation at the cellular level. Whatever the cause, intestinal ischemia has the same results which vary from completely reversible functional alterations to total necrosis of portions or all of the bowel.

In spite of the great attention given to acute mesenteric ischemia, this condition still has a high mortality rate which is mainly due to failure to diagnose ischemia before intestinal gangrene occurs. A high index of suspicion is needed in patients who are fibrillating or who have evidence of arterial pathology elsewhere, and who present with acute symptoms in the abdomen.

Clinical presentation
Acute mesenteric ischemia develops mainly in patients with heart disease, longstanding congestive heart failure, cardiac arrhythmias, recent myocardial infarction, hypovolemia or hypotension. The development of abdominal pain in patients with one of these conditions should suggest the possibility of acute mesenteric ischemia. Abdominal pain is present in 75–98% of patients with intestinal ischemia, although it varies in severity, nature and location [37–41].

Patients affected by superior mesenteric artery thrombosis suffer from postprandial abdominal pain for several weeks or months before the acute episode. A characteristic early clinical feature of acute mesenteric ischemia is a disparity between the severity of the pain and the paucity of significant abdominal findings. The only indication of acute intestinal ischemia is sometimes unexplained abdominal distension or gastrointestinal bleeding. In the early course of an ischemic episode there are no abdominal findings, but, as infarction develops, increasing tenderness, rebound tenderness, and muscle guarding reflect the progressing intestinal changes. Nausea, vomiting, fever, rectal bleeding, hematemesis, intestinal obstruction, back pain, shock and increasing abdominal distension are other late signs.

Among the earliest findings are a neutrophilic leukocytosis above 15 000 cells/mm^3. An increase in hemoglobin concentration and hematocrit reflect the hemoconcentration produced by plasma loss into the gut. Metabolic acidosis supervenes. Hypoamylasemia is noted early after the onset of acute mesenteric vascular insufficiency; amylase levels later return to normal and then rise. Late in the course of mesenteric infarction, the enzymes LDH, SGOT, SGPT and creatine phosphokinase are markedly elevated.

Chronic intestinal ischemia

Clinical manifestation
The diagnosis of abdominal pain caused by mesenteric ischemia is difficult because the clinical presentation and physical findings are nonspecific. The patients always present a history of mid-abdominal or epigastric pain, usually severe, related to ingestion of food, and as the pain episodes increase in frequency and severity, the patient develops a food aversion resulting in weight loss, which is the most common physical finding. Physical findings are rarely diagnostic: nausea, vomiting, episodic diarrhea and bowel disturbance are often present.

Seventy-five percent of patients have an epigastric bruit, but this is a common finding and not a diagnostic abnormality. Laboratory studies are nonspecific, though occasionally there is occult blood in the stool. Both vague presentation and insidious progression of symptoms often mimic visceral malignancy or are mistaken for functional bowel disease.

Celiac band syndrome

The median arcuate ligament can sometimes compress the origin of the celiac artery and it has been suggested that this may be responsible for postprandial pain and weight loss [42, 43].

The syndrome of celiac axis compression was first described by Dunbar *et al.* [44]. Compression of the celiac artery by the diaphragmatic crura is a common abnormality that has been demonstrated on lateral angiography in 50% of asymptomatic subjects [45]. Compression at the origin of the vessel could rarely give rise to symptoms of intestinal ischemia when the other two vessels are lesions-free; the existence of the celiac artery compression syndrome is therefore in doubt.

Acute and chronic intestinal ischemia are clinical syndromes produced by the reduction of visceral blood flow by one of several pathologic processes. Acute intestinal ischemia remains a serious and often fatal problem because of the delayed diagnosis; chronic ischemia is uncommon and the presence of collateral pathways, and of nonspecific symptoms, renders the pathology unknown.

References

1. Maxwell MH, Bleifer KH, Franklin SS, Varady PD. Cooperative study of renovascular hypertension. Demographic analysis of the study. J Am Med Assoc 1972;220:1195–204.
2. Holley KE, Hunt JC, Brown AL Jr, Kincaid OW, Sheps SG. Renal artery stenosis: A clinical-pathologic study in normotensive and hypertensive patients. Am J Med 1964;37:14–22.
3. Eyler WR, Clark MD, Garman JE, Rian KL, Meininger DE. Angiography of the renal areas including a comparative study of renal artery stenosis in patients with and without hypertension. Radiology 1962;78:879–91.
4. Brewster DC, Retana A, Waltman AC, Darling RC. Angiography in the management of aneurysms of the abdominal aorta: Its value and safety. N Engl J Med 1975;292:822–5.
5. Brewster DC, Buth J, Darling RC. Combined aortic and renal artery reconstruction. Am J Surg 1976;131:457–63.
6. Bauer GM, Porter JM, Eidemiller LR. The role of arteriography in abdominal aortic aneurysm. Am J Surg 1978;136:184–9.
7. Choudhri AH, Cleland JGF, Rowlands PC, Tran TL, McCartey M, Al-Kuubi MAO. Unsuspected renal artery stenosis in peripheral vascular disease. Br Med J 1990;301:1197–8.
8. Olin JW, Melia M, Young JR. Prevalence of atherosclerotic renal artery stenosis in patients with atherosclerosis elsewhere. Am J Med 1990;88:46–51.
9. Barral X, Delorme JM, Favre JP, Farcot M, Berthoux F. Lesions arterielles renales et anevrysmes de l'aorte abdominale sous-renale. In: Les anevrysmes de l'aorte abdominale sous-renale. Paris: AERCV, 1990:337–48.
10. Speziale F, Massucci M, Giannoni MF et al. Stenoses des arteres renales et restauration aorto-iliaque. Faut-il faire un bilan extensif? J Mal Vasc 1994;19(Suppl.A):68–72.
11. Wallenweber J, Sheps SG, Davis GD. Clinical course of atherosclerotic renovascular disease. Am J Cardiol 1968;21:60–71.
12. Hunt JC, Strong CG. Renovascular hypertension: Mechanisms, natural history and treatment. In: Laragh JH, (ed.), Hypertension Manual. New York: Yorke, 1976:509–36.
13. Novick AC, Khauli RB, Vidt DG. Diminished operative risk and improved results following revascularization for atherosclerotic renovascular disease. Urol Clin North Am 1984;11:435–49.
14. Dean RH. Renovascular hypertension. Curr Probl Surg 1982;22:1–67.
15. Meany TF, Dustan HP, McCormack LJ. Natural history of renal artery disease. Radiology 1968;91:881–7.
16. Tollefson DFJ, Ernst CB. Natural history of atherosclerotic renal artery stenosis associated with aortic disease. J Vasc Surg 1991;14:327–31.
17. Schreiber MJ, Pohl MA, Novick AC. The natural history of atherosclerosis and fibrous renal artery disease. Urol Clin North Am 1984;11:383–92.
18. D'Addato M. La malattia renovascolare. G Ital Chir Vasc 1994;1:3–20.
19. Goncharenko V, Gerlock AJ, Shaff MI. Progression of renal artery fibromuscular dysplasia in 42 patients as seen on angiography. Radiology 1981;139:45–51.
20. Dean RH, Kieffer RW, Smith BM et al. Renovascular hypertension. Anatomic and renal function changes during drug therapy. Arch Surg 1981;116:1408–15.
21. Hricik DE, Browning PJ, Kopelman R, Goorno WE, Madias NE, Dzau VS. Captopril induced functional renal insufficiency in patients with bilateral stenosis or renal artery stenosis in a solitary kidney. N Engl J Med 1983;373:308–11.
22. Haimovici H, Zinicola N. Experimental renal artery stenosis. Diagnostic significance of arterial hemodynamics. J Cardiovasc Surg 1962;3:259–62.
23. Bjorno L, Pettersson H. Hydro- and haemodynamic effects of catheterization of vessels. V. Experimental and clinical catheterization of stenoses. Acta Radiol (Diagn) 1977;18(2):193–209.

24. Bookstein JJ, Abrams HL, Buerger RE. Radiologic aspects of renovascular hypertension. Part 2. The role of urography in unilateral renovascular disease. J Am Med Assoc 1972;220:1225–31.
25. Gifford RW Jr. Epidemiology and clinical manifestation of renovascular hypertension. In: Stanley JC, Ernst CB, Fry WJ, Renovascular hypertension. Philadelphia: Saunders, 1984:77–99.
26. Dean RH. Management of renovascular hypertension due to atherosclerosis. In: Rutherford R (ed.), Vascular surgery. Philadelphia: Saunders, 1989:1245–53.
27. Freeman RH, Davis JO. The control of renal secretion and metabolism: In: Genest *et al* (eds), Hypertension: physiopathology and treatment. New York: McGraw-Hill, 1977:210–40.
28. Vander AJ. Renin–angiotensin system. In: Stanley JC, Ernst CB, Fry WJ (eds), Renovascular hypertension. Philadelphia: Saunders, 1984:20–45.
29. Goldblatt H, Lynch J, Hanzal RF, Summerville WW. Studies on experimental hypertension. I. The production of persistent elevation of systolic blood-pressure by means of renal ischemia. J Exp Med 1934;59:347.
30. Pickering TG, Laragh JH, Sos TA. Renovascular hypertension. In: Schrier RW, Gottscholk CW (eds), Disease of the kidney. Boston: Little Brown, 1987:1597.
31. Hoobler SW. History of experimental renovascular hypertension. In: Stanley JC, Ernst CB, Fry WJ. Renovascular hypertension. Philadelphia: Saunders, 1984:12–20.
32. Smolens P, Stein JH. Pathophysiology of acute renal failure. Am J Med 1981;70:479–82.
33. Weibull H. Renovascular occlusive disease: Aspects of reconstructive options. Malmoe, 1992.
34. Bengtsson U, Bergentz SE, Norback B. Surgical treatment of renal artery stenosis with impending uremia. Clin Nephrol 1974;2:222–9.
35. Hansen KJ, Dean RH. Renal revascularization in the azotemic patient: Diagnostic and therapeutic implications. In: Veith FJ (ed.), Current critical problems in vascular surgery. St Louis; UMP, 1990:197–203.
36. Moskowitz M, Zimmerman H, Felson B. The meandering mesenteric artery of the colon. Am J Roentgenol 1964;92:1088.
37. Boley SJ, Borden EB. Acute mesenteric vascular disease In: Wilson SE, Veith FJ, Hobson RW, Williams RA (eds), Vascular surgery: principles and practice. McGraw-Hill, 1987:659–71.
38. Stoney RJ, Wylie EJ. Recognition and surgical management of visceral ischemia syndromes. Ann Surg 1966;164:174.
39. Stoney RJ, Wylie EJ. Surgery of celiac and mesenteric arteries. In: Halmovici H (ed.), Vascular surgery: principles and techniques (2nd edition). New York: McGraw-Hill, 1976:668–79.
40. Hertzer NR, Beven EG, Humphries AW. Chronic intestinal ischemia. Surg Gynecol Obstet 1977;145:321.
41. Stoney RJ, Reilly LM, Ehrenfeld WK. Chronic mesenteric ischemia and surgery for chronic visceral ischemia. In: Wilson SE, Veith FJ, Hobson RW, Williams RA (eds), Vascular surgery: principles and practice. McGraw-Hill, 1987:672–84.
42. Lord R, Tracy GD. Coelic artery compression. Br J Surg 1980;67(8):590–3.
43. Stanley JC, Fry WJ. Median arcuate ligament syndrome. Arch Surg 1971;103:252–8.
44. Dunbar JD, Molnar N, Beman FF, Maradle SH. Compression of the celiac trunk and abdominal angina: Preliminary report of 15 cases. Am J Roentgenol Radium Ther Nucl Med 1965;95:731–6.
45. Szilagyi DE, RiAn RL, Elliott JP, Smith RF. The coeliac artery compression syndrome: Does it exist? Surgery 1972;72:849–63.

24. Management of diseases of the renal, celiac and mesenteric arteries

PAOLO FIORANI, FRANCESCO SPEZIALE, MARCO MASSUCCI, LUIGI RIZZO and ALVARO ZACCARIA

Renovascular occlusive disease has two important clinical manifestations:

- *renovascular hypertension*, i.e. hypertension caused by renal artery disease, which can potentially be cured or improved with renal revascularization or nephrectomy; and
- *renovascular renal insufficiency* which can be defined as a renal insufficiency caused by a reduction of renal blood flow.

It is essential to distinguish the problem of hypertension from that of renal function.

Evaluation of renovascular hypertension

There are three main issues in the management of renovascular hypertension (RVH):

1. Detection of patients in the population of hypertensive patients.
2. Selection of patients with renal artery stenosis who will benefit from revascularization.
3. Choice of either percutaneous transluminal angioplasty (PTA) or surgery of the renal artery.

A number of screening diagnostic studies have been advocated for recognition of the patient with RVH: these have included plasma renin determination, rapid sequence intravenous pyelogram, isotope renography, renal duplex echography and renal arteriography.

Plasma renin determination

As the pathophysiology of renovascular hypertension is considered to be due to an increased renin output in the presence of a decreased renal arterial perfusion, it would seem that renin measurements should be valuable in establishing the diagnosis of renovascular hypertension; the relationship between renin activity elevation and hypertension is not however a simple one.

Currently, renin determination is performed in one of three ways:

1. peripheral plasma renin activity (PRA);
2. renal vein renin ratio (RVRR); and
3. renal vein renin/systemic renin index (RSRI).

Peripheral plasma renin levels are often normal and a literature review reported a 44% incidence of elevated PRA among RVH patients [1]. Determination of baseline peripheral vein renin is influenced by several circumstances such as upright position, antihypertensive drugs, sodium depletion etc. [2]. These observations suggest that peripheral PRA measurement is a poor diagnostic test for RVH.

A second approach to the use of renin measurements is the determination of (RVRR), comparing the ischemic with the normal kidney. Currently a ratio exceeding 1.5:1 is considered positive. The cure rate of patients with a positive test approaches 95%, but the false negative rate is high, ranging from 21 to 57% [3–5]. Stanley's group [6] has found the RSRI to be a more reliable prognosticator of operative response. The ischemic kidney RSRI was significantly greater than the contralateral kidney RSRI in both cured and improved patient groups but it was the degree of contralateral suppression of renin production that discriminated between patients who were subsequently cured and those who were only improved by revascularization.

The role of renin measurement in the evolution of renal ischemia can be summarized as follows: in unilateral disease when there is an elevated peripheral PRA, contralateral suppression of renin production, and lateralization of increased renin production to the ischemic kidney (RVRR > 1.5:1 or RSRI > 0.48) there is a reasonable likelihood that renovascular hypertension is present and the beneficial response from revascularization is probable.

Combining test modalities increases the sensitivity, but does not eliminate false negative results. Bilateral disease significantly reduces the diagnostic accuracy and prognostic reliability of all modalities.

Intravenous urogram

The rapid sequence intravenous urogram is the classic method of screening for renovascular hypertension. It was proposed in the early 1960s as a test to detect clinically significant renal artery stenosis [7]. The characteristic features are: a delayed excretion of dye in the 1- and 2-minute films; a difference in kidney size; delay and hyperconcentration in caliceal filling; a weak nephrogram; and ureteral notching due to collateral blood supply along the ureteric artery. A literature review shows a sensitivity of 75% and specificity of 86% [8].

Radionucleotide renography/scintigraphy

Isotopic renal blood flow has been considered as a noninvasive means of diagnosis of renovascular hypertension [9, 10]. The classic renogram, based on ^{131}I-labeled

Hippuran excretion, is no more accurate than intravenous urography with a high level of false negative results. The use of ^{99m}Tc-labeled dimercaptosuccinic acid (^{99m}Tc-DMSA) and ^{99m}Tc-labeled diethyltriaminepentaacetic acid (^{99m}Tc-DTPA) scans with computed analysis of the uptake and excretion of the isotope has increased the accuracy of this investigation considerably; Hippuran is a marker for plasma flow, DMSA a marker for parenchymal function with an unknown mechanism, and DTPA is a marker for glomerular filtration rate. Using these substances in combination with captopril and with diuretic enhancement, sensitivities and specificities of over 90% have been obtained in significant unilateral stenosis [11–13]. Angiotensin-converting enzyme (ACE) inhibition improves the sensitivity of renography and scintigraphy for unilateral renal artery stenosis [14].

Renal sonography and renal duplex Doppler sonography

Renal ultrasound examinations only provide anatomical information, such as whether the patient has one or two kidneys, the size of the kidney, differences in size, and alteration of the cortico-medullary index.

Renal duplex sonography is under development: diagnosis of renal artery stenosis depends on the velocity changes detected along the course of the renal arteries; Taylor et al. [15] report a sensitivity of 84% and a specificity of 97% for detection of a stenosis higher than 60%.

Renal angiography

Aortorenal angiography continues to be the definitive study in the evolution of renovascular disease: it is the preferred diagnostic method for evaluation of the anatomy of the renal circulation, as well as the extent of the disease and its morphologic characteristics. Two methods of angiography are usually utilized: conventional arteriography and intra-arterial digital subtraction renal angiography.

The disadvantages of arteriography are twofold. It is an invasive test requiring, in the case of conventional arteriography, hospitalization, and exposes patients to the risks of arterial catheterization and contrast-related complications. Moreover it diagnoses renovascular disease and not renovascular hypertension. The overall complication rate is however low: 0.06–0.11% mortality and 0.2–0.9% major complications [16]; complications due to the contrast medium occur with a frequency of 1–40% [17–19].

Treatment of renovascular disease

The objectives in management of diseases of the renal artery are to control blood pressure and prevent the progressive deterioration of renal function.

Pharmacological treatment, since the advent of new drugs, namely converting enzyme inhibitors, is effective in lowering blood pressure; but preoperative studies show that hypertensive patients with renal arterial occlusive disease medically treated will progress toward an arterial occlusion while renal function continues to deteriorate, in many cases despite the effectiveness of the antihypertensive therapy [20]. These observations stress the importance of renal revascularization in lowering blood pressure and preserving renal function [21, 22].

However in recent years percutaneous transluminal angioplasty (PTA) has been proposed as the technique of choice and effective method of treatment for renal revascularization [23–30], thus again questioning the role of surgery in hypertensive patients.

Pharmacological therapy

During the 1970s several studies reported disappointing results from the treatment of renovascular hypertension with various types of antihypertensive drugs [31–34]. These results were reconsidered when captopril, an ACE inhibitor, was introduced [35–38]. Use of this drug has improved the hypertension in 75% of patients with renovascular hypertension without azotemia [38]. There is a risk of acute renal failure during use of ACE inhibitors, and Hollenberg [38] reported that it occurred in 6% of cases. In a large percentage of cases, however, despite the effectiveness of the pharmacological therapy, renal function continues to deteriorate and the renal artery stenosis progresses toward occlusion [20].

Surgical therapy

The choice of surgery must be tailored according to the site of the lesion, its etiopathogenesis, the presence of associated aortoiliac lesions, renal function, and the condition of the patient.

A variety of operative techniques have been used to correct renal artery stenosis. From a practical standpoint, two basic operations have been most frequently utilized: aortorenal bypass and thromboendarterectomy. With regard to aortorenal bypass, various possibilities exist to use venous, arterial or synthetic grafts which adapt well to both technical requirements and those of the surgeon.

Termino-lateral aortic anastomosis is generally used on the antero-lateral wall of the aorta after longitudinal aortotomy; the anastomosis between the graft and the renal artery is performed using a termino-terminal type suture since this technique is hemodynamically effective.

When the infrarenal aorta cannot be used for proximal anastomosis because it is involved in atherosclerotic or inflammatory disease, an alternative site for proximal anastomosis is the supraceliac aorta which is generally free from atherosclerotic lesions [39]. Other authors prefer to perform extra-anatomical renal revascularization in the presence of an aorta with widespread atherosclerotic lesions and in high-risk patients. A popular technique is iliorenal bypass [40]. Splenorenal bypass for left renal revascularization [41, 42] and hepatorenal bypass for right renal revascularization [43] represent the most commonly used alternative methods.

When concomitant lesions of the aorta and renal artery exist, the indication for simultaneous surgery is still controversial. The increased morbidity and mortality reported in combined surgery, owing to the more complex nature of the operation [44–46], may underlie the nonaggressive approach adopted to aortoiliac lesions. Because of the high surgical risk, some authors have proposed the use of concomitant treatment only for aneurysmatic lesions or in symptomatic aortoiliac obstructive disease [39]. Some recent studies report a gradual but progressive reduction in the mortality rate that, at present, is 2–12% [45, 46].

Results of surgery
Renal revascularization may provide satisfactory long-term relief or improvement of hypertension in 80% of patients over follow-up of 48 months [47] with minimum mortality and morbidity rates [41, 45, 47–51]. This is obtained more frequently in patients with dysplastic lesions, while in patients with atherosclerotic disease the likelihood of good results decreases according to how widespread are the arterial lesions [52]. These different results of surgery may be related to a long-lasting previous mild hypertension frequently seen in atherosclerotic patients [53] which may cause diffuse arteriolar lesions or lesions in the contralateral kidney, which prevent relief of hypertension after revascularization. These data are confirmed by the observation that good long-term results are in proportion to the shortness of duration of the hypertension and also, the more immediate is the normotensive response to the renal revascularization, the longer this result will be maintained. However, these arteriolar lesions are not a contraindication to renal artery revascularization, because the passage from a state of severe hypertension, difficult to control by medical therapy, to a less hypertensive state, easily controlled by minimal doses of hypotensive drugs [47, 54] is still feasible.

The overall operative mortality ranges between 2 and 6.1% in patients with atherosclerotic lesions [47, 51, 54]. The long-term improvement or relief of hypertension can reduce the late mortality which was related in many cases to cardiovascular complications. In fact, the survival curve of patients operated on with success shows a better survival probability after five and ten years, than in patients remaining hypertensive and who did not benefit from operation [47].

These data suggest renal revascularization is a safe procedure, able to reduce arterial hypertension and preserve renal function, providing the patency is long lasting. The patency rate of renal revascularization in the immediate perioperative period is around 97% [47]. The overall late patency rate is around 95% [47, 51] when directly evaluated by angiography or indirectly tested by repeated clinical examinations of normotension associated with normal response of renal functional studies [55].

Percutaneous transluminal angioplasty

After the introduction of renal artery transluminal angioplasty by Gruntzig [23], this method has been proposed by many authors as the treatment of choice for renal artery lesions [24–29]. In addition to the successful results obtained, the advantages of the method, which account for its widespread use, also include the possibility of avoiding surgery, a short period of hospitalization and the possibility of repeating the procedure if necessary.

Several studies have been reported but the results of percutaneous transluminal angioplasty (PTA) are difficult to compare due to the varying parameters of evaluation such as percentage of stenosis, type of lesion, localization, clinical response to arterial hypertension, renal function, and follow-up.

Selection criteria for patients undergoing PTA vary considerably. Indications for PTA are dysplastic lesions uncomplicated by lesions of segmentary branches or anastomotic lesions, and unilateral non-ostial lesions.

Results of renal PTA
The results obtained with PTA in cases of dysplastic lesions seem to be equal to those obtained with surgical revascularization [16, 28, 29] with a positive outcome in 76% and 98% of cases, measured by technical or functional results.

The role of PTA in atherosclerotic lesions, especially in ostial localization, is controversial. Successful results have been reported in 34–94% [16, 26–28, 56, 57] and, with regard to the localization of lesions, the success rate, in the case of ostial localization, is approximately 30% [16, 51, 58]. With regard to the results of renal PTA on renal function, a positive outcome was reported in 65–85% of cases of non-ostial lesions [58, 59].

This procedure is not without complications, varying between 1 and 10%: dissection of the intima, embolization, perforation, rupture and thrombotic occlusion of the renal artery [58] have been reported. Restenosis following PTA has been reported with an incidence of 5–8% [56]; it usually occurs within one year of PTA [27] and some authors report levels as high as 22% [60].

Investigations in mesenteric ischemia and surgical revascularization

Detection of mesenteric arterial insufficiency is clinically difficult and diagnosis requires angiography. In recent years advances in duplex scanning have made this method an ideal technique for noninvasive screening of patients for chronic mesenteric arterial occlusive disease, with a 96% accurate for predicting a greater than 70% superior mesenteric artery and celiac axis stenosis [61].

The definitive investigation of chronic mesenteric ischemia is angiography with selective views of the visceral vessels. For symptomatic patients the indications for surgical revascularization are influenced by the extent of disease, the severity of symptoms and the patient's general condition.

There are three basic procedures for visceral revascularization:

1. Reimplantation, which consists of transection of the artery distal to the orifice lesion and reimplantation of the normal vessel into an adjacent segment of aorta.
2. Bypass with autogenous tissue or prosthetic graft constructed for retrograde flow, running cephalad from the ventral surface of the infrarenal aorta to the

side of the superior mesenteric artery distal to the diseased area, or anterograde flow with grafting from the undiseased supraceliac aorta to the visceral branch.
3. Endarterectomy, which is advantageous because it is entirely autogenous and anatomic; but the extensive nature of dissection restricts its use to patients with a good prognosis.

Acute intestinal ischemia is a serious, often fatal problem because it is usually diagnosed too late. Laparotomy is indicated during the course of acute mesenteric ischemia, either to restore intestinal flow, after an embolus or thrombosis, or to resect damaged bowel, but the mortality rate is 70–90% [62].

References

1. Marks LS, Maxwell MH. Renal vein renin value and limitations in the prediction of operative results. Urol Clin N Am 1975;2:311.
2. Wise KL, McCann RL, Dunnick NR, Paulsson DF. Renovascular hypertension. J Urol 1988;140:911–24.
3. Russell RP. Renal hypertension. Surg Clin N Am 1974;54:349.
4. Dean RH, Foster JH. Criteria for the diagnosis of renovascular hypertension. Surgery 1973;74:926.
5. Marks LS, Maxwell MH, Varady PD, Lupu AN, Kaufman JJ. Renovascular hypertension: Does the renal vein renin ratio predict operative results? J Urol 1976;115:365–8.
6. Stanley JC, Gewertz BL, Fry WJ. Renal systemic renin indices and renal vein renin ratios as prognostic indicators in remedial renovascular hypertension. J Surg Res 1976;20:149.
7. Maxwell MH, Gonick HC, Wittar V, Kantman JJ. Use of the rapid sequence intravenous pyelogram in the diagnosis of renovascular hypertension. N Engl J Med 1964;270:213–20.
8. Havey RJ, Krumlovsky F, Del Greco F, Martin HG. Screening for renovascular hypertension: Is renal digital subtraction angiography the preferred noninvasive test? J Am Med Assoc 1985;254:388–93.
9. Maxwell MH, Lupu AN, Viskoper RJ, Aravena LA, Waks VA. Mechanisms of hypertension during acute and immediate phases of the one-clip, two-kidney models in dogs. Circ Res 1977;40:24–8.
10. Velchik MG. Radionucleotide imaging of the urinary tract. Urol Clin N Am 1985;12:603–31.
11. Sfakianakis GN, Bourgoignie JJ, Jaffe D, Kyriakides G, Perez-Stable E, Duncan RC: Single-dose captopril scintigraphy in the diagnosis of renovascular hypertension. J Nucl Med 1987;28:1383–92.
12. Fommei E, Ghione S, Palla L et al. Renal scintigraphic captopril test in the diagnosis of renovascular hypertension. Hypertension 1987;10:21:2–20.
13. Geyskes GG, Oei HY, Puylaert CB, Mees EJ. Renovascular hypertension identified by captopril-induced changes in the renogram. Hypertension 1987;9:451–8.
14. Setaro JF, Saddler MC, Chen CC et al. Simplified captopril renography in diagnosis and treatment of renal artery stenosis. Hypertension 1991;18:289–98.
15. Taylor DC, Ketier MD, Moneta GL et al. Duplex ultrasound scanning in the diagnosis of renal artery stenosis: A prospective evaluation. J Vasc Surg 1988;7:363–9.
16. Weibull H. Renovascular occlusive disease: Aspects of reconstructive options. Malmo: Hyppomed AB, 1992.
17. Schwartz RD, Rubin JE, Leeming BV, Silvia P. Renal failure following angiography. Am J Med 1978;65:31–7.
18. Mason RA, Arbeit AL, Giron S. Renal dysfunction after arteriography. J Am Med Assoc 1985;253:1000–4.
19. Jacobson HR. Ischemic renal disease: An overlooked clinical entity? Kidney Int 1988;34:729–43.
20. Dean RH, Kleffer RW, Smith BM et al. Renovascular hypertension. Anatomic and renal function changes during drug therapy. Arch Surg 1981;116:1408–15.

21. Dean RH. The effect of renal revascularization on kidney function. J Surg Res 1977;22:443–7.
22. Sicard GA, Etheredge EE, Maeser MN, Anderson CB. Improved renal function after renal artery revascularization. J Cardiovasc Surg 1985;26:157–62.
23. Gruntzig A, Vetter W, Meier B, Kuhlmann U, Lutolf U, Siegenthaler W. Treatment of renovascular hypertension with transluminal dilatation of a renal artery stenosis. Lancet 1978;1:801–2.
24. Katzen BT, Chang J, Knox WJ. Percutaneous transluminal angioplasty with the Gruntzig balloon catheter. A review of 70 cases. Arch Surg 1979;114:1389–93.
25. Grim CE, Yune HY, Donohue JP, Weimberger MH, Dilley R, Klatte EC. Renal vascular hypertension. Surgery vs dilatation. Nephron 1986;44(Suppl.1):96–100.
26. Cicuto KP, McLean GK, Oleaga JA, Freiman DB, Grossman RA, Ring EJ. Renal artery stenosis. Anatomic classification for percutaneous transluminal angioplasty. Am J Roentgenol 1981;137:599–601.
27. Colapinto RF, Stronell RD, Harries-Jones EP. Percutaneous transluminal dilatation of the renal artery. Follow-up studies on renovascular hypertension. Am J Roentgenol 1982;139:727–32.
28. Council on Scientific Affairs. Percutaneous transluminal angioplasty. J Am Med Assoc 1984;251:764–8.
29. Flechner SM. Percutaneous transluminal dilatation. A realistic appraisal in patient with stenosing lesions of the renal artery. Urol Clin N Am 1984;11:515–27.
30. Melki JP, Riche MC, Dutemple C et al. Traitement des stenose de l'artere renale par angioplastic transluminale percutanee. A propos de 106 observations. VI Congres SALF, Lyon, 10–12 October 1986.
31. Owen K. Results of surgical treatment in comparison with medical treatment of renovascular hypertension. Cli Sci Mol Med 1973;45(Suppl. 1):95–8.
32. Buhler FR, Laragh JH, Vaughan ED. The antihypertensive action of propranolol. Specific antirenin responses in high and normal renin forms of essential, renal renovascular and malignant hypertension. In: Laragh JH (ed.), Hypertension manual. New York: Yorke, 1973;873–98.
33. Hunt JC, Strong CG. Renovascular hypertension: Mechanisms, natural history and treatment. In: Laragh JH (ed.), Hypertension manual. New York: Yorke, 1976;509–36.
34. Streeten DHP, Anderson GH. Outpatient experience with saralasin. Kidney Int 1979;15:44–52.
35. Rubin B, Laffan RJ, Kotler DG, O'Keefe EH, Demaio DA, Goldberg ME: SQ 14,255 (D-3-mercapto-2-methylpropanoyl-1-proline), a novel orally active inhibitor of angiotensin l-converting enzyme. J Pharmacol Exp Ther 1978;204:271–80.
36. Case DB, Lynch J, Hanzal RF. Clinical experience with blockade of the renin–angiotensin–aldosterone system by oral enzyme inhibitor (SQ 14,255, captopril) in hypertensive patients. Prog Cardiovasc Dis 1978;21:195–206.
37. Zweifler AJ, Julius S. Medical treatment of renovascular hypertension. In: Stanley JC, Ernst CB, Fry WJ (eds), Renovascular hypertension. Philadelphia: Saunders, 1984:231–53.
38. Hollenberg NK. Medical therapy for renovascular hypertension: A review. Am J Hypertens 1988;1:338–43.
39. Novick AC, Stewart R. Use of the thoracic aorta for renal revascularization. J Urol 1990;143:77–9.
40. Bergentz SE, Berquist H. Optimal reconstruction of the renal arteries. Acta Chir Scand 1990;555:227–35.
41. Brewster DC, Darling RC. Splenorenal arterial anastomosis for renovascular hypertension. Ann Surg 1979;189:353–8.
42. Kauli R, Novick AC, Ziegelbaum W. Splenorenal bypass in the treatment of renal artery stenosis: Experience with 69 cases. J Vasc Surg 1985;2:547–51.
43. Chibaro EA, Libertino JA. Use of hepatic circulation for renal revascularization. Ann Surg 1984;199:406–11.
44. Franklin SS, Young JD, Maxwell MH et al. Operative morbidity and mortality in renovascular disease. J Am Med Assoc 1975;231:1148–53.
45. Brewster DC, Buth J, Darling RC, Austen WG. Combined aortic and renal artery reconstruction. Am J Surg 1976;131:457–63.
46. Speziale F, Massucci M, Giannoni MF et al. Stenoses des arteres renales et restauration aortoiliaque: faut-il faire un bilan extensif? J Mal Vasc 1994;19(Suppl. A):68–72.

47. Fiorani P, Faraglia V, Aissa N et al. Late results of reconstructive surgery for renovascular hypertension. Int Angiol 1989;8:81–91.
48. Meaney TF, Dustan HP, McCormack LJ. Natural history of renal arterial disease. Radiology 1968;9:877–87.
49. Perona PG, Baker WH, Fresco R, Hano JE: Successful revascularization of an occluded renal artery after prolonged anuria. J Vasc Surg 1989;9:917–21.
50. D'Addato M, Mirelli M. Pontages aorto-renaux. In: Kieffer E (ed.), Chirurgie des arteres renales. Paris: AERCV, 1993:155–67.
51. D'Addato M. La malattia renovascolare. G Ital Chir Vasc 1994;1:3–20.
52. Fry RH, Fry WJ. Renovascular hypertension in the patients with severe atherosclerosis. Arch Surg 1982;117:938–42.
53. Dean RH. What is new in renal revascularization? In: Greenhalgh RM, Jamieson CW, Nicolaides AN (eds), Vascular surgery: Issues in current practice. 1986.
54. Hallet JW, Fowl R, O'Brien PC et al. Renovascular operations in patients with chronic renal insufficiency: Do the benefits justify the risk? J Vaso Surg 1987;5:622–7.
55. Cox DR. Regression models and life tables. J R Stat Soc 1972;34:187–220.
56. Tegtmeyer CJ, Kellum CD, Ayers C. Percutaneous transluminal angioplasty of the renal artery. Results and long-term follow-up. Radiology 1984;153:77–84.
57. Canzanello VJ, Millan VG, Spiegel JE, Ponce SP, Kopelman RI, Madias NE. Percutaneous transluminal renal angioplasty in management of atherosclerotic renovascular hypertension: results in 100 patients. Hypertension 1989;13:163–72.
58. Sos TA, Pickering PG, Snidermann KW et al. Percutaneous transluminal renal angioplasty in renovascular hypertension due to atheroma of fibrous dysplasia. N Engl J Med 1983;309:274–9.
59. O'Donovan RM, Guterres OH, Izzo JL. Preservation of renal function by percutaneous renal angioplasty in high-risk elderly patients: short-term outcome. Nephron 1992;60:187–92.
60. Schwarten DE. Percutaneous transluminal angioplasty of the renal arteries: Intravenous digital subtraction angiography for follow-up. Radiology 1984;150:369–73.
61. Harward JRS, Smith S, Seeger JM. Detection of celiac axis and superior mesenteric artery occlusive disease with use of abdominal duplex scanning. J Vasc Surg 1993;17:738–45.
62. Boley SJ, Borden ED. Acute mesenteric vascular disease. In: Wilson SE, Veith FJ, Hobson RW, Williams RA (eds), Vascular surgery, principles and practice. New York: McGraw-Hill, 1987:659–71.

25. Classification, epidemiology, risk factors, and clinical manifestations of hypertension

LUIGI COREA and MAURIZIO BENTIVOGLIO

Introduction

A wide range of blood pressure values is found among populations, and their distribution has no natural break separating normal from abnormal values. Therefore the definition of hypertension is empirical.

Several prospective studies have shown that the risk of cardiovascular morbidity and mortality increases with the level of blood pressure throughout the entire range of pressures found. A review of the observational studies shows a continous relation between a wide range (even within the 'normal' range) of diastolic blood pressure values (particularly when corrected for the regression dilution bias) and cardiovascular morbidity and mortality [1]. Therefore 'normality' in the sense of freedom from risk has no meaning in relation to blood pressure, and the border between 'normotension' and 'hypertension' is arbitrary. As a consequence, those blood pressure levels whose treatment reduces the cardiovascular risk for the patient have been considered 'hypertensive levels' [2].

However, the cardiovascular risk for the patient also depends on other conditions, which include age, sex, race, family history of premature coronary heart disease or stroke, smoking, left ventricular hypertrophy, dyslipidemia, diabetes mellitus, patient history or symptoms of cardiovascular, cerebrovascular or renal disease, microalbuminuria, obesity, and sedentary life. In clinical practice, these conditions do not modify the diagnosis of arterial hypertension, but do influence the therapeutic approach.

According to the WHO–ISH memorandum, systolic blood pressure values < 140 mmHg and diastolic blood pressure values < 90 mmHg define 'normotension', whereas ≥ 140 mmHg and/or ≥ 90 mmHg are in the 'hypertensive' range [3].

Classification of arterial hypertension

According to WHO–ISH, arterial hypertension is classified as: mild hypertension – diastolic blood pressure (DBP) between 90 and 104 mmHg (in the subgroup 'borderline hypertension', DBP values range between 90 and 95 mmHg); moderate hypertension – DBP values between 105 and 114 mmHg; severe hypertension – DBP values ≥ 115 mmHg.

With regard to systolic blood pressure (SBP), values between 140 and 180 mmHg define mild hypertension (in the subgroup 'borderline hypertension', SBP values range between 140 and 160 mmHg); values ≥ 180 mmHg define moderate or severe hypertension.

With DBP levels < 90 mmHg, SBP levels between 140 and 160 mmHg are in the 'systolic borderline hypertension' range, while SBP values ≥ 160 mmHg define 'isolated systolic hypertension', as detailed in Table 25.1 [3].

The Joint National Committee on Detection, Evaluation and Treatment of High Blood Pressure, however, classified blood pressure values as 'normal', 'high normal' and stage 1 (mild) hypertension, stage 2 (moderate), stage 3 (severe) and stage 4 (very severe hypertension) [4]. This classification is given in Table 25.2.

In the WHO–ISH experts' opinion, the definition 'high normal' blood pressure does not have sufficient scientific support, and encompasses too many subjects. Furthermore, the word 'stage' of hypertension is reserved to indicate the absence, or the presence and severity of complications, rather than to classify blood pressure values, as detailed in Table 25.3 [3].

Table 25.1. Classification of arterial hypertension (based on blood pressure levels).

	SBP (mmHg)		DBP (mmHg)
Normotension	< 140	and	< 90
Mild hypertension	140–180	and/or	90–105
Borderline hypertension	140–160	and/or	90–95
Moderate–severe hypertension	≥ 180	and/or	≥ 105
Isolated systolic hypertension	≥ 160	and	< 90
Borderline systolic hypertension	140–160	and	< 90

SBP = Systolic blood pressure
DBP = Diastolic blood pressure

Table 25.2. Classification of blood pressure for adults aged 18 years and older according to the Joint National Committee on Detection, Evaluation, and Treatment of High Blood Pressure.

Category[a]	SBP (mmHg)	DBP (mmHg)
Normal	< 130	< 85
High normal	130–139	85–89
Hypertension	≥ 140	≥ 90
Stage 1 (mild)	140–159	90–99
Stage 2 (moderate)	160–179	100–109
Stage 3 (severe)	180–209	110–119
Stage 4 (very severe)	≥ 210	≥ 120

[a] When systolic and diastolic blood pressure fall into different categories, the higher category should be selected to classify the individual's blood pressure status.
SBP = Systolic blood pressure
DBP = Diastolic blood pressure

Table 25.3. Classification of arterial hypertension according to target organ damage.

Stage	Target organ damage (TOD)
Stage I	No TOD
Stage II	At least one of the following signs of TOD: – Left ventricular hypertrophy (radiology, ECG, echocardiography) – Arterial narrowing (fundoscopy) – Proteinuria and/or serum creatinine levels 1.2–2.0 mg/dl – Documented (echocardiography, radiology) atherosclerotic plaque (carotid, aorta, iliofemoral artery)
Stage III	Both signs and symptoms of TOD: – Heart: angina pectoris, myocardial infarction, left ventricular failure – Brain: transient ischemic attacks, stroke, hypertensive encephalopathy – Retina: hemorrhages, exudates with or without papilledema – Vessels: dissecting aneurysm, symptomatic peripheral vascular disease

These classifications of arterial hypertension are appropriate for casual or basal blood pressure readings obtained by the indirect method with a mercury sphygmomanometer. Ambulatory blood pressure monitoring and home readings are frequently several mmHg lower than conventional measurements. At the present time these measurements cannot be used for diagnostic purposes or to classify arterial hypertension. However in some situations ambulatory blood pressure monitoring may be very useful in the clinical setting [3] (see Table 25.4).

Hypertensive crises: Emergencies and urgencies

Hypertensive emergencies are those situations that require immediate blood pressure reduction (not necessarily to normal range) to prevent or limit target organ damage, such as hypertensive encephalopathy, intracranial hemorrhage, acute left ventricular failure with pulmonary edema, dissecting aortic aneurysm, eclampsia or

Table 25.4. Situations in which automated noninvasive ambulatory blood pressure monitoring devices may be useful.

'Office' or 'white-coat' hypertension: blood pressure repeatedly elevated in office setting but repeatedly normal out of office
'White-coat' effect: blood pressure repeatedly higher in office setting than out of office
Evaluation of drug resistance
Evaluation of nocturnal blood pressure changes
Episodic hypertension
Hypotension symptoms associated with antihypertensive medications or autonomic dysfunction
Carotid synus syncope and pacemaker syndromes

severe hypertension associated with pregnancy, unstable angina pectoris and acute myocardial infarction.

Hypertensive urgencies are those situations in which it is desirable to reduce blood pressure within hours (no more than 24), and include accelerated or malignant hypertension without severe symptoms or progressive target organ complications, non-hemorrhagic cerebrovascular accidents with severe hypertension, severe perioperative hypertension, severe hypertension after renal transplant, severe burns, hypertensive rebound after sudden interruption of antihypertensive treatment.

Although the incidence of malignant hypertension is rapidly decreasing, this condition remains the most frequent cause of hypertensive emergency or urgency [5]. A list of hypertensive emergencies is given in Table 25.5

Table 25.5. Hypertensive emergencies.

Brain	Hypertensive encephalopathy
	Parenchymatous cerebral hemorrhage
	Subarachnoid hemorrhage
Heart	Dissecting aneurysm of the aorta
	Acute left ventricular failure
	Acute myocardial infarction
	After coronary artery bypass grafts
Catecholamines	Pheochromocytoma
	Interaction with MAO-inhibitors
Pregnancy	Eclampsia
Bleeding	Postoperatively from vascular sutures
	Massive epistaxis

Hypertension in special situations

Hypertension in children

In children, arterial hypertension is defined as systolic blood pressure and/or diastolic blood pressure ≥ 95° percentile per age and sex in three separate measurements. According to The Second Task Force on Blood Pressure Control in Children, arterial hypertension in the juvenile age groups may be classified as 'significant' and 'severe', as detailed in Table 25.6 [6].

Hypertension in the elderly

Mean values of systolic blood pressure increase with age among adults in most populations [7]. Systolic hypertension is a well-established independent risk factor for cardiovascular diseases. In all industrialized countries, the prevalence of arterial hypertension in an aged population approaches or even exceeds 50%, and the prevalence of isolated systolic hypertension increases after age 60 years. Therefore,

Table 25.6. Classification of arterial hypertension in children[a]

Age (years)	Significant hypertension		Severe hypertension	
	SBP (mmHg)	DBP (mmHg)	SBP (mmHg)	DBP (mmHg)
< 2	> 112	> 74	> 118	> 82
3–5	> 116	> 76	> 124	> 84
6–9	> 122	> 78	> 130	> 86
10–12	> 126	> 82	> 134	> 90
13–15	> 136	> 86	> 144	> 92
16–18	> 142	> 92	> 150	> 98

[a] DBP values measured at K4 in children < 13 years old.
SBP = Systolic blood pressure
DBP = Diastolic blood pressure

arterial hypertension is the most frequent of the chronic health problems of the elderly. One of the more important advances in cardiovascular medicine during the past decade is the evidence that antihypertensive therapy is especially effective in reducing overall cardiovascular morbidity in older people [8].

Hypertension in pregnancy

Arterial hypertension develops in more than 5% of all pregnancies, and may result in life-threatening consequences for both mother and fetus [9].

The criteria for diagnosing hypertension in pregnancy are: SBP increase ≥ 30 mmHg and DBP increase ≥ 15 mmHg compared with the average values before 20 weeks' gestation. When previous blood pressure values are not known, a reading ≥ 140 and/or ≥ 90 mmHg is considered abnormal.

It is important to differentiate chronic hypertension (that antedates pregnancy) and transient hypertension (characterized by a blood pressure increase during the last gestational weeks and which persists up to ten days after delivery), from a pregnancy-induced or -worsened hypertension. Pregnancy-induced hypertension occurs primarily in primigravidas after the twentieth week of gestation, and may be associated with proteinuria and edema (preeclampsia), and even convulsions and coma (eclampsia).

The National High Blood Pressure Education Program's 'Working Group Report on High Blood Pressure in Pregnancy' recommends a simple classification of hypertension in pregnancy, as detailed in Table 25.7 [10].

Secondary forms of arterial hypertension

One of the goals of the initial evaluation of the hypertensive patient is to detect a non-idiopathic (or primary, or essential) form of arterial hypertension. A secondary cause of arterial hypertension is present in roughly 5% of the hypertensive population; the absolute number of such patients is therefore not small [11]. It is important

Table 25.7. Classification of arterial hypertension in pregnancy.

Chronic hypertension in pregnancy
Preeclampsia–eclampsia
Chronic hypertension with superimposed preeclampsia
Transient hypertension in pregnancy

to recognize secondary forms of hypertension which can often be corrected or cured by surgical or specific medical therapy.

Surgical cure of hypertension is possible in patients with renovascular hypertension, primary hyperaldosteronism, and pheochromocytoma. Clues to the presence of a secondary cause of hypertension are: hypertension presenting at an atypical age, poor response to drug treatment, sudden appearance of severe hypertension at any age, and significant accompaning symptoms. The more common secondary causes of hypertension are detailed in Table 25.8.

For the clinician, after exclusion of the drug-induced forms of hypertension, it is useful to focus on three major correctable causes: renal artery stenosis, pheochromocytoma and primary aldosteronism. The clinical clues suggesting renovascular hypertension are detailed in Table 25.9, the clinical features and the differential diagnosis of pheochromocytoma are detailed in Tables 25.10 and 25.11, respectively.

Table 25.8. Secondary causes of high blood pressure.

Renal:	Bilateral or focal renal parenchymal disease Renovascular (atherosclerotic, fibrous, thromboembolic)
Endocrine:	Adrenal (pheochromocytoma, primary aldosteronism, Cushing's syndrome, adrenocortical enzyme deficiencies) Extra-adrenal (hypothyroidism, hyperthyroidism, hyperparathyroidism, acromegaly, carcinoid syndrome, diabetes)
Drug induced:	Oral contraceptives, alcohol, corticosteroids, nonsteroidal antiinflammatories, sympathomimetics, sympatholytic agent withdrawal, monoamineoxidase/ tyramine ingestion, amphetamines, cocaine, narcotics (and their withdrawal), ergotamine, glycyrrhizic acid (licorice), cyclosporin, erythropoietin
Neurologic:	Increased intracranial pressure, peripheral neuropathies
Post-lithotripsy	
Post-cardiac surgery:	Post-coronary bypass, post-cardiac transplant, post-aortic valve replacement

Table 25.9. Clinical clues suggesting renovascular hypertension.

Systolic/diastolic epigastric, subcostal, or flank bruit
Accelerated (malignant) hypertension
Unilateral small kidney
Sudden development or worsening of hypertension at any age
Hypertension and unexplained impairment of renal function
Sudden worsening of renal function in hypertensive patient
Hypertension refractory to appropriate three-drug regimen
Impairment in renal function in response to ACE inhibitor
Extensive occlusive disease in coronary, cerebral, and peripheral circulation

Table 25.10. Individual features suggesting pheochromocytoma.

Pallor
Excessive sweating
Flushing
Episodes of tremor, anxiety, feeling of malaise
Headaches
Tachycardia and palpitations
Postural hypotension
Nausea, abdominal discomfort
Weight loss
Impaired glucose tolerance or diabetes mellitus
Polycythemia
Neurofibromatosis
Multiple endocrine adenomatosis syndrome (types II and III)
Von-Hippel–Lindau syndrome

Table 25.11. Differential diagnosis of pheochromocytoma.

Anxiety
Hyper-beta-adrenergic circulatory state
Hyperthyroidism
Paroxysmal tachycardia
Autonomic neuropathies
Sympatholytic agent withdrawal
Monoamineoxidase inhibitor–tyramine interaction
Menopausal syndrome
Migraine and cluster headache
Carcinoid syndrome
Hypovolemia
Acute coronary insufficiency
Diencephalic seizure syndrome

Epidemiology

Arterial hypertension is the most common risk factor for cardiovascular events in Western countries, with a prevalence in the general population ranging from 10 to 40% [4, 12].

The most complete data have been collected in the United States. The prevalence of arterial hypertension in the USA has increased dramatically over the past decades, probably not because of any real increase in the numbers of patients, but because definitions of arterial hypertension have changed over the years. According to the data of the National Center for Health and Nutritional Examination Surveys, about 60 million Americans are hypertensive, including 25 million borderline hypertensives [13]. In particular, in the age group between 18 and 74 years, 33% of males and 26.8% of females are affected by arterial hypertension. The prevalence of arterial hypertension increases with age (Table 25.12). In the Systolic Hypertension in the Elderly Program, increased blood pressure values were found in 60% of subjects aged 65–74 years and in 68% of subjects aged 75 years or over

Table 25.12. Prevalence of arterial hypertension in relation to age[a].

Age (years)	Prevalence of hypertension (%)
18–29	4
30–39	11
40–49	21
50–59	44
60–69	54
70–70	64
≥ 80	65

[a] Data from NHANES III, 1991.

[14]. The greater prevalence of hypertension among older versus younger persons had been emphasized by the Framingham Study, which found that 39% of men and 48% of women aged 65 years and older were hypertensive [15].

Risk factors

It is commonly accepted that blood pressure level is a function of both genetic and enviromental factors (originating either early *in utero* or later during adult life). Genetic analyses have demonstrated that blood pressure is a quantitative trait in which several genes may be involved. From 20% to 49% of blood pressure variation in the general population can be attributed to genetic factors [16]. To date, some genetic markers that permit an early detection of subjects at risk for developing arterial hypertension have been identified. The tools of molecular biology will provide the means to define the genetic basis of hypertension. However, hypertension may represent the result of the action of various inherited biochemical abnormalities. In fact, essential hypertension has been considered as a heterogeneous group of disorders [17]. Specific subtypes of essential hypertension might be categorized according to age, gender, race, sodium sensitivity, insulin sensitivity, plasma renin activity, lipid profile and obesity [17]. The association of hypertension and obesity has been well recognized for decades: in the Framingham Study the incidence of hypertension among the obese approached 50%, and obesity was very prevalent among hypertensive patients [18].

Pathophysiologic factors that have been implicated in the genesis of arterial hypertension include inappropriate renal sodium retention, increased sympathetic activity, chronic high-sodium intake, overproduction of a sodium-retaining hormone, inadequate dietary intakes of potassium and calcium, increased renin secretion, decreased endothelium derived relaxing factor, increased activity of vascular growth factors with increased vasocostriction of resistance vessels, altered membrane ion transport and membrane receptor structure, diabetes mellitus, insulin resistance and obesity. The association of high blood pressure and overweight, high plasma insulin levels and elevated serum cholesterol and triglycerides is considered to be the result of interaction between genetic predisposition and enviroment. Therefore, the challenge for a primary prevention of hypertension is to identify

Table 25.13. Risk factors for arterial hypertension.

Familial and genetic factors
Ethnic and racial factors
Physical inactivity
Psychosocial factors
Overweight and obesity
High sodium intake
Inadequate potassium and calcium intake
Excessive alcohol consumption
Cigarette smoking

genetic markers such as family history of hypertension, dyslipidemia or diabetes mellitus, so as to recognize the individual at risk, and to undertake suitable methods of intervention, such as body weight control by means of a proper diet, increased physical exercise, reduction of dietary sodium and alcohol intake, increased potassium intake and reduction in psychosocial stress. Furthermore, cigarette smoking should be strongly discouraged [19]. A list of the factors which increase the risk of developing arterial hypertension is detailed in Table 25.13.

Clinical manifestations

Although in patients with severe hypertension common symptoms include headache, dyspnea, dizzines, blurred vision, depression and nocturia, in most patients with mild to moderate hypertension there are no clinical manifestations other than the elevated blood pressure. It is obvious that the measurement of blood pressure requires precision and consideration of a number of factors to avoid erroneous labeling of a normotensive patient as hypertensive. Hypertension should not be diagnosed on the basis of a single measurement. Initial elevated readings should be confirmed on at least two subsequent visits with an interval of at least one week. Before measurement patients should be seated several minutes (at least five) in a quiet room. They should have their arm bared and supported at the heart level. The patients should not have smoked or ingested caffeine within 30 minutes before measurement. The appropriate cuff size must be used (height: 13–15 cm, length: 30–35 cm for a middle-sized arm). The disappearance of sounds (phase V) should be commonly used for the diastolic readings. The measurement should be read to the nearest 2 mmHg. Two or more readings separated by two minutes should be averaged. In the initial visit, blood pressure should be measured in both arms, and both in sitting (or lying) and standing position [3, 4].

In the baseline evaluation of hypertensive patients, efforts should be made to detect clinical clues to secondary causes of hypertension and to assess target organ damage as well as other risk factors for cardiovascular disease. The clues which point to the possibility of secondary hypertension may be related to age, history, physical examination and laboratory results. For example, an arterial hypertension which develops before age 30 or after age 50, an abdominal bruit, the presence of severe retinopathy, or the sudden onset of severe hypertension are usual clues to renovascular hypertension (see Table 25.9). Some patients with primary aldosteronism may present nocturia, polydipsia, weakness, paresthesias or tetany resulting from hypokalemia. The multiple symptoms of pheochromocytoma, which include hypertension (usually paroxysmal in character), palpitations, tachycardia, apprehension and excessive sweating are detailed in Table 25.10, while the differential diagnoses are listed in Table 25.11. A palpable kidney may signify polycystic disease, while coarctation of the aorta is suggested by diminished and delayed leg pulses as well as by a systolic murmur at the left sternal border and at the back. The general appearance of the patient may direct the diagnosis to acromegaly, hyperthyroidism, hypothyroidism, Cushing's syndrome and alcoholism. Isolated systolic hypertension is associated with atherosclerosis, aortic regurgitation, coarctation of the aorta, arterio–venous fistulas and diabetes mellitus.

The diagnosis of target organ damage includes clinical, laboratory and instrumental examinations. Hypertension is the most common cause of congestive heart failure. Therefore, the clinician should search for the related clinical signs. Simple laboratory tests can exclude renal damage. Furthermore, the diagnosis of target organ damage is based on fundoscopic examination, to evaluate the absence or the presence and the stage of hypertensive retinopathy, as well as on the screening for coronary heart disease and hypertensive heart disease. Noninvasive diagnostic techniques that provide assessment of left ventricular hypertrophy include the physical examination, chest X-ray, electrocardiogram and echocardiogram. Echocardiography is now considered the technique of choice to calculate left ventricular mass and to detect left ventricular hypertrophy, but its cost precludes a generalized use in all hypertensive patients. Expense reasons also limit the use of carotid duplex ultrasonography, which, however, is justified in patients with a carotid artery bruit or history of transient ischemic attacks. For the same reasons, specific diagnostic tests to explore renal function are not indicated without clinical suspicion, when urine sediment, blood urea nitrogen and creatinine are normal, and proteinuria is absent. However, it is worthwhile to mention that microalbuminuria (urinary albumin excretion 15–200 μg/minute), which may be present with a normal dipstick test, may be an early marker of hypertensive nephropathy [20].

References

1. MacMahon S, Peto R, Cutler J et al. Emidemiology. Blood pressure, stroke, and coronary heart disease. Part I, prolonged differences in blood pressure: Prospective observational studies corrected for the regression dilution bias. Lancet 1990;335:765–74.
2. Rose GA. The hypertensive patient. In: Marshall AJ, Barrit DW (eds), Kent, England: Pitman Medical Press, 1980.
3. Linee guida per il trattamento dell'ipertensione arteriosa lieve: memorandum del Meeting OMS/ISH 1993. VI Meeting OMS/ISH sull'ipertensione lieve; 1993 March 28–31; Chantilly. Chantilly: ISH Hypertension News, 1993.
4. The Fifth Report of the Joint National Committee on Detection, Evaluation, and Treatment of High Blood Pressure (JNC V). Arch Intern Med 1993; 153:154–83.
5. Ferguson RK, Vlasses PH. How urgent is 'urgent' hypertension? Arch Intern Med 1989;149:257–8.
6. Report of the Second Task Force on Blood Pressure Control in Children. Pediatrics 1987;79:1–25.

Classification and epidemiology of hypertension 353

7. Rodriguez BL, Labarthe DR, Huang B, Lopez-Gomez J. Rise of blood pressure with age. New evidence of population differences. Hypertension 1994;26:779–85.
8. Hollenberg NK. Hypertension in an aging population: Problems and opportunities. Am J Med 1991;90(Suppl.4B):1s–2s.
9. Kaplan NM. Hypertension with pregnancy and the pill. In: Clinical hypertension. Baltimore: Williams & Wilkins, 1986:345.
10. National High Blood Pressure Education Program Working Group. Report on high blood pressure in pregnancy. Am J Obstet Gynecol 1990;163:1689–712.
11. Venkata C, Ram S. Secondary hypertension: Workup and correction. Hosp Prac 1994;4:137–50.
12. National High Blood Pressure Education Program Working Group. Report on primary prevention of hypertension. Arch Intern Med 1993;153:186–208.
13. Horan MJ, Lenfant C. Epidemiology of blood pressure and predictors of hypertension. Hypertension 1990;15(Suppl.I):20–4.
14. Hulley SB, Furberg CD, Gurland B et al. Systolic Hypertension in the Elderly Program (SHEP): Antihypertensive efficacy of chlorthalidone. Am J Cardiol 1985;56:913–20.
15. Volkonas PS, Kannel WB, Cupples LA. Epidemiology and risk of hypertension in the elderly: The Framingham Study. J Hypertens 1988;6(Suppl.1):s3–s9.
16. Ward R. Familial aggregation and genetic epidemiology of blood pressure. In: Laragh JH, Brunner BM (eds), Hypertension: Pathophysiology, diagnosis, and management. New York: Raven Press, 1990:81–100.
17. Iwai N, Ohmichi N, Hanai K, Nakamura Y, Kinoshita M. Human SA gene locus as a candidate locus for essential hypertension. Hypertension 1994;23:375–80.
18. Kannel WB, Brand N, Skinner JJ, Dawber TR, Mc Namara PM. The relation of adiposity to blood pressure and development of hypertension. Ann Intern Med 1967;67:48–59.
19. Conclusions from a joint WHO/ISH Meeting: Prevention of hypertension and associated cardiovascular disease: 1991 statement. Clin Exper Hyper Theory Prac 1992;A14:333–41.
20. Yudkin JS, Forrest R, Jackson CA. Microalbuminuria as predictor of vascular disease in non-diabetic subjects. Islington diabetic survey. Lancet 1988;2:530–3.

26. Diagnosis, complications and management of hypertension

GIUSEPPE LICATA, ROSARIO SCAGLIONE and ANTONIO PINTO

Introduction

Evaluation and treatment of hypertension require training and experience. Since the start of the National High Blood Pressure Education Program (NHBEP) in 1972 [1], remarkable progress has been made in detecting, treating and controlling hypertension. In the last two decades the number of hypertensives has increased dramatically, as has the percentage of hypertensives taking medication. Diagnosis of hypertension includes evaluation of current blood pressure, according to methodology suggested by the Joint National Committee on Detection, Evaluation and Treatment of High Blood Pressure or WHO, and determination of whether the hypertension is primary or secondary [2]. Management of hypertension includes assessment of other cardiovascular risk factors associated with high blood pressure and the evaluation of complications related to hypertensive disease. Therapeutic management of hypertension includes lifestyle modification and pharmacological treatment.

Documenting blood pressure

Blood pressure shows a consistent variability depending on awake-versus-asleep and active-versus-resting status, position (supine, sitting, standing), changes in body weight, emotional status, sodium level, and intake of antihypertensive drugs. Most information on the relationship of blood pressure to certain outcomes (i.e., fatal and nonfatal cardiovascular, cerebrovascular, and renovascular events) is related to blood pressure measured using mercury or calibrated aneroid sphygmomanometers [3, 4].

Office blood pressure measurement

The fifth report of the National Committee on Detection, Evaluation and Treatment of High Blood Pressure (JNC V) recommends the use of a mercury sphygmomanometer, a recently calibrated aneroid manometer, or a calibrated electronic device [2]. JNC V states that blood pressure should be measured with the patient

---

The authors appreciate the support of Tiziana Di Chiara, MD, for her contribution to the drawing up of this manuscript.

seated and the arm bared at heart level. Patients should have no coffee or cigarettes within 30 minutes of the reading. After a minimum of a five-minute wait, two or more measurements separated by two-minute intervals should be averaged to derive the *'casual office blood pressure'*. Both systolic and diastolic pressures should be recorded. The disappearance of sound (Korotkoff phase V) should be used for the diastolic reading. Additional readings are recommended if the difference is 6 mmHg or more. If there is arrhythmia six or more readings should be taken. In addition, an appropriate size cuff must be used, especially in obese subjects. The bladder should nearly (at least 80%) or completely encircle the arm.

Moreover, before hypertension is diagnosed in persons 18 years and older, initially elevated levels should be averaged with findings at two or more follow-up visits separated by one to several weeks [2–4].

Home and ambulatory monitoring

Home blood pressure monitoring is often helpful in evaluating hypertension, but portable automated ambulatory monitoring is recommended only in the following specific situations [5, 6]:

1. Office or white coat hypertension.
2. Suspected drug resistance.
3. Nighttime blood pressure change.
4. Episodic hypertension.
5. Hypotensive episodes and carotid sinus syncope and pacemaker syndromes.

Training of patients and family members who are to measure blood pressure at home is required and it is better that someone other than the patient take the measurements. Home blood pressure measurements should be taken in the same manner as casual office measurements [6].

Several studies have suggested that findings from home monitoring and automated ambulatory monitoring correlate better with outcome and presence of target-organ disease than those detectable from casual office blood pressure monitoring [3–7].

The dividing line between normotension and hypertension is not fixed but reflects present judgment on the level at which intervention is justified. However, clinical evaluation of patients with confirmed hypertension should help answer the following questions:

1. Does the patient have primary or secondary hypertension?
2. Are cardiovascular risk factors present in addition to hypertension?
3. Are complications present?

For these reasons screening procedures are necessary.

Screening procedures

Identifiable causes of hypertension, particularly surgically curable forms, are rare even in the population attending a specialized blood pressure clinic. Therefore, detailed screening and extensive investigations of all subjects with raised blood pressure are useful [8].

History

History indicates the duration of hypertension and other relevant information, for example presence of diabetes mellitus, smoking habits, salt and alcohol consumption, usual exercise and weight gain. It is important to investigate family history of hypertension, premature cardiovascular and cerebrovascular diseases or death, since offspring of parental hypertensives have a higher risk of cardiovascular events [3, 4, 7, 8]. Drug history should pay particular attention to nonsteroidal antiinflammatory drugs, but use of nasal decongestants and other cold remedies, appetite suppressants, monoamineoxidase inhibitors, cyclosporin, oral contraceptive steroids and hormone replacement therapy are also relevant. Endocrine hypertension is occasionally revealed by history [8].

Patients with pheochromocytoma may complain of attacks characterized by throbbing headache, sweating, palpitations and nervousness. Primary hyperaldosteronism has few symptoms but there is sometimes nocturia and muscle weakness. Cushing's syndrome is characterized by rapid weight gain, increased skin fragility and headache. In addition, history may reveal sleep-apnea through investigation of the presence of early morning headaches, daytime somnolence, loud snoring and erratic sleep [3, 4, 8].

Clinical examination

The physical examination includes a number of tests to distinguish primary from secondary hypertension (Table 26.1). Indications of secondary hypertension include abdominal aortic aneurysm, delayed or absent femoral pulses and central obesity with abdominal striae. In renal artery stenosis it is possible to recognize a systolic–diastolic bruit lateral to midline or in the flank. Delayed femoral pulses in younger patients point to coarctation of the aorta. Distinctive physical appearance may suggest acromegaly or Cushing's syndrome. Palpable kidneys may indicate polycystic kidneys. Clinical examination in patients with pheochromocytoma is

Table 26.1. Important aspects of the physical examination.

Accurate measurement of blood pressure
General appearance: distribution of body fat, skin lesions,
    muscle strength, alertness
Funduscopy
Neck: palpation and auscultation of carotids, thyroid
Heart: size, rhythm, sounds
Lung: rhonchi, rales
Abdomen: renal masses, bruits over aorta or renal arteries,
    femoral pulses
Extremities: peripheral pulses, edema
Neurologic assessment

often not very helpful but sometimes there is neurofibromatosis or postural hypotension [3, 4, 7, 8].

Bilateral flame-shaped retinal hemorrhages indicate malignant hypertension and the need for prompt treatment and their presence correlates with fibrinoid necrosis in the arterioles of the kidneys, the pathogenic hallmark of malignant hypertension. In addition, papilledema is detectable in malignant hypertension [3, 4, 7, 8].

Urine tests

Proteinuria or *hematuria* in the absence of malignant hypertension suggest renal pathology, such as glomerulonephritis, although concentrated or highly buffered alkaline urine may give false positive strip tests for protein. About 10% of middle-aged patients with hypertension have positive tests. Strongly positive paper strip tests for protein should always be confirmed by quantification of protein excretion on a timed urine collection over 24 h and results may be expressed in relation to creatinine [3, 4, 8].

Hypertensive patients with impaired renal function due to hypertensive nephrosclerosis may show proteinuria, but the amount excreted rarely exceeds 2 g/day. Some patients with untreated unilateral renovascular disease and severe hypertension have quite marked proteinuria which may be in the nephrotic range (> 3.5 g/24 h). About 25% of middle-aged patients with essential hypertension have *microalbuminuria* with urinary albumin in the range of 30–300 mg/24 h, but negative or weakly positive dipstick tests. There are some correlations between microalbuminuria and indices of target organ damage, but obesity and factors related to insulin resistance seem also to be relevant. As in normal subjects, upright posture and exercise tend to increase the rate of albumin excretion [9].

A 24-h collection of urine for sodium may be suitable as a measure of *sodium intake* in selected subjects once it has been established that diet is relatively stable [7]. Routine measurement of urinary excretion of catecholamines or metabolites as a screening test for pheochromocytoma is not worthwhile. Only very rarely is concomitant glucose intolerance caused by endocrine disease such as pheochromocitoma, Cushing's syndrome and acromegaly.

Blood tests

Measurements of serum concentrations of *creatinine* and *urea* are performed routinely. Renovascular disease now quite often comes to attention during monitoring of serum creatinine concentrations in patients on ACE inhibitors. Serious declines in overall renal function are most likely in patients with bilateral disease and the risk is increased if loop diuretics are also given [3, 4, 8].

Total serum cholesterol is measured in all patients but a fasting lipid screen is only indicated when random cholesterol is markedly and persistently elevated. Serum urate should be measured.

Serum potassium is a simple screening test for primary hyperaldosteronism but false negative results are found in up to 20% of patients. In primary hyperaldosteronism or in other rare forms of mineralocorticoid hypertension (such as 11β-hydroxylation deficiency, 17α-hydroxylation deficiency and carbenoxolone or licorice ingestion), hypokalemia, mild alkalosis and slightly increased serum concentration of sodium are present. Hypokalemia in mineralocorticoid hypertension is more evident if high dietary intake of sodium or diuretic treatment are associated [3, 4, 8].

Primary hyperparathyroidism may be suspected if *serum calcium* concentrations are raised, but a proportion of patients with essential hypertension also have slightly raised serum levels of total calcium. Although more severe hyperparathyroidism undoubtedly causes hypertension, the relationship between high blood pressure and mild primary hyperparathyroidism is not clear [10].

Electrocardiography

ECG is helpful to detect left ventricular hypertrophy. If left ventricular hypertrophy is associated with ST and T-wave changes in the leads overlying the left ventricle, the patient is at great risk. If there is doubt about end organ damage, echocardiography is a much more sensitive and specific marker of left ventricular hypertrophy [11]. ECG stress testing should be performed only if there are symptoms suggestive of angina.

Chest X-ray

Routine chest X-ray is of limited value. An enlarged heart is more likely to represent chamber dilation than increased ventricular wall thickening. Chest X-ray is helpful in patients over 70 years who are more likely to have heart enlargement or heart failure [12]. Notching on the underside of ribs caused by collateral vessels and loss of the aortic knuckle may indicate aortic coarctation.

Specialized investigations

The frequencies of various causes of secondary hypertension are shown in Table 26.2. In addition, Table 26.3 indicates an overall guide to work-up for secondary

Table 26.2. Frequency of various diagnoses in hypertensive subjects

	Frequency of diagnosis	
Number of patients	10 476	
Essential hypertension	9782	(93.4%)
Renovascular disease	147	(1.4%)
Chronic renal disease	462	(4.4%)
Coarctation of the aorta	43	(0.4%)
Primary aldosteronism	22	(0.20%)
Pheochromocytoma	10	(0.1%)
Cushing's syndrome	10	(0.1%)

Adapted from Kaplan (1994) [3].

Table 26.3. Guidelines for secondary hypertension

Diagnosis	Diagnostic screening	
	Initial	Additional
Renovascular disease	PRA	Isotopic renogram
	Captopril test	Arteriography
Chronic renal disease	Urinalysis	Isotopic renogram
	Serum creatinine	Renal biopsy
	Renal sonography	
Aortic coarctation	BP in legs	Aortogram
Primary aldosteronism	Plasma K$^+$, PRA	Urinary K$^+$ and
	Plasma aldosterone	aldosterone after
		saline load
		Adrenal computer
		tomography (CT)
		Scintscans
Cushing's syndrome	Plasma cortisol	Urinary cortisol
		Adrenal CT
		Scintscans
Pheochromocytoma	Urinary catecholamines	Plasma catecholamines
		Clonidine test
		Adrenal CT
		Scintscans

causes of hypertension. These indicate that the incidence of secondary hypertension is low.

Renovascular disease

Renovascular hypertension is due more to atheroma than to fibromuscular hyperplasia. Intravenous urography is now obsolete as a screening test: sensitivity in detecting unilateral renal artery stenosis is only 75% and the test gives little information on bilateral disease. If urography is performed in unilateral renal artery stenosis the characteristic findings on the affected side are increased pyelographic density and delay in washout of contrast, often associated with reduced renal size [3, 4, 8].

The best screening test for renovascular hypertension is probably the measurement of plasma renin activity, especially with concomitant measurement of urinary sodium excretion over 24 h to detect individuals taking unusually low or high intakes of salt. In some centers screening measurements of plasma renin activity are performed after a single dose of 25 mg captopril which gives a sensitivity of about 75% and specificity of about 90%: others still use the stimulus of upright posture and ambulation. Patients with marked blood pressure elevation and high or high-normal plasma renin values which are not explained by low dietary sodium should have captopril renography [13].

Isotope renography as a screening test for unilateral renal artery stenosis is positive in 80–90% of cases. Sensitivity is too low for effective screening, but can be greatly enhanced by prior treatment with an ACE inhibitor. For untreated patients several protocols have been used with renography after oral captopril or an intravenous ACE inhibitor. Renography is performed with ^{99m}Tc-DTPA or labeled iodohippurate often in combination with measurement of glomerular filtration rate. Labeled hippuran provides an estimate of renal plasma flow. Where renography has been done before and after an ACE inhibitor a difference in the renogram curve is a very specific finding but less sensitive. In all high-risk patients it is best to perform angiography with digital vascular imaging. Arteriography with fine gauge catheters is the preferred technique.

Other renal conditions

The most frequent causes of renal parenchymal disease are chronic glomerulonephritis, chronic pyelonephritis, and polycystic kidneys. In young women and patients with suspected parenchymal renal disease, ultrasonography is a useful non-invasive test able to diagnose polycystic kidney disease, hydronephrosis, and significant asymmetry in renal size. Ultrasonography has a role in the assessment and monitoring of abdominal aortic aneurysms which often coexist with atherosclerotic renovascular disease, especially in older men [3, 4, 7, 8, 13].

Mineralocorticoid hypertension

Routine screening for primary hyperaldosteronism and other forms of mineralocorticoid excess includes measurement of forearm venous concentrations of potassium. Patients with mineralocorticoid hypertension often have a slightly high or high-normal serum concentration of sodium, and plasma renin activity is characteristically markedly suppressed. Plasma aldosterone is best measured in blood samples taken at around 08.00 h because the diurnal rhythm of aldosterone secretion in primary aldosteronism follows ACTH rather than angiotensin II. Urinary aldosterone may be measured but is generally less sensitive than plasma estimates. The association of mineralocorticoid hypertension with suppressed levels of renin and aldosterone should prompt consideration of other rare syndromes. In view of this, licorice may produce this pattern by inhibiting the renal 11β-hydroxysteroid dehydrogenase shuttle enzyme [3, 4, 7, 8].

Pheochromocytoma

When there is reason to suggest this condition, measurement of urinary excretion of noradrenaline is a good initial test, but some physicians continue to use tests based on catecholamine metabolites with vanillylmandelic acid. The most sensitive and specific tests involve plasma or urine catecholamine measurements before and after suppression of sympathetic nerve activity with drugs. Plasma concentrations of noradrenaline and adrenaline can be measured using either radioenzymatic or HPLC methods before and after a single oral dose of clonidine (300 μg). The ratio of noradrenaline and adrenaline to creatinine in an overnight sample of urine after clonidine administration can also be used, the so-called '*sleep-clonidine test*' [14].

Clonidine testing readily separates patients with pheochromocytoma from patients with hypertension and raised catecholamine levels secondary to overactivity of the sympathetic nervous system, but can cause quite marked falls in blood pressure in patients not affected by pheochromocytoma especially with the overnight test.

Interaction of hypertension with other risk factors

Because hypertension is only one risk factor for cardiovascular disease, appropriate management requires an integrated approach to identification and modification of other reversible risk factors. In fact, epidemiological data and clinical experience indicate an association with cigarette-smoking, type A personality and sedentary lifestyle, hyperlipoproteinemia, diabetes and central obesity (Table 26.4) [3, 4, 11, 15].

In hypertension clinic attenders, the risk of developing cardiovascular event is enhanced by the concomitant presence of other risk factors. Different factors have a cumulative effect on risk. In fact, the risk of coronary heart disease increases if there is associated hypercholesterolemia, hypertriglyceridemia, diabetes mellitus, cigarette-smoking, left ventricular hypertrophy and central obesity. Central obesity also promotes increased total cholesterol, reduced HDL-cholesterol, increased LDL/HDL cholesterol, left ventricular hypertrophy and diabetes mellitus. Heavy alcohol drinkers are less compliant with antihypertensive treatment and have a drop-out rate among heavy drinkers of almost 50% at one year [3, 4, 7, 8].

Cigarette-smoking contributes to coronary heart risk but is particularly hazardous when combined with other risk factors or in women taking oral contraceptive steroids. Smoking is common in hypertensive patients, has at least an additive effect with other risk factors, and more than doubled mortality in the MRC trial. Hypertensives who smoke are also more likely to develop malignant hypertension [15].

Estrogen-containing oral contraceptive steroids worsen atherogenic traits attributable to blood pressure and glucose intolerance. Estrogen as hormone replacement therapy may also increase risk of coronary heart disease in post-menopausal smoking women. Behavior promoting emotional stress appears to influence risk factor or is directly associated with coronary heart disease incidence. Type A behavior is particularly associated with coronary disease [3, 4, 8, 15].

Table 26.4. Prevalence of obesity in normotensive and hypertensive subjects (unpublished personal data).

	Normotensive		Hypertensive	
Number of cases	8.847		867	
Lean	3.982	(45%)	206	(23.7%)
Overweight	2.654	(30%)	313	(36.1%)
Moderate obese	1.769	(20%)	302	(34.8%)
Severe obese	442	(4%)	46	(5.3%)

Pearson chi-square test $p < 0.001$.

Diabetes mellitus often coexists with hypertension. The existence and progression of diabetic microvascular disease is worsened by hypertension. About 40% of insulin-dependent diabetics go on to develop proteinuria or persistent microalbuminuria with a progressive decline in glomerular filtration rate [3, 4].

Complications of hypertension

The translation of high BP into vascular damage involves three mechanisms: pulsatile flow, endothelial cell changes, and the remodeling and growth of smooth muscle cells. These alterations involve the well-known 'target organ' with specific clinical manifestations (Table 26.5) [3, 4, 7, 16].

Specific organ involvement

In general complications of hypertension can be considered either 'hypertensive' or 'atherosclerotic' (Table 26.6). Those listed as hypertensive are caused more directly by the increased blood pressure *per se*, whereas the atherosclerotic complications have multiple causes, hypertension playing a variable role. However, the relevant contribution of hypertension to atherosclerotic disease is shown by epidemiological data [2, 3, 4, 7].

Manifestations of target-organ disease are summarized in Table 26.5. They include clinical manifestations of cardiac, cerebrovascular, lower limbs, renal, and retina involvement [2, 3, 4, 7, 16].

Hypertensive heart disease
The most common effect of hypertension on the heart is left ventricular hypertrophy (LVH). In normotensive adults, LV mass is directly related to the risk of developing subsequent hypertension suggesting that LVH may be involved in genetic or other factors responsible for the pathogenesis of hypertension [17].

Table 26.5. Manifestations of target-organ disease.

Organ system	Manifestations
Cardiac	Clinical, electrocardiographic, or radiologic evidence of coronary artery disease
	Left ventricular hypertrophy of 'strain' by electrocardiography or left ventricular hypertrophy by echocardiography
	Left ventricular dysfunction or cardiac failure
Cerebrovascular	Transient ischemic attack or stroke
Peripheral vascular	Absence of one or more major pulses in the extremities (excepts for dorsalis pedis) with or without intermittent claudication; aneurysm
Renal	Serum creatinine ≥ 130 μmol/L (1.5 mg/dl)
	Proteinuria (1+ or greater)
	Microalbuminuria
Retinopathy	Hemorrhages or exudates, with or without papilledema

Table 26.6. Complications of hypertension

Hypertensive
Accelerated malignant hypertension (III and IV retinopathy)
Left ventricular hypertrophy
Congestive heart failure
Aortic dissection
Renal insufficiency
Encephalopathy
Cerebral hemorrhage

Atherosclerotic
Myocardial infarction
Coronary artery disease
Claudication syndromes
Cerebral thrombosis

The basic signals that initiate and maintain myocardial hypertrophy probably include a number of growth factors whose effects may be transmitted via the α_1 adrenergic receptor to activate intracellular transducing proteins and ribonucleic acid transcription factors. An important role of the renin–angiotensin system is suggested by the clear-cut effect of angiotensin-converting enzyme inhibitors in causing regression of LVH and preventing remodeling after a myocardial infarction, particularly since all components of the system are in cardiac tissue [18, 19].

Hypertensives with LVH are more likely to experience cardiovascular morbidity and mortality than those without LVH [20]. Since LVH may promote a number of deleterious effects of hypertension on cardiac function, one of the goals of treatment of hypertension is to reverse LVH. Moreover, the various abnormalities of systolic and diastolic function related to LVH obviously could progress into LV pump failure or cardiac heart failure (CHF). Hypertension is present in 75% of patients who develop CHF, tripling the risk of normotensives [21].

Most episodes of CHF in hypertensive patients are associated with dilated cardiomyopathy and a reduced ejection fraction. However, about 40% of episodes of CHF are associated with preserved LV systolic function but with diastolic dysfunction induced by LVH, fibrosis, and ischemia and increased afterload [22].

The development of myocardial ischemia reflects an imbalance between myocardial oxygen supply and demand. Hypertension, by reducing the supply and increasing the demand, can easily change this balance. It has been well documented that hypertension is associated with multiple factors that accelerate coronary artery disease [3, 4, 7, 8, 11, 15].

Vessels disease
Hypertension is a risk factor for the development of peripheral vascular disease which is usually characterized as intermittent claudication [23]. Other large vessels disease, often associated with hypertension, are abdominal aortic aneurysm, aortic dissection, and Takayasu's disease. Recently, it has been demonstrated that alterations in small arteries could influence peripheral hemodynamics so profoundly that all blood pressure excess might be explained, provided that the alterations

occurred downstream in small resistance-sized vessels. For example, several reports indicated that a decline occurs in the coronary vascular reserve in essential hypertension and that this can be sustained by abnormalities in small intramyocardial arteries. This predisposes the heart to the possibility of periods of ischemia during times of increased oxygen demand [3, 4].

Cerebrovascular disease
Even more so than with heart disease, hypertension is the major cause of stroke. The risk of stroke is even greater in hypertensives with other risk factors including diabetes, smoking, previous cardiovascular disease, atrial fibrillation, and left ventricular hypertrophy [24]. Elderly hypertensives often also have silent cerebrovascular disease, which eventually may lead to brain atrophy and vascular dementia [3]. Atherosclerotic disease in extracranial carotid arteries, often identified by bruits, is associated with a greater likelihood of transient ischemic attacks and other cerebrovascular events. As identified by ultrasonography, both geometric and functional changes within the common carotid artery are often associated with left ventricular hypertrophy, reflecting a higher risk of cardiovascular complications.

Renal involvement
Renal dysfunction is almost always demonstrated in hypertensives. The main changes are hyalinization and sclerosis of the walls of the afferent arterioles, referred to as 'arteriolar nephrosclerosis' [3, 4, 7].

Microalbuminuria, which reflects intraglomerular hypertension, is the earliest manifestation of this and it may be detectable in normotensive subjects with higher risk to develop hypertension (Figure 1) [25, 26]. The loss of renal function rises progressively as BP increases but only a minority of hypertensives die as a result of renal failure. Nonetheless, hypertension remains a leading risk for end-stage renal disease.

Retinopathy
The retina is one of the principal target organ of hypertension [3, 4, 7]. Funduscopy often reveals some alterations in retinal vessels according to the conventional Keith–Wagener–Barker classification, especially related to duration and severity of hypertension. The most important lesions of the retina are detectable in severe hypertension. Bilateral flame shaped retinal hemorrhages indicate malignant hypertension and their presence correlates with fibrinoid necrosis in the arterioles of the kidneys. Cottonwool spots due to infarction of the nerve fiber layer of the retina tend to occur in patients with papilledema. Papilledema does not seem to influence adversely the prognosis in hypertension already complicated by bilateral retinal hemorrhages and exudates. Hard exudates which cluster around the macula may also be seen especially in the healing phase of malignant hypertension.

Therapeutic management

The goal of treating patients with hypertension is to control blood pressure and to prevent morbidity and mortality associated with high blood pressure. This should

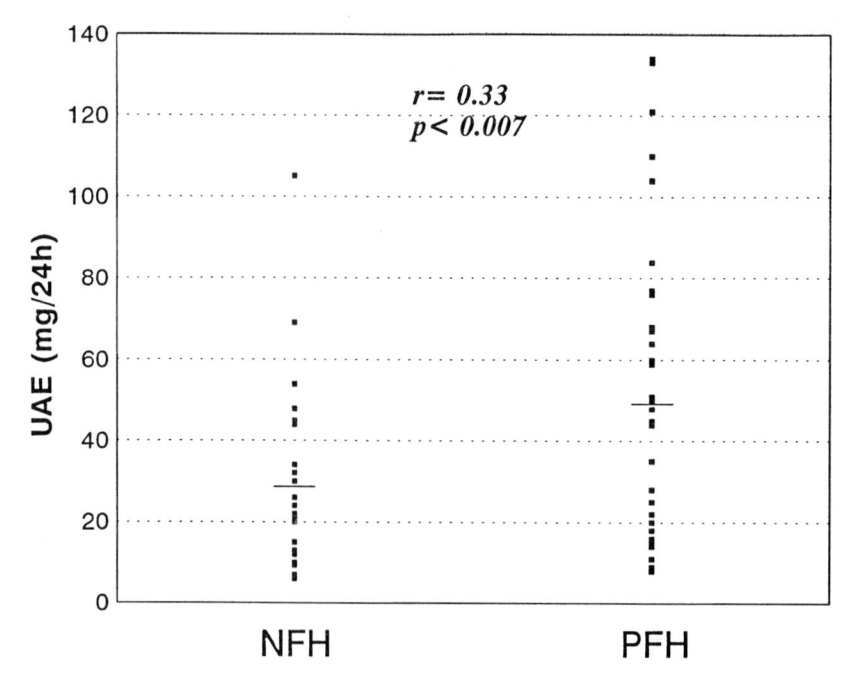

Figure 26.1. Relationship between microalbuminuria (UAE) and family history for cardiovascular disease in centrally obese subjects (unpublished personal data). NFH = negative family history; PFH = Positive family history

be accomplished by achieving and maintaining arterial pressure below 140 mmHg SBP and 90 mmHg DBP, while concurrently controlling other modifiable cardiovascular risk factors. Further reduction to levels of 130/85 mmHg may be achieved, but with particular regard for cardiovascular function, especially in older persons. How far the DBP should be reduced below 85 mmHg is still unclear. Treatment of hypertension includes lifestyle modification (previously termed nonpharmacologic therapy) and pharmacologic treatment [27–30].

Lifestyle modification

Hygienic strategies are recommended as a first step in the management of hypertensives, and also a way to prevent hypertension. The underlying assumption is that a lowered blood pressure, however achieved, will diminish the risk of cardiovascular disease [25, 27, 29]. The following procedure has been suggested by various experts:

- Stop smoking.
- Maintain near-ideal body weight.
- Restrict dietary sodium intake to 100 mmol/day (2–3 g sodium or 6 g sodium chloride) with caution not to reduce the intake of calcium-rich foods.
- Increase dietary potassium intake by replacing processed foods with natural foods.

- Supplement with calcium and magnesium only if deficient.
- Increase fiber and restrict saturated fat.
- Limit alcohol to 1 ounce per day, as contained in two usual portions of wine, beer or spirits.
- Increase physical activity.
- Use relaxation therapy, if indicated.

Pharmacologic therapy

The antihypertensive drugs available are summarized in Table 26.7. The class of antihypertensive should be chosen according to the particular patient demographics and the presence or absence of target-organ and concomitant disease. Physicians should be familiar with the various agents in terms of blood pressure reduction, adverse reactions, and cost-effectiveness.

Table 26.7. Antihypertensive drugs

Thiazide and related diuretics
Loop diuretics
Potassium-sparing diuretics
Beta-adrenergic blockers
Alpha$_1$-adrenergic blockers
Central nervous system-acting adrenergics
Peripheral nervous system-acting adrenergics
Angiotensin-converting-enzyme (ACE) inhibitors
Calcium antagonists
Direct vasodilators

Therapeutic approach

It is necessary to emphasize that there are major differences in the opinion of experts in the United States and the rest of the world, especially regarding the treatment of mild hypertension.

Initial agent
JNC V recommends either a diuretic or a beta blocker as the preferred first choice for monotherapy [2]. This recommendation was based on documented effectiveness in control of blood pressure, safety, and reduction in the incidence of fatal and non-fatal cardiovascular events (e.g., stroke, ischemic heart disease, congestive heart failure) with these two classes of antihypertensive drugs. This indication has been recently criticized by several North American researchers. They recommend the use of ACE-inhibitors and calcium antagonists as initial agents to treat hypertension [31, 32].

Pharmacologic intervention
This may be approached in four ways:

1. Start with the minimum dose of one initial antihypertensive agent and increase the dose to maximum. If goal blood pressure is not achieved, prescribe an additional one or two antihypertensive agents of different classes, up to the maximum dose. When goal blood pressure is achieved, continue all agents.
2. Follow steps in No. 1, but when goal blood pressure is achieved, discontinue the initial or added drug to minimize the number of antihypertensive agents being used.
3. Follow steps in No. 1 or 2 but use only half the maximum doses of each class to minimize adverse reactions.
4. If goal blood pressure is not achieved with initial drug at half-maximum or maximum dose, discontinue and try another class of antihypertensive.

After initiation of a treatment regimen (even if no antihypertensives are prescribed), casual office blood pressure should be monitored during at least two visits separated by two or more weeks for each change in dose or drug class. In addition, effects on target-organ disease and other concomitant disorders, such as diabetes mellitus, dyslipidemia, airways diseases, and arthritis, must be considered and monitored.

Special populations
Among hypertensive patients with ischemic heart disease (i.e., angina pectoris, post-myocardial infarction, silent ischemia on electrocardiography), beta blockers are preferred and diuretics probably should be avoided. If a beta blocker cannot be used, a calcium antagonist is preferred.

Large decreases in diastolic blood pressure should be considered with caution in patients with ischemic heart disease of the J-curve phenomenon [33]. This is because in hypertensive patients, ischemic heart disease may be caused by obstructive atherosclerotic epicardial coronary artery disease, abnormal regulation of coronary blood flow resulting from hypertensive heart disease, or both. Thus, higher perfusion pressure (i.e. diastolic blood pressure), may be necessary to maintain myocardial blood flow.

In hypertensive patients with congestive heart failure and a dilated left ventricle, reduced ejection fraction, or both, an ACE inhibitor is preferred, with or without a diuretic and digoxin. Those with diastolic dysfunction, normal ejection fraction, thick ventricular walls, and a small left ventricular cavity mass respond well to a calcium antagonist or beta-adrenergic blocker.

A diuretic or beta blocker alone or a combination of the two is effective for control of blood pressure and reduction of cardiovascular events, especially stroke, in older patients and those with isolated systolic hypertension [3, 4, 7, 27].

In patients with gout, arthritis, ventricular ectopic activity, dyslipidemia, or diabetes mellitus, diuretics should be avoided, if possible. In patients with diabetes mellitus and dyslipidemia, beta blockers should also be avoided. Whether a diuretic or a beta blocker or a combination of both allows progression of early or late atherosclerosis (especially among those with dyslipidemia or diabetes mellitus) when blood pressure control is maintained has not been documented in humans [3, 4, 7, 27].

Hypertensive patients with a history of asthma, obstructive airways disease, or claudication should not receive a beta blocker. Among hypertensive patients with renal failure, an ACE inhibitor or calcium-antagonist may slow progression, especially in the presence of diabetic nephropathy. However, physicians must be alert to the possibility of hyperkalemia induced by ACE inhibitors and worsening of renal failure. Nonsteroidal antiinflammatory drugs may accelerate renal failure in the presence of an ACE inhibitor [3, 4, 7, 27].

Black hypertensive patients respond less well to ACE inhibitors and beta blockers and better to diuretics than white hypertensive patients. Calcium antagonists and $alpha_1$ adrenergic blockers are equally effective in both groups [34].

References

1. National High Blood Pressure Education Program Working Group. Report on primary prevention of hypertension. Arch Int Med 1993;153:186–208.
2. The Fifth Report of the Joint National Committee on Detection, Evaluation and Treatment of High Blood Pressure. Arch Int Med 1993;153:154–83.
3. Kaplan NM. Clinical hypertension. Sixth edition. Baltimore: William and Wilkins, 1994.
4. Laragh JH, Brenner BM. Hypertension. Pathophysiology, diagnosis and management. Second edition. New York: Raven Press, 1994.
5. Bottini PD, Prisant LM, Carr AA. Automated blood pressure monitoring. Should it be used routinely in managing hypertension? Post Grad Med 1994;95:89.
6. American College of Physicians. Automated ambulatory blood pressure device and self-measured blood pressure monitoring devices: Their role in the diagnosis and management of hypertension. Ann Int Med 1993;118(11):889.
7. Licata G Manuale di Malattie dell'Apparato Cardiovascolare. Palermo, Italy: Ragno, 1991.
8. McInnes GT, Semple PF. Hypertension: Investigation, assessment and diagnosis. Br Med Bul 1994;50(2):443.
9. West JNW, Gosling P, Dimmitt SB, Littler WA. Non diabetic microalbuminuria in clinical practice and its relationship to posture, exercise and blood pressure. Clin Sci 1991;81:373–7.
10. Dominiczak AF, Lyall F, Morton JJ. Blood pressure, left ventricular mass and intracellular calcium in primary hyperparathyroidism. Clin Sci 1990;78:127–32.
11. Devereux R. Cardiac involvement in essential hypertension. Med Clin N Am 1987;71:813.
12. Sever P, Beevers G, Bulpitt C. Management guidelines in essential hypertension: Report of the Second Working Party of British Hypertension Society. Br Med J 1993;306:383–7.
13. Mann SJ, Pickering TG, Sos TA. Captopril urography in the diagnosis of renal artery stenosis: Accuracy and limitations. Am J Med 1991;90:30–40.
14. Macdougal JC, Isles CG, Stuart H. Overnight clonidine suppression test in the diagnosis and exclusion of pheochromocytoma. Am J Med 1988;84:993.
15. Stamler R, Stamler J, Gosch FC. Primary prevention of hypertension by nutritional–hygienic means: Final report of a randomized controlled trial. J Am Med Assoc 1989;262:1801–7.
16. Prisant LM, Houghton JL, Bottini BP, Carr AA. Hypertensive heart disease. How does blood pressure affect left ventricular mass? Post Grad Med 1994;95:59.
17. De Simone G, Devereux RB, Roman MJ, Alderman MH, Laragh JH. Echocardiographic LV mass and electrolyte intake predict arterial hypertension. Ann Int Med 1991;114:202–9.
18. Paul M, Ganten D. The molecular basis of cardiovascular hypertrophy: The role of the renin–angiotensin system. J Cardiovasc Pharmacol 1992;19(Suppl.5):51.

19. Pfeffer MA, Braunwald E. Effect of captopril on mortality and morbidity in patients with LV dysfunction after myocardial infarction. Results of the survival and ventricular enlargement trial. N Engl J Med 1992;327:669.
20. Ghali JK, Liao Y, Simmons B, Castaner A, Cao G, Cooper RS. The prognostic role of LV hypertrophy in patients with or without coronary artery disease. Ann Int Med 1992;117:831.
21. Levi D, Ho KKL, Kannel WB. The progresson from hypertension to overt heart failure. J Am Coll Cardiol 1993;21:101A.
22. Bonow RO, Udelson JE. LV diastolic dysfunction as a cause of congestive heart failure. Mechanisms and management. Ann Int Med 1992;117:502.
23. Perry IJ, Wannamethee G, Shaper AG. Haematocrit BP and stroke in middle-aged men. J Hypertens 1992;10:1430A.
24. Pinto A, Scaglione R, Galati D *et al.* Evaluation of regional haemodynamics and alterations of vascular wall of the lower limbs in hypertensive patients. Eur Heart J 1995;16:1692–7.
25. Licata G, Corrao S, Parrinello G, Scaglione R. Obesity and cardiovascular disease. Ann Ital Med Int 1994;9:29.
26. Harvey JM, Howie AJ, Lee SJ, Beevers DG. Renal biopsy findings in hypertensive patients with proteinuria. Lancet 1992;340:1435.
27. Ramsay LE, Yeo WW, Chadwick IG, Jackson PR. Non-pharmacological therapy of hypertension. Br Med Bull 1994;50:494.
28. World Hypertension League. WHL workshop: Economics of hypertension control. World Hypertens News 1991;20:4.
29. Subcommittee on Nonpharmacologic Therapy of the 1984 Joint National Committee on Detection, Evaluation, and Treatment of High Blood Pressure. Nonpharmacological approaches to the control of high blood pressure. Hypertension 1986;8:444–67.
30. Treatment of Mild Hypertension Research Group. The treatment of Mild Hypertension Study: A randomized, placebo-controlled trial of a nutritional–hygienic regimen along with various drug monotherapies. Arch Intern Med 1991;151:1413–23.
31. Alderman MH. A review of the JNC 1993. Am J Hypertens 1993;7:896–8.
32. Tobian L, Brunner HR, Cohn JN. Modern strategies to prevent coronary sequelae and stroke in hypertensive patients differ from the JNC V consensus guidelines. Am J Hypertens 1994;7:859–72.
33. Farnett L, Mulrow CD, Liner WD *et al.* The J-curve phenomenon and the treatment of hypertension: Is there a point beyond which pressure reduction is dangerous? J Am Med Assoc 1991;265:489.
34. Rutdlege DR. Race and hypertension. What is clinically relevant? Drugs 1994;47:914.

27. Varicose veins and varicose ulcers

CLAUDIO ALLEGRA, MARISA BONIFACIO, ANITA CARLIZZA, ANTONIO FREZZOTTI, MICHELE BARTOLO, BRUNA CARIOTI and DANIELA CASSIANI

Varicose veins are one of the most widespread and ancient diseases in the world. Ancient Egyptian hieroglyphics, Aztec illustrations and Greek bas-reliefs reported this disease in ordinary people in its different stages of evolution from tortuous venous dilation, to edema and trophic lesions. It is a disease which has been treated over time with ever more sophisticated techniques all aimed at a single result, namely elimination of escape routes.

The actual innovations in the therapeutic field are the result of different anesthetic techniques and of the study of the repercussion of the pressure in the large venous trunks on microcirculation. It took 300 years to distinguish outgoing and return circulation (Harvey), so it can be safely said that if the therapy is ancient, knowledge of the pathogenesis is relatively recent.

For such an affection to be represented in basreliefs since ancient times means that it must have been widespread even at that time. To attribute varicose vein disease to a modern lifestyle and associated risk factors (sedentary habits, overweight and so on) appears to be overreaching. In the past, as in the present, varicose disease has always been categorized among the minor affections despite its diffusion, even though it entails a heavy social burden due to ensuing chronic disability. Is this because of underestimation or because of low cultural interest? Lately some studies have been published with titles that invariably included the words 'practical', 'in daily practice', 'phlebology in clinical practice' and the like.

Classification and epidemiology

Definition

Etymologically, the word 'varicose' is derived from the Latin root 'varix', which means tortuous. According to such definition, therefore, a varicose vein should mean a tortuous vein; by convention, WHO has defined varicose veins as 'sack-like dilations of the veins which are frequently tortuous' [1]. There are therefore two characteristics of varicose veins: dilation and tortuousness.

The Basel study [2] employs a topographic criterion to distinguish varicose veins into three types, according to the district they belong to:

1. Truncal varicose veins if they are in the saphenous district.
2. Reticular if they are in the extra-saphenous superficial district.
3. Telangiectasias.

The classification of primitive and secondary varicose veins according to whether a direct causal factor can be identified or not is based on etiopathologic criteria. A description of the symptoms which a subject with varicose veins will present cannot be determined from the latter classification, which includes evolutional and therapeutic characteristics associated with etiopathogenesis.

Whether varicose veins fit into the framework of an 'obstructive phlebopathy' or 'dilatative phlebopathy' merits separate consideration. The distinction is important because it places emphasis on the pathogenesis of valvular reflux, which invariably constitutes the basic element of the onset, development and therapy of varicose veins. Furthermore, this distinction allows us to account for dolicho-mega veins and varicose veins from hypoplasia or valvular agenesia [3] which has appeared with greater frequency since echographic exploration of the venous system has been practiced routinely.

Epidemiology

The prevalence and incidence of varicose disease are not well known inasmuch as all studies report data with significant discrepancies according to the method of inquiry and the classification employed by a researcher in identifying the disease. Prevalence is defined as the frequency of the disease observed in a sample population at a given moment. Incidence is defined as the estimated number of patients in which the disease has developed in a sample population over a longer period of time. In varicose vein disease the confusion between the two concepts produces a so-called prevalence that varies from 15 to 56% [4].

Another cause of the discrepancies lies in the diversity among personnel who collect epidemiological data. The data available so far have been collected on a national and regional level and recorded by both medical and non-medical personnel through questionnaires and clinical examinations. The significant difference in approach is the reason for the discrepancies in the data reported.

A European survey has reported a percentage frequency of patients with venous insufficiency of 35% in the working population and over 50% among retired persons. From a survey conducted by the Italian Society of Vascular Desease (SIPV) it emerges that the percentage of patients with venous insufficiency, measured among other general medical pathologies, is 12.9% in cities with over 300 000 inhabitants and 10.4% in cities with less than 60 000 residents.

If the epidemiological data are uncertain, there is even more uncertainty as to the costs of the disease. The costs include the following:

1. Days of hospitalization.
2. Specialized outpatient visits.

3. Instrumental examinations.
4. Lost work days.
5. Drugs taken and non-pharmacological therapeutic treatments utilized.

The lack of consistency in the data also relates to the type of health-care system, which varies from country to country. Furthermore, case studies do not specify whether varicose veins surveyed are primitive or secondary to phlebothrombosis; this distinction is important, not only from the epidemiological standpoint, but also because secondary varicose veins entail greater treatment requirements for examination, therapy and hospitalization, and often involve systemic disease.

Anatomy and physiology of the venous system of the lower limbs

The returning blood flow system in the lower limbs consists of veins identified according to their position with respect to the aponeurotic fascia.

1. *Superficial saphenous system*, constituted by the great and small saphenous veins and their collaterals, which run above the aponeurotic muscle fascia in a sort of 'fibroadipose bed'. This is located under the 'subcutaneous pseudo-fascia' of connective tissue that is thin but rather resistant and protects them from accidental lesions and dilation forces, and anchors them to the muscular plains.
2. *Deep venous system*, under the aponeurotic fascia.
3. *System of communicating veins* or perforating veins that cross the aponeurotic fascia and connect the two systems either directly, by *direct communicants*, or by the interposition of muscular veins, by *indirect communicants.*

In addition to the communicants, the superficial and deep systems anastomose at junction points or at the *saphenopopliteal cross* and *saphenofemoral cross.*

In addition to the collaterals, the *subcutaneous venous network* feeds into the internal and external saphenous system, with variable distribution between the epidermis and hypodermis, which is more superficial with respect to the large veins of the saphenous system, which run above the pseudo-fascia of fibrous connective tissue that protects the saphenous axes and their collaterals.

The *superficial venous system* mainly consists of the great, internal or long saphenous vein, or safena magna, and the small, external or short saphenous vein, or safena parva. The great saphenous vein is the longest vein in the body; it commences approximately 15 mm from the anterior border of the inner malleolus, a fixed reference point, as a prolongation of the external marginal vein of the foot, and runs medially, accompanied by the saphenous nerve, the terminal branch of the femoral nerve, and flows into the femoral vein in the inguinal region crossing the fascia in the oval fossa of the thigh (Figure 27.1).

Before entering the oval fossa it is joined by at least seven small superficial tributaries and the following veins: *superficial circumflex iliac, inferior superficial epigastric* and *superficial external pudendal*, occasionally by the *internal pudendal* which usually terminates in the common femoral vein.

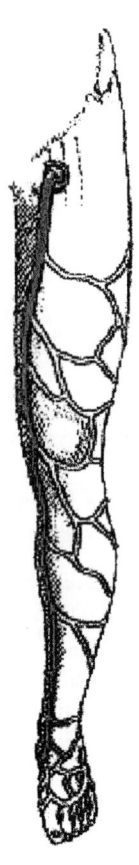

Figure 27.1. Internal saphena or great saphena: schematic course. Antero-medial projection of the lower limb.

Along its course it emits collateral branches, among which the most constant in the leg are the *anterior collateral of the leg* which originates at the dorsum of the foot and reaches the great saphenous at the medial third–upper third of the leg and the *posterior collateral, or Leonardo's vein*, that originates at the apex of the internal malleolus and, after emitting numerous and important perforating veins, connects to the internal saphena at the height of the anterior collateral. At the level of the thigh there are two important affluents, the *antero-lateral of the thigh*, sometimes called the *anterior saphenous of the thigh* and the *postero-medial of the thigh, or Cruveilhier's vein*, which, especially if of significant caliber, may substitute the great saphena on the operating table.

An inconstant collateral, *Giacomini's anastomotic vein*, connects the great saphena of the upper third of the thigh with the small saphena, running along the external posterior region of the thigh and flowing into the external saphena at a variable level of the leg (Figure 27.2).

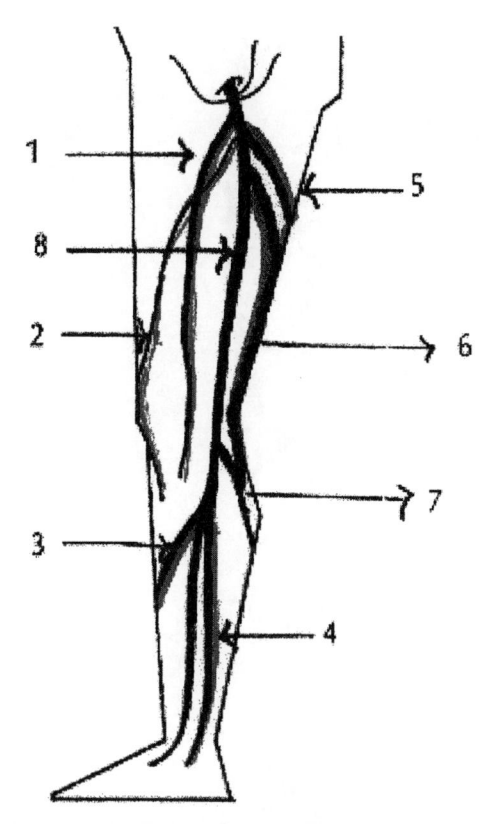

Figure 27.2. Diagram of the collaterals and the great and small saphena: medial projection of the lower limb. (1) anterior collateral vein of the internal saphena of the thigh; (2) antero-lateral collateral vein of the internal saphena of the thigh; (3) anterior collateral vein of the internal saphena of the leg; (4) posterior collateral vein of the internal saphena or Leonardo's vein of the leg; (5) posterior collateral vein of the internal saphena of the thigh; (6) Giacomini's anastomotic vein; (7) external saphena vein; (8) internal saphena vein.

The *external saphena* commences at the outer side of the foot as a continuation of the dorsal venous arch and ends in the popliteal vein, between the two heads of the gastrocnemius muscle, after a subfascial course in the intermediate tract (Figure 27.3).

Unlike the great saphena, duplication of the external saphena is rare (approximately 25%), while it is common to find anatomic variances of the termination, which may not be in the popliteal, but may flow through an intermediate branch into the great saphena or even into the deep femoral vein, usually within the first 3 cm above the bend of the knee, but can be found up to 7 cm cranially from the bend (Figure 27.4).

The *deep venous system* consists of satellite veins of the tibial and peroneal arteries of the leg and superficial and deep femorals of the thigh, in a ratio of 2:1 or rarely, 3:1 for veins of small or medium caliber and 1:1 for large-caliber vessels.

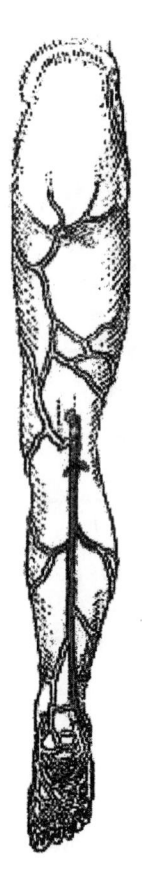

Figure 27.3. External or small saphena: schematic course. Posterior projection of the lower limb.

There are therefore two anterior tibial veins, two posterior tibial veins, two peroneal veins, one popliteal vein, one superficial femoral vein, not rarely double, and one deep femoral vein. In addition to the tibial and peroneal in the leg, which are intermuscular veins, the muscular veins of the soleus, which are sinusoidal in the adult, and the gastrocnemius, which is avalvular, have considerable importance; they number from two to four and are tributaries of the popliteal; running inside the muscle fascia, they are the most compressed during muscular contraction. The deep veins contribute in pairs to form individual trunks which join in the superior part of the calf to form the popliteal vein.

The *communicant veins* are divided into medial, lateral and posterior communicants of the leg and thigh; a medial communicant in the leg can be found just under the medial malleolus and three to four other communicants are located above the malleolus, behind the tibia. This group, commonly called Cockett's group, does not directly drain the great saphena but connects the vein of the posterior arch, or Leonardo's vein, with the posterior tibial veins. In addition to the more or less constant communicants, located at approximately 7, 12 and 18 cm from the medial

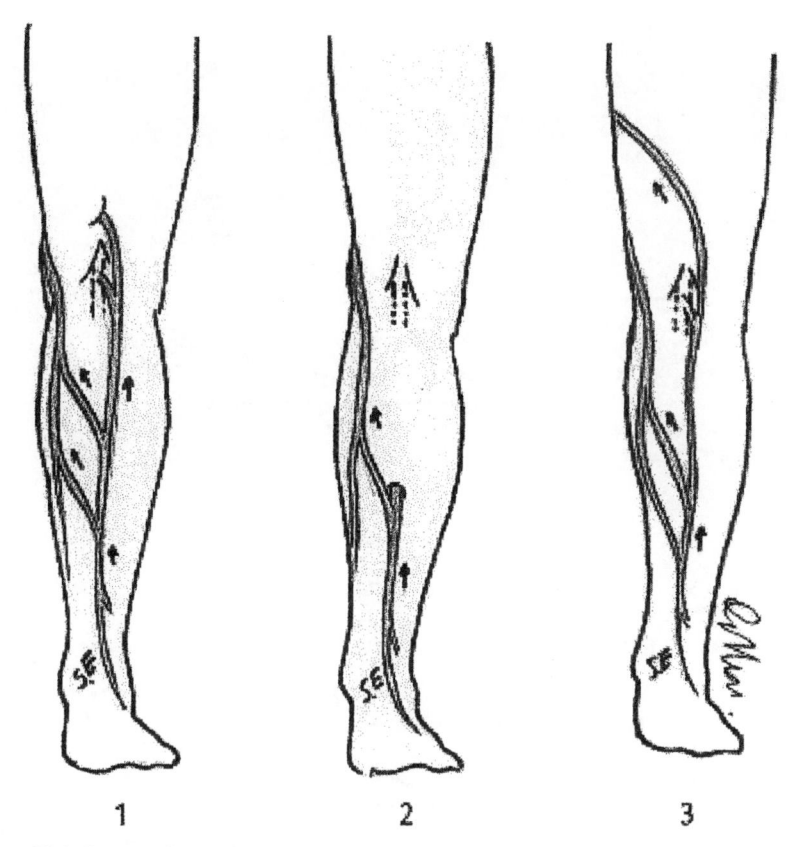

Figure 27.4. Some variants of the termination of the small saphenous vein: (1) bifid termination; (2) low outflow; (3) bifid termination with confluence of the higher lateral branch in the internal saphenous vein.

malleolus, one of the most constant (Boyd's communicant), found at approximately 10 cm below the knee joint, is a point of confluence with the anterior and posterior collaterals of the great saphena of the leg and connects the main saphena trunk with the posterior tibial veins. The lateral communicant veins do not have constant reference points and connect the small saphena with the peroneal veins at variable points.

More constant points of reference exist for the posterior communicants, at approximately 4 and 12 cm from the heel along the medial line in correspondence with the soleus and gastrocnemius points and they connect the small saphena with the muscle veins of the soleus and gastrocnemius muscles. In the thigh, the most constant connecting group between the saphena trunk and the femoral trunk is Dodd's group, composed of several veins that pass through Hunter's canal. The most surgically important and often described communicant veins are only a part of a system of over one hundred veins per limb (Figure 27.5) [4].

378   *Claudio Allegra* et al.

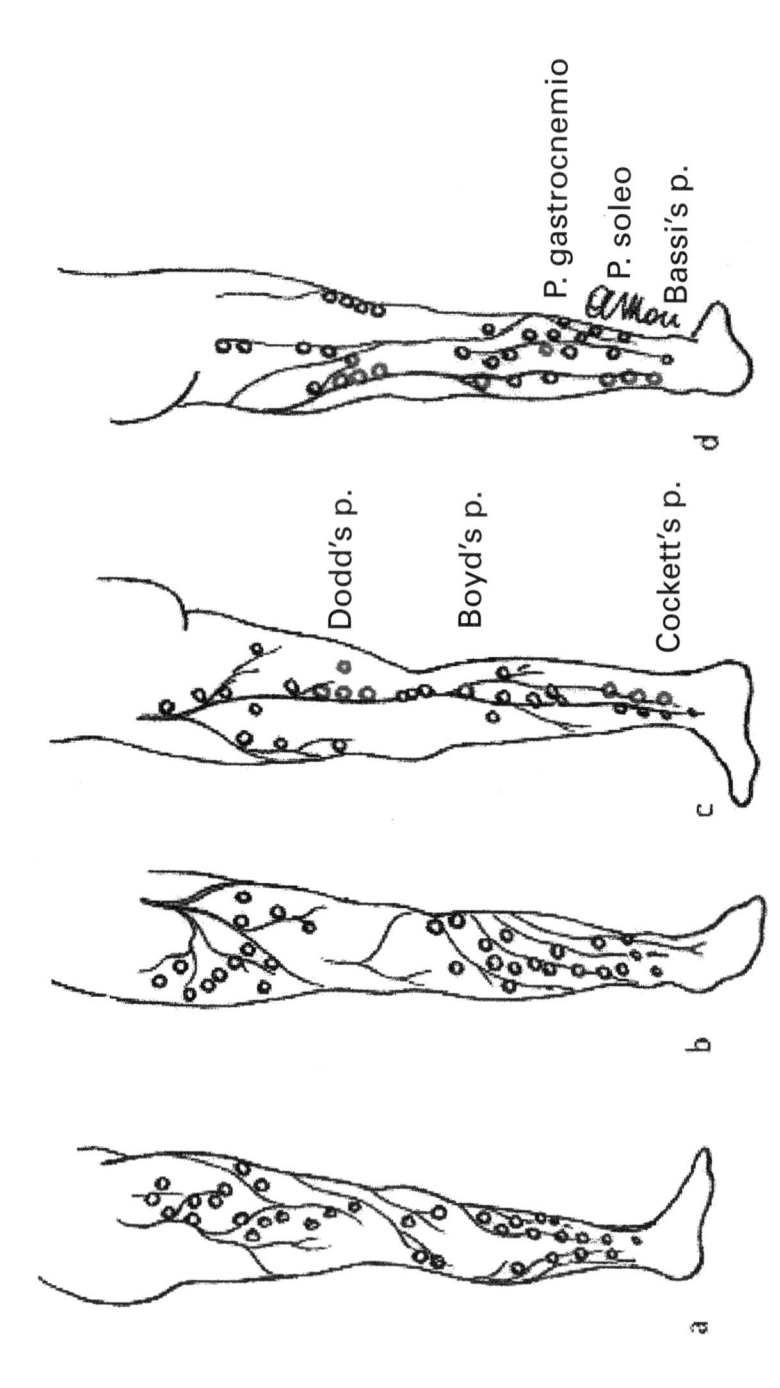

Figure 27.5. Communicant or perforating veins of the lower limb: (a) lateral aspect; (b) anterior aspect; (c) medial aspect; (d) posterior aspect.

The direction of the blood flow is assured by the integrity of the *valves*, constituted by duplications of the venous endothelium with elements of the media. The number of valves varies from person to person and from district to district; in the lower extremities they are numerous in deep veins, located below the fascia with respect to the superficial veins, and the number decreases in the cranial direction, there being a small number or none at all in 25% of subjects in the common femoral, few or none at all in 75% of subjects in the iliac veins, and none in the cava. Under physiological conditions, the proper play of the valves in the lower extremities, the cusps of which at rest fluctuate along the longitudinal axis of the vein, orients the direction of the blood from the superficial to the deep circulation and from down upwards.

Varicose veins

Topographically, we distinguish saphena varicose veins if caused by reflux from a cross or a saphena perforating vein, constituting the so-called *truncal* varicose veins if derived from the axes of the internal or external saphena or both, from the *saphena collateral varicose veins*, if caused generally by osteal refluxes directed toward the collaterals. Varicose veins are defined as *extrasaphena* if they originate from refluxes of extrasaphena origin (gluteal veins and external pudendal veins not fed by crosses). Despite the fact that the system of the great saphena is the most frequently involved in the varicose disease, its affluents are the most frequently dilated, in all likelihood because they are not protected by the layer of fibrous tissue that attaches it to the deep fascia [5].

Etiopathogenetic hypotheses and risk factors for primitive varicose veins

The most accredited etiopathogenetic hypothesis of primitive varicose disease identifies a congenital or at least familial structural and metabolic anomaly of the connective tissue of the venous wall in which there seems to be a lower content of elastin and collagen [4, 6] to which are added predisposing or risk factors which in order of importance are the following:

- Gender: the prevalence is two to three times greater in women than in men; the difference diminishes with age. In developing countries, perhaps because of the change in lifestyle imposed by type of work, men seem to be affected before women.
- Postural habits and work habits: all studies conducted on the disease have considered such variables, confirming a direct correlation between prolonged standing or sitting positions and the appearance of varicose veins.
- Body weight and diet: all studies confirm a correlation between excess weight and varicose veins. Excess weight reduces the front pressure induced by the diaphragm in the inspiratory position and, by compressing the intestinal packet on the iliac veins, causes centrifugal refluxes. Such refluxes have a direct effect on the saphenofemoral juncture since the cava lacks valves and the iliac veins have few of them. Excess weight is often associated with poor diet.

- Pregnancy: in addition to compression of the iliac and pelvic veins by the pregnant uterus, a predisposing factor can also be seen in modifications in the tone of the venous wall caused by progesterone. Both the number of pregnancies and the interval between them seem to play a role.
- Race: while the influence of race is in itself insignificant, various factors associated with race have an effect, including environmental, genetic, diet, constitutional and other factors such as clothing and occupation.
- Medication: the estrogen–progesterone drugs constitute a predisposing factor, as does pregnancy.

The microcirculation in venous disease

Venous diseases can be divided into acute and chronic. Acute venous disease, in turn, can be divided into superficial and deep phlebothrombosis and thrombophlebitis, and varicophlebitis. Chronic venous disease includes primary varicose veins and postphlebitic syndrome, which is the sequela of the acute inflammatory forms. To simplify, the clinical signs of chronic venous disease are grouped together under the name chronic venous insufficiency (CVI) [7, 8]. CVI is a condition that progresses over time from intermittent edema to trophic lesions (phlebostatic venous ulcer).

Classification of CVI

There are various classifications of the natural history of CVI, which differ depending on whether the evolutionary clinical aspect of the anatomical and functional involvement of the return circulation is taken into consideration. Varices are a constant feature of CVI and may be either primary (idiopathic varices) or secondary (following postphlebitic syndrome). These two forms are distinguished by their clinical course: rapidly worsening with the early appearance of trophic lesions in the secondary forms, slowly developing in the primary forms. Varicose veins are characterized by venous stasis, whose hemodynamic expression is reflux (reversal of the flow in the centrifugal direction). In primary varicose veins, reflux is caused by valvular incompetence, whereas in the secondary forms (phlebothrombosis) reflux is initially caused by the thrombotic occlusion which impedes venous return, and later by the destruction of the valves following recanalization.

Development of CVI

Two stages can be distinguished in venous insufficiency. The first stage is represented by avalvulation of the large venous trunks with reversal of the flow centrifugally through the perforator veins. Clearly, this phenomenon will be most evident where the gravitational force of the foot – heart water column is greatest, i.e., at the level of the lower third of the leg and, more specifically, of the Cockett perforator veins. At this level two flows meet: the large flow from above, drained

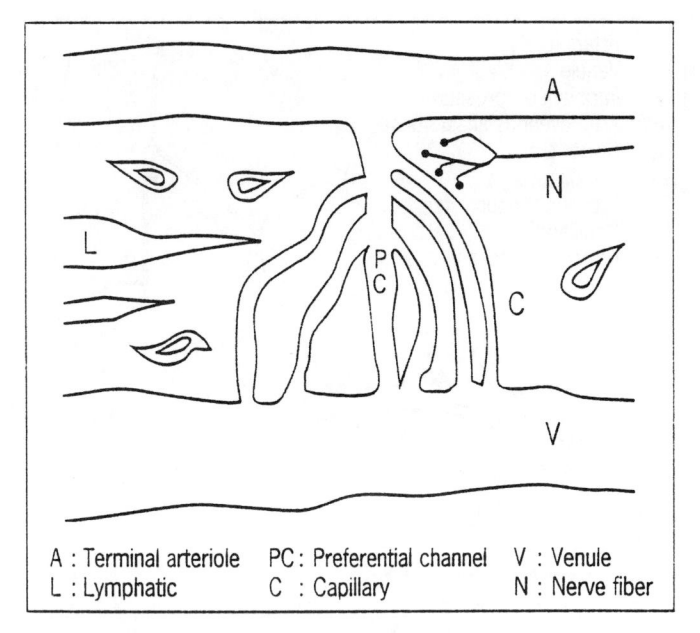

```
A : Terminal arteriole   PC : Preferential channel   V : Venule
L : Lymphatic            C  : Capillary              N : Nerve fiber
```

Figure 27.6. Schematic representation of the microcirculatory unit.

by the saphena system, and the short, horizontal flow from the perforator veins. The converging of these two flows results in blood stasis and increased venous pressure; this effect is greater during walking, due to the increase in deep venous pressure.

The second stage is reached when repercussions occur at the microcirculatory level. The microcirculatory unit consists of an afferent arteriole and several efferent venules. The arterial and venous elements are interconnected by a preferential channel from which the capillary network originates, and which thus represents the fulcrum of the two systems (Figure 27.6).

Upstream of the capillary system are the arteriovenous anastomoses, which are responsible for maintaining the pressure balance of drainage [9–11]. When stasis induces active or passive venous hypertension, the arteriovenous anastomoses become functional 'venalizing' the arteriole, thus relieving intraluminal venular pressure and avoiding an increase in capillary hydrostatic pressure [12]. The chemical mediators which are released during stasis may cause the closing of the precapillary sphincters (Figure 27.7).

If the disorder is not reversed, the affected microcirculatory unit is shunted in favor of others. The summation of the excluded units results in ischemia and stasis with overflow into the interstitial connective tissue and initial lymphatics. The lymphatic capillaries can only partially and not totally compensate for the dysfunction of the microcirculatory unit, since they are fewer in number than the blood capillaries. Hence the phlebolymphedema of CVI. From the above, it can be clearly seen how an initially purely macrocirculatory hemodynamic phenomenon becomes, via a

382 *Claudio Allegra* et al.

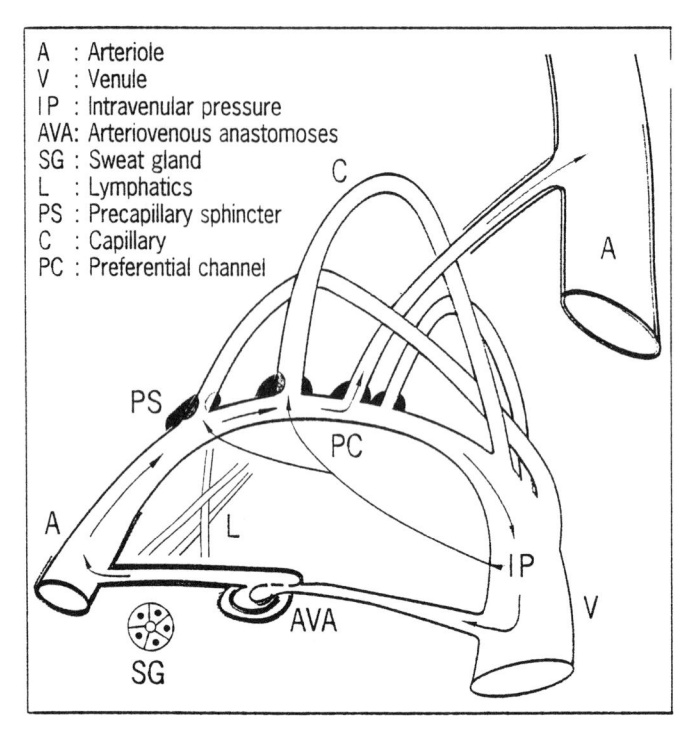

Figure 27.7. Aspect during venous hypertension with arteriolar venalization and closure of precapillary sphincters.

cascade effect, a microcirculatory one (Figure 27.8) [13]. With regard to the above-mentioned succession of the three fundamental clinical signs of CVI: edema, stasis pigmentation, and venous ulcer, the question arises as to how these three symptoms relate to the hemodynamic cascade of events characterizing CVI. We should remember the now classic distinction of the circulatory apparatus into conduction, distribution, exchange, and capacitance vessels: it is at the level of the exchange vessels (capillary network) that the key to these symptoms can be found [14].

Edema is classically attributed to a disequilibrium between intracapillary hydrostatic and oncotic pressure, and interstitial pressure. The trophic alterations, *stasis pigmentation* and *venous ulcer*, are related to the thickening of the basement membrane of the capillary as a result of endothelial damage, with disappearance of Copley's membrane and depolymerization of the glycosaminoglycans (GAGs) present in the lymphatic spaces of the basement membrane and in the pericapillary surface (pericapillary fibrin cuff phenomenon).

The above may be considered the 'traditional interpretation' of the mechanism of microcirculatory hemodynamic decompensation resulting from venous stasis.

Recent acquisitions

We shall now focus on the more recent acquisitions in the understanding of the mechanism of venous stasis. These may be summed up by four microcirculatory

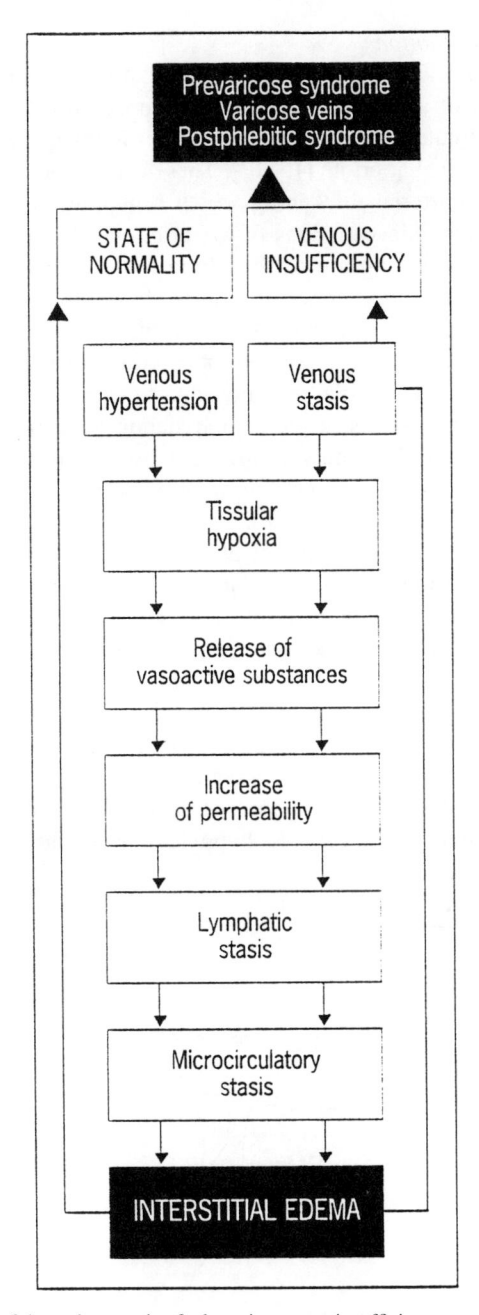

Figure 27.8. Diagram of the pathogenesis of edema in venous insufficiency.

phenomena: vasomotion and flowmotion; leukocyte activation; variation in functional capillary density; variation in pressure and permeability of the lymphatic microvessels.

Vasomotion and flowmotion

The term *vasomotion* designates rhythmic, oscillating movements resulting from successive periods of arteriolar dilatation and constriction (oscillation frequency 20±3 cycles per minute), the frequency of which is inversely proportional to the diameter of the terminal arteriole [15–17]. These oscillations appear to originate in a sphincter-like endarterial thickening which functions as a pacemaker (Figure 27.9) [18]. Such rhythmic variations of the arteriolar diameter are thought to be responsible for: a redistribution of the blood mass circulating in the capillary network; variations of blood concentration in the capillaries, thus changing the oncotic pressure/hydrostatic pressure ratio. In turn, the variations of frequency and the periods of arteriolar vasoconstriction or vasodilatation seem to be determined by the variations of the interstitial pressure and of the PO_2 through adenosine.

The term *flowmotion* refers to the hemodynamic outcome of vasomotion, i.e., the way in which capillary flow is affected by the fluctuations of arteriolar diameter. From a rheological standpoint, flowmotion obeys a stochastic law (Casson's law: $\sigma 1/2 = A\gamma 1/2 + B$) [7, 8].

On the basis of these new physiological acquisitions, a description of the actual succession of events triggered by stasis can be given. When stasis induces active or passive venous hypertension, the arteriole is shunted in order to reduce intraluminal venular pressure and avoid an increase in the capillary hydrostatic pressure. This defence mechanism causes upstream modifications of vasomotion, resulting in a prevalence of the phases of opening of the precapillary sphincters over those of closing at the arteriolar level (Figure 27.10) [19]. This in turn affects flow in the capillary network, avoiding capillary/tissue overflow and causing capillary hemoconcentration. This phenomenon, on the one hand, draws fluid from the interstitial spaces and, on the other hand, prevents hypoxic injury to the endothelium and sub-

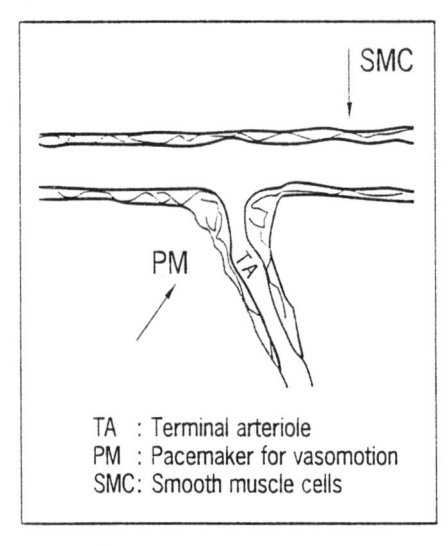

TA : Terminal arteriole
PM : Pacemaker for vasomotion
SMC: Smooth muscle cells

Figure 27.9. Schematic representation of the terminal bed with pacemaker sphincter.

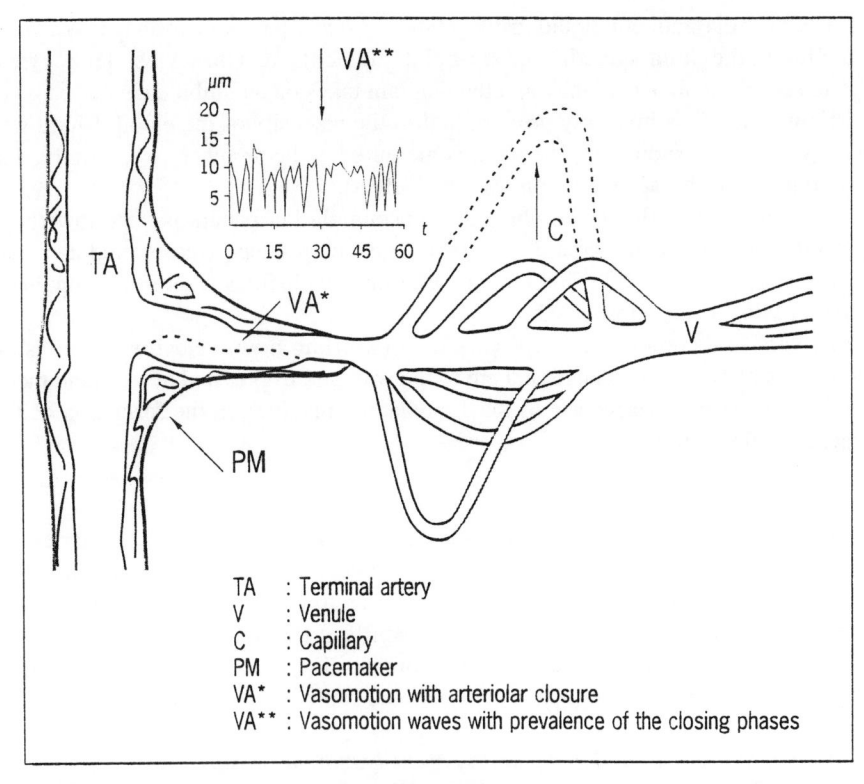

Figure 27.10. Schematic representation of the microcirculatory defense mechanism during venous stasis (from Allegra [12]).

TA : Terminal artery
V : Venule
C : Capillary
PM : Pacemaker
VA* : Vasomotion with arteriolar closure
VA** : Vasomotion waves with prevalence of the closing phases

sequent blood – tissue barrier alterations. In this respect, the capillary endothelium, which is characterized by the presence of a basement membrane without any underlying muscle cells, can be considered as an important organ playing a major role in microcirculation autoregulation.

The degree of continuity of the endothelium is of great importance in diffusion, which takes place through various direct and indirect mechanisms. When the continuity of this barrier is altered in the presence of stasis or perfusional ischemia, massive outflow of liquids and corpuscles into the interstitial spaces occurs, resulting first in edema, then in tissue necrosis [17–20].

Leukocyte activation
Blood is not a Newtonian, i.e. perfect, liquid, as it is pseudoplastic and thixotrophic as far as dispersion is concerned (corpuscular part dispersed and serous) and its viscosity varies depending on flow velocity. The fluid layer directly in contact with the wall (endothelium) has a flow velocity nearly equal to zero due to cohesive forces [21]. Velocity increases progressively as the fluid layer moves away from the periphery so that at the center the velocity is highest (coaxial velocity).

The flow diagram of a liquid inside a tube is usually parabolic in shape. When, as in blood, the fluid contains corpuscular elements (erythrocytes, leukocytes, platelets), these flow coaxially and the diagram takes on an umbilicate shape.

Flow velocity is inversely proportional to the viscosity of the blood. Blood viscosity varies depending on whether it is measured at the periphery or centrally, due to axial corpuscles accumulation (Magnus effect).

The minimum velocity at which axial accumulation occurs is very low (high tolerability index) and increase in velocity does not produce greater axial accumulation (Haynes) [21, 22]. This remains true up to velocities where the propulsion pressure/flow ratio is respected.

At very low (venous stasis) or very high (whirling flow) velocities, there is an axial loss of corpuscles. These adhere to the wall and trigger leukocyte phenomena which give rise to the release of local mediators, resulting in the formation of the capillary fibrin cuff.

Functional capillary density
Functional capillary density (FCD) indicates the number of perfused capillaries per tissue volume unit. FCD is a function of the critical closing pressure, which, at the capillary level, is itself a function of the interstitial pressure. Any increase in interstitial pressure (venous stasis with capillary overflow) accompanied by a reduction of capillary perfusion due to precapillary sphincter closure (venous hypertension) leads to a reduction of functional capillary density.

Variation in pressure and permeability of the lymphatic vessels
The initial lymphatic capillaries originate from fissures of the interstitial tissue, which open and close through the action of anchoring fibers according to variations in interstitial pressure. Interstitial pressure, in turn, is determined by the capillary oncotic and hydrostatic pressure ratio. The initial lymphatic capillaries consist

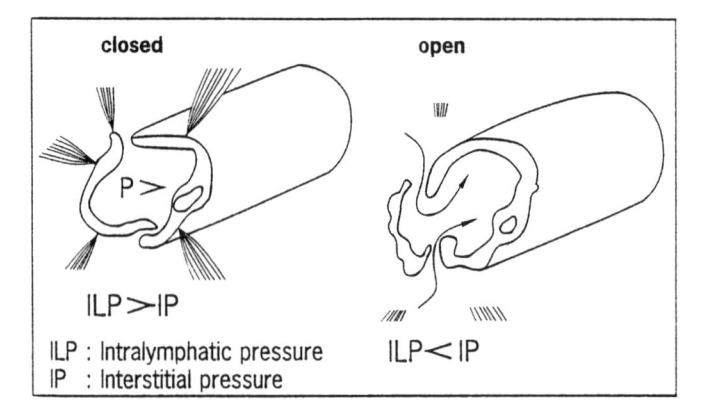

Figure 27.11. Opening and closing of the initial lymphatic capillaries depending on the interstitial pressure/intralymphatic pressure ratio.

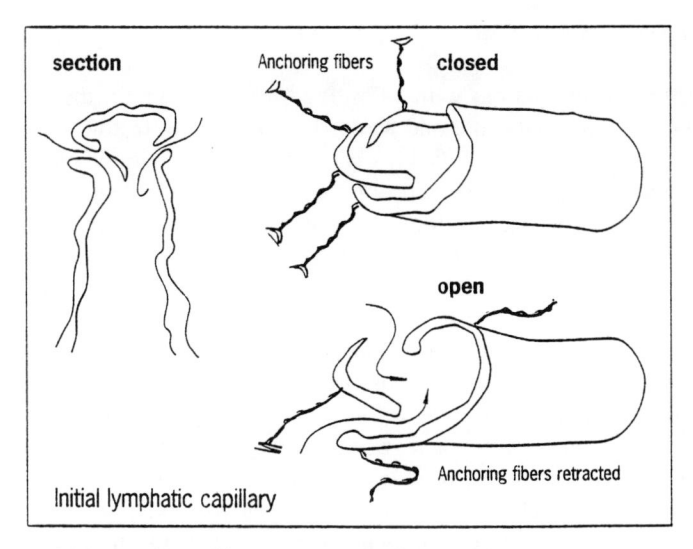

Figure 27.12. Initial lymphatic capillary with anchoring fibers and filaments.

exclusively of an endothelial layer. At very low interstitial pressures (4.0 ± 4.5 mmHg) the endothelial layer is continuous, and at high interstitial pressures the endothelial layer becomes permeable and the anchoring fibers retract, thereby making the virtual lymphatic capillary lumen become real (Figures 27.11 and 27.12).

Conclusion

These recent pathophysiological acquisitions highlight the major role played by the microcirculatory unit and give a clearer understanding of the mechanism through which initially purely macrocirculatory disorders – stasis and venous hypertension – cause well-known clinical manifestations of venous disease.

Clinical implications of varicose veins

Clinical examination

A careful patient history and a proper objective examination must establish in the physician's mind the physiopathological and hemodynamic cause of a varicose syndrome which will almost never appear exactly the same from patient to patient. Unless clinical examination has yielded the pathogenic cause, even the most advanced instrumental test can be misleading: how often have recidivist varicose veins brought to mind Shakespeare's words, 'there are more things in heaven and earth, Horatio, than I dreamt of in your philosophy'.

A first approach: patient history

In the history of the patient with primitive varicose veins in the lower limbs, variously combined congenital and acquired predisposing factors may be found. The first group comprises family history, female gender and altered statics. The second group comprises work activities and a sedentary lifestyle, overweight, estrogen–progestogen preparations and pregnancies, especially if close to one another. The appearance of varicose veins is reported in 20% of first pregnancies, while a family history of varicose veins is reported in 60% of cases. Increased weight and altered statics, which are often interrelated, are present in 40% of cases [23]. The results of surgical or accidental traumas, prolonged breastfeeding, discoagulopathies, hemopathologies, mesenchymal pathologies and neoplasias have an effect on the patient history as far as secondary varicose syndromes are concerned, since they are a more or less delayed sequela of postphlebitic syndrome. Among subjective symptoms, pain is reported to the physician with the greatest anxiety and frequency. However, in many cases, varicose veins are merely innocent bystanders in painful conditions of some other nature. Thus, the characteristics of the pain should be investigated as part of the patient history. Intensity, onset, extent, duration and, if present, variations while lying down and during muscular activity should be examined.

Varicose syndrome pain is described as a feeling of weight or tension often localized in the calf or the medial area of the leg or thigh. It is rarely of such intensity as to completely impede the patient's work activity. It develops progressively throughout the day and diminishes with rest or upon lying down in a supine position.

Neuralgic pain may be continuous or intermittent and is described as dull, acute, piercing or burning, and may be intense to the point of hampering normal activities. The pain and paresthesias are localized in the area of the interested nerve. Often the symptoms are more acute at night and basically independent of body position, or they may force the patient to assume an 'antalgic' position.

The characteristics of radicular pain conform with the above but have a dermatomeric distribution. In some cases, osteoarticular and muscular pain may improve with rest, but usually worsen with exertion and walking, and at any rate betray their causal and topographic relationship with activation of the affected muscle or articular groups.

In primitive varicose veins, and even more in secondary ones, pain may be particularly intense during the phase of hemodynamic district failure, with the involvement of venular and capillary districts, and coincident with the appearance of areas of tissue hypoxia and then ulceration.

Described as burning, it is localized in the lesion area and may not subside promptly when the patient lies down.

Common symptoms of varicose syndrome also include muscular cramps in the lower limbs while at rest. They are easily distinguished from arterial claudication since they have no relation to exertion. Lastly itching, which is often associated with dermatoepidermatitis, should be mentioned.

The objective examination

The examination should be performed with the patient standing and the lower limb semi-flected, that is, in the 'Greek statue' position. Edema, if present, appears while standing during the day. Usually it is not symmetrical and recedes with night rest. Edema not caused by pressure or heart dysfunction is always symmetrical and accompanied by other patient history and clinical elements such as hepatopathology, steatorrhea, dyspnea following exertion, orthopnea, etc. Lymphatic edema may be mono- or bilateral; it is usually more extensive and pronounced than edema from varicose veins, is cold and pale, less regressible and tends to stabilize.

Evaluation of the location of varicose veins may be very important. Primitive varicose veins are the result of an infelicitous combination between hydrostatic pressure, parietal hypotonia and valvular incompetence. Thus, they have a centrifugal flow and may be present exclusively in the lower limbs.

Secondary varicose veins are due to obstructed drainage or, more rarely, to hyperflow; thus they have a centripetal flow and edema may be present wherever the above-mentioned hemodynamic conditions subsist. For example, a varicose syndrome limited to the lower limb may lead one to suppose an 'essential' form. However, if suprapubic varicose veins are also present, an iliac obstruction with collateral intersaphena or contralateral saphenofemoral circulation should be sought.

When the patient is lying down with the ankle at the height of the right atrium, there is a complete, prompt abatement of phlebectasias in primitive varicose syndromes. In secondary varicose syndrome this often does not occur. The instrumental equivalent of this phenomenon occurs during the echographic examination: a very evident, distended saphena vein when lying down always indicates obstructed drainage of the DVC (deep venous circulation).

Based on caliber and anatomic site, varicose veins are classified as truncal, collateral, reticular, or corymbose. The first concern the large collectors of the superficial venous circulation and usually have a greater caliber and less tortuous path. Collateral varicose veins are generally of lesser caliber, but this is not a rule since they may reach large dimensions in some cases. Their course may have a complex configuration that is coiled, scallop or sponge-like. The collateral veins originate in the main trunks or the perforating veins. Varicose veins in the anteromedial area of the thigh may originate from the great saphena, its anterior collateral branch, the suprarotular branch, or Dodd's perforating veins. In the posterior and lateral areas, the veins may originate from the posterior collaterals, Giacomini's anastomotic vein or the posterior perforating veins of the thigh. The varicose veins of the lateral surface of the leg usually originate from the small saphena; posterior varicose veins originate from the latter or, as in the case of medial varicose veins, from the internal saphena, its collaterals or the perforating veins of the leg. Unfortunately, in this distribution, field invasions are not uncommon. The presence of isolated 'suspended' varicose veins is often due to the incompetence of one or more perforating veins. These therefore should be carefully sought through palpation. Pressing gently and alternatively with the fingertips on the varicosity, the examiner can follow its course upwards as if scrolling a keyboard. In many cases, at the origin of the varicosity there is a small tender area that is more or less round in shape and often painful, which is the site of the fascial interruption where the incompetent perforating vein is located. In these cases, with the patient lying down, a tourniquet is applied a few centimeters below the origin of the varicosity. The patient is then asked to rise, while the physician keeps the perforating vein compressed with the fingertips. Subsequent release of the two ends allows observation of the direction of the filling. Palpation also allows determination of the venous tone and the possible presence of thrombi in the varicose veins. In these cases, the examiner will also evaluate whether it is warm or painful to the touch. Palpation also determines the competence of the saphenofemoral and saphenopopliteal junctions. While palpating the two confluences with the patient in a standing position and the leg semi-flected, the physician should ask the patient to cough vigorously. In case of incompetence the physician will feel the expansion of the saphena wall, accompanied in some cases by vascular thrill.

The tests of Schwarz, Trendelemburg, and Perthes are the points of reference in phlebological semiotics.

Schwarz's test is carried out with the fingertips of both hands placed at a distance along the projection of the venous axis. One hand feels the reflux wave elicited by light percussions of the other hand. Performing the test in both directions can yield information on the continuity of the segments explored and on valvular competence.

The Trendelemburg test is begun with the patient supine, lifting the limb in order to empty completely the superficial venous circulation. With a tourniquet applied to the base of the thigh, the patient is asked to stand. Upon removal of the tourniquet, the physician may observe the direction of filling of the varicosity, which may occur from the bottom up, through the perforator veins, or rapidly from the top down due to incompetence of the saphenofemoral junction. In many cases, the filling will occur in both directions, showing a brief and a long reflux respectively of the perforating veins and the saphena junction. Repetition of the test with the tourniquet placed at several levels will allow the physician to identify with greater precision the loci of the incompetent perforating veins.

Perthes' test is carried out in a standing position by placing a tourniquet above the knee. Asking the patient to walk, the physician will witness the emptying of the varicose veins if deep venous circulation is pervious and the perforating veins are competent. In many cases of post-phlebitic syndrome there is no emptying but an accentuation of the varicosity.

Surgical treatment of primitive varicose syndromes

Surgical strategies may be summarized as follows:

1. Stripping along the great saphena vein; phlebectomy of the collaterals.
2. Short stripping of the great saphena; phlebectomy of the collaterals.
3. Stripping of the small saphena; phlebectomy of the collaterals.
4. Combinations of 1 and 3 or 2 and 3.

5. Phlebectomy of the collaterals.
6. Strategic ligature of veno-venous shunts in the context of superficial venous circulation (SVC) and between SVC and DVC (CHIVA).

The purpose of surgical strategy in essential varicose syndrome is to eliminate the long reflux paths (e.g. saphena) and short reflux paths (e.g. perforating and collateral veins).

Conceptually this may be obtained by the more or less extended removal of the superficial circulation and its connections with the subfascial circulation or by multiple ligatures and phlebectomies of the SVC and perforating veins, aimed at decreasing the number of reflux paths and restoring venous drainage. The latter solution, conceived by Claude Franceschi, is called CHIVA. Since it is conservative and less traumatic it is viewed favorably by many authors [24].

At this point it should be pointed out that whatever strategy is used, the clinical examination should include a careful anatomical and functional evaluation of the SVC and DVP through Doppler probe and color flow Doppler scanning. Precise echosonographic mapping of the escape routes and venous flow reentry is indispensable in CHIVA. Indeed, while in ablative therapy a dermatographic pencil is used to indicate the path of venous dilations and the site of any incompetent perforating veins, in CHIVA, hemodynamic references are indicated in addition to the morphological points of reference [25].

Stripping of the great saphenous vein

Short stripping has the advantage of making available a segment of vein for arterial grafts that may be needed in the future and is less harmful to the saphena nerve [26]. This strategy is acceptable so long as there is sufficient anatomic and functional integrity of the saphena vein in the leg. An ectatic, tortuous vein is a poor choice for an arterial graft.

Phlebectomy of collateral veins and ligature of perforating veins

Stripping the internal or external saphena vein is completed by phlebectomy of the collateral veins. In cases in which the saphena vein is competent at the cross, only phlebectomy of the collaterals need be performed, since usually under such conditions only a small number are ectatasic.

Performing a phlebectomy using Muller's technique at the point of varicosity found in prior mapping entails making small incisions of 3–4 mm at a distance from each other that allow extraction of the longest possible segment of vein. The collateral is grasped and extracted from the skin with hooks of various sizes [27]. The extroflected vein is thus sectioned between two mosquitoes. Perforating veins are tied as deeply as possible above the muscular fascia using microincisions [28]. Suprafascial ligature may not be effective in some cases, particularly when it is difficult to identify and follow the perforating vein for a sufficient length. However, in surgery on primitive varicose veins, suprafascial ligature is preferable to subfascial ligature since the latter produces unesthetic results and, depending on the technique used, may cause cutaneous necroses and muscular, arterial and nerve trauma. Before finishing up skin suturing it is a good idea to squeeze gently along the course of the ablations to allow clots to escape. Lastly, a compressive bandage is applied from the foot to the inguinal region. The patient is mobilized immediately after the surgery and the stitches removed on the fifth or sixth day.

Stripping of the small saphena vein

Stripping the external saphena vein should not be considered an obligatory complement to stripping the great saphena; it is justified only if the small saphena vein is incompetent. Valvular incompetence of the external saphena can be ascertained with certainty by clinical examination in only a small number of confirmed cases. In all cases it will be necessary to perform an ultrasonographic examination. It allows determination of valvular incompetence, the course and the confluence, which is often the site of anatomical variations. In 57% of cases the small saphena vein joins the popliteal vein a few centimeters above the fold of the popliteal fossa. In 10% of cases the saphena vein may have a shorter course and terminate in the subfascial veins of the calf. In 25% of cases it may anastomose with the great saphena above the knee. If the exact position of the external saphena and its junction cannot be determined by ultrasonography, phlebography is indicated [28].

CHIVA (Cure Conservatrice et Hemodynamique de l'Insuffisance Veineuse en Ambulatoire)

CHIVA surgery on varicose veins is based on two main hemodynamic elements: correction of veno-venous shunts (more commonly defined as short and long refluxes) and reduction of transmural venous pressure through segmentation of the hydrostatic column in the superficial-perforating veins circulation system. Figure 27.10 shows the concept of a veno-venous shunt schematically. In reality the reflux path can be very complex and involve several perforators and collaterals [24].

CHIVA provides for the exclusion of the main avenue of long reflux, through ligature of the saphenofemoral junction, respecting the more declivous reentry paths. This is accomplished by interrupting the short shunts and performing ligatures below the intermediate perforating veins. It is obvious that a strategy like this requires careful hemodynamic ultrasonographic study of the function of the DVC, of the perforating veins, of the escape and reentry routs, and adaptation of the intervention to the anatomical and functional framework. An imprecise hemodynamic strategy, sometimes fostered by the insurmountable complexity of the varicose architecture, may result in postoperative phlebitis from stasis.

Final considerations

Varicose vein syndrome is not life threatening. Therefore any condition that increases the risks associated with surgery may be a sufficient cause to forgo an ablative intervention. The threshold beyond which surgical risks caused by other pathological conditions outweighs the potential benefits of surgery on varicose veins should be clear in the mind of the physician and surgeon and should come naturally as a result of knowledge of the other diseases. The study of morphology and, more important, the hemodynamics of venous dysfunction will dictate the surgical strategy to be followed. Stripping the saphena is pointless if the saphena is competent at the cross. The small saphena need not necessarily share the fate of the great saphena. If the morphological and especially the functional evaluation is performed correctly the strategy to be followed will be obvious. Since the morphology of varicose veins is evident and unsightly, it may tempt the physician to neglect function and hemodynamics, which are the real but hidden causes of the morphology; these should be carefully sought out and studied.

Medical therapy

Varicose veins, in the sense of anatomical lesions, are not the target of medical treatment *per se*; treatment is aimed at the multiplicity of physiopathological and clinical conditions that constitute 'varicose disease'. The objectives of medical treatment of varicose veins are:

- to impede the progress of venous dilations;
- to correct or reduce venous and tissue stasis in order to avoid inundation of interstitial tissue, of which edema is the clinical expression;
- to reduce the symptomatology; and
- to prevent or treat complications.

These objectives are achievable through two types of treatment:

1. *Physical therapy*, which is the application of a number of measures aimed at reducing passive large-vessel venous hypertension, that is, intervention at the physiopathological moment that causes the onset and evolution of the disease. These measures consist of the prescription of *lifestyle and health guidelines*, and *compressive therapy* through bandages or compression hosiery. Lifestyle guidelines include a number of measures and habits aimed at improving the performance of organs or apparatuses involved in the dynamics of venous return; or at the reactivation or strengthening of all physiological antigravitational mechanisms, such as the muscular pump, through adequate physical or perhaps rehabilitative activity, proper squeezing of the plantar venous sole and the diaphragm pump to strengthen front pressure.

    Elastic-compressive therapy, which utilizes elastic bandages or compression hosiery with gradually decreasing pressure from the bottom up. To be effective it must achieve a sort of centripetal squeezing of the venous system, exercising a decreasing antigravitational counterpressure which, according to Laplace's equation, is directly proportional to the tension of the material utilized and inversely proportional to the curvature radius of the surface to be compressed.
2. *Pharmacologic therapy*, which is aimed at correcting morphofunctional alterations of the microcirculation caused by stasis, understood as the slowing down

of the return circulation, if possible before the onset of interstitial fibrosis. Pharmacologic substances currently in use are subdivided into the following:
Bioflavonoids:
- *Extracts*: present in certain plants, known since the medicine of Phoenician times: rutin, Troxerutin, whortleberry anticyanocides, diosmin.
- *Synthetics*: diosmin.
- *Associated*: part extract and part synthetic [4].

Non-bioflavonoids: dihydroergotamine, centella asiatica, pure or in association.

Varicose veins and varicose ulcers – instrumental testing

Noninvasive macrocirculatory and microcirculatory instrumental tests such as Doppler ultrasound, echography, reflected light rheography, laser Doppler, transcutaneous oxymetry and capillaroscopy, and invasive tests such as phlebography and microlymphography can be used. The characteristics, purposes and clinical utility of these are described below.

Doppler ultrasonography

A directional Doppler probe is used to study the venous system. With the patient lying down and still, venous pressures in the deep venous circulation and superficial circulation are measured. In the healthy subject venous pressure at the ankle averages 20 mmHg. In subjects with post-phlebitic syndrome (secondary varicose veins), there is an increase of 20–40 mmHg in venous pressure, usually with a greater burden on the posterior tibial vein compared to the internal saphena. In primitive varicose veins with long and/or short refluxes, venous pressure is increased in the internal saphena. Spontaneous venous noises are usually not detected in the superficial circulation. Examination of the deep venous system is performed with the patient lying on his/her back. This is an essentially dynamic examination whose interpretation is based mainly on subjective analysis of the sound signal [29]. Examination is carried out at the following levels:

- suprainguinal (inferior vena cava and iliac axes);
- femoral (common and superficial);
- popliteal; and
- sural.

The purpose of studying the deep venous system is to depict any obstructions and the collateral circulation and evaluate valvular competence [29–32]. In the normal subject, venous flow from the lower limbs is characterized by a continuous sound like a howling wind, which is modulated by respiratory acts. This sound, called the 'S-sound' (spontaneous), is caused by movement of the diaphragm that acts as a sort of venous valve. Above it, venous return to the heart is favored during inspiration inasmuch as it reduces intrathoracic pressure; below it, venous hemodynamics depend on the position of the subject: it is favored during inspiration in a standing position, while it is impeded in the supine position for opposite reasons. In forced inspiration, venous velocity tends toward zero and, during performance of the Valsalva maneuver, it ceases for the entire duration of the maneuver and resumes upon its termination. The 'A' sound (from acceleration) is a broad, sharp sound with decreasing tonalities resulting from compressive maneuvers on the muscles of the limbs which cause rapid acceleration of blood circulation in the event the probe is positioned below the point of compression. If the probe is placed above, there will be a drop in the curve (arrested flow) followed by a rapid peak of acceleration due to rehabilitation of the venous bed which had been previously emptied by compression. Lastly, the study of the sural venous system is carried out at the distal level by placing the probe on the posterior tibial vein and compressing the plantar venous sole; proximally the probe is placed at the level of the popliteal fossa. In case of venous occlusion (obstructive syndrome) [30–32], normally signal cannot be detected at the level of the occluded vessel; on the venous vessels above, velocity is detected and it is reduced in relation to the amount of collateral circulation, it is continuous and not modulated by respiratory acts and modified barely or not at all by the Valsalva maneuver. This is caused by venous hypertension as a result of the obstruction. At the point of collateral circulation, a high flow velocity is also detected. In case of rechanneling of the main venous trunk, an unmodulated high flow velocity can be detected; in order to differentiate it from the collateral circulation, a slight compression should be carried out with the probe that will interrupt the superficial collateral circulation without modifying the velocity graph of the principal vein. Valvular competence should be analyzed with respiratory acts, the Valsalva maneuver and compressions. The amount and duration of any reflux may yield qualitative information on the seriousness of valvular insufficiency [29].

Real-time echotomography

High-resolution real-time echotomography associated with a continuous or pulsed-wave Doppler ultrasound system permits study of the morphology and function of venous vessels. This examination must always be preceded by a conventional Doppler ultrasound examination of the venous circulation of the limb. The instrument must be capable of emission frequencies of 7.5 or 10 MHz that yield maximum spatial resolution on relatively superficial planes, permitting examination of the superficial venous system. For deep planes (iliac veins and, venae cavae), frequencies of 5 MHz are preferable [33, 34]. The examination should always be based on a comparison of the two limbs. The saphena veins along their courses, the main communicating veins, the saphenofemoral and saphenopopliteal crosses, and the deep venous circulation are examined. Under normal conditions the venous lumen is without echoes since circulating blood is normally nonechogenic [35]. Static examination shows a normal vein as a nonechogenic structure delimited by a thin homogenous layer of echoes. It is not very mobile spontaneously and at times it presents spontaneous caliber variations with respiratory acts and rhythmic movements transmitted from contiguous arteries. Inside the lumen, the venous valves can be detected as hyperechogenic mobile structures, which are more visible when open than shut. Venous walls, unlike arterial walls, may not be parallel inasmuch as they adhere to nearby anatomical structures. The postphlebitic venous wall is generally hyperechogenic, thicker and more rigid than normal, and rarely shows spontaneous movement. There are often irregularities in the endoluminal echogenic profile, with nonhomogeneous echo absorption caused by old thrombotic formations adhering to the walls.

The perforating veins may be studied in their course and caliber, and often their course can be followed until termination in the deep vein. The dynamic examination includes the compression test, the dilation test and the transmitted parietal mobility test. The compression test is performed by exercising slight pressure with the probe on the vein under examination; in normal conditions the vein is compressible until the walls touch; in the presence of a recent thrombus the occlusion is partial; in the presence of an old thrombus the vein cannot be compressed. The dilation test is performed by increasing venous pressure below the point of examination, by compression of the muscles or by the Valsalva maneuver; normally the vein dilates until it doubles in diameter; in case of an old thrombosis the test has no effect, while there is little change if the thrombosis is recent. The test outcome is significantly altered in the case of previous thrombophlebitis (sclerotic venous wall), but the vein can be squeezed shut by the compression test. The duplex examination, aiming the sample volume of the Doppler at a selected area, clarifies any remaining doubts. The study of thrombi requires particular care. A recent thrombus can be echogenic, nonechogenic or scarcely homogeneous. An old thrombus often appears hyperechogenic, nonhomogeneous and dilates the vein. The thrombus can occlude the lumen homogeneously with the wall; lastly it may present a floating tail, the movement of which can be detected during the dynamic examination. Thrombi in the internal saphena vein are very important and it is important to establish whether or not they extend to the crosses because, in the event that they do, there is a high risk of mobilization through the deep circulation [36]. Examination of the saphenofemoral and saphenopopliteal crosses respectively at the inguinal fold and the popliteal fossa is carried out with axial and transverse scanning. The anatomical structure of the crosses, any venous collaterals of the saphena that terminate in the vicinity of the crosses, and whether there are thrombotic formations near the termination of the saphena into the deep circulation should be examined [37].

Reflected light rheography (RLR)

This is a noninvasive testing method of the peripheral venous system suitable for evaluating variations in filling of the subcutaneous venous plexus. It is based on variations in skin luminosity caused by fixed components (cutaneous structures) and mobile components (blood). RLR records variations in skin luminosity based on venous flow [37]. The most important parameter is the venous filling time in seconds, which is over 25 seconds in the normal subject. In phlebopathic subjects the time is reduced, since reflux of incompetent vessels significantly affects venular filling time. The advantage of RLR in diagnosis of varicose vein pathology is its ability to discriminate between primitive varicose veins and those resulting from post-phlebitic syndrome (or deep venous hyperplasia) [38]. In the case of primitive varicose veins, venous filling time can be essentially superimposed on the time measured in a normal subject. In post-phlebitic syndrome, venous filling time is shortened in relation to the seriousness of the venous insufficiency [39, 40]. The advantages of the method consist in its noninvasiveness, repeatability, simplicity, and rapid execution.

Laser Doppler

Laser Doppler is an instrumental method that measures velocity, exploiting the Doppler effect of a low-power beam of laser light which, penetrating subcutaneous tissues, records nutritional capillary flow, which represents only 15% of the microcirculatory flow of the skin at rest, and derivative flow, which constitutes 85% of the total, provides thermoregulation and is the site of hemodynamic regulation and modulation [41]. The beam of coherent light penetrates the tissue, undergoes slight variations in frequency due to moving structures, mainly blood cells, and is then retrodiffused. The signal has a nondirectional amplitude and is a function of the average velocity multiplied by the concentration of blood cells then present in the target tissue. Values are expressed in relative terms as the difference between a zero signal and the actual signal. The amplitude of the signal is measured in perfusion units (PU) or arbitrary units of perfusion. The volume that can be measured, as a consequence of the depth of penetration of the laser beam, depends on the optical characteristics of the tissues. In the skin it is equal to a hemisphere with a radius of 1 mm. The patient should be examined in an environment with a constant temperature (23°C), avoiding other sources of thermal and emotional stimuli which may induce vasomotor reflexes. The probe is attached to the skin through a probe holder equipped with a double-adhesive ring and a thermostat. The examination begins with a spontaneous baseline signal and is usually accompanied by microcirculatory stimulation functional tests that analyze the functional reserve of the microcirculation. The tests most often used are reactive hyperemia, thermal stimulation, the postural test and venous occlusion test. In phlebology the most interesting data are provided by the postural test, which is based on the fact that in the standing position there is greater evidence of phlebopathy. The following parameters are considered: baseline, or resting flow (RF); flow variation after standing up, or standing flow (SF); their relationship expressed as VAR (RF–SF/RF × 100); and the microangiopathy index (VAR/RF) [42].

The VAR is a vasoconstriction response of precapillary arterioles in the transition from lying down, to the sitting position, to a standing position, aimed at protecting the microcirculation from hyperflow and limiting the increase in capillary pressure as a result of gravity. A normal subject who stands up experiences a 40% reduction in microflow in less than 3–5 min. In severe chronic venous insufficiency, the RF increases approximately three-fold and vasomotion is minimal, indicating that most of the capillaries are open. In a standing position the VAR is minimal [42, 43].

Transcutaneous oxymetry

This is a noninvasive complementary examination that evaluates the metabolic status of the tissue by recording the partial tension of O_2 and CO_2 extracted from the skin. The sensor consists of an electrode with a platinum cathode and a silver anode and incorporates an electrical resistor connected to a thermostat that maintains it at a constant temperature. The sensor is applied to cleansed skin and kept there for 20 minutes, enough time to read the values of PO_2 of the system at equilibrium. The sensor is brought to 44°C, the value at which there is a massive arteriolar dilation and consequent capillary arterialization with an increase in flow and the amount of O_2. The quantity of O_2 measured by the sensor is conditioned by capillary density and therefore by the amount of O_2 delivered by the arteriola through vasomotion, by use by the cutaneous cells, and by the thickness of the vessel walls of the derma and the epidermis [44].

In phlebology, measurements are carried out in the internal malleolar region which is most affected by stasis in proximity of the ulcer if present. In microangiopathy from stasis there is an increase in O_2 use and a defect in O_2 diffusion from the capillary to the tissue as a consequence of increased venular-capillary permeability due to venous hypertension, accompanied by edema, interstitial accumulation of macromolecules such as fibrinogen, formation of a perivasal fibrin cuff, fibroblastic activation, hypertrophy and collagen sclerosis. These all contribute to ulceration and atrophy.

Simultaneously with the fall in transcutaneous PO_2, there is an increase in transcutaneous PCO_2, which shows a metabolic tendency toward anaerobiosis, but it does not reach the critical levels of non-return found in critical ischemia and can be corrected with appropriate physical and pharmacologic therapy. In phlebology, transcutaneous oxymetry is useful during transitional phases to detect tendencies toward the subsequent stage and to evaluate the functional recovery of the microcirculation in response to therapy [45, 46].

Dynamic capillaroscopy

Microcirculatory alterations can be studied directly through dynamic capillaroscopy [13]. The system consists of a microscope that allows magnification of 10–40 times with a filter (515 nm is used) to visualize fluorescence and in a system of illumination with a mercury vapor lamp. The microscope is connected to a camera which in turn is connected to a videorecorder and a monitor that displays the field explored and records the images. Software allows morphological analysis of the images and calculation of various parameters such as:

- erythrocyte flow velocity;
- relative hematocrit;
- capillary diameter; and
- transcapillary diffusion of intravital tracers such as fluorescin 20%.

Measurement of the velocity (cross-correlation) indicates the velocity of RBC flow in the capillaries in mm/sec. The relative hematocrit is measured with a densitometric method, measuring the percentage difference in optical density between the two photometric windows. The densitometric method is also used to calculate the quantity of fluorescence inside and outside the capillary in arbitrary units.

According to the Widmer classification, stage I of chronic venous insufficiency (CVI) is characterized by slight edema and phlebectasic corona at the capillaroscopic level and shows microcirculatory alterations which are not very evident since there are still reactive mechanisms to combat the initial stages of stasis. Stage II is characterized by severe edema, hyperpigmentation and hyperkeratosis. The appearance of cutaneous capillaries changes profoundly since microcirculatory decompensation is underway. The capillaries appear dilated with a glomerular aspect and a pericapillary halo is present due to microedema; its edges however are still defined. In stage III, which is characterized by trophic lesions, the pericapillary halo is much more extensive and indistinct between adjacent capillaries, thus indicating the presence of a pericapillary edema which alters the blood–tissue exchange causing tissue hypoxia and cutaneous ulcerations [47, 48].

The flow velocity of red blood cells in stage II is less than in healthy subjects, while in stage III the reduction in velocity is even more marked. The relative microhematocrit instead increases significantly in both stage II and stage III with respect to healthy control subjects, losing the direct correlation between the trend in velocity and that of the capillary micro-hematocrit [49].

Capillary diffusion, evaluated through the injection of 1–1.5 ml NaF 20%, shows in stage III a faster escape of the tracer into the interstitial space compared with stage II [15] and therefore a greater luminous intensity throughout the explored range, at different measurement times form the appearance of fluorescence, probably due to increased endothelial permeability.

Microlymphography

It is now possible to visualize and study initial lymphatics in any body district and analyze important factors such as morphology, diameter, and permeability of microlymphatic vessels, and extension of the halo of the microcirculation in the inoculation zone. The microlymphatic images are obtained, under microscopic control with fluorescent light, by injecting 0.01 ml Dextran FICT 150 000 in the subepidermis utilizing a micro-needle with a diameter of 0.2 ml. Intramicrolymphatic pressure is measured using the Servo Nulling System linked to a computer. To enter the microlymphatic system, glass micropipettes that have a tip of 7–9 Tm and are filled with a 2M solution are utilized. The micropipette is mounted on a micromanipulator and, under microscopic guidance, penetrates the fluorescent microlymphatic vessel allowing measurement of endolymphatic pressure. Lasting venous stasis causes a functional overload of the lymphatic system that can lead over time to dynamic insufficiency by exceeding the transport capacity of the lymphatic vessels. Lymphoangiopathy will then ensue which will contribute to edema from venous as well as lymphatic hypertension [50, 51].

References

1. Prerovskly I. Diseases of the veins. World Health Organisation, Internal comunication. Mho- Pa 10964.
2. Widmer LK. Perpheral venous disorders. Prevalence and social-medical importance. Observations in 4529 apparently healthy persons. Basel III Study. Bern Hans Huber, 1978.
3. Bartolo M, Di Fortunato T, Antigniani PL. Epidemiologia delle flebopatie. Min Ang 1989;14:3–14.
4. Allegra C. Appunti di flebologia. Arti Grafiche Istaco, 1990:10–1.
5. Thompson H. The surgical anatomy of the superficial and perforating veins of the lower limb. Ann R Coll Surg Engl 1979:61–198.
6. Roose SS, Ahmed A. Some thoughts on the aetiology of varicose veins. J Cardiovasc Surg 1986:27–534.
7. Allegra C. Endotelio come Organo. Pragma, March 1991.
8. Allegra C. Comparison of investigation techniques in chronic venous insufficiency In: Raymond P Martimbeau, Prescott R, Zummo M (eds), Phlebology'92, Vol. 1, 11th World Congress of the Union Internationale de Phlébologie. Montreal, 30 August–4 September 1992. Paris: John Libbey Eurotext.
9. Curri SB. Correlazioni microvasculo-tessutali e stasi venosa = alterazioni dei microvasi e dei tessuti cutaneo, adiposo e muscolare. 4th Italian Phlebology Congress, Naples, 30 November–3 December 1987. Bologna: Monduzzi, 1987:265.
10. Merlen JF. Relations histo-angéiques en phlébologie. Phlebologie 1974; 27(4):427–31.
11. Merlen JF. Les modalités réactionelles a l'étage du lit vasculaire. Congres Anesthésiologie, Evian 1967.
12. Allegra C. Fino a che punto la stasi venulare e un fenomeno reversibile senza sequele? 5th National Congress of the Italian Clinical and Experimental Phlebology Society, Palermo, 7–10 December 1988. Monduzzi.
13. Bollinger A, Fagrell B. Clinical Capillaroscopy. Toronto: Hogrefe & Huber, 1990.
14. Allegra C, Carlizza A. Rheoplethysmography and laser Doppler velocimetry in the study of microcirculatory flow variability. Symposium on vasomotion and flowmotion. Rome, October'91. Prog Appl Microcirc 1991:20.
15. Allegra C, Intaglietta M, Messmer K. The role of the microcirculation in venous ulcers. Phlebolymphology 1994;2:3–8.
16. Intaglietta M, Allegra C. Vasomotion and flowmotion. Minerva Med 1992;17(Suppl.2).
17. Intaglietta M. La vasomotion comme activité microvasculaire normale et comme réaction a une perturbation de l'homéostasie. Prog Appl Microcirc 1989;15:1–9.
18. Colantoni A, Bertuglia S, Intaglietta M. Variations of rhythmical diameter changes at the arterial microvascular bifurcation. Pflugers Arch 1985;403:289–95.
19. Allegra C, Carioti B. Diffusione endoteliale capillare *in vivo*. Minerva Angiol 1993;18(Suppl.1):245–51.
20. Haynes RH. The rheology of blood. PhD thesis. University of Western Ontario, Canada, 1957.
21. Haynes RH, Burton AC. Proc 1st Nat Biophys Conf, 1959. Am J Physiol 1959;197:943–50.
22. Dormandy J, Thomas P. The role of leucocytes in chronic venous insufficiency and venous leg ulceration. Stemmer DR, London: John Libbey Eurotext Ltd. Phlebology 1989:113–5.
23. Schadeck M, Vin F. Varices des membres inferieures et grossesses. Phlebologie 1984;37:(4)561–9.
24. Franceschi C. Theorie et pratique de la cure conservatrice et hemodynamique de l'insuffisance veineuse en ambulatoire. L'Amarcon October 1988.
25. Browse NL, Burnard KG, Thomas ML. Malattie delle vene. Momento Med 1988; 1:209–50.
26. Bilancini S, Lucchi M. Le varici nella pratica quotidiana. Min Med 1991;333.
27. Muller R, Bacci PA. La flebectomia ambulatoriale. Salu Ed Intern 1987: 1–76.
28. Koffoed H. Peripheral nerve blocks at the knee and ankle in operations for common foot disorders. Clin Orthop 1982;168:97–101.
29. Bartolo M, Nicosia PM, Antignani PL, Todini AR. Rilievo delle pressioni Doppler: 10 anni di esperienza. Ultradiagnostica 1985;6:65.

30. Dauzat M. Pratique de l'ultrasonographie vasculaire, Doppler-echographie. Paris: Editions Vigot, 1986.
31. Sigel B. Diagnosis of the lower limb venous thrombosis by Doppler ultrasound technique. Arch Surg 1972;104–74.
32. Strandeness DE Jr, Summer DS. Ultrasonic velocity detector in the diagnosis of thromboplebitis. Arch Surg 1972;104–80.
33. Yao ST, Gourmos C, Hobbs JT. Detection of proximal vein thrombosis by Doppler ultrasound flow detection method. Lancet 1972;1–1.
34. Dauzat M. Pratique de l'ultrasonographie vasculaire, Doppler-échographie. Paris: Vigot, 1986.
35. Franceschi C, Franco G, Luizy F, Tanitte M. Precis D'echotomographie vasculaire. Paris: Vigot, 1986.
36. Larouche JP, Dauzat M. Echotomographie des veins: Proposition d'une methodologie et illustration des premiers resultats pour le diagnostic des thromboses veinouses profondes. J Imag Med 1983;2:193–7.
37. Tanitte M, Bonneton G, Morzol B, Aubert M. L'echographie veineuse en pratique angeologique courante. J Mal Vasc 1985;10:165–71.
38. Allegra C. La RLR nello studio dell' attivita sfigmica del plesso subpapillare. Atti del XIII Congresso Nazionale della Soc. It. Microcirc. Monduzzi, 1987.
39. Andreozzi GM. et al. La RLR. Impostazione metodologica. Atti del XIII Congresso Nazionale della Soc. Ital. Microcirc. Monduzzi, 1987.
40. Wieneirt V. et al. Eine neue apparative nichtinvasive diagnostik der chronisch-venosen insuffizienz. Phlebol U Proctol 1982;11–110.
41. Sheperd A, Oberg P. Laser Doppler blood flowmetry. Boston: Kluwer Academic Publishers, 1990:73.
42. Nilsson GE et al. Evaluation of a Laser Doppler flowmeter for measurement of tissue blood flow. IEEE Trans Biomed Eng 1989;27:597.
43. Belcaro GE et al. Blood flow in the perimalleolar skin in relation to posture in patients with venous hypertension. Ann Vasc Surg 1989;1:5–7.
44. Allegra C et al. TcPO2-TcPCO2: Topographie du pied et de la main chez des sujets sains. Angiologie 1988;84:535–8.
45. Belcaro G et al. The role of PCO_2 measurements in association with laser Doppler flowmetry in venous hypertension.
46. Franzeck U et al. Transcutaneous oxygen tension, capillary morphology and density in patients with chronic venous incompetence (CVI). Circulation 1984;70:6.
47. Speiser DE, Bollinger A. Microangiopathy in mild chronic venous incompetence (CVI): Morphological alterations and increased transcapillary diffusion detected by fluorscence videomicroscopy. Int J Microcirc Clin Exp 1991;10:55–66.
48. Allegra C, Carioti B, Cassiani D, Bartolo M, Jr. Relationship between relative haematocrit and blood cell velocity in blood human capillaries in chronic venous insufficiency. Int J Microcirc Clin Exp 1994;14:52.
49. Allegra C, Carioti B, Cassiani D, Bartolo M, Jr. Intravital capillaroscopy in subjects with mild and severe chronic venous insufficiency. Int J Microcirc Clin Exp 1994;14(Suppl.1):52.
50. Bartolo M, Todini AR, Antignani PL. Fisiopatologia del circolo linfatico. Atti del 5th Congresso nazionale della Societa Italiana di Patologia Vascolare. Cagliari, 8–11 December 1983.
51. Bassi G. Compendio di terapia flebologica. Minerva Medica, 1986.

28. Deep vein thrombosis

SERGIO COCCHERI

Definition

Deep vein thrombosis (DVT) results from formation and propagation of a thrombus, or multiple thrombi, along the lumen of veins situated under the muscular fascia of the lower, or less frequently, the upper limbs.

In the lower limbs, the thrombus frequently but not invariably originates in the deep veins of the calf (distal DTV), namely the tibial, peroneal and gastrocnemial veins, or in the soleal sinuses. Although DVT can initiate at any level of the deep vein system, 'proximal' DVT often results from centripetal propagation of a calf vein thrombus to more proximal veins, such as the popliteal, superficial and deep femoral, and iliac veins, and in some instances up to the vena cava.

Prevalence and natural history

The prevalence of DVT is difficult to evaluate as it is known that only one-third or less of all the cases are symptomatic. According to creditable epidemiological studies, the overall prevalence of DVT occurring in outpatients, or 'extra hospital', is evaluated to be around 0.3%. To this figure, many more cases of in-hospital (post-surgical or 'medical') DVT must be added. For instance, the frequency of postoperative DVT, when diagnosed with an objective method such as phlebography, can be expected to be around 30% (10–50%), especially if adequate prophylaxis is not provided. Thus, the overall prevalence of DVT can be estimated to be about 1–2% of the total population: DVT appears therefore to be a frequent disease.

Lone calf vein thrombosis is often asymptomatic, but it can progress into the proximal veins (popliteal and further cranially) in 20–30% of cases, thus becoming more frequently symptomatic.

Pulmonary embolism, the major complication of DVT, is more often a consequence of proximal rather than distal DVT, although not invariably so. The prevalence of symptomatic pulmonary embolism (PE) among patients with DVT not properly treated with anticoagulants may be as high as 4–8% (a quarter of them fatal). In properly treated DVT patients, symptomatic PE occurs in less than 1% of cases, but asymptomatic pulmonary microembolism diagnosed by means of lung scanning may be as frequent as 30–50% of DVT cases despite treatment. In a retrospective assessment it was calculated that, during 1968, around 200 000 fatalities due to PE occurred in the US, a figure that would indicate around 600 000 cases of symptomatic pulmonary embolism.

Etiology and risk factors

Surgery is the main risk factor for DVT in hospitalized patients. By the use of objective diagnostic techniques it has been demonstrated that more than two-thirds of all cases of post-surgical DVT are asymptomatic. In orthopedic surgery, and especially in elective hip or knee operations, phlebographically diagnosed DVT occurs as frequently as in 40–50% of cases if no prophylaxis is performed. Fatal pulmonary embolism appears to occur in 1–6% of cases after total elective hip replacement. During this operation, a specific additional thrombogenic factor is represented by intraoperative dislocation and torsion of the operated limb: thus, femoral vein thrombi are more frequent in the operated limb while calf vein thrombi are equally distributed in the two limbs.

DVT prevalence is also high in gynecological surgery, but especially after Wertheim's hysterectomy (27%), an operation usually performed for pelvic tumors. Regarding urological surgery, open prostatectomy has a DVT rate of 35% while in transurethral resection the DVT rate does not exceed 10%. General abdominal and thoracic surgery (14–33%) and neurosurgery also bear thrombotic complications.

Trauma, and especially lower limb fractures and their conservative or surgical treatment, are also frequently complicated by DVT (up to 50%). Peritrochanteric fractures are highly thrombogenic; the incidence of pulmonary embolism in these conditions is even higher (4–12%) than after elective hip surgery. Polytrauma is also often complicated by DVT.

Pregnancy *per se*, despite its physiological clotting activation state, does not appear to be associated with increased prevalence of DVT in the antepartum period, except in cases with primary thrombophilic conditions (see later). However, the *postpartum period*, where an additional traumatic, or sometimes surgical component must be considered, bears a high risk of DVT.

In other cases, DVT is a complication of typically 'medical' conditions: in cardiac disease, DVT complications of acute myocardial infarction (AMI) (34–38% with the fibrinogen leg scan) and pulmonary emboli have been found at autopsy in 7–8% of the fatal cases of AMI. Congestive heart failure is also associated with an increased risk of DVT and pulmonary embolism.

Malignancy is an important risk factor for DVT, both considered *per se*, and especially during cancer chemotherapy and oncologic surgery. Moreover, an episode of apparently 'idiopathic' DVT, in the absence of other known causes, can be associated with subsequent development of cancer. The relationship between malignancy and DVT is attributed to procoagulant substances (for example, the 'cancer procoagulant', a cysteine protease acting as a direct activator of Factor X) that are produced by tumor cells and especially released during chemotherapy and after surgery.

Other important risk conditions are neurological diseases with limb paralysis and immobility, as in stroke and paraplegia due to spinal injury.

Additional risk factors are: advanced age; obesity; diabetes; the nephrotic syndrome; some chronic inflammatory diseases such as ulcerative cholitis; varicose veins (dubious); prolonged immobilization and bed rest; and a history of previous thromboembolism.

With regard to blood groups, it has been suggested that DVT is less frequent in subjects belonging to O group, but this finding has not been proved. Some studies also suggest changes in prevalence according to geographical or ethnic factors, but this issue also is unresolved.

Oral contraceptives are associated with a higher incidence of DVT, with an increase in risk of 4–10 times in users of the pill. However, although a hypercoagulable state while on the pill is a common finding, clinical thrombosis is still a rare event. With use of the more recent, low-estrogen pills, the incidence of thrombosis appears to have been reduced. In many of the women affected by DVT during low-dose oral contraceptive use, factors of primary thrombophilia (see below) are often found: thus the pill seems to trigger thrombosis in the presence of an underlying primary thrombophilic disorder. Estrogen replacement therapy appears to bear no risk of DVT, or, in some studies, a risk lower than that of contraceptive estrogens. High-dose estrogens, as used in treatment of prostatic cancer and in suppression of lactation, increase the incidence of DVT.

Primary thrombophilic conditions are defined as biochemical blood abnormalities, congenital or acquired, which strongly predispose to thrombosis, and especially to DVT.

Among these states, congenital deficiencies of the main blood coagulation inhibitors, such as antithrombin III, protein C and protein S, are strongly associated with familial, juvenile, and recurrent DVT. Other factors of this group are: qualitative alterations in fibrinogen, and a defective fibrinolysis due to qualitative alterations in the plasminogen molecules, or to an increase in tissue activator inhibitor PAI 1 (the latter being more frequently acquired than congenital). Recently, a new abnormality has been described in the protein C pathway, the so-called 'activated protein C resistance' (APCR), a coagulation inhibition defect in which protein C and S are normal. This defect has been recently attributed to a mutation in Factor V (Factor V Leiden) that makes this factor less sensitive than normal Factor V to the inhibiting action of protein C. Increased APCR appears to represent the single most frequent abnormality among the primary thrombophilic conditions: its suggested prevalence is about 21% in series of thrombotic patients and about 3–6% in the general population.

With regard to acquired thrombophilic conditions, lupus-like anticoagulant (LAC), associated or not with anticardiolipin antibodies is often, but not invariably associated with recurrence of venous thrombosis.

Primary thrombophilic conditions should always be suspected in cases of apparently idiopathic and juvenile (under 45 years) DVT; especially if familial. However, the presence of other established risk factors such as pregnancy, oral contraceptives, surgery and trauma at young age, and even malignancy, does not exclude the presence of one of the primary thrombophilias.

Pathogenesis

The mechanisms of venous thrombogenesis are, in order of importance, disturbances of venous flow (stasis), activation of blood coagulation, and vessel wall damage. Venous thrombi usually form in regions of slow blood flow, as the large venous sinuses of the calf, valvular pockets of different deep veins, but also in avalvulated veins especially if exposed to trauma. Venous thrombi are usually predominantly composed of fibrin and red cells, with variable amounts of white blood cells and platelets.

Stasis favors formation of a venous thrombus by hampering the washing out and dilution of locally activated clotting factors, thus also preventing proper contact between coagulation activators and inhibitors. The main factor producing stasis is immobility: lack of a proper pump function of the calf muscles is especially severe in extreme cases, such as a paralyzed limb, but also occurs in other conditions, such as prolonged bed rest, or treatment of a fracture with plaster casts. Stasis is particularly marked in conditions of mechanical venous obstruction, either extrinsic as in pelvic tumors, or intrinsic, as after a first or recurrent episode of DVT.

Venous dilatation may be a contributory factor to stasis, occurring, for example, during pregnancy, contraceptive treatment, or as a consequence of release of venulo-dilating factors, such as leukotrienes, cytokines and tumor necrosis factor (TNF), after operations or during malignancy.

Hyperviscosity of blood, either due to a high hematocrit as in polycythemia vera, or to red blood cell rigidity as in spherocytosis and sickle cell anemia, or finally to dysproteinemic conditions and hyperfibrinogenemia (increased plasma viscosity), may act as a contributing factor to venous stasis.

Activation of blood coagulation occurs especially through the release of tissue factor and the formation of the tissue factor–Factor VII complex. This complex in turn activates both Factor X, directly, forming Factor Xa or prothrombinase, and Factor IX, recruiting the so-called intrinsic system that also contributes to the formation of prothrombinase. Release of tissue factor is not necessarily caused only by gross damage of the vessel wall, but can also result from endothelial cell 'perturbation' due to cytokines, TNF, and traces of thrombin; or from activation of inflammatory cells, such as leukocytes and especially monocytes, or malignant cells. Some types of malignant cells also produce a cysteine protease capable of directly activating Factor X to Xa. Activation of the intrinsic pathway through Factors XII and XI and activation of platelets seem to be a less important mechanisms in venous thrombogenesis. Activation of blood coagulation leads to cleavage of the prothrombin molecule and formation of thrombin, which in turn triggers transformation of fibrinogen into fibrin. These processes are especially relevant in areas of blood flow retardation (see above).

The rate by which Factor Xa, thrombin and fibrin are formed also depends on the power of the counter-regulatory mechanisms, such as the coagulation inhibitors antithrombin III, protein C and protein S, and the fibrinolytic system. Congenital deficiencies of these systems are known to favor venous thrombogenesis. Acquired deficiency of antithrombin III, such as occurs in liver disease and nephrotic syndrome, and during oral contraceptive use, may also favor venous thrombosis, as does increased production of the tissue fibrinolytic activator inhibitor PAI I, a consequence of endothelial cell perturbation.

A number of markers of blood clotting activation and ongoing coagulation can be measured in the laboratory, including the prothrombin fragment F1 + 2, reflecting cleavage of prothrombin by factor Xa; the fibrinogen fragment fibrinopeptide A (FPA), reflecting cleavage of fibrinogen by thrombin; and the fibrin degradation product 'D-dimer', reflecting the presence of cross-linked fibrin undergoing fibrinolysis.

Defective fibrinolysis is also a pathogenic factor for DVT. Physiologically, tissue fibrinolytic activity is lower in the leg veins compared with the arm veins. Reduced fibrinolytic activity was found to be associated with recurrent superficial and deep vein thrombosis, and with occurrence of DVT after hip surgery. The 'fibrinolytic shutdown' observed after surgical operations is probably an important contributory factor for postoperative DVT.

Vascular wall damage is generally considered less relevant in venous than in arterial thrombogenesis. However, overt venous wall injury has a definite role in thrombosis after direct mechanical trauma, and after hip or knee surgery. More discrete endothelial lesions or endothelial 'perturbation' can be brought about by cytokines, such as interleukin I and TNF, produced by inflammatory or malignant cells, even at remote sites, or by traces of preformed thrombin. Thus the endothelium loses its antithrombotic potential and becomes thrombogenic, by releasing tissue factor, activating the intrinsic Factors XII and XI, and triggering blood cell – endothelial interactions, leading to platelet and leukocyte activation and aggregation.

Diagnosis

Clinical signs and symptoms of DVT, when present, are as follows. The patient first complains of discomfort and pain at the calf, or, less frequently, the thigh. Ankle swelling occurs early, and edema quickly progresses to the calf, and also to the thigh in DVT involving femoral or more proximal veins. Distension of superficial veins can be observed and the affected limb appears red or cyanotic, or less frequently pale. Pain persists for a few days even under proper treatment, especially, but not only, in the upright position. Forced dorsiflexion is painful or increases pain (Homan's sign). Differential diagnosis on a clinical basis must include consideration of many affections causing a swollen or painful leg. Among them, chronic venous insufficiency and postphlebitic syndrome, lymphedema and especially musculoskeletal condition, or an inflamed popliteal cyst (Baker's cyst) should be considered. A recently proposed standardized clinical model was shown to improve accuracy of diagnosis significantly [1].

Clinical suspicion of DVT, when compared with the results of phlebography, turns out to be incorrect in more than half the cases. It has been reported [2] that in a series of 87 cases with clinical suspicion of DVT but a normal phlebogram, musculoskeletal affections were the most frequent underlying condition (42.5%), whereas 13.8% of patients had venous or lymphatic insufficiency, and 4.6% an inflamed Baker's cyst.

On the other hand, DVT is often clinically asymptomatic [3, 4]: data on postoperative DVT showed that only one-third or less of DVTs proven with objective methods had been clinically suspected. This observation is extremely important, especially in view of the fact that the main complications of DVT, namely pulmonary embolism and post-thrombotic syndrome, can occur during and after asymptomatic as well as symptomatic cases of DVT.

It is therefore clear that objective instrumental methods are mandatory for a correct diagnosis of DVT, both in clinical trials, to warrant disclosure of asymptomatic cases, and in clinical practice, in order to allow confirmation of the clinical suspicion, considering the potential hazards of effective antithrombotic treatment [5].

Despite progress in other less invasive diagnostic techniques, ascending phlebography still stands as the diagnostic 'gold standard' for DVT. Phlebography, especially if performed by the method of Rabinov and Paulin, correctly detects symptomatic and asymptomatic DVTs both in the distal and in the proximal districts. Phlebography has however a few pitfalls: a certain degree of technical and operator-related variability in the evaluation of the filling of minor distal veins; a few uncomfortable side-effects, including chemical thrombophlebitis, mostly superficial (in 2% of all phlebographic procedures); and the costs of the procedure. However, the risk–benefit and cost–benefit ratios of phlebography are favorable in all cases in which absolutely accurate and thorough diagnosis is required: asymptomatic patients, as in postoperative DVT prevention trials; distal DVT with contraindications for antithrombotic therapy; suspected recurrent DVT; or recurrent DVT in the course of a postphlebitic syndrome. For the diagnosis of more proximal thromboses of the pelvis and abdomen, computer assisted phlebography is superior to conventional phlebography.

Real time B-mode echotomography is a validated alternative to phlebography in the diagnosis of symptomatic proximal DVT. Doppler venous flow detection improves the performance of echotomography, but is not essential in this indication. The main diagnostic criterion for echotomographic assessment of proximal DVT is failure of the explored vein (popliteal or femoral) to collapse under compression exerted by gentle pressure with the ultrasonographic probe (Figures 28.1 and 28.2). Direct detection of intravascular echogenic material is useful but not essential. In symptomatic patients compression ultrasonography has a high sensitivity and specificity for proximal DVT (Table 28.1). Compression ultrasonography is however non-validated for distal DVT, and inadequate for all asymptomatic thromboses, even those proximal, as these forms are usually due to small non-occlusive thrombi that may not affect vein compressibility.

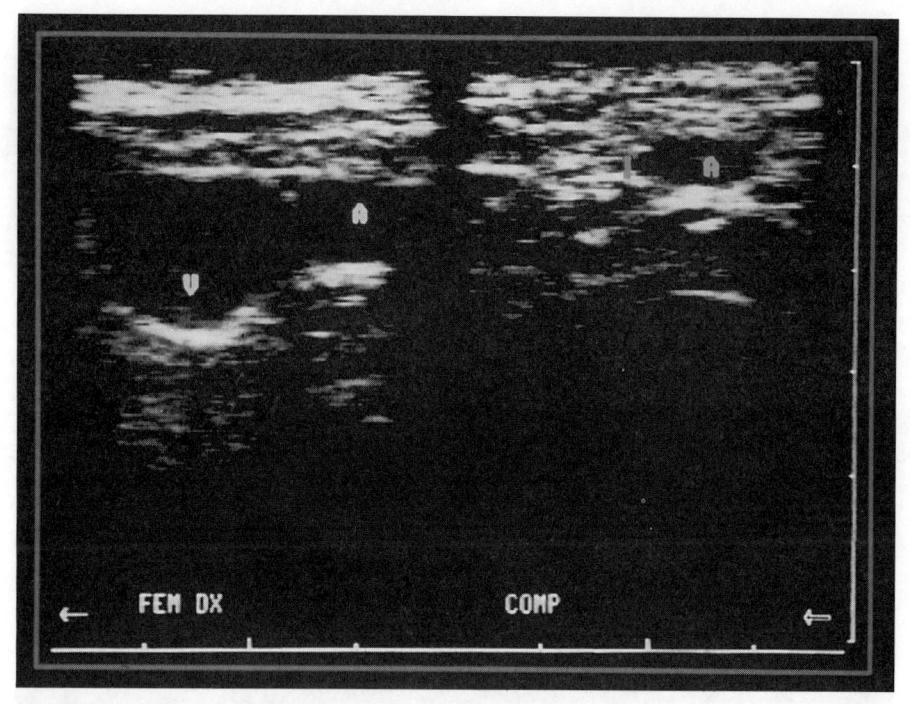

Figure 28.1. Healthy control. Compression echotomography of the right common femoral vein. See, in the right side of figure, complete collapse of the vein after compression. No femoral DVT.

Impedance plethysmography measures the electrical impedance between two electrodes placed around the calf. Venous obstruction and blood engorgement proximal to the measurement site decrease the limb's impedance (blood being a good conductor) or rather prevent the fall of impedance occurring in normal limbs after deflation of a cuff. Impedance plethysmography is not very sensitive to calf vein thrombosis but performs well in proximal DVT. However, its sensitivity has recently been questioned, and found especially inadequate in asymptomatic DVT.

Radio-iodinated fibrinogen scanning has been the most widely used method in clinical studies of postoperative DVT prophylaxis. This method is very sensitive to calf-vein thrombosis, but rather insensitive to the more proximal thigh thromboses. Fibrinogen scanning has now been abandoned because of the theoretical risk of viral transmission by hemoderivates.

More recently developed methods, such as radionuclide venography and magnetic resonance venography, have been studied in some centers. Magnetic resonance venography has recently been validated against traditional phlebography in proximal DVT [6].

The main contribution of the clinical laboratory to the diagnosis of DVT is the measurement of D-dimer, a fibrin degradation product specific for cross-linked fibrin. D-dimer has a high sensitivity for DVT and pulmonary embolism, coupled with a poor specificity (Table 28.2). Therefore, it should be considered only for its

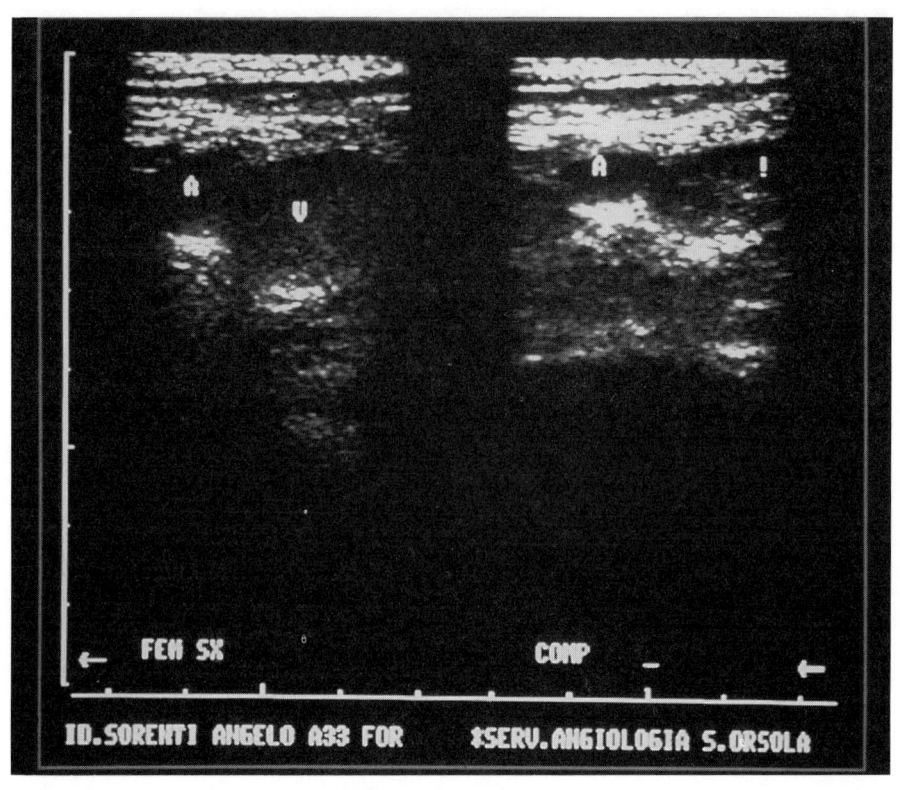

Figure 28.2. Case with suspected proximal DVT. Compression echotomography of left common femoral vein. See, in the right side of figure, no collapse of the vein under compression. Femoral DVT.

Table 28.1. Sensitivity and specificity of noninvasive instrumental procedures in diagnosis of proximal symptomatic DVT versus ascending phlebography. Notice the high values for compression echotomography, with no additional advantage from 'color' devices.

Procedure	Sensitivity (%)	Specificity (%)
Impedance plethysmography	92	95
Doppler flowmetry	88	88
Compression echotomography	97	97
Echo-color Doppler	97	97

Table 28.2. High sensitivity and low specificity of D-dimer test (ELISA or EIA methods) in ascertained DVT, in five recent studies.

Study and year		Sensitivity (%)	Specificity (%)
Elias	1990	98	29
Kroneman	1991	92	21
Boneu	1991	94	51
Heijboer	1992	100	25
DVT Enox	1993	97	?

negative predictive value and always in combination with imaging techniques. Coupling of compression phlebography and D-dimer test gives optimal results.

To summarize, ascending phlebography is still the gold standard for both symptomatic and asymptomatic, proximal and distal DVT. However, in symptomatic patients, compression ultrasonography is diagnostic for proximal DVT, and echotomographic follow-up can determine the patients in which an initial calf thrombosis progresses to more proximal veins, thus selecting the cases deserving immediate full-dose anticoagulation. D-dimer can be useful, if negative, to exclude DVT, but should always be combined with imaging techniques.

Prophylaxis

Because of the serious complications of DVT and the potential hazards of an effective antithrombotic therapy, prevention of DVT in patients at risk is preferable to the necessity of treating the acute condition. Most of the experience collected over the last 20 years refers to prevention of postoperative DVT. Postoperative DVT is an ideal model for clinical trials of prevention, as it offers a condition of medium- to high-risk concentrated in a well identifiable and rather short period of time. The information on prevention of DVT in medical conditions is more limited.

Studies of postoperative DVT prophylaxis must consider all types of DVT, either proximal or distal, symptomatic or asymptomatic, occurring after operation. Therefore, only those studies in which objective instrumental diagnosis of DVT was performed can be considered. Unfortunately, compression echotomography is rather insensitive both to asymptomatic and to distal DVT. Therefore, only the studies carried out with radioactive fibrinogen scanning or, even better, with phlebography, can be considered.

Non-pharmacologic measures of prophylaxis are especially designed to counteract venous stasis, a major pathogenic factor of DVT. Intermittent bilateral pneumatic compression of the calf muscles with a special mechanical device has proved to be effective in several forms of postoperative DVT, especially in medium-risk patients, and can be preferred in certain types of surgery at high bleeding risk (e.g. neurosurgery). However, pneumatic compression is a costly procedure as it involves logistic and human resources. Another apparatus, the so-called 'foot pump', which exerts intermittent compression on the plantar venous sinuses, is presently undergoing final stages of evaluation. Graduated elastic stockings with 18 mm Hg compression at the ankle, gradually decreasing proximally (so-called 'antiembolism stockings'), are effective in low-risk patients, and, together with pharmacological therapy, in medium- to high-risk patients.

Pharmacological agents include standard heparin, low molecular weight (LMW) heparin, oral anticoagulants, dextran, and the antiplatelet drug aspirin.

Low-dose subcutaneous heparin (calcium or sodium salt) at the standard dose of 5000 U every 12 or 8 hours, begun preoperatively and continued to the seventh of eight postoperative day, is still the first choice treatment in the majority of medium-risk surgical conditions. The same doses of heparin given for variable durations have been shown to be effective in medical conditions, such as after myocardial infarction, stroke, etc. According to a meta-analysis the protective effect of subcutaneous low-dose heparin can be quantified as a 50–66% reduction of the relative risk of DVT and a 40–64% reduction of the rate of pulmonary embolism. The relative risk of major hemorrhage, especially represented by wound hematoma requiring reintervention, increased by 2%, but no increase in fatal bleedings was recorded.

Although the effectiveness of low-dose heparin has been proved beyond any doubt [7], it is evident that in high thrombotic risk surgery (such as orthopedic and oncologic), the quoted relative risk reduction is not satisfactory in absolute terms, as a considerable number of DVT episodes could not be prevented. In order to obtain pharmacological preparations of heparins with a better ratio between the antithrombotic activity (simplistically identified with Factor Xa effect) versus the prohemorrhagic activity (simplistically attributed to the antithrombin activity, revealed by APTT prolongation), a number of low molecular weight heparin fractions have been prepared and made available for therapy.

Thorough clinical testing has demonstrated that LMW heparins are more effective, and also more cost-effective, than standard heparin in the prevention of DVT after orthopedic surgery, and probably also in other high-risk operations and patients. The benefit of LMW heparins versus standard heparin is only marginal in general surgery and in low- to medium-risk patients. LMW heparins have two other important advantages: they can be administered once or twice a day because of their long bioavailability; and they are marginally safer in terms of hemorragic risk, and definitely safer in terms of heparin-induced thrombocytopenia [8, 9].

Low-dose oral anticoagulants have been proved to be effective in selected series of patients at high thrombotic risk, as in orthopedic surgery, hip fractures, and in women with advanced breast cancer treated with chemotherapy.

Low molecular weight dextran is also effective in DVT prevention: however, its use is limited by: the volume overload, hazardous especially in the elderly; some described allergic reactions; and the high costs.

A recent meta-analysis has shown that aspirin may also be effective. However, given the contradictory results of the trials, there is currently no rational ground to recommend aspirin or other antiplatelet drugs instead of heparin or LMW heparins in prevention of DVT.

The evaluation of thrombotic risk in surgical or medical patients is essential for a correct prophylactic choice. Clinical criteria related to the patients are: any disease predisposing to thrombosis (e.g. tumors, diabetes, chronic inflammation), age, obesity, previous thromboembolism, varicose veins, pregnancy, and oral contraceptives. Criteria related to the type of surgery are: the surgical procedure (e.g., hip surgery, pelvic and urologic surgery), its duration, the type of anesthesia etc.

Despite many studies, it has up to now proved non-beneficial, and certainly non-economical, to rely on laboratory tests to evaluate the risk, especially in relation to postsurgical thrombosis. Evaluation of the risk of postoperative thrombosis is therefore a clinical problem.

Thus a low-risk can be attributed to patients younger than 40 years, undergoing general surgery operations of less than 60 minutes duration; or to a medical condition such as pregnancy – graduated compression stockings and early ambulation will be sufficient. A medium or moderate risk is attributed to patients aged over 40 years undergoing general surgery operations of more than 60 minutes duration, or to frankly thrombogenic medical conditions such as myocardial infarction, congestive heart failure, and the postpartum period. In moderate-risk cases, low-dose heparin twice daily, possibly associated with elastic stockings, or pneumatic compression, is recommended. High-risk allocation is reserved for elderly patients with additional risk factors (e.g. tumors) and long-lasting operations, or for elective hip or knee arthroplasty, major fractures or polytrauma, and, in medical patients, stroke and paraplegia. In these cases, LMW heparins, or sometimes low- to medium-dose warfarin, are the treatments of choice.

Therapy

The immediate goal of therapy of DVT is to reduce thrombus volume and length and to restore the hampered venous discharge in the affected limb. The clinical objectives are the following:

1. Healing of the acute inflammatory and edematous clinical picture (in symptomatic DVT).
2. Prophylaxis of recurrent DVT.
3. Prophylaxis of pulmonary embolism.
4. Prevention of the post-thrombotic syndrome.

A correct therapeutic strategy first requires validation of the clinical suspicion, and confirmation of diagnosis of proximal DVT (see above). In proximal DVT, more frequently complicated by pulmonary embolism than distal disease, aggressive antithrombotic treatment is compulsory. There is no general agreement with regard to the treatment of ascertained or suspected distal DVT. Distal DVT, if confirmed with phlebography, can also be submitted to full-dose antithrombotic treatment although not all centers will agree on this point. Suspected distal DVT not confirmed with phlebography is treated in several centers only with supportive therapies or moderate-dose heparin, under follow-up with serial compression echotomography in order to detect proximal extension of the thrombus.

With regard to pharmacological treatment, full-dose heparin therapy is the standard choice in proximal DVT [10] and is also recommended by a number of authors in confirmed distal DVT. Treatment is usually started as soon as possible, with an intravenous bolus of sodium heparin (1 ml, corresponding to 5000 IU), followed by continuous intravenous infusion at doses of 400–450 IU/kg/24h, or 1000–1400 IU/h. Adjustment of the dose by means of the activated partial thromboplastin time (APTT) is essential: the therapeutic range of the APTT ratio (the ratio between the APTT of the patient and the laboratory control value, or the patient's pretreatment value when available) is between 1.5 and 2.5 and there is evidence that values under 1.5 or above 2.5 are associated with, respectively, high rates of DVT recurrence, or of hemorragic complications.

Subcutaneous heparin (calcium or sodium) can substitute for continuous intravenous heparin and is equally effective, provided that therapeutic doses of heparin properly adjusted with APTTs performed six hours after injection are administered. Subcutaneous heparin is more practical, and is mostly used in non-extensive proximal, or in distal DVT. Administration of subcutaneous heparin is usually performed every 8 hours (initially 10–12 500 IU per dose) or every 12 hours (initially 17 500 IU per dose). It is also recommended that therapy is initiated with the intravenous bolus when the subcutaneous route is selected for further treatment. The ideal duration of heparin therapy is 5 to 7 days, as a longer duration is associated with side-effects, both hemorrhagic and, in rare cases, related to heparin induced thrombocytopenia.

Oral anticoagulants are started during the first three days of heparin treatment. It usually takes 3 to 4 days to achieve the desired prolongation of the prothrombin time, as expressed by a PT international normalized ratio (INR) of between 2 and 3.5. As soon as this level is reached, heparin therapy can be discontinued; this usually happens between the fourth and seventh day. At this time the patient, also submitted to elastic supportive treatment with adequate bandage, or graduated elastic stockings with a pressure of 30 mmHg or more at the ankle ('class 2 compression'), can be discharged as soon as he or she is able to walk, and oral anticoagulants are continued for at least three months, which is the high-risk period for thromboembolic recurrences. In cases with persistence of risk factors for thrombosis, such as malignancy, primary thrombophilias and others, oral anticoagulants can be continued for longer periods of time (6–12 months or more). It has recently been reported that six months is better than six weeks, but no conclusive study is available on the ideal duration of oral anticoagulation after DVT. It has been demonstrated that low- or moderate-dose subcutaneous heparin cannot substitute for oral anticoagulants in the secondary prevention of recurrent venous thromboembolism.

Heparin therapy followed by oral anticoagulation achieves excellent clinical results in terms of healing of the acute process, partial restoration of venous flow and, even more important, effective prevention of pulmonary embolism. However, significant recanalization of an occlusive thrombus, which could result from inhibition of thrombus growth associated with spontaneous fibrinolysis, can be objectvely demonstrated in less than 25% of the cases treated with heparin. It must be stressed that echotomographic follow up of the evolution of the thrombus does not supply validated criteria for the regulation of the length of anticoagulant treatment or of its different phases.

Recently, LMW heparins have been introduced into the treatment of DVT. The advantages of these new compounds with respect to unfractionated heparin, are a longer bioavailability that allows subcutaneous administration once or twice a day, and a better predictability of the anticoagulant effect of the injected dose that makes laboratory control non-mandatory. LMW Heparins do not greatly influence APTT as they act mainly on Factor Xa. Another advantage is the lower hemorrhagic risk which has been demonstrated with some of the preparations [11].

In the trials which have been performed, initial therapy of DVT with LMW heparin followed by oral anticoagulants in the same fashion codified for standard heparin treatment, was associated with equivalent or better outcomes in terms of short- and medium-term thromboembolic recurrences, and better results in terms of phlebographic score [12].

Given the practical advantages of the LMW heparins, the possibility of treating at least some types of DVT cases as outpatients became practical, and indeed two recent large multicenter trials have shown that initial treatment at home with LMW heparin is as effective and safe as initial in-hospital treatment with infusional unfractionated heparin (both treatments being followed by oral anticoagulants).

The cost-effectiveness of an 'at home' treatment of DVT is self-evident. However, outside a clinical trial, the psychological impact, the clinical outcome, and the possible legal consequences of a pulmonary embolism or a major bleeding occurring at home must be considered before adopting home treatment of DVT as a generalized policy. Home treatment might first be restricted to confirmed distal DVTs or generally to compliant patients with good home assistance.

Thrombolysis is an effective treatment for DVT, as it is capable of inducing a rapid clinical improvement of the affected limb similarly to heparin, but is associated with a recanalization rate of 60–75%, much higher than that obtained with heparin. However, it must be considered that, due to the size and length of many deep venous thrombi, thrombolytic treatment has to be maintained for 24 to 72 hours for optimal results. Only recent thrombi are sensitive to thrombolytic therapy. Durations and dosages of thrombolytic agents in DVT are therefore much higher than those used, for example in acute myocardial infarction. This makes thrombolytic treatment potentially hazardous in the present indication. An overview of the available studies showed that hemorrhagic complications during thrombolysis in DVT are three to four times more frequent than with heparin [13].

It has been surmised that early and effective recanalization as obtained with thrombolysis may be advantageous in terms of prophylaxis of the post-thrombotic syndrome. This statement has not been conclusively demonstrated but is likely to be true. Some authors however maintain that the degree of post-thrombotic syndrome is poorly predictable from the results of the acute phase treatment, and that an early onset of treatment is more important than which therapeutic agent is used.

Thrombolytic treatment should therefore be performed in selected patients, e.g. young patients with thrombosis of recent onset less than 7 days, at low hemorrhagic risk, with gangrenous DVT, or extensive proximal DVT in which occurrence of a severe post-thrombotic syndrome would induce lifelong disability.

Steptokinase (SK) or urokinase (UK) are the drugs of choice. The suggested schedule for SK is a loading dose of 250 000 IU (rapid infusion), followed by 100 000 IU per hour for 3–4 days. Thrombin time (TT) should be 3–5 times the control value: if TT is more than five times the control value, the dose should paradoxically be increased, and decreased when TT is lower than two times, as higher doses of SK increase preferentially the SK–plasminogen complex rather than circulating plasmin. With regard to UK, a loading dose of 4000 U/kg is first given in 15–30 minutes, followed by 4000 U/kg/hour for 3–5 days. Control with TT is less mandatory: in this case an excessively prolonged TT calls for a reduction of the dose and vice versa.

Tissue plasminogen activator (rtPA or Alteplase) has been tested in doses of 0.25–0.50 mg/kg daily for 3–7 days, but with no evidence of superiority versus SK and UK [14].

Surgical treatment of DVT consists of thrombectomy. Indications for thrombectomy are rather limited: isolated proximal DVT especially iliac, gangrenous DVT, and phlegmasia coerulea dolens. Recurrency is frequent and anticoagulant treatment is necessary.

Caval filters are special devices that are placed into the inferior vena cava with the aim of blocking the centripetal migration of venous emboli. Several models of filter are currently available and the most recent ones bear a lesser risk of complications related to placement or permanence *in situ*.

The indications for caval filters are limited to: contraindications to anticoagulant or thrombolytic therapy of DVT; recurrence of pulmonary emboli despite correct antithrombotic treatment; and severe cardio-respiratory insufficiency where superimposed pulmonary embolism or even microembolism could be lethal. Removable caval filters can be very useful in special conditions, such as protection of patients with DVT that must undergo emergency high – risk surgery, for example neurosurgery, that could not be performed during anticoagulant or thrombolytic therapy.

References

1. Wells Ph S, Hirsh J, Anderson DR *et al.* Accuracy of clinical assessment of deep-vein thrombosis. Lancet 1995;345:1326–30.
2. Hirsh J, Hull RD. Venous thromboembolism: Natural history, diagnosis, and management. Boca Raton: CRC Press, 1987.
3. Kakkar VV. Venous Thrombosis today. Haemostasis 1994;24:86–104.
4. Weinmann EE, Salzman EW. Deep vein thrombosis. New Engl J Med 1994;331:1630–41.
5. Buller HR, Lensing AWA, Hirsh J, Ten Cate JW. Deep vein thrombosis – new non-invasive diagnostic tests. Thromb Haemost 1991;66:133–7.
6. Dupas B, El Kouri D, Curtet C *et al.* Angiomagnetic resonance imaging of iliofemorocaval venous thrombosis. Lancet 1995;346:17–9.
7. Collins R, Scrimgeour A, Yusuf S, Peto R. Reduction in fatal pulmonary embolism and venous thrombosis by perioperative administration of subcutaneous heparin. N Engl J Med 1988;318:1162–73.
8. Clagett GP, Salzman EW, Wheeler HB, Anderson FA, Levine MN. Prevention of venous thromboembolism. Chest 1992;102(4,Suppl.):391S–407S.
9. Nurmohamed MT, Rosendaal FR, Buller HR *et al.* Low-molecular-weight heparin versus standard heparin in general and orthopaedic surgery – a meta-analysis. Lancet 1992;340:152–6.
10. Hyers ThH, Hull RD, Weg JG. Antithrombotic therapy for venous thromboembolic disease. Chest 1992;102(4,Suppl.):408S–25S.
11. Coccheri S. Low molecular weight heparins: An introduction. Haemostasis 1990;20(Suppl.1):74–80.
12. Hull RD, Pineo GF. Therapeutic use of low molecular weight heparins – the knowledge to date as applied to therapy. Semin Thromb Hemost 1993;19:111–5.

13. Goldhaber SZ, Buring JE, Lipnick RJ, Hennekens CH. Pooled analysis of randomized trials of streptokinase and heparin in phlebographically documented acute deep vein thrombosis. Am J Med 1984;76:393–7.
14. Bounameaux H, Banga JD, Coccheri S et al. Double-blind, randomized comparison of systemic continuous infusion of 0.25 versus 0.50 mg/kg/24 h of Alteplase over 3 to 7 days for treatment of deep venous thrombosis in heparinized patients: Results of the European Thrombolysis with rt-PA in Venous Thrombosis (ETTT) Trial. Thromb Haemost 1992;67:306–9.

29. Cardiovascular manifestations and complications of diabetes mellitus

JAFFAR ALLAWI

The survival rate among patients with diabetes mellitus has increased substantially, largely in response to: the discovery of insulin, which reduced the mortality related to ketoacidosis; and the development of antibiotics for effective treatment of infections. These developments have resulted in a significant increase in macrovascular (cardiovascular) and microvascular (nephropathy, neuropathy, retinopathy) complications [1–3].

Despite our best efforts, these complications continue to be responsible for significant morbidity and mortality. Indeed, the complications of both insulin-dependent diabetes mellitus (IDDM) and noninsulin-dependent diabetes mellitus (NIDDM) are that it is: the leading cause of blindness in adults; the most common cause of end-stage renal disease, accounting for 30–40% of this population; responsible for 40% of all nontraumatic amputations of the lower extremities in adults; and a major risk factor for cardiac and cerebrovascular disease [4].

Cardiovascular disease therefore remains a major cause of morbidity in diabetes, with considerable cost to the individual and society [5], and also contributing to a significant increase in premature mortality, particularly in the middle-aged. The risk is substantial, not only for those with IDDM, especially women, but even more so for those with NIDDM.

Epidemiology

The incidence and prevalence of the major manifestations of coronary heart disease (angina, myocardial infarction, and sudden death) are increased in patients with diabetes mellitus [6, 7]. Ischemic heart disease is about twice as prevalent among diabetics as nondiabetics. Because of the impact of mortality, however, prevalence rates may underestimate the actual rate of occurrence of heart disease. Incidence rates more accurately reflect the risk of developing this complication. Most reports [2, 6, 7] suggest that the incidence of ischemic heart disease among diabetic patients is two to three times that among nondiabetic individuals, that the relative risk for ischemic coronary heart disease increases with age at diagnosis of diabetes mellitus, and that the relative risk for ischemic heart disease is greater for women with diabetes than for men with the disorder.

In stroke populations form every region of the world, patients with diabetes mellitus or impaired glucose tolerance are represented in greater numbers than expected by chance alone [8–10]. It has also been established that the risk of thromboembolic infarction but not cerebral hemorrhage is greater in the diabetic population than in comparable nondiabetic subjects [10]. Also, atherosclerotic disease in the bulb of carotid arteries is an important determinant of propensity to stroke that can be identified by noninvasive testing. The likelihood of stroke in patients with asymptomatic carotid bruits according to three different studies is about 15–19% over the next 7–13 years, and probability of transient ischemic attacks varies from 11 to 27% over the same period [11].

The toll of peripheral vascular disease (PVD) in diabetes mellitus is enormous. It has been estimated to be 30 times more common in diabetic than in nondiabetic individuals, and the risk of gangrene is increased markedly in diabetic patients. In hospital studies of diabetic patients, PVD may account for 25% of their admission, and hospital stays are typically very long. Whether conservative medical management, bypass surgery or angioplasty, or amputation is chosen, prolonged hospitalization is usually necessary [12]. Several recent studies using improved noninvasive diagnostic techniques have shown that both incidence and prevalence of PVD are much higher in the diabetic population compared to the nondiabetic [13, 14].

Pathology

The hallmark of macrovascular disease is the atherosclerotic plaque which is the same in diabetic and nondiabetic subjects [15, 16]. The Atherosclerosis Project demonstrated that the extent of raised lesions was greater in diabetic than in nondiabetic subjects [17]. Diabetics patients have an excess of atherosclerotic lesions with ulceration, thrombosis or hemorrhage [18].

Diabetic patients have been reported to have more atherosclerotic arterial wall changes [19]. They have also been reported to have more vessels involved: in one study 43% of diabetic subjects had three-vessel disease compared to 25% of nondiabetics [20]. Diabetic patients have been reported to have atherosclerotic changes that extend more peripherally [21, 22]. A statistically increased prevalence of left main coronary artery disease has also been reported in diabetic subjects [13%] compared to nondiabetic controls (6%) [23].

Abnormalities of the small blood vessels, including microaneurysms of the coronary vessels, capillary membrane thickening, perivascular and interstitial fibrosis, scarring of adjacent tissues and myocytolysis, have been found within the heart [24]. These changes are similar to those observed in skeletal muscle, kidney, and the retina of patients with diabetes [25]. Proliferative lesions have been reported in all sizes of arterial branches and venules. In addition, arteriosclerosis-like lesions of small arteries and arterioles were 2–2.5 times more frequent among diabetic patients than nondiabetics [26].

Postmortem examination of the brain in persons with known history of diabetes has revealed many findings [27, 28]. Two major differences have been noted between diabetic and nondiabetic patients: the unlikely occurrence of cerebral hemorrhage; and the substantial increase in frequency and number of lacunes, small foci of infarction that usually cavitate. The lacunar state is conventionally associated with hypertension, although lacunes have been discovered in the absence of a history of hypertension. It is not surprising that the propensity to lacunes should be associated with diabetes, since hypertension occurs more commonly in diabetics. A synergistic effect between hypertension and diabetes in the occupancy of lacunes has been suggested [28, 29].

Putative cardiovascular risk factors

Several variables have been shown to have a significant statistical association with a morbid or mortal macrovascular event in diabetics and nondiabetics. These variables or risk factors may either be modifiable risk factors such as hypertension [30], central obesity [31], smoking [32], dyslipidemia [33], or non-modifiable risk factors such as male gender [34] and age above 40 [35].

The literature available indicates that the effect of risk factors on macrovascular complications is similar in both diabetic and nondiabetic populations [36]. Moreover, the increased risk factors for coronary artery disease in diabetic populations is not solely because of the increased prevalence of risk factors for coronary vascular disease [9]. Only part of the increased prevalence of coronary artery disease in diabetic patients can be explained by the high rate of risk factors in this group [37].

Microalbuminuria (an increased urinary albumin excretion which is above the normal but below the range normally detected by routine urinalysis with Albustix) is not a risk factor, but a possible marker of vascular injury. Microalbuminuria, which shows different prevalence in different populations [38], is a well-known predictor of cardiovascular mortality in NIDDM [39, 40]. Microalbuminuria in its early stages, has been shown to be amenable to interventional maneuvers, such as improving diabetes control and hypertension if present. Also, angiotensin-converting enzyme inhibitors, aspirin and low-animal protein diets have all been found to have a beneficial effect on diminishing microalbuminuria [41]. Such interventional maneuvers may reduce the rate of diabetic renal deterioration [41]; whether such maneuvers have a similar beneficial effect on future development of macrovascular complications is still not clear. Well-designed studies to address and clarify this issue are urgently required.

A plethora of data are available to show that putative cardiovascular risk factors profoundly influence the prevalence and severity of diabetic cardiovascular complications. In this chapter, the impact of asymptomatic hyperglycemia, glycemic control, hyperinsulinemia and autonomic neuropathy, on the cardiovascular system of the diabetic patients will be reviewed.

Asymptomatic hyperglycemia

The relation of asymptomatic hyperglycemia to cardiovascular risk has been addressed by the Paris Prospective Study [42], the Tecumseh Study [43], and the Chicago Heart Association Detection Project [44]. These studies strongly suggest that asymptomatic hyperglycemia is an independent risk factor for coronary artery disease. In the Tecumseh Study, 921 men and 937 women aged 40 years and older who were without coronary artery disease at entry were followed for a minimum of 12 years. Although diabetes was a statistically significant independent risk factor for a mortality due to coronary artery disease for both sexes (17.8 deaths per 1000 persons with diabetes as opposed to 5.9 per 1000 persons without diabetes), an elevated blood glucose (1 hour after a 100-g oral glucose challenge) in those individuals without a diagnosis of diabetes was also associated with excess mortality due to coronary artery disease. It is of interest that this study showed no excess mortality in women over that in men. It was concluded that hyperglycemia following glucose challenge may identify individuals who have other cardiac risk factors, such as obesity, high blood pressure, hyperlipidemia, and hyperinsulinemia.

Similar findings were noted in the Chicago Heart Association Detection Project, which compiled nine-year follow-up data for 11 230 white men and 8030 white women aged 35–64 years at entry [44]. Both diabetes and asymptomatic hyperglycemia were associated with increased mortality from coronary artery disease. The extent of association was greater in women than in men with regard to relative risk, while absolute excess risk for both diabetes and asymptomatic hyperglycemia was greater for men.

More, recently, Wilson *et al.* reported on the relation of non-fasting blood glucose levels to the incidence of coronary artery disease in the Framingham Heart Study [45]. Age-adjusted incidence of coronary artery disease was associated with blood glucose levels in nondiabetic women who did not develop diabetes during follow-up. No such association was seen in men. Multivariate analysis confirmed the independent association of blood glucose levels with subsequent coronary artery disease in nondiabetic women. This study suggests that hyperglycemia in the original Framingham cohort is an independent risk factor for coronary artery disease in women but not in men.

Glycemic control

A relationship between hyperglycemia and the development of long-term complications of diabetes has long been suspected, based on the results of animal studies and epidemiological observations in people with diabetes. These important early observations provided the justification for the initiation of prospective controlled randomized trials designed to test 'the glucose hypothesis', namely, that treatment that reduces hyperglycemia will prevent or delay the long-term complications of diabetes. The largest study of this kind was the Diabetes Control and Complications Trial (DCCT) [4, 46]. The DCCT study has shown that good glycemic control can prevent microvascular complications i.e. retinopathy, nephropathy and neuropathy, but the effect of tight glycemic control on macrovascular complications was non-conclusive and non-significant. Whether tight glycemic control reduces cardiovascular morbidity and mortality remains a subjects of debate.

The Framingham Study [47] has shown that a reduction in risk of coronary artery disease in the patient with diabetes depends more on the control of obesity, correction of hypertension, cessation of cigarette smoking, and improvement in the ratio between low-density lipoprotein (LDL) and high-density lipoprotein (HDL) than on the control of hyperglycemia. Waller *et al.* studied the extent of atherosclerosis in the coronary arteries of 229 patients with diabetes and found that the type of treatment received by patients (diet, insulin, or oral agents) or their adherence to the therapeutic regimen did not correlate with the number of severely narrowed coronary arteries [48]. The results of three prospective studies [42–44] suggest a nonlinear relationship between atherosclerosis with a threshold phenomenon (relationship between atherosclerosis and response to oral glucose is not linear) in the upper range of the distribution of blood glucose values after an oral glucose load. Multivariate analysis showed that the association of blood glucose levels with cardiovascular disease was not independent of the major risk variables. Hence, it is not clear whether stringent control of blood glucose levels directly reduces the risk of the development of cardiac disease in persons with diabetes.

Hyperinsulinemia

Hyperinsulinemia, abdominal obesity and hypertension in the NIDDM patient is the diabetologist's syndrome – X [49]. Hyperinsulinemia, which is particularly common in patients with NIDDM, especially with central obesity, appears to be a risk factor for macrovascular complications [31]. Hyperinsulinemia, even in the presence of normal glucose tolerance, is associated with other risk factors for coronary artery disease, including low HDL levels and hypertension [50, 51]. Hyperinsulinemia may also play a role in promoting atherosclerosis by causing proliferation of smooth muscle cells and synthesis of cholesterol, as well as by increasing levels of growth hormone [52].

Autonomic neuropathy

Several noninvasive tests [53, 54] assessing autonomic control of the cardiovascular system have extensively been evaluated and were found to be reliable and of great clinical application:

1. Heart rate variation with: deep breathing; Valsalva maneuver; and postural change; and
2. Blood pressure changes with: sustained hand grip; and postural changes.

These tests were frequently found to be abnormal in diabetic patients with symptoms of autonomic dysfunction (postural hypotension–dizziness, diarrhea, hypoglycemia unawareness, abnormal sweating, disturbed bladder function, impotence, gastric fullness). Although the same tests were occasionally found to be abnormal in the diabetic patients with asymptomatic autonomic neuropathy, especially if there was evidence of microvascular disease [55, 56] the development of symptoms in these patients is an ominous sign, with mortality over 50% three years after its onset [53]. Sudden death, presumably cardiac-related, is responsible for up to one-third of these deaths. Autonomic neuropathy may lead to ischemia or infarction by several routes: increasing myocardial demand for oxygen by increasing resting heart rate; reducing myocardial blood flow by increasing coronary vascular tone at the site of a coronary stenosis; and by reducing coronary perfusion pressure during orthostatic hypotension [57].

The importance of intact autonomic function during cardiovascular stress (as during a myocardial infarction) is exemplified in diabetic patients undergoing general anesthesia. Page and Watkins [58] reported that cardiorespiratory arrest occurred commonly amongst diabetics with autonomic neuropathy, particularly after anesthesia, and recommended careful monitoring of such patients after surgery or during illnesses which might interfere with respiratory drive. The increased morbidity seen in diabetic patients during general anesthesia may be due to an inability to counteract the hemodynamic effects of the induction of anesthesia because of impaired cardiovascular reflexes. Burgos et al. [59] has shown that 35% of diabetic patients required a vasopressor intraoperatively compared with only 5% of nondiabetic patients ($p < 0.05$). Furthermore, the diabetic patients who required vasopressor support had significantly greater autonomic impairment than did those who did not require it.

Sudden death in diabetics with autonomic neuropathy may be due to arrhythmia secondary to a silent myocardial infarction; autopsy studies have demonstrated a surprising absence of significant coronary artery disease in some diabetic patients who died unexpectedly [60, 61]. A relation exists between diabetic cardiac autonomic neuropathy and a prolonged QT-interval on the electrocardiogram [62–64], which may predispose to life-threatening ventricular arrhythmia. It has been proposed that the combination of relatively heightened sympathetic tone and the prolongation of QT-interval might increase the likelihood of arrhythmias leading to sudden death [65, 66]. Although a search for other causes of prolongation of QT interval in these patients is not well documented, it is quite possible that other factors such as acute ischemia, electrolyte disturbances (hypokalemia), metabolic abnormalities (hypomagnesemia, hypocalcemia, hypophosphatemia), and drug toxicity (digoxin) could have contributed to the sudden death in these patients by altering the threshold for life threatening arrhythmia.

Presentation

Autonomic neuropathy may result in blunted appreciation for pain among diabetics [67], myocardial ischemia or infarction may be associated with only mild symptoms and go unrecognized or may be entirely asymptomatic and thus truly silent. Although 25% of the myocardial infarctions in the Framingham Study were 'silent', symptoms referable to the unrecognized infarction could be elicited in nearly one-half of these cases [68]. The remaining infarctions (or approximately 12% of the total) were considered truly asymptomatic. Unrecognized infarction tends to be more common in persons with diabetes [69] and accounts for 39% of their infarctions as compared with 22% of those in persons without diabetes [70]. As might be inferred from the above, persons with diabetes may also lack angina during ischemia. The incidence of painless ST depression during exercise tolerance tests in diabetic patients is more than double that seen in nondiabetic patients. (75% vs. 35%) [71]. Also, angina is less common in diabetic than nondiabetic patients during ischemia assessed by exercise thallium scintigraphy [72].

Atypical symptoms such as confusion, dyspnea, fatigue, or nausea and vomiting may be the presenting complaint in 32–42% of diabetic patients with myocardial infarction as compared with 6–15% of nondiabetic patients [73]. In some cases such symptoms may mimic those associated with either hypo- or hyperglycemia and result in a delay in the patient's treatment [74]. The unusual presenting symptoms seen in the diabetic patient may influence the clinician's suspicion of infarction, leading to a reduction in the level of care [75], and may alter the patient's perception of the nature of his or her illness and interfere with the decision to seek medical care [76]. It is therefore possible that these atypical symptoms may lead to a delay in receiving appropriate care, and could contribute to the observed increase in morbidity and mortality in diabetic patients with myocardial infarction.

The clinical presentation of diabetic patients with PVD is somewhat altered by the frequent presence of neuropathy. The important point to be made here is that diabetic patients may present with foot ulcer or small areas of gangrene when relatively mild ischemia is present. Because of the neuropathy, it is necessary to maintain a high arterial perfusing pressure to prevent ulceration at pressure points in the foot. When skin necrosis occurs, it should not be ascribed solely to neuropathy until the possibility of coexisting ischemia has been carefully evaluated. A thorough physical examination is essential in the diabetic with lower extremity complaints. The peripheral pulses at all levels should be palpated. Although diabetics have a propensity toward atherosclerotic occlusion of the tibial arteries, it is not unusual to encounter atherosclerosis of the aorto-iliac region, as evidenced by diminished femoral pulses. Patients who have only tibial vessel disease present with normal femoral and popliteal pulses but no foot pulses (dorsalis pedis or posterior tibial) [77]. Examination of peripheral pulses is still the single most important step in the evaluation for ischemia. It is also important to examine both lower limbs neurologically. The skin should be examined carefully, and all ulcers and the tissue surrounding it. Probing the base of an ulceration will give some indication as to the involvement of bone structures in the infectious and ischemic process.

Plain radiographs of any lower extremity that has an ulcer or has a history of a healed ulcer but remains symptomatic should be undertaken as part of the initial evaluation. A number of noninvasive techniques have been developed to measure arterial pressure in the lower extremity. Measurement of arterial pressures at different levels of extremity, using a pneumatic cuff and a flow sensor, usually, a Doppler ultrasound sensor, is the most commonly used technique [78]. Less compressible arteries due to medial calcinosis is a peculiar anatomical finding in the diabetic and requires other methods to assess perfusing pressure. The most popular of these is pulse volume recording a form of plethysmography [79]. Other noninvasive techniques have been used with some success, such as transcutaneous oxygen tension measurement [80, 81]. Once surgery has been selected, confirmation of the presumptive diagnosis with angiography must be considered. An accurate arteriogram of the entire lower extremity, including the foot vessels, is essential to successful arterial reconstruction in the diabetic.

The clinical presentation of stroke in diabetics differs in no way from that of nondiabetic patients. In the diabetic receiving insulin or a sulfonylurea, hypoglycemia must always be considered because its features are protean and may occur concomitantly with a stroke syndrome in patients with a preexisting ischemic focus. Lacunar infarcts, on the other hand, are much more common in diabetic patients than in nondiabetics. It is possible that the clinical manifestation of multiple lacunes varies from the asymptomatic to a florid encephalopathic state, although the latter is rare. Considering the high prevalence of lacunes determined by several studies, subtle clinical abnormalities may not be identified. Indeed, lacunes are considered to account for a variety of states, such as:

1. Pure motor hemiparesis.
2. Pure sensory stroke.
3. Ataxic hemiparesis.
4. Pure motor hemiparesis with motor aphasia.

It is also important to remember that in the lacunar state, hypertension is an important confounding factor.

Finally, morbidity and mortality following a stroke is much higher in the diabetic patient than in the nondiabetic [82]. This is probably attributed to the influence of hyperglycemia on cerebral metabolism [83]. Hyperglycemia has been postulated to predispose to cerebral edema [83].

Conclusion

As the population ages, the macrovascular complications of diabetes become more prevalent. Diabetic subjects, especially women, have increased morbidity and mortality from coronary artery disease. Diabetic patients have an increased incidence of risk factors which predispose to vascular atherosclerosis. In addition, hyperglycemia, hyperinsulinemia, abdominal obesity, altered coagulation and other metabolic changes all contribute to the atherosclerotic process. Ischemic heart disease, PVD and cerebrovascular disease are all more prevalent in the diabetic, and the prognosis from these complications is poorer than for nondiabetic patients. The DCCT study has proved that improving hyperglycemia control can reduce the risk of microvascular disease. Also, it showed a small but nonsignificant reduction in major vessel disease. Although the reduction may not be significant, it is a trend, and a trend that may require a much longer study period to prove.

References

1. Kessler II, Mortality experience of diabetic patients: A twenty-six year follow up study. Am J Med 1971;51:715–24.
2. Garcia MJ, McNamara PM, Gordon T, Kannell WB. Morbidity and mortality in diabetics in the Framingham population: Sixteen year follow-up study. Diabetes 1974;23:105–11.
3. Kannel WB, Hjortland M, Castelli WP. Role of diabetes in congestive heart failure: The Framingham study. Am J Cardiol 1974,34:29–34.
4. Zinman B. The Diabetes Control and Complications Trial: Implications for the Management of Type 1 Diabetes Mellitus. In the 1994 Syllabus, 46th Postgraduate Assembly, The Endocrine Society Publications 1994:1–4.
5. Laing WJ, Williams R (eds), Diabetes: A Model for Health Care Management. OHE report 1989 No. 92.
6. Palumbo PJ, Eleveback LR, Connolly DC. Coronary heart disease and congestive heart failure in the diabetic: Epidemiological aspects. The Rochester Diabetes Project. In: Scott RC, (ed.), Clinical cardiology and diabetes, Vol. 1. Part 1: Fundamental considerations in cardiology and diabetes. Mount Kisco, NY: Futura Publishing, 1981:13–28.
7. Barrett-Connor E, Orcchard T. Diabetes and heart disease. In: Diabetes in America, Diabetes Data compiled 1984. Bethesda, MD: NIH Publication No. 85–1468, August 1985.
8. Barrett-Connor E, Khaw KT. Diabetes Mellitus: An independent risk factor for stroke? Am J Epidemiol 1988;128:116–23.
9. Kannel WB, McGee DL. Diabetes and cardiovascular disease. The Framingham Study. J Am Med Assoc 1979;241:2035–8.
10. Abbot RD, Donahue RP, MacMahon SW, Reed DM, Yano K. Diabetes and the risk of stroke. The Honolulu Heart Program. J Am Med Assoc1987;257:949–52.
11. Dorazio RA, Ezzet F, Nesbitt NJ. Long-term follow up of asymptomatic carotid bruits. Am J Surg 1980;140:212–3.
12. Colwell JA. Peripheral vascular disease in diabetes mellitus. In: Davidson JK (ed.), Clinical diabetes mellitus, a problem-oriented approach. 2nd edition. Thieme Medical Publishers, 1991:486–95.
13. Beach KW, Brunzell JD, Conquest LL. The correlation of arteriosclerosis obliterans with lipoproteins in insulin dependent and noninsulin dependent diabetes. Diabetes 1979;28:836–40.
14. Janka HU, Standl E, Mehnert H. Peripheral vascular disease in diabetes mellitus and its relation to cardiovascular risk factors: Screening with the Doppler ultasonic techique. Diabetes Care 1980;3:207–13.
15. Keen H, Jarrett RH, Fuller JH, McCartney P. Hyperglycemia and arterial disease. Diabetes 1981;30(Suppl.2):49–53.
16. Steiner G. Atherosclerosis: The major complication of diabetes. Adv Exp Med Biol 1985;189:277–89.
17. Robertson WB, Strong JP. Atherosclerosis in persons with hypertension and diabetes mellitus. Lab Invest 1968;18:538–51.
18. Woolf N. Diabetes and atherosclerosis. Acta Diab Lat 1971;8:14–42.
19. Hamby RI, Sherman L. Duration and treatment of diabetes; relationship to severity of coronary artery disease. NY State J Med 1979;79:1683–8.
20. Dortimer A, Shenoy P, Shiroff R et al. Diffuse coronary artery disease in diabetic patients: Fact or fiction? Circulation 1978;57:133–6.
21. Vigorita V, Moore G, Hutchins G. Absence of correlation between coronary arterial atherosclerosis and severity or duration of diabetes mellitus of adult onset. Am J Cardiol 1980;46:535–41.
22. Salomon NW, Page US, Okies JE. Stephens J, Krause AH, Bigelow JC. Diabetes mellitus and coronary artery bypass; short term risk and long term prognosis. J Thorax Cardiovasc Surg 1983;85:264–71.
23. Waller B, Palumbo P, Lie J, Robert W. Status of the coronary arteries at necropsy in diabetes mellitus with onset after 30 years: Analysis of 229 diabetic patients with and without clinical evidence of coronary heart disease and comparison to 183 control subjects. Am J Med 1980;69:498–506.

24. Crall F, Robert W. The extramural and intramural coronary arteries in juvenile diabetes mellitus – analysis of nine necropsy patients aged 19–38 years with onset of diabetes before age 15 years. Am J Med 1978;64:222–30.
25. Factor S, Okun E, Minase T. Capillary microaneurysms in the human diabetic heart. N Engl J Med 1980;302:384–8.
26. Blumenthal HT, Alex M, Goldenberg S. A study of lesions of the intramural coronary artery branches in diabetes mellitus. Arch Pathol 1960;70:27–40.
27. Alex M, Baron EK, Goldenberg S, Blumenthal HT. An autopsy of cerebrovascular accident in diabetes mellitus. 1962;25:663–73.
28. Aronson SM. Intracranial vascular lesions in patients with diabetes mellitus. J Neuropathol Exp Neurol 1973;23:183–96.
29. Mohr JP. Lacunes. In: Barnett HJM, Stein BM, Mohr JP, Yatsu FM (eds), Stroke pathophysiology, diagnosis, and management, Vol. 1. New York: Churchill Livingstone, 1986:475–96.
30. Ganda P. Pathogenesis of macrovascular disease in human diabetic. Diabetes 1980;29:931–42.
31. Allawi J, Jarrett RJ. Male-type fat distribution is associated with cardiovascular risk factors and the prevalence of cardiovascular disease in non insulin treated diabetics. J Diabetic Complications 1990;4:150–3.
32. Muhlhauser I. Smoking and diabetes. Diabetic Med 1990;7:10–5.
33. Winocour PH, Laker MF. Drug therapy for diabetic dyslipidemia: A practical approach. Diabetic Med 1990;7:292–8.
34. Ellison HW, Antonio MG. Clinical features of ischemic heart disease in diabetes mellitus. In: Alberti KGMM, DeFronzo RA, Keen H, Zimmet P (eds), International textbook of diabetes mellitus. Chichester: Wiley, 1992;1487–507.
35. Pirart J. Diabetes mellitus and its degenerative complications: A prospective study of 4400 patients observed between 1947 and 1973. Diabetes Care 1978;1:252–61.
36. Pyorala K. Diabetes and coronary heart disease. Acta Endocrinol 1985;110 (Suppl.272):11–9.
37. Kannel W. Diabetic–atherogenic connection: A continuing puzzle. Cardiology 1987;74:333–4.
38. Allawi J, Rao PV, Gilbert R et al. Microalbuminuria in non-insulin dependent diabetes: Its prevalence in Indian compared to Europid patients. Br Med J 1988;296:462–4.
39. Allawi J, Jarrett RJ. Microalbuminuria and cardiovascular risk factors in type 2 diabetes mellitus. Diabetic Med 1990;7:115–8.
40. Jarrett RJ, Viberti GC, Argyropolous A. Microalbuminuria predicts mortality in non insulin dependent diabetics. Diabetic Med 1984;1:7–19.
41. Gilbert RE, Cooper ME, McNally PG, O'Brieen RC, Taft J, Jerums G. Mircoalbuminuria prognostic and therapeutic implication in diabetes mellitus. Diabetic Med 1994;11:636–45.
42. Eschwege E, Richard JL, Thibult N et al. Coronary heart disease mortality in relation with diabetes, blood glucose and plasma insulin levels. The Paris Prospective Study, ten years later. Horm Metab Res Suppl 1985;15:41–6.
43. Butler WJ, Ostrander LD Jr, Carman WJ, Lamphiear DE. Mortality from coronary heart disease in the Tecumseh study. Long-term effect of diabetes mellitus, glucose tolerance and other risk factors. Am J Epidemiol 1985;121:541–7.
44. Pan WH, Cedres LB, Liu K et al. Relationship of clinical diabetes and asymptomatic hyperglycemia to risk of coronary heart disease mortality in men and women. Am J Epidemiol 1986;123:504–16.
45. Wilson PWF., Cupples LA, Kannel WB. Is hyperglycemia associated with cardiovascular disease? The Framingham Study. Am Heart J 1991;121:586–90.
46. Diabetes Control and Complications Trial Research Group. The effect of intensive treatment of diabetes on the development and progression of longterm complications in insulin-dependent diabetes mellitus. N Engl J Med 1993;329:977–86.
47. Kannel WB, Lipids, diabetes and coronary artery disease: Insights from the Framingham Study. Am Heart J 1985;110:1100–17.
48. Waller BF, Palumbo PJ, Lie JT. Roberts WC. Status of the coronary arteries at necropsy in diabetes mellitus with onset after 30 years: Analysis of 229 diabetic patients with and without clinical evidence of coronary heart disease and comparison to 183 control subjects. Am J Med 1980;69:498–506.

49. Raven G. 'The Banting Lecture': Role of insulin resistance in human disease. Diabetes 1988;37:1595–607.
50. Modan M, Halkin H, Almog S et al. Hyperinsulinemia: A link between hypertension, obesity and glucose intolerance. J Clin Invest 1985;75:809–18.
51. Orchard TJ, Becker DJ, Bates M et al. Plasma insulin and lipoprotein concentration – an atherogenic association. Am J Epidemiol 1983;118:326–47.
52. Stout RW. Insulin and atheroma: An update. Lancet 1987;1:1077–9.
53. Ewing DJ, Campbell IW, Clarke BF. The natural history of diabetic autonomic neuropathy. Q J Med 1980;49:95–108.
54. Clarke BF, Ewing DJ. Cardiovascular reflex test. NY State J Med 1982;82:903–8.
55. Mackay JD, Page MMcB, Cambridge J. Diabetic autonomic neuropathy. Diabetologia 1980;18:471–8.
56. Dryberg T, Benn J, Christiansen JS. Prevalence of diabetic autonomic neuropathy measured by simple bedside tests. Diabetologia 1981;20:190–4.
57. Almog C, Pik A. Acute myocardial infarction as a complication of diabetic neuropathy. J Am Med Assoc 1978;239:2782.
58. Page MMcB, Watkins PJ. Cardiorespiratory arrest and diabetic autonomic neruopathy. Lancet 1978;i:14–6.
59. Burgos LG, Ebert TJ Assiddao C et al. Increased intraoperative cardiovascular morbidity in diabetics with autonomic neuropathy. Anesthesiology 1989;70:591–7.
60. Ewing DJ, Campbell IW, Clarke BF. Mortality in diabetic autonomic neuropathy. Lancet 1976;1:601–3.
61. Ewing DJ, Campbell IW, Clarke BF. Assessment of cardiovascular effects in diabetic automatic neuropathy and prognostic implications. Ann Intern Med 1980;92:308–11.
62. Ewing DJ, Boland O, Neilson JM et al. Autonomic neuropathy, QT interval lengthening and unexpected deaths in male diabetic patients. Diabetologia 1991;34:182–5.
63. Bellavere F, Ferri M. Guarini L et al. Prolonged QT period in diabetic automatic neuropathy: A possible role in sudden cardiac death? Br Heart J 1988;59:379–83.
64. Jermendy G, Toth L, Voros P et al. Cardiac autonomic neuropathy and QT interval length. A follow-up study in diabetic patients. Acta Cardiol 1991;46:189–200.
65. Khan JH, Sisson JC, Vinik AL. QT interval prolongation and sudden cardiac death in diabetic autonomic neuropathy. J Clin Endocrinol Metab 1987;64:751–4.
66. Bernardi L, Ricordi L, Rossi M et al. Impairment of modulation of sympathovagal activity in diabetes: An explanation for sudden death? (Abstract) Circulation 1989;80(Suppl. 2):1564.
67. Watkins PJ, Mackay JD. Cardiac denervation in diabetic neuropathy. Ann Intern Med 1980;2:304–7.
68. Kannel WB, Abott RD. Incidence and prognosis of unrecognised myocardial infarction. N Engl J Med 1984;311:1144–7.
69. Niakan E, Harati Y, Rolak LA et al. Silent myocardial infarction and diabetic cardiovascular autonomic neuropathy. Arch Intern Med 1986;146:2229–30.
70. Margolis JR, Kannel WB, Feinleib M et al. Clinical features of unrecognised myocardial infarction – silent and symptomatic: Eighteen year follow-up: The Framingham Study. Am J Cardiol 1973;32:1–7.
71. Murray DP, O'Brien T, Mulrooney R, O'Sullivan DJ. Autonomic dysfunction and silent myocardial ischaemia, on exercise testing in diabetes mellitus. Diabetic Med 1990;7:580–4.
72. Nesto RW, Phillips RT, Kett KG et al. Angina and exertional myocardial ischemia in diabetic and nondiabetic patients: Assessment by exercise thallium scintigraphy. Ann Intern Med 1988;108:170–5.
73. Nesto RW, Phillips RT. Asymptomatic myocardial ischemia in diabetic patients. Am J Med 1986;80(Suppl. 4C):40–7.
74. Pladziewicz DS, Nesto RW. Hypoglycemia-induced silent myocardial ischemia. Am J Cardiol 1989;63:1531–2.
75. Soler NG, Bennett M, Pentecost BL et al. Myocardial infarction in diabetics. QJ Med 1975;173:125–32.
76. Uretsky BF, Farquhar DS, Berizin AF, Hood WB Jr. Symptomatic myocardial infarction without chest pains: Prevalence and clinical course. Am J Cardiol 1977;40:498–503.

77. Sidawy AN, Menzoian JO, Cantelmo NL, LoGerfo FW. Effect of inflow and outflow sites on the results of tibioperoneal vein grafts. Am J Surg 1986;152:211–4.
78. Allen JS, Terry HJK. The evaluation of ultrasonic flow detector for assessment of peripheral vascular disease. Cardiovasc Res 1969;3:503.
79. Rains J. In: Rutherford RB (ed.), Vascular surgery. 2nd edition. Philadelphia: Saunders, 1984:59–64.
80. Wyss CR, Matsen FA, Simmons CW, Burgess EM. Transcutaneous oxygen tension measurements on limbs of diabetic and nondiabetic patients with peripheral vascular disease. Surgery 1984;95:339–45.
81. Franzech UK, Talke P, Bernstein EF, Glbranson FL, Fronek A. Transcutaneous PO_2 measurements in health and peripheral arterial occlusive disease. Surgery 1982;91:156–63.
82. Oppenheimer SM, Hoffbrand BI, Oswald GA, Yudkin JS. Diabetes mellitus and early mortality from stroke. Br Med J 1985;291:1041–15.
83. Berger I, Hakim AM. The association of hyperglycemia with cerebral edema in stroke. Stroke 1986;17:865–71.

30. Autonomic dysfunction and hypotension

GIUSEPPE NUZZACI and I. NUZZACI

'Le malade d'Hypotension Orthostatique est comparable à Antée le quel terrassé par Hercule, retrouvait toutes ses forces au contact de la Terre, sa mère' [1].

The major clinical evidence of autonomic system dysfunction is closely related to missing postural control of the systemic arterial pressure (AP) in which the sympathetic nervous system (SNS) plays the principal role through its direct regulation of the cardiac output and of the systemic vascular resistance.

Anatomic and chemical organization of the sympathetic nervous system

The SNS is considered mainly as an efferent system with center areas, located in the hypothalamus and in the brain stem in very close association with each other and with the limbic cortex, paravertebral and prevertebral ganglia (the celiac and hypogastric), sympathetic nerves, whose cell body lies in the intermediolateral horn of the spinal cord (preganglionic fibers), emerging from the thoracic and upper two or three lumbar spinal segments, which synapse in ganglia from which postganglionic fibers supply every organ. Finally the preganglionic fibers arrive to the adrenal medulla and synapse with epinephrine (E) and norepinephrine (NE) secreting cells, embriologically derived from the neural crest and therefore to be considered as postganglionic cells. The preganglionic fibers secrete acetylcholine (ACh) and are said to be cholinergic, the postganglionic fibers secrete NE and are said to be adrenergic.

Synthesis of NE begins in the axoplasm of the terminal nerve endings of adrenergic nerve fibers but is completed inside the vesicles. ACh and NE are synthesized at the terminal nerve endings of the adrenergic nerve fibers and stored inside the vescicles, which are bulbous enlargements located over or near the effector cells, and where there are large numbers of mitocondria, to supply the ATP required to energize ACh or NE synthesis. The basic steps are:

1. Tyrosine → DOPA.
2. DOPA → dopamine.
3. Transport of dopamine into the vesicles.
4. Dopamine → norepinephrine.
5. Norepinephrine → epinephrine.

All these compounds are said to be catecholamines as they possess the catechol ring which is a benzene ring with two hydroxyl radicals and one aminic group. The step between tyrosine and DOPA (dihydroxyphenylalanine) depends on the availability of tyrosine hydroxylase which is a specific enzyme of the catecholamine-producing tissues. Its lack, therefore, is necessarily associated with a fall in catecholamine synthesis. The step between DOPA and dopamine is under the control of DOPA aminodecarboxylase which is also available in the liver and stomach. Dopamine is transformed into NE by dopamine betahydroxylase. When this enzyme is lacking this pathway may be bypassed by dihydroxyphenylserine [2]. The final step takes place in the adrenal medulla where about 80% of the NE is transformed into E by means of phenylethanolamine N-methyltranferase.

The plasma E concentration, depending almost exclusively on the adrenal medulla secretion, is closely related to the adrenal medulla activity. Plasma NE concentration depends mainly on its secretion at the terminal nerve endings, yet its plasma level may not be considered closely related to the sympathetic activity as only 20% of its secretion passes into the peripheral circulation. Plasma levels of catecholamines change after upright posture, physical activity, cold, diet sodium content, tea, coffee, smoking, mental and physical stress. A catecolamine circadian rhythm is detectable with the lowest level in the night and the highest in the morning. After secretion by the terminal nerve endings, NE is removed in two different ways:

1. Reuptake into the adrenergic nerve endings themselves by an active transport process, accounting for removal of 50–80% of the secreted NE (neural uptake).
2. Diffusion away from the nerve endings into the surrounding body fluid and then into the blood, accounting for removal of the remainder of the NE (extraneuronal uptake).

In neural uptake, the principal pathway of metabolism, NE may be either stored in the vesicles and then secreted again or destroyed by enzymes. One of these enzymes is monoamineoxidase which is found in the nerve endings themselves; another is catechol-O-methyltransferase which is present diffusely in all tissues. The NE secreted directly into a tissue remains active for only a few seconds. The NE and E secreted into the blood by the adrenal medulla remain active until they diffuse into some tissue where they are destroyed. They remain very active for 10–30 seconds, and less active for 1 to several minutes [3]. In the urine vanylmandelic acid, methoxyhydroxyphenylglycol, normetanephrine and metanephrine represent the final products respectively of the neural and extraneural metabolism. To stimulate the effector organ NE and E must firstly bind with highly specific receptors of the effector cells. There are two major types of adrenergic receptor: alpha receptors and beta receptors, according to the different affinity for isoproterenol (IS), NE and E. Recently dopaminergic receptors for dopamine and purinergic receptors for ATP have been found [4, 5]. Beta-adrenergic receptors (affinity $IS > E \geqslant NE$) in turn are divided into beta-1 and beta-2 according to their affinity for E and NE.

Beta-1 receptors are chiefly located in the postsynapsis area; there are many of them in the heart where they influence the frequency, excitability and contractility. Beta-2 receptors are located in the presynapsis area and in extraneural sites, chiefly in the wall of the arterioles and veins; their stimulation is associated with vasodilatation.

Alpha-adrenergic receptors (affinity E > NE ≫ IS) in turn are divided into alpha-1 and alpha-2 receptors. Alpha-1 receptors (NE > E) are chiefly located at the postsynapsis junction at the level of the vascular media. Their excitatory effects are associated with vasoconstriction. Alpha-2 receptors (E > NE) are prevalent at the extrasynapsis but also in the presynapsis site where they control NE release. Their stimulation causes vasoconstriction. D_1 dopaminergic receptors are prevalent in the mesenteric and renal arteries (postsynapsis site); their stimulation is associated with vasodilatation. D_2 dopaminergic receptors are present at the level of central and peripheral sympathetic neurons, and at the level of the adrenal medulla and cortex where they control, in the inhibitory sense, the release of E and of aldosterone respectively.

Purinergic receptors are located in the presynaptic site where they control, in the inhibitory sense, NE release. The presynaptic receptors are known as autoreceptors because they bind with their own neurotransmitter. They function according to a feedback mechanism with minor response (desensitization) when the neurotransmitter or the agonist is present in excess or with major response (hypersensitization) when they are lacking (denervation syndrome). In this situation there is an increase of the number of receptors on the axon membrane.

Concerning the events following neurotransmitter uptake, the hypothesis generally accepted is that there is a conformational change in the structure of the protein molecule which in turn excites or inhibits the cell by causing a change in the cell membrane permeability with rapid influx of sodium and/or calcium with excitatory effect. At other times the potassium channels are open, allowing potassium ions to diffuse out of the cell with inhibitory effect. Another mechanism is the activation or inactivation of an enzyme inside the cell (i.e. activation of the enzyme adenyl cyclase), causing production of cAMP (the second messenger), which in turn can initiate any one of many different cellular actions [3].

Anatomic and chemical organization of the parasympathetic nervous system

The parasympathetic fibers leave the central nervous system through cranial III, VII, IX, and X, the second and third sacral nerves and occasionally the first and fourth sacral nerves.

The parasympathetic system, like the sympathetic one, has both preganglionic and postganglionic neurons. Except in the case of a few cranial parasympathetic nerves, the preganglionic fibers pass uninterrupted all the way to the organ that is to be controlled, where the postganglionic neurons are located. The preganglionic fibers synapse with these and short postganglionic fibers leave the neurons to spread through the organ [3].

Acetylcholine is synthesized in the terminal endings of cholinergic nerve fibers. Most of this synthesis occurs in the axoplasm outside the vesicles; the ACh is then transported inside the vesicles where it is stored in a highly concentrated form until it is released.

The basic chemical reaction of ACh synthesis is:

$$\text{Acetyl-CoA + Choline} \xrightarrow{\text{Choline acetyltranferase}} \text{Acetylcholine.}$$

After secretion ACh persists in the tissue for a few seconds, then is destroyed by the enzyme acetylcholinesterase. The choline formed is in turn transported back into the terminal nerve ending where it is used again for synthesis of new ACh.

ACh activates two different types of receptor: muscarinic and nicotinic receptors. The former are present in all effector cells stimulated by postganglionic neurons of the parasympathetic nervous system. The latter are present in the synapses between the pre- and postganglionic neurons.

Atropine blocks muscarinic cholinergic receptors. It increases heart rate and enhances atrioventricular conduction; in addition atropine reverses cholinergically mediated bronchoconstriction and diminishes respiratory tract secretion.

Parasympathetic stimulation causes excitation in some organs but inhibition in others. When sympathetic stimulation excites a particular organ, parasympathetic stimulation sometimes inhibits it, showing that the two systems occasionally act reciprocally to one another.

Parasympathetic effects on the heart are mediated by the vagus nerve. ACh reduces the rate of spontaneous depolarization of the sinoatrial node and decreases heart rate which, in different physiological states, is the result of coordinated interaction between sympathetic stimulation, parasympathetic inhibition and the intrinsic activity of the sinoatrial pacemaker. ACh also delays impulse conduction within the atrial musculature and at the atrioventricular node, reduces conduction velocity, and increases the effective refractory period, thus diminishing the ventricular response during atrial flutter or fibrillation. ACh-induced decreased inotropy, is related to the prejunctional inhibitory effect on sympathetic nerve endings as well as to a direct inhibitory effect on the atrial myocardium. The ventricular myocardium is not greatly affected since innervation by cholinergic fibers is minimal.

Parasympathetic stimulation has virtually no effect on total peripheral resistance since parasympathetic innervation of the vasculature is not extensive. The usual effect is a slight fall in pressure. The parasympathetic nervous system may influence peripheral resistance indirectly by inhibiting NE release from sympathetic nerves. However, very strong vagal stimulation may occasionally stop the heart entirely and cause loss of all arterial pressure [6].

In the last 25 years much data has been accumulated suggesting that the sympathetic and parasympathetic nervous system should not be considered as a reciprocal antagonist system.

The sympathetic fibers in mammals can release both NE and ACh. This capacity, which is very high at birth, becomes lower during the following years but some neurons retain this capacity throughout their life [7–9].

Besides monoamines, many other substances, such as ATP, serotonin, GABA, dopamine, and peptides are present within the autonomic nerves and may work either as neurotransmitters or neuromodulators at the pre- or postsynaptic level [10–12].

The autonomic nervous system operates in the regulation of arterial pressure by means of visceral reflexes whose afferent limbs arise in the stretch receptors located in the aortic arch, the carotid sinuses, ventricles, and atria. Impulses are transmitted through the afferent fibers of glossopharyngeal and vagus nerves, to the central connections located in the medulla. Synapses connect not only the sympathetic and parasympathetic nuclei and efferent arches but also the cerebral cortex and hypothalamus nuclei which control hormonal secretion via the pituitary gland [13]. This arterial pressure control system, called the 'pressure buffer system', represents a rapidly acting pressure control mechanism that becomes active within seconds. When there is a sudden fall of pressure, the baroceptor impulses decrease and the reflex activation of sympathetic outflow associated with inhibition of parasympathetic activity results.

The net effects are: vasoconstriction of arterioles and veins, increased heart rate and strength of myocardial contraction along with increased medullary secretion, increased output of antidiuretic hormone (ADH), adrenocorticotrophic hormone (ACTH), renin, and aldosterone. Therefore inhibition of the baroreceptors by hypotension reflexly causes arterial pressure to increase. Conversely, high pressure has opposite effects, reflexly causing the pressure to fall back toward normal [3].

Assumption of the upright posture imposes gravitational forces that raise the intravascular pressure and cause pooling of blood in the vessels below the 'hydrostatically indifferent point' [14]. The venous pooling is approximately 500–700 ml blood in the legs [15, 16] and is associated with a fall in venous return and a drastic reduction of systemic blood pressure, cerebral ischemia, and loss of consciousness, unless the pressure buffer system does not intervene immediately. Due to this compensatory mechanism the change from recumbent to standing posture in a normal person is usually associated with: a rise in diastolic pressure; no change in systolic pressure; an invariable diminution of pulse pressure; and an invariable increase of pulse rate [17–20]. Impairment of any element of the pressure buffer system results in hypotension.

Classification of the causes of postural hypotension is usually made according to the site of the lesion along the baroreceptors reflex arch:

1. Baroreceptor failure (tumors, irradiation, surgical operations).
2. Disorders of the afferent nerves (IX and X neuralgia, age-related orthostatic hypotention).
3. Central disorders (preganglionic):
   – Shy–Drager syndrome.
   – Familial dysautonomia (Riley–Day syndrome).
   – Parkinson's disease.
   – Infection, trauma, neoplasms, vascular accidents, hydrocephalus, craniopharyngioma, demyelinating disease, Werniche encephalopathy.

4. Peripheral dysfunction of the sympathetic nerves (postganglionic):
   - Primary autonomic hypotension (Bradbury–Eggleston syndrome).
   - General disorders: diabetic, alcoholic, amyloid and other polyneuropathies, Guillain–Barré syndrome, porphyria, beri-beri.
   - Spinal cord disorders: syringomyelia, subacute combined sclerosis, tabe dorsalis, pernicious anemia, spinal cord trauma, autochthonous neoplasms, and metastatic tumors from pulmonary, breast and pancreatic carcinoma.
   - Surgical sympathectomy.
5. Pharmacological causes (the most frequent causes of orthostatic hypotension) such as:
   - Ganglionic blocking drugs (pentolinium).
   - Drugs blocking NE release from noradrenergic neurons (guanethidine, bethanidine etc.).
   - Alpha-1 adrenergic receptor antagonists: prazosin.
   - Alpha-1 and alpha-2 adrenergic antagonists: phentolamine and phenoxybenzamine.
   - Alpha-2 adrenergic agonists: clonidine, methyldopa and guanabenz.
   - Dopamine antagonists: phenothiazines and haloperidol.
   - Tricyclic psychotropic drugs: imipramine and others.
   - L-dopa.
   - Vincristine.
   - Angiotensin-converting enzyme inhibitors (captopril, enalapril, lisinopril). (Adapted from Streeten, 1987 [20]).

Conditions in which there is primary chronic autonomic failure include Bradbury–Eggleston syndrome (1925), Shy–Drager syndrome (1960) or multiple system atrophy (MSA), dopamine beta-hydroxylase (DBH) deficiency, and familial dysautonomia.

Bradbury–Eggleston syndrome [21] appears to be a degenerative disorder, involving both the sympathetic and parasympathetic branches of the autonomic nervous system, which clinically spares other neurological systems. In the Shy–Drager syndrome [22] there is a widespread autonomic failure associated with impairment of cerebellar, extrapyramidal and neuromuscular or cerebral systems. Sympathetic and parasympathetic postganglionic neurons appear however to be intact.

Patients with Bradbury–Eggleston syndrome have in recumbent posture low levels of plasma NE (generally less than 200 pg/ml and often less than 100 pg/ml), which does not increases after standing or exercise. Plasma E levels are also reduced, but to a lesser extent, and dopamine levels are usually around 50% of normal.

In contrast, patients with Shy–Drager syndrome have normal plasma levels of NE while recumbent and which fail to increase normally after standing or exertion. These data suggest that in the first group of patients, without signs of central nervous system disease, the defect affects peripheral sympathetic nerves, whereas in patients of the second group, the lesion is central so that they are unable to activate appropriately an otherwise intact peripheral sympathetic nervous system [23].

Dopamine beta-hydroxylase (DBH) deficiency, recognized in the 1980s by Robertson et al. (1986) [24] and by Man in't veld (1987) [25] is characterized by the virtual absence of plasma, urinary and cerebrospinal NE and E, together with greatly increased plasma dopa and dopamine levels. NE metabolites are absent while dopamine metabolites are increased. There is no evidence of other neurological defects, either cerebral or peripheral.

Familial dysautonomia (Riley–Day syndrome) is a progressive disorder, inherited in a pattern consistent with the autosomal recessive trait, and is limited primarily to Ashkenazi Jews [26]. It is characterized by the appearance at birth or soon afterward of autonomic instability with both postural hypotension and hypertensive episodes due to defective reflex control of vascular tone. Tissue NE stores are normal or elevated. Plasma catecholamine concentrations are normal in patients who are recumbent and at rest, but fail to increase normally with exercise or assumption of the upright posture. The specific abnormality responsible for this syndrome remains unidentified. Defective release of NE from nerve endings is a prominent pathophysiological component, but demonstrable degeneration of the reticular formation of the brain stem suggests a primary abnormality in the central nervous system [27, 28].

Chronic diabetes mellitus is one of the most frequent conditions associated with secondary autonomic failure. In this disorder all the symptoms of autonomic insufficiency may be present, especially hypotension associated with meals and insulin administration. Pathologically there are lesions located at the level of the intermediolateral horn of the spinal cord, such as loss of myelin, axonal degeneration, vacuolar degeneration and loss of myelinic fibers.

Other endocrine disorders, such as adrenocortical insufficiency, leading to reduction of plasma volume, hypoaldosteronism and altered vascular response to catecholamines (Addison's disease) are primary causes of hypotension. Also pheochromocytoma may be a primary cause of postural hypotension, due to plasma volume depletion, and of E-induced vasodilatation in some patients with E-secreting tumors [13].

Another important aspect of the pressure buffer system dysfunction is syncope, which is defined a sudden temporary loss of consciousness associated with a deficit of postural tone with spontaneous recovery. Most syncopal attacks result from sudden transient reduction of blood flow to those parts of the brain subserving consciousness (brain stem reticular activating system). Typically syncopal attacks are characterized by hypotension, pallor, diaphoresis and loss of consciousness. Syncope is frequently a manifestation of hypotension and in that case consciousness is promptly restored when the patient falls or is placed in horizontal position.

There are three principal mechanisms leading to syncope: vasomotor instability associated with decreased systemic vascular resistance or venous return or both; heart diseases associated with reduction of cardiac output; and cerebrovascular disease with decreased cerebral perfusion.

Vasodepressor syncope (Vasovagal syncope, VVS) is the most common form of syncope accounting for more than 55% of cases in some series [29]. It may occur as a response to fear, anxiety, pain or in the setting of real threatened or phantasized injury. Surgical manipulation, the sight of blood, and receiving frightening news represent common precipitating factors. Vasodepressor syncope may also occur without any identifiable predisposing factors. The attack most characteristically develops in the erect position and is relieved by lying down, but in severe cases symptoms may persist or even develop in the recumbent position. In the early phase there is a general sense of muscular weakness followed by discomfort in the epigastrium, sweating, nausea, restlessness, facial pallor, sighing respiration and yawning. These symptoms are usually relieved by lying down, but they may persist and grow more intense, to be followed by lightheadedness, blurring of vision and sudden loss of consciousness. If the period of unconsciousness exceeds 15–20 seconds clonic convulsive movements often ensue [30]. The pathophisiology of VVS has not yet been elucidated definitively. Engel [30], on the basis of clinical and psychological observations, suggests that VVS is a reaction which may result during experiencing of fear or anxiety when action is inhibited or impossible. Vasodepression syncope is preceded by evidence of an increase in sympathetic activity and a decrease in vagal activity immediately before loss of consciousness. During this phase blood pressure and heart rate increase abruptly followed by hypotension and often bradycardia. The major reason for hypotension is vasodilatation in the skeletal muscles as well as in the cutaneous, mesenteric, renal, and cerebral districts. This appears to be due to the inhibition of sympathetic vasoconstriction activity. While in normal individuals the fall in peripheral vascular resistance induced by vasodilatation would be compensated for by a compensatory increase in heart rate and cardiac output which would limit the reduction of arterial pressure, in patients with VVS cardiac output and heart rate fail to rise, perhaps because of failure of normal venous constriction, diminished rise in plasma renin and angiotensin-mediated vasoconstriction [31–35].

Vasodepressor syncope is generally considered a benign entity, however it may be associated with sudden death and cardiac arrest [36]. Engel [37] suggests that psychophysiological processes responsible for VVS may also be those leading to sudden death such as that which occurrs after loss of loved ones, humiliation, and other psychological stress.

Other syncopes related to reflex-mediated vasomotor instability occur in syndromes such as carotid sinus hypersensitivity (CSH) [38, 39]. This syndrome is manifested in two principal forms [40]. The vagal or cardioinhibitory type, occurring in approximately 70% of patients, is characterized by sinus bradycardia, sinus arrest, atrioventricular block or asystole; the vasodepressor type is manifested by marked hypotension without bradycardia or atrioventricular block. The two forms may be present in the same patient. CSH usually occurs in the elderly. Arteriosclerosis, hypertension, diabetes mellitus, and scars, lymph nodes and tumor involving the carotid body may be associated with the syndrome.

Fainting due to hypersensitivity of the vagal carotid sinus reflex is most likely to occur in the sitting or standing positions since reflex asystole long enough to produce loss of consciousness in the recumbent position is rare. It is important to emphasize that when asystole and/or hypotension arise from a hypersensitive carotid sinus reflex, the sinus is usually found to be exquisitely sensitive to touch.

Only the slightest pressure for a few seconds is sufficient to elicit the cardioinhibitory response. Episodes are often precipitated by turning the head or simply stretching the skin of the neck in preparation for shaving. On the contrary, when vigorous or prolonged massage is necessary to provoke slowing or asystole, it is unlikely that the spontaneus reflex has originated in the carotid sinus. It must be appreciated however that the response is very variable, and hence the examination should be carried out repeatedly if the clinical history is suggestive of this syndrome [30]. Disease involving other afferents to the vagus center, such as biliary tract disease, may also be associated with carotid sinus hypersensitivity which disappears when the biliary tract disease is successfully treated [41]. The risk of complications of carotid sinus stimulation is potentially catastrophic and includes carotid standstill and hemiplegia, especially in the elderly [42].

To avoid these complications manual pressure should be applied, only lightly at first on one side and for a maximum of 20 seconds while the electrocardiogram and blood pressure are monitored. In most cases in which no anatomical cause is recognizable, precautions to avoid rapid movements and avoidance of tight collars usually constitute effective therapy. When severe bradycardia is associated with ventricular or atrioventricular pacing, administration of alpha-adrenergic agents, cholinergic antagonists or both can improve symptoms. Surgical resection or denervation of the hypersensitive carotid sinus may be required for refractory cases [40, 43–46].

In micturition or post-micturition syncope, patients, healthy young or middle-aged men, faint while standing before, during or immediately after urinating. It has been suggested that many factors act together leading to syncope such as sudden decompression of the bladder, decreased peripheral resistance during sleep, vagal stimulation associated with micturition, or Valsalva maneuvre leading to decreased venous return. In cough syncope [47] the patient, typically a middle-aged man who is large-chested, mildly obese, and a heavy smoker with chronic pulmonary disorders and chronic cough, presents with syncope after paroxysms of severe cough. Syncope in this syndrome results not only from reflex-mediated mechanisms but also from hydraulic factors. Coughing in these patients produces extremely high intrathoracic and intrabdominal pressure, at times reaching 300 mmHg, resulting in an exaggerated Valsalva response with decreased venous return and cardiac output. This high pressure is transmitted virtually undiminished to the cerebrospinal fluid compartment with squeezing of blood from the cranium so that the brain rapidly becomes 'bloodless', anoxia develops and syncope ensues [48–50].

Swallow syncope occurs in patients who have been found to have esophageal disorders such as diverticula, spasm, achalasia and stricture, and also cardiac disorders including acute rheumatic carditis treated with digitalis, and acute myocardial infarction. Sinus arrest or asystole, complete AV block, and nodal or sinus bradycardia have been demonstrated as the cause of swallow syncope. Use of vagolytic agents or insertion of a cardiac pacemaker have abolished symptoms. Swallow syncope is due to dysfunction of the afferent–efferent loop between the brain stem and the heart [51]. Patients who have syncope with glossopharyngeal neuralgia suffer paroxysms of intense pain along the glossopharyngeal nerve – the base of the tongue, tonsillar region, soft palate or throat, ear, angle of the jaw – lasting a few seconds to a few minutes, during which faintness, unconsciousness or convulsion may ensue [52]. The syndrome may be completely cured by intracranial section of the glossopharyngeal nerve.

The oculovagal reflex syndrome occurs through a reflex whose afferent portion is located in the orbital branches of the trigeminal nerve. Pressure over the eyeballs may induce bradycardia, AV dissociation and higher degrees of AV block, chiefly in patients with cardiac disease and digitalis treatment [53]. Spontaneous syncope of this origin is very rare.

The 'long QT syndrome' [54] is characterized by the occurrence of syncope or heart standstill attacks usually associated with physical and/or emotional stresses in children with marked lengthening (at least 450 ms in males and 460 ms in females) of the QT electrocardiographic interval. This disorder has been ascribed to the congenital predominance of the left over right cardiac sympathetic supply. This hypothesis has been supported by the significant decrease (from 99% to 45%) of morbidity and mortality obtained after left cardiac sympathetic denervation [55].

References

1. Trocme'. Un cas d'hypotension orthostatique à évolution grave. Arch Mal Coeur January 1938.
2. Biaggioni I, Robertson D. Endogenous restoration of noradrenaline by precursor therapy in dopamine beta-hydroxylase deficiency. Lancet 1987;ii:1170–2.
3. Guyton AC. Textbook of medical physiology. 8th ed., Philadelphia: Saunders, 1991:3.
4. Burnstock G, Buckley N. The classification of receptors for adenosine and adenine nucleotides. In: Paton DM, ed., Methods used in adenosine research. Methods in pharmacology. Vol. 6, New York: Plenum Press, 1985:193.
5. Burnstock G, Kennedy C. Is there a basis for distinguishing two types of P_2-purinoreceptors? Gen Pharmacol 1985;16:433.
6. Landsberg L, Young JB. in: Harrison's principles of internal medicine, 13th ed. New York: McGraw–Hill, 1994:424–5.
7. Burnstock G. Evolution of the autonomic innervation of visceral and cardiovascular systems in vertebrates. Pharmacol Rev 1969;21:247.
8. Burnstock G. Do some sympathetic neurones release both noradrenaline and acetylcholine? Prog Neurobiol 1978;11:205.
9. Schotzinger RJ, Landis SC. Cholinergic phenotype developed by noradrenergic sympathetic nervous after innervation of a novel cholinergic target *in vivo*. Nature 1988;335:637.
10. Cuello AC, (ed.). Co-transmission. London:MacMillan, 1982.
11. Hoyle CHV, Burnstock G. Evidence that ATP is a neurotransmitter in the frog heart. Eur J Pharmacol 1986;124:285.
12. Hokfelt T. *et al*. Coexistence of neuronal messengers: A new principle in chemical transmission. Progr Brain Res 1986;68:24.
13. Sobel BE, Roberts R. In: Braunwald E. (ed.), Heart Disease. Philadelphia: Saunders, 1988:884–7.
14. Vagner E. Fortgesetzte undersuchungen uber den einfluss der schwere auf den kreislauf. Arch Ges Physiol 1886;39:371.
15. Hickam JB, Pryor WW. Cardiac output in postural hypotension. J Clin Invest 1951;30:410.
16. Folkow B. Nervous control of the blood vessels. Physiol Rev 1955;35:629.
17. Akesson S. Uber veranderungen des elecktrokardiogramms bei orthostatischer zirkulationsstorung. Ups Lakareforens Forhandl 1936;41:381.
18. Hammarstrom S. Arterial hypertension. I. Variability of blood pressure. II. Neurosurgical treatment, indications and results. Acta Med Scand. 1947;192:(Suppl.) 1–301.

19. Frohlich ED, Tarazi RC, Ulrych M et al. Tilt test for investigating a neural component in hypertension. Its correlation with clinical characteristics. Circulation 1967;36:387–93.
20. Streeten DHP. Orthostatic disorders of the circulation. Mechanisms, manifestations and treatment. New York and London: Plenum Medical Book Company, 1987:117–29.
21. Bradbury S, Eggleston C. Postural hypotension: A report of three cases. Am Heart J 1925;1:73–86.
22. Shy GM, Drager GA. A neurological syndrome associated with orthostatic hypotension. Arch Neurol 1960;2:511–27.
23. Ziegler MG, Lake CB, Kopin IJ. The sympathetic nervous system defect in primary orthostatic hypotension. N Engl J Med 1977;296:293.
24. Robertson D, Goldberg MR, Onrot J et al. Isolated failure of anatomic noradrenergic neurotransmission. Evidence for impaired beta-hydroxylation of dopamine. N Engl J Med 1986;314:1494–7.
25. Man in't veld AJ, Boomsma F, Moleman P et al. Congenital dopamine beta-hydroxylase deficiency. A novel orthostatic syndrome. Lancet 1987;i:183–7.
26. Riley CM, Day RL, Greeley DM et al. Central autonomic dysfunction with defective lacrimation. I. Report of 5 cases. Pediatrics 1949;3:468–78.
27. Dancis J, Smith AA. Familial dysautonomia. N Engl J Med 1966;274:207.
28. Ziegler MG, Lake CR, Kopin IJ. Deficient sympathetic nervous response in familial dysautonomia. N Engl J Med 1976;294:630.
29. Wayne HM. Syncope, physiological considerations and an analysis of the clinical characteristcs of 510 patients. Am J Med 1961;30:418.
30. Engel GL. Fainting. Springfield, Illinois: Charles C. Thomas 1962:7.
31. Barcroft H, Edholm OG, McMichael J et al. Posthemorrhagic fainting. Study by cardiac output and forearm flow. Lancet 1944;I:489.
32. Weissler AM, Warren JV, Estes EH Jr et al. Vasopressor syncope. Factors influencing cardiac output. Circulation 1957;15:875.
33. Aviado DM, Jr, Schmidt CF. Cardiovascular and respiratory reflexes from the left side of the heart. Am J Physiol 1959;196:726.
34. Glick G, Y PN. Hemodynamic changes during spontaneus vasovagal reactions. Am J Med 1963;34:42.
35. Epstein SE, Stampfer M, Beiser GD. Role of the capacitance and resistance vessel in vasovagal syncope. Circulation 1968;37:524.
36. Schraeder PL, Pontzer R, Engel TR. A case of being scared to death. Arch Int Med 1983;143:1793.
37. Engel GL. Psychologic stress, vasodepressor (vasovagal) syncope, and sudden death. Ann Int Med 1978;89:403.
38. Weiss S, Baker J.P. The carotid sinus reflex in health and disease. Its role in the causation of fainting and convulsion. Medicine 1933;12:297.
39. Leatham A. Carotid sinus syncope. Br Heart J 1982;47:409.
40. Gardner RS, Magovern GJ, Park SB et al. Carotid sinus syndrome. New surgical considerations. Vasc Surg 1975;9:204.
41. McLemore Ga, Levine SA. The possible therapeutic value of cholecystectomy in Adams–Stokes disease. Am J Med Sc 1955;229:386.
42. Coplan NL, Schweitzer P. Carotid sinus hypersensitivity. Case report and review of the literature. Am J Med 1984;77:561.
43. Trout HH, Brown LI, Thompson JE. Carotid sinus syndrome: Treatment by carotid sinus denervation. Am Surg 1979;189:575.
44. Morley CA, Dehn TCB, Perrins EJ, et al. Baroreflex sensitivity measured by the phenylephrine pressor-test in patients with carotid sinus and sick sinus syndrome. Cardiovasc Res 1984;18:752.
45. Almquist A, Gornick C, Benson W Jr et al. Carotid sinus hypersensitivity. Evaluation of the vasodepressor component. Circulation 1985;71:927.
46. Murphy AL, Rowbothan BJ, Boyle RS et al. Carotid sinus hypersensitivity in elderly nursing home patients. Aust NZ J Med 1986;16:24.
47. Charcot J. 1876. In: Engel GL. Fainting, Springfields, Illinois: Charles C. Thomas, 1962:105.
48. McCann WS, Bruce RA, Lovejoy FW et al. Tussive syncope observations on the disease formerly called laryngeal epilepsy with a report of two cases. Arch Int Med 1949;84:845.
49. Sharpey-Schafer EP. Mechanism of syncope after coughing. Br Med J 1953;2:860.

50. McIntosh HE, Estes EH, Warren JV. The mechanism of cough syncope. Am Heart J 1956;52:70.
51. Weiss S Ferris EB. Adams Stokes syndrome with transient complete heart block of vagovagal reflex origin. Arch Int Med 1934;54:931.
52. Kjellin K, Muller R, Widen L. Glossopharyngeal neuralgia associated with cardiac arrest and hypersecretion from ipsilateral parotid gland. Neurology 1959;9:527.
53. Schamroth L. Electrocardiographic effects of eyeball compression. Am J Cardiol 1958;2:321.
54. Schwartz DJ. Idiopathic long QT syndrome. Progress and questions. Am Heart J 1985;109:399–411.
55. Schwartz DJ, Locati EH, Moss AJ *et al*. Left cardiac sympathetic denervation in the therapy of congenital long QT syndrome: A worldwide report. Circulation 1991;84:503–11.

31. Hemostatic defects and venous thromboembolism

CATHERINE OZANNE and HANNAH COHEN

Normal hemostasis

The normal hemostatic mechanism depends on several overlapping and sequential events including the vessel response to injury, platelet activation and aggregation, and the activation of the coagulation system leading to formation of a stable fibrin thrombus. This leads to activation of fibrinolysis which results in clot dissolution, enabling repair of vessel damage.

The coagulation system is a finely balanced network of interacting procoagulant and anticoagulant factors. Recent evidence suggests that the major initiator of blood coagulation is the tissue factor/activated factor VII (VIIa) complex [1]. Human tissue factor is a single chain integral transmembrane protein, MW 45 kDa. Under normal circumstances there is little or no tissue factor in the plasma, but it is released locally into the circulation in response to tissue or vessel injury. The tissue factor/VIIa complex activates factors X and IX. Tissue factor pathway inhibitor (TFPI), a 40-kDa glycoprotein, binds to and inhibits the generated activated factor X (Xa); this complex then binds to and inhibits the tissue factor/factor VIIa complex. TFPI-mediated negative feedback inhibition limits further generation of thrombin via activated factor X [2]. Further generation of thrombin occurs via the tissue factor/factor VIIa activation of factor IX with its cofactor, factor VIII. The tenase and prothrombinase complex interactions occur on the negatively charged platelet membrane phospholipids, exposed following platelet activation. The final events in the procoagulant system are the cleavage of fibrinogen to fibrin by thrombin. The formed fibrin monomer polymerizes and is cross-linked by thrombin activated factor XIII, to form a stable fibrin thrombus. Fibrinogen is a dimeric glycoprotein, MW 340 kDa, synthesized in the hepatocyte. It has a half-life of 4 days, and consists of two identical subunits, each containing three dissimilar polypeptide chains: $A\alpha$, $B\beta$ and γ joined near the N-terminal by disulfide bonds. In addition to formation of fibrin, fibrinogen binds specifically to platelet membrane glycoprotein IIb/IIIa and is an acute phase reactant that influences blood flow properties and is a major determinant of blood and plasma viscosity.

Procoagulant activity is balanced by the naturally occurring anticoagulant mechanisms, antithrombin and the protein C system. Antithrombin (AT) (hitherto called antithrombin III), a 58-kDa glycoprotein, synthesized in the liver and possibly vascular endothelium, is the principal inhibitor of thrombin in adult life with a half-life of 45–65 hours. The gene for antithrombin is located on chromosome 1 [3]. Antithrombin has two reactive sites, a heparin binding site and a site that reacts with serine residues. The action of AT is accelerated at least 1000-fold in the presence of heparin, which induces a conformational change in the AT molecule facilitating binding to thrombin and other serine proteases [4]. The endothelial cell synthesizes the sulfated proteoglycans dermatan, chrondroitin and heparin sulfates, which bind to AT and neutralize locally generated thrombin. This system is highly efficient, with a capacity for thrombin neutralization fivefold greater than of commercial heparin.

Protein C, a 62-kDa glycoprotein synthesized in the liver, is a vitamin K dependent inactive zymogen of a serine protease which is converted to activated protein C (APC) by proteolytic cleavage. This cleavage, catalyzed by thrombin, is accelerated at least 20 000-fold by thrombomodulin [5], a high affinity binding site for thrombin within the endothelial cell membrane. Activated protein C inactivates activated coagulation factors V (Va) and VIII (VIIIa), a cell membrane phospholipid associated process that requires the presence of a cofactor, protein S [6]. Activated protein C, in animal studies and *in vitro*, has been shown to enhance fibrinolysis by increasing levels of plasminogen activator [7] and by inactivation of plasminogen activator inhibitor-1 (PAI-1) [8], the major physiological inhibitor of tissue plasminogen activator (t-PA). However, the profibrinolytic effect of protein C *in vivo* is uncertain. The level of APC activity is regulated by specific inhibitors: protein C inhibitor and alpha 1-antitrypsin [9]. Protein S is a 70-kDa vitamin K dependent glycoprotein, synthesized in the liver, endothelial cells [10] and a variety of other tissues. It exists in plasma in two forms: free protein S (the active form) and bound to C4b binding protein (C4b BP), the free fraction representing 40% of the total [11]. Protein S, a cofactor for activated protein C [12], appears to bind protein C to the platelet surface [13]. Protein S has a half-life of 42.5 hours whilst the half-life of protein C is 6 hours. The gene for protein C is found on chromosome 2 [14]. There are two genes for protein S, the active PSα gene and the pseudogene PSβ, both on chromosome 3 [15].

The fibrinolytic mechanism consists of a complex enzyme system which serves to generate localized proteolysis. The essential reaction of fibrinolysis is the conversion of the proenzyme plasminogen to the active plasmin. Fibinolysis activation pathways can be divided into extrinsic (t-PA mediated) and intrinsic (contact factor mediated), which interact. The major physiological activator of fibrinolysis is believed to be t-PA, synthesized and released by vascular endothelial cells. Factor XII is an important component of the intrinsic system and its action has been shown to account for 23% of the total plasma fibrinolytic activity. Activated factor XII converts prekallikrein to kallikrein; both factor XII and kallikrein may directly activate plasminogen to plasmin, and kallikrein activates prourokinase to urokinase which also activates plasminogen. In addition, kallikrein releases kinins, including bradykinin, from high molecular weight kininogen. Bradykinin stimulates release of t-PA from the vascular endothelium, indirectly activating fibrinolysis. Inhibitors are essential components of the fibrinolytic system and include PAI-1 synthesized and released by vascular endothelial cells, PAI-2 released by the placenta, alpha-2-antiplasmin and histidine rich glycoprotein.

Hemostatic defects predisposing to venous thromboembolism (thrombophilia)

It is well recognized that advancing age and certain situations including surgery, immobilization, pregnancy, the combined oral contraceptive pill, and malignancy, are associated with an increased risk of venous thromboembolism. However, individuals may develop thrombosis at a relatively young age, or in the absence of an obvious risk factor. In these patients, an underlying hemostatic defect should be sought. Thrombophilia may be defined as the presence of a familial or acquired disorder of hemostasis which predisposes to thrombosis. Potential thrombophilic defects may be caused by the following: increased coagulation system activity, increased platelet activity, decreased fibrinolysis and endothelial damage or dysfunction. The characterization of defects of endothelial or platelet activity is limited. Investigation in the clinical situation is largely confined to identification of defects in the coagulation and fibrinolytic systems.

A candidate risk factor for familial thrombophilia should fulfil the following criteria: it should be heritable, and cosegregate with thrombotic manifestations. Association between the laboratory abnormality and thrombosis should be statistically significant and significance should persist even after the proband has been eliminated. Using these criteria there are five established risk factors: antithrombin deficiency, protein C deficiency, protein S deficiency, activated protein C resistance, and defects of fibrinogen. Other possible thrombophilic defects include deficiencies of heparin cofactor II, plasminogen, factor XII, decreased fibrinolysis and inborn errors of metabolism (e.g. homocystinuria). A major cause of acquired thrombophilia is the presence of antiphospholipid antibodies. Acquired deficiencies of the naturally occurring anticoagulants also occur and may predispose to thrombosis.

Antithrombin deficiency

Antithrombin deficiency predisposing to thrombosis was first described in 1965 [16]. It is perhaps the most severe of the heterozygous thrombophilic defects with 85% of those possessing the genetic abnormality having had a thrombotic event by the age of 55 years with a peak incidence between 15 and 40. Children tend to be less often affected in the heterozygous state as they are afforded protection by higher levels of alpha-2 macroglobulin [17]. The risk of a thromboembolic event in heterozygotes has been estimated to be 12% per annum [18]. Antithrombin deficiency may be divided into type I, in which both antigenic and functional activity is reduced equally, and type II, where there is reduced activity but relatively normal antigen levels. Type I accounts for 80–90% of deficiencies [19]. The type II deficiencies can be further subdivided according to which of the active sites are affected: type IIa is characterized by defects of both the reactive and the heparin binding sites. In type IIb, only the reactive site is affected and in type IIc, the heparin binding site is abnormal [20]. Patients with type IIc deficiencies have a significantly lower risk of venous thrombosis of approximately 6% as compared with 50–60% in individuals with type IIb [21]. The genetic defects giving rise to antithrombin deficiency are heterogeneous and include deletions, insertions and single base pair substitutions.

Defects of the protein C system

Protein C and S deficiency

Defects of proteins C and S causing familial thrombophilia were described in the early 1980s [22, 23]. There are two types of protein C deficiency; type I in which both antigenic and functional activity is reduced equally, and type II, where there is reduced activity but relatively normal antigen levels. The genetics are heterogenous but the clinical manifestations do not appear to differ with the type of deficiency. Protein S deficiencies are subdivided into three types: type I in which levels of total and free protein S are reduced as well as the reduction in the activity of protein S; type II in which there is reduced activity but normal levels of free and total protein S [24] and type III (the least common) which is characterized by normal levels of total protein S but reduced free levels and reduced activity [25]. The risk of thrombosis in asymptomatic carriers of protein C or S deficiency has been estimated at approximately 3% per annum with a 0% incidence in nondeficient relatives [26]. Patients with protein C and S deficiencies tend to present at an older age than those with AT deficiency. By the age of 50, 80% of those with protein S deficiency and 50% of those with protein C deficiency will have had their first thrombotic episode [27].

Activated protein C resistance

This recently defined autosomal dominant thrombophilic defect is due to an abnormality of factor V which renders factor Va relatively resistant to inactivation by protein C [28]. In the majority of patients (90–95%) this is due to a single base pair substitution – the factor V Leiden mutation – which results in a CGA to CAA transition which leads to Gln being substituted for Arg at position 506, within the N-terminal APC cleavage site. Factor Va is normally cleaved sequentially at three sites by activated protein C; the 506 site is cleaved first and leads to the exposure of the other two sites (Arg 306 and Arg 679). In addition intact factor V acts as a cofactor for activated protein C [29]. Activated protein C resistance is the most common recognized cause of inherited thrombophilia. It is usually a relatively mild abnormality; however owing to its high prevalence (see below), it may occur in association with other thrombophilic defects leading to a more severe phenotype often with patients being affected at a younger age [30]. The incidence of thrombosis is also markedly affected by other risk factors including combined oral contraceptive usage, pregnancy, surgery and immobilization. Indeed the risk of a thrombotic event in a heterozygous woman has been estimated to increase 35-fold if she is taking the oral contraceptive pill [31]. In addition, APCR is associated with second trimester fetal loss [32].

Clinical manifestations of antithrombin deficiency and defects of the protein C system

Patients with the heterozygous form of these defects share certain clinical manifestations. Deep vein thromboses, mainly of the lower limb, and pulmonary emboli are the commonest clinical manifestations. Thromboses may also occur in cerebral, mesenteric, portal, hepatic, axillary, inferior caval, renal, and retinal veins, and may be recurrent. Superficial thrombophlebitis also occurs quite frequently, mainly in patients with deficiencies of proteins C and S. Arterial occlusions (coronary, femoral, splanchnic, and cerebral) occur less commonly in this group of conditions but have been reported. Thrombosis may present in situations of increased risk such as pregnancy or prolonged immobilization or may be spontaneous.

An unusual complication of deficiencies of protein C [33] and S [34] is coumarin induced skin necrosis which occurs on initiation or escalation [35] of warfarin therapy. This is due to thrombosis in the subcutaneous microcirculation leading to necrosis of the dermis and subcutaneous fat. It is hypothesized that the levels of protein C fall rapidly on initiation of warfarin due to its short half-life (6 hours), whilst the anticoagulant effect of warfarin does not occur until the level of factor II, half-life 60 hours, falls. Thus, in the initial phase of warfarin anticoagulation, protein C levels in the heterozygote may fall to those seen in the homozygous state. Purpura fulminans neonatorus is a potentially lethal complication of homozygosity or compound heterozygosity for defects of the protein C system. In a process similar to coumarin skin necrosis there is widespread microvascular thrombosis in the subcutaneous tissues evident shortly after birth in these infants who have very low or undetectable levels of either protein C or S [36]. There may be an associated disseminated intravascular coagulation. In some cases fetal thrombosis (cerebral or ophthalmic) or neonatal thrombosis of large vessels may occur. The severity of clinical manifestations varies with the levels of the deficient protein C or S.

Venous thromboembolic events in patients with thrombophilia are often precipitated by a specific additional challenge to the hemostatic mechanism such as immobilization, surgery, pregnancy, or use of estrogen-containing combined oral contraceptive preparations. The incidence of thrombosis per patient year on the combined oral contraceptive pill in AT and protein C deficiency is reported to be 27.5% and 12% respectively compared with 6.9% and 3.4% in the control patient groups, but the risk in protein S deficient patients appears to be unaffected [37]. The pattern of inheritance of the thrombophillic defects is usually autosomal dominant, however some more complex inheritance patterns are recognized, for instance there are examples of particularly mild heterozygous defects that are only expressed in homozygotes [38] or in compound heterozygotes.

Defects of fibrinogen
Congenital fibrinogen defects may be classified into three groups: hypofibrinogenemia (or afibrinogenemia), dysfibrinogenemia and hypodysfibrinogenemia. The latter two may predispose to thrombosis [39]. Congenital dysfibrinogenemia is due to synthesis of a functionally defective fibrinogen. Many molecular defects are described, most are autosomal dominant. Congenital dysfibrinogenemia may be asymptomatic in 55% of cases; 25% have a bleeding tendency. Twenty percent are associated with arterial and/or venous thromboembolism due either to defective binding of thrombin to abnormal fibrin or impaired stimulation of t-PA. Hypodysfibrinogenemia may also be associated with thrombosis.

Prevalence of inherited thrombophilic defects

Although there are many published studies of the prevalence of the various thrombophilic defects, these vary considerably, and depend on the population studied, the selection criteria applied and the test methodology employed. The true prevalence of these defects remains unknown.

Estimates of the prevalence of thrombophilic defects in the general population are derived from studies in healthy blood donors. The prevalence of antithrombin deficiency (excluding type IIc) in Scottish blood donors is approximately 1:1500 [40]. A further study by Tait et al. showed an observed prevalence of protein C deficiency of 1:750 [41]. This contrasts with the reported prevalence in North American blood donors of 1:250 [42]. There are no reliable studies of the prevalence of protein S deficiency in the general population. The prevalence of activated protein C resistance is variable within different population groups. In healthy Dutch controls the prevalence is 4.7% [43] but the defect has not been found in certain populations including Afro-Caribbeans.

The prevalence of thrombophilic defects in individuals with a history of venous thromboembolism depends on selection criteria, which include age range, presence of a family history or recurrent episodes. In unselected DVT cases, Heijboer et al. reported 6.5% prevalence of antithrombin, protein C and S deficiencies [44], whereas in a study of selected cases, the prevalence was 26% [45]. Congenital dysfibrinogenemia is very rare; 250 cases are reported, and of these, 10% have hypodysfibrinogenemia. Prior to the discovery of activated protein C resistance (APCR), an underlying hemostatic defect was found in only a relatively small proportion of individuals with venous thromboembolism. APCR is by far the most common heritable thrombophilic defect with a reported prevalence in patients with DVT between 21% [43] to 64% [46].

Acquired thrombophilia

Acquired deficiencies of the naturally occurring anticoagulants

Acquired deficiencies of the naturally occurring anticoagulants, proteins C and S and AT, occur in liver disease, disseminated intravascular coagulation (DIC), and acute thrombosis, and in association with treatment with some chemotheraputic agents. In addition antithrombin deficiency may be seen in heparin therapy, estrogen administration, major surgery, protein losing enteropathy and nephrotic syndrome. Protein C and S deficiency occurs in patients receiving warfarin, the antiphospholipid syndrome and systemic lupus erythematosus [47]. Protein C deficiency also complicates cardiopulmonary bypass and hemodialysis, whilst protein S deficiency is associated with pregnancy. A recently described autoimmune protein S deficiency has been reported in children with postinfectious purpura fulminans, particularly following varicella zoster infection [48].

Antiphospholipid antibodies

Antiphospholipid (aPL) antibodies are a heterogenous group of immunoglobulins directed against different protein–phospholipid complexes. They include lupus anticoagulants (LA) and anticardiolipin (aCL) antibodies. The LA recognize the prothrombin–phospholipid complex and thereby inhibit phospholipid-dependent coagulation reactions *in vitro* [49]. Anticardiolipin antibodies are directed toward β_2-glycoprotein 1 (β_2GP1) bound to an anionic lipid surface [50]. They can be divided into two groups: aCL-type A which inhibit *in vitro* coagulation reactions by enhancing the binding of β_2GP1 to the procoagulant phospholipid surface; and aCL-type B which do not exhibit anticoagulant properties *in vitro*.

Antiphospholipid antibodies are associated with recurrent miscarriage, thrombosis, and thrombocytopenia – the primary antiphospholipid syndrome (PAPS) [51]. Other clinical associations include neurological and dermatological manifestations. Antiphospholipid antibodies are also found in about 40% of patients with systemic lupus erythematosus (SLE) [52] as well as in other autoimmune disorders, and in about 2% of apparently healthy individuals [53]. Not all antiphospholipid antibodies are pathogenic. IgM antibodies are often detected following viral infections, such as syphilis, adenovirus, chickenpox, mumps, and human immunodeficiency viral infection. They are not associated with thrombotic complications and do not bind β_2GP1 [54]. Non-pathogenic antibodies may also occur in association with administration of drugs including chlorpromazine, hydrazine and procainamide.

Retrospective studies suggest that cessation of warfarin treatment in individuals with aPL antibodies is associated with a high incidence, 53% [55] and 69% [56], of recurrent thromboembolic events. Approximately half the thrombotic events are arterial. In patients with SLE thromboembolic events occur in 42% of those with antiphospholipid antibodies; however, 12% of patients with SLE who do not have aPL antibodies also suffer thrombotic events [52]. A prospective study of patients with antiphospholipid antibodies has estimated the risk of a thrombotic event to be 2.5% per annum [57].

The precise mechanism by which thrombosis occurs in aPL antibody positive patients remains unclear. It has been suggested that aPL antibodies may predispose to thrombosis by inhibiting prostacyclin production from vascular endothelial cells [58], but *in vitro* studies on prostacyclin release using sera from patients with LA have been contradictory [59, 60]. Other suggested mechanisms include platelet activation, endothelial cell damage leading to increased procoagulant activity or impaired fibrinolytic responses [61], or inhibition of the protein C/S anticoagulant system [62]. It has also been proposed that inhibition of ATIII activity on endothelial cell surfaces may predispose patients with aPL to vascular thrombosis [63].

Approach to the patient with suspected thrombophilia

Guidelines for the selection of patients in whom thrombophilia screening should be performed have been proposed by the British Society for Hematology (BSH) by the

Haemostasis and Thrombosis Task Force [64]. It should be recognized that some patients with a thrombophilic defect will not be investigated using these criteria. Thrombophilia screening tests are expensive and labor intensive. Criteria for testing should be locally established. Our practice is to offer thrombophilia screening to the following patient groups: venous or arterial thrombosis before the age of 45 years; recurrent venous thromboembolism or thrombophlebitis; thrombosis in an unusual site; family history of thrombosis; or relatives of patients with a known thrombophilic defect. In addition, patients with the following conditions are screened for the presence of antiphospholipid antibodies: recurrent pregnancy loss; unexplained thrombocytopenia; systemic lupus erythematosus; and prolonged activated partial thromboplastin time (APTT). The recently defined high prevalence of APCR has prompted the suggestion that all women should perhaps be screened for this defect prior to administration of combined oral contraceptive preparations. The cost-effectiveness of this approach has not been evaluated.

Patients referred for thrombophilia screening should have a comprehensive clinical assessment. A full history should be taken with particular reference to the following: previous thrombotic events and their circumstances; documentation of exposure to situations associated with an increased risk of thrombosis; drug history; and family history. It is essential to ascertain the certainty with which the diagnosis of venous thromboembolism has been made, as this has important implications for future management. Clinical diagnosis of deep venous thrombosis and pulmonary embolism is notoriously unreliable with a false positive diagnosis being made in up to 80% of patients on clinical history and signs alone [65]. Thus, objective diagnostic tests are mandatory. The timing of thrombophilia testing may influence the results obtained. For this reason, investigation should if possible be avoided under the following circumstances: the acute post-thrombotic period; whilst on heparin or warfarin; within six weeks of pregnancy; and whilst on or within six weeks of stopping the combined oral contraceptive pill. The practice of stopping anticoagulant treatment for the purpose of performing thrombophila screening is potentially dangerous.

Laboratory investigation for thrombophilia

Standardization of test conditions is critical for assessment of fibrinolytic parameters which may be affected by several factors including venostasis, serum lipid levels, and diurnal variation. The importance of standardized conditions for assessment of other thrombophilic defects has not been established. Careful sample collection and processing, as well as standardization of laboratory tests is essential to ensure the validity of results. The initial thrombophilia screen should include certain general investigations to exclude non-hemostatic defects which may predispose to thrombosis; a peripheral blood count to exclude myeloproliferative disease; creatinine and liver function tests; and a screen for the presence of paraproteinemia (erythrocyte sedimentation rate or serum protein electrophoresis). Fasting blood lipid and blood glucose levels should be performed as part of risk assessment, as certain thrombophilic defects may predispose to arterial as well as venous thrombosis.

It is our practice to perform the following tests for thrombophilia: coagulation screen (prothrombin time, APTT, and thrombin time), fibrinogen (Clauss), antithrombin and protein C activities (chromogenic assay), and protein S (total and free) by ELISA. Testing for antiphospholipid antibodies includes a screening and specific test for the presence of lupus anticoagulant (80:20 mix of patient:normal plasma and a dilute Russell's viper venom time test with a platelet neutralization procedure) and IgG and IgM anticardiolipin antibodies by standardized ELISA. There is a considerable degree of overlap between the results obtained with the clotting test for APCR and the presence of the factor V Leiden mutation, detected by PCR analysis. Therefore, both techniques should be employed. In addition in our laboratory we assay factor XII activity, plasminogen activity, and fibrin plate lysis, a screening test for fibrinolytic activity. If fibrinolytic activity is reduced, pre- and post-venous occlusion (20 minutes at 80 mmHg) assessment is done. Specific assays for t-PA and PAI-1 may be performed.

If a specific thrombophilic defect is identified, repeat confirmatory testing is necessary in all cases. In addition further investigation is usually required to characterize the abnormality; antigen assays by ELISA in the case of functional antithrombin or protein C deficiencies; C4b binding protein in patients with protein S deficiency; and high performance liquid chromatography of fibrinopeptides released by thrombin for the dysfibrinogenemias. DNA analysis to delineate the genetic basis of the defect is largely restricted to research laboratories. In patients on warfarin, levels of protein C and S are reduced. A low protein C:factor VII ratio in patients stable on warfarin treatment has been shown to be highly suggestive of protein C deficiency. Testing for the presence of the lupus anticoagulant is also affected by coumarin therapy and requires careful interpretation of results. Antiphospholipid antibodies may be transient, and in order to make the diagnosis of the antiphospholipid syndrome, persistence of aPL antibodies should be demonstrated. Confirmatory testing should therefore be deferred for at least two months.

Management

The management of the initial acute thromboembolic episode should be along standard lines. Prior to investigation for thrombophilia, the purpose, limitations and implications of testing need to be explained to the patient. Whether or not a thrombophilic defect is identified, the patient is given specific advice on risk reduction measures against thrombosis, including advice to avoid dehydration and maintain mobility on long airflights. Contraception must be addressed. Estrogen-containing oral contraceptive preparations should be avoided, but progesterone-only preparations are suitable [66]. Low intensity warfarin cover may be considered for patients requiring hormone replacement therapy. Advice should be given on the potential symptoms of thrombosis and the need to seek medical attention should they occur. Thromboprophylaxis is required for surgery, prolonged immobilization and pregnancy. Screening of family members for the presence of thrombophilic defects needs to be undertaken for all those in whom an abnormality is identified.

The major dilemmas in the management of patients with a history of a thromboembolism and/or a defined thrombophilic defect surround the indications for long-term anticoagulation and the timing of anticoagulation in situations of high risk particularly pregnancy. There is a lack of prospective randomized controlled trials to guide treatment decisions in patients with thrombophilia. In making these decisions, the personal history (including site and severity of thromboembolism), family history, possible contraindications to therapy, conditions under which the thrombosis took place, other risk factors and nature of the thrombophilic defect(s) all have to be considered. An individualized treatment stategy is then defined for each patient. It is generally accepted that patients who have had two thromboembolic events would normally be offered lifelong anticoagulation regardless of whether or not they had an identified defect.

Antithrombin deficiency

This is the most severe deficiency and carries the highest risk of thromboembolism in pregnancy [67]. In view of the high incidence of thromboembolism, a case could be made for long-term warfarinization in the asymptomatic patient in those with type I, and type 2a and 2b antithrombin deficiency after the age of 15; however this is not currently standard practice and would be unlikely to influence survival [68]. It is probably reasonable to institute long-term anticoagulation after a single thrombotic event particularly if the event is spontaneous or life-threatening.

Anticoagulation with heparin initially followed by coumarins is usually safe and effective. Specific antithrombin concentrates are available. These products are virally inactivated [69], as are all currently available concentrates. They are useful in congenital antithrombin deficiency associated with extensive venous thromboembolism, and prophylactic usage should be considered for major surgery or complicated operative obstetric deliveries as an adjunct to anticoagulation. Concentrates are administered intravenously; antithrombin levels should be monitored with a functional assay and the dose adjusted to keep the antithrombin level in the normal range. The risk of a thromboembolic event during pregnancy and the puerperium associated with antithrombin deficiency has been estimated to be 18% and 33% respectively [67]. Therefore, asymptomatic as well as symptomatic individuals with antithrombin deficiency should receive prophylactic anticoagulation as soon as pregnancy is confirmed and for 6–12 weeks postpartum. Antithrombin concentrates may be useful around the time of delivery. Paternal testing should be undertaken in the case of all thrombophilic abnormalities to identify potential neonates with homozygous or compound heterozygous deficiencies.

Protein C deficiency

Asymptomatic heterozygotes are offered counseling, thromboprophylaxis and long-term follow-up. Long-term warfarin is usually only initiated if there is a history of recurrent thromboembolic events but may be considered after a single spontaneous event where this was severe and life or limb threatening. Heterozygotes have a substantially increased risk of thrombosis associated with surgery or immobilization compared with their unaffected relatives [70]. Therefore vigorous thromboprophylaxis at times of high risk is warranted. The use of protein C concentrates may be valuable to cover major surgery, initiation of warfarin therapy in certain situations or in severe homozygous inherited deficiency states.

Pregnancy and the postpartum period carry a risk of thrombosis of 7% and 19% respectively. Hence if a woman has no thrombotic history it would be reasonable to administer anticoagulation in the final trimester and for 6–12 weeks postpartum. A history of a thromboembolic episode outside pregnancy probably warrants anticoagulation throughout pregnancy. If the history of the thromboembolic event was during pregnancy or in the puerperium, then anticoagulation should start 4–6 weeks before the gestation at which the previous event occurred. Protein C concentrate may be useful around the time of delivery.

Protein S deficiency

The management of patients with protein S deficiency is similar to that of those with protein C deficiency. However, no specific protein S factor concentrate is commercially available. Fresh frozen plasma may be used as a source of protein S in severe deficiency situations. The risk of thromboembolism in pregnancy is low and is estimated to be 17% in the postpartum period [67]. Therefore in the absence of a thrombotic history women should only be anticoagulated in the postpartum period.

Treatment of purpura fulminans and warfarin skin necrosis

When purpura fulminans is due to severe protein C deficiency, protein C concentrate should be given to maintain the protein C level in the normal range [71] and full dose intravenous heparin instituted and monitored to maintain an APTT ratio of 1.5–2.5, although the effectiveness of heparin has not been demonstrated. Fresh frozen plasma 10–15 ml/kg 12-hourly should be given to those children with protein S deficiency or where the defect is unknown. Long-term these children are usually maintained on coumarin therapy [72].

The main aim of management of warfarin skin necrosis must be to prevent this serious complication of treatment. Patients with deficiencies of protein S and C should be heparinized prior to the institution of therapy and warfarin introduced slowly; protein C concentrate may be useful particularly if the patient gives a past history of skin necrosis. The patient needs to be instructed to report any skin lesions which are usually red and painful. If skin lesions appear warfarin must be immediately discontinued, vitamin K_1 given intravenously, with full dose heparinization and either protein C concentrate or fresh frozen plasma.

Activated protein C resistance

Long-term anticoagulation should be considered for recurrent thrombosis. In addition it may be considered after one event if the patient is homozygous for the factor V Leiden mutation, has an additional risk factor such as coinheritance of another thrombophilic defect, or has suffered a life-threatening thrombosis. Thromboprophylaxis for risk situations should be recommended for patients, including those who are asymptomatic, and avoidance of combined oral contraceptives stressed. Clinical experience of this recently described defect is limited. However, careful consideration must be given to thromboprophylaxis during pregnancy as 60% of women who develop a first episode of venous thrombosis during pregnancy are APC resistant [73].

Defects of fibrinogen

The management of patients with these rare defects depends on the clinical spectrum of disease. Special consideration must be given to these patients, who may suffer bleeding as well as thrombotic manifestations, with regard to long-term anticoagulation. In the event of acute thromboembolim or bleeding, fibrinogen should be administered preferably as the concentrate or as cryoprecipitate. Fibrinogen levels should be monitored using a functional assay and levels maintained above 1 g/L.

Antiphospholipid antibodies

Patients who are asymptomatic should be followed up and offered thromboprophylaxis in high-risk situations. Following a single thrombotic event long-term high intensity warfarin (INR > 3.0) should be considered [74], in view of the high recurrence rate. However, prospective studies are needed. Addition of aspirin may further reduce the thrombotic risk. The risk of bleeding with high intensity warfarin is 0.071 per patient year, including a 0.017 per patient risk of severe bleeding [56]. In pregnancy the risks to mother and fetus include recurrent fetal loss and thrombocytopenia in addition to the thromboembolic risk. Management in pregnancy should be based on the past medical and obstetric history. In patients with recurrent miscarriages (three or more pregnancy losses) there is a 90% fetal loss rate in pregnancies where no specific treatment is given [75]. Anecdotal reports state that a variety of treatments including corticosteroids, intravenous immunoglobulin, aspirin and heparin may be beneficial. In a prospective randomized trial low-dose subcutaneous heparin plus low-dose aspirin yielded a significantly higher live birth rate of 70% compared with 40% for low-dose aspirin alone [76]. Patients with a history of thromboembolism require prophylactic heparin throughout pregnancy and for 6–12 weeks postpartum.

Anticoagulant treatment in pregnancy

Coumarins are associated with fetal malformations, mainly of the central nervous system, when administered in the first trimester, and fetal bleeding, particularly intracranial hemorrhage, throughout pregnancy. Heparins are effective and safe for the fetus [77] but cause maternal osteoporosis although this is usually reversible. Both are associated with an increased risk of maternal bleeding and require frequent out patient attendance for monitoring. It is our practice to anticoagulate appropriate patients with low molecular weight heparin throughout pregnancy and institute warfarin immediately after delivery for 6–12 weeks. Patients on low molecular weight heparins are monitored monthly in the first two trimesters and fortnightly in the last trimester, aiming for an anti-factor Xa level of 0.15–0.3 IU/ml. In the case of AT deficiency and aPL antibodies associated with a history of thromboembolism, we usually maintain the anti-factor Xa level at 0.2–0.3 IU/ml. Patients on long-term warfarin should have the risks of conceiving on warfarin discussed. The risks of teratogenesis are small at conception but maximal, 25%, at 6–12 weeks of gestation [78]. It is preferable to avoid heparin preconceptually to limit the period of heparinization required because of the risk of osteopenia with prolonged usage. Patients on warfarin are advised to report as soon as pregnancy is confirmed to enable institution of prophylactic subcutaneous heparin before six weeks of gestation.

References

1. MeVey JH. Tissue factor pathway. Clin Haematol 1994;7(3):469–484.
2. Broze GJ. The role of tissue factor pathway inhibitor in a revised coagulation cascade. Seminars Haematol 1992;29:159–69.
3. Bock SC, Harris JF, Balazs I, Trent JM. Assignment of the human antithrombin III gene to chromosome 1q23–25. Cytogenetics Cell Genetics 1985; 39:67–9.
4. Choaty J, Petitou M, Lormeau JC. Structure activity relationship in heparin: A synthetic pentasaccharide with high affinity for antithrombin III and eliciting anti-factor Xa activity. Biochem Biophy Res Commun 1983;116:492–9.
5. Esmon CT. Owen WG. Identification of an endothelial cell cofactor for thrombin-catalyzed activation of protein C. Proc Nat Acad Sc USA 1981;78:2249–52.
6. Walker FJ. Regulation of activated protein C by a new protein. J Biol Chem 1980;255:5521–4.
7. Comp PC, Esmon CT. Generation of fibrinolytic activity by infusion of activated protein C in dogs. J Clin Invest 1981;68:1221–8.
8. Sakata Y, Loskutoff DJ, Gladson CL, Hekman CM, Griffin JH. Mechanism of protein C dependent clot lysis: Role of plasminogen activator inhibitor. Blood 1986;68:1218–23.
9. Heeb MJ, Espana F, Griffin JH. Inhibition and complexation of activated protein C by two major inhibitors in plasma. Blood 1988;78:2283–90.
10. Fair DS, Marlar RA, Levine EG. Human endothelial cells synthesize protein S. Blood 1986;67:1168–71.
11. Dahlbäck B. Purification of the human C4b-binding protein and formation of its complex with vitamin K-dependent protein S. Biochem J 1983;261:1168–171.
12. Walker FJ. Regulation of activated protein C by protein S. The role of phospholipid in factor Va inactivation. J Biol Chem 1981;258:11128–31.
13. Harris KW. Esmon CT. Protein S is required for bovine platelets to support activated protein C binding and activity. J Biol Chem 1985;260:2007–10.
14. Plutzky J, Hoskins JA, Long GL et al. Evolution and organization of the human protein C gene. Proc Nat Acad Sci USA 1986;83:546–50.
15. Ploos van Amstel HK, van der Zanden AL, Bakker E et al. Two genes homologous with human protein S cDNA are located on chromosome 3. Thromb Haemostasis 1987;62:897–901.
16. Egeberg O. Inherited antithrombin deficiency causing thrombophilia. Thromb Diathesis Haem 1965;13:516–30.

17. Hirsh J, Piovella F, Pini M. Congenital antithrombin III deficiency. Incidence and clinical features. Am J Med 1989;87:34S–38S.
18. Finazzi G, Barbui T. Different incidence of venous thrombosis in patients with inherited deficiencies of antithrombin III, protein C, and protein S. Thromb Haemostasis 1994;71:15–8.
19. Prochownik EV. Molecular genetics of inherited antithrombin II deficiencies. Am J Med 1989;87(Suppl.3B):15–18.
20. Lane DA. Olds RR, Thien SL. Antithrombin III and its deficiency states. Blood Coag Fibrinolysis. 1992;3:315–42.
21. Finazzi G, Caccia R, Barbui T. Different prevalance of thromboembolism in the subtypes of congenital antithrombin III deficiency: Review of 404 cases. Thromb Haemostasis 1987;58:1094.
22. Griffin JH, Evatt B, Zimmerman TS et al. Deficiency of protein C in congenital thrombotic disease. J Clin Invest 1981;68:1370–3.
23. Schwartz HP, Fischer M, Hopmeier P, Batard MA, Griffin JH. Plasma protein S deficiency in familial thrombotic disease. Blood 1984;64:1297–300.
24. Mannucci PM, Valsecchi C, Krachmalnicoff A et al. Familial dysfunction of protein S. Thrombo Haemostasis 1989;62:763–6.
25. Comp PC, Forristall J, West CD et al. Free protein S levels are elevated in familial C4b-binding protein deficiency. Blood 1990;76:2527–9.
26. Pabinger I, Kyrle PA, Heistinger M, Kichinger S, Wittmann K, Lechner K. The risk of thromboembolism in asymptomatic patients with protein C and protein S deficiency: A prospective cohort study. Thromb Haemostasis 1994;71:441–5.
27. Allaart CF, Brieët E. Familial venous thrombophilia. In: Bloom AL, Forbes CD, Thomas DP, Tuddenham EGD (eds), Haemostasis and thrombosis. London: Churchill Livingstone, 1994:1349–60.
28. Dahlbäck B. Carlsson M, Svensson PJ. Familial thrombophilia due to a previously unrecognized mechanism characterized by poor anticoagulant response to activated protein C: Prediction of a cofactor to activated protein C. Proc Nat Acad Sci USA 1993;90:1004–8.
29. Dahlbäck B, Hildebrand B. Inherited resistance to activated protein C is corrected by anticoagulant cofactor activity found to be a property of factor V. Proc Nat Acad Sci USA 1994;91:1396–400.
30. van Boven HH, Reitsma PH, Rosendaal FR et al. Interaction of factor V Leiden with inherited antithrombin deficiency. Thromb Haemostasis 1995;74:94–100.
31. Hellgren M, Svensson PJ, Dahlbäck B. Resistance to activated protein C as a basis for venous thromboembolism associated with pregnancy and oral contraceptives. Am J Obstet Gynecol 1995;173:210–13.
32. Rai R, Regan L, Hadley E, Dave M, Cohen H. Second trimester pregnancy loss is associated with activated protein C resistance. Br J Haematol 1996;92:489–90.
33. McGehee WG, Klotze TA, Epstein DJ et al. Coumarin skin necrosis associated with hereditary protein C deficiency. Ann Intern Med 1984;101:59–60.
34. Goldberg SL. Orthner CL, Yalisove BL et al. Skin necrosis following prolonged administration of coumarin in a patient with inherited protein S deficiency. Am J Hematol 1991;38:64–6.
35. Teepe RG, Broekmans AW, Vermeer BJ et al. Recurrent coumarin-induced skin necrosis in a patient with an acquired functional protein C deficiency. Arch Dermatol 1986;122:1408–12.
36. Sills RH, Marlar RA, Montgomery RR et al. Severe homozygous protein C deficiency. J Paediat 1984;105:409–13.
37. Pabinger I, Schneider B. Thrombotic risk of women with hereditary antithrombin II, protein C and protein S deficiencies taking oral contraceptive medication. Thromb Haemostasis 1994;71:548–52.
38. Tripodi A, Franchi F, Krachmalnicoff A et al. Asymtomatic homozygous protein C deficiency. Acta Haematol (Basel) 1990;83:152–5.
39. Koopman J, Haverkate F, Briët E et al. A congenitally abnormal fibrinogen (Vlissingen) with a 6-base deletion in the gamma-chain gene, causing defective calcium binding and impaired fibrin polymerization. J Biol Chem 1991;266:13456–61.
40. Tait RC, Walker ID, Perry DJ et al. Prevalence of antithrombin III deficiency subtypes in 4000 healthy blood donors. Thromb Haemostasis 1991;65:534 (Abstract).
41. Tait RC, Walker ID, Reitsma PH et al. Prevalence of protein C deficiency in the healthy population. Thromb Haemostasis 1995;73:87–93.

42. Miletich J, Sherman L, Broze G. Absence of thrombosis in subjects with heterozygous protein C deficiency. N Engl J Med 1987;87:991–6.
43. Koster T, Rosendaal FR, de Ronde F, Briët E, Vandenbroucke JP, Bertina RM. Venous thrombosis due to poor response to activated protein C: (Lieden thrombophilia study). Lancet 1993;342:1503–6.
44. Heijboer H, Brandjes DPM, Buller HR, Sturk A, ten Cate JW. Deficiencies of coagulation inhibiting and fibrinolytic proteins in outpatients with deep vein thrombosis. N Engl J Med 1990;323:1512–6.
45. Briët E, Engesser L, Brommer EJP, Broekmans AW, Bertina RM. Thrombophilia: Its causes and a rough estimate of its prevalence. Thromb Haemostasis 1987;58:39 (Abstract).
46. Griffin JH, Evatt H, Wideman C, Fernandes JH. Anticoagulant protein C pathway is defective in the majority of thrombophilic patients. Blood 1993;82:1989–93.
47. Greaves M, Preston FE. Clinical and laboratory aspects of thrombophilia. In: Poller L (ed.), Recent advances in blood coagulation 5. Edinburgh: Churchill Livingstone; 1991:119–40.
48. Levin M, Eley BS, Louis J, Cohen H, young L, Heyderman RS. Postinfectious purpura fulminans caused by an autoantibody directed against protein S. J Paed 1995;127:355–63.
49. Bevers EM, Galli M, Barbui T et al. Lupus anticoagulant IgGs (LA) are not directed to phospholipids only but to a complex of lipid-bound human prothrombin. Thromb Haemostasis 1991;66:629–32.
50. McNeil HP, Simpson RJR, Chesterman CN et al. Anticardiolipin antibodies are directed against a complex antigen that includes a lipid-binding inhibitor of coagulation: β2-glycoprotein I (apolipoprotein H). Proc Nat Acad Sci USA 1990;87:4120–4.
51. Asherson RA. A primary antiphospholipid syndrome? J Rheumatol 1988;15:1742–6.
52. Love PE, Santoro SA. Antiphospholipid antibodies: Anticardiolipin and the lupus anticoagulant in systemic lupus erythematosus (SLE) and in non-SLE disorders. Ann Intern Med 1990;112:682–98.
53. Manoussakis MN, Gharavi AE, Drosos AA, Kitridou RC, Moutsopoulous HM. Anticardiolipin antibodies in unselected autoimmune rheumatic patients. Clin Immunol Immunopathol 1987;44:297–307.
54. Hunt JE, McNeil HP, Morgan GJ, Crameri RM, Krilis SA. The phospholipid-β2 glycoprotein I complex is an antigen for anticardiolipin antibodies occurring in autoimmune disease but not infection. Lupus 1992;1:83–90.
55. Roscove MH, Brewer PM. Antiphospholipid thrombosis: Clinical course after the first thrombotic event in 70 patients. Ann Intern Med 1992;117:303–8.
56. Khamashta MA, Cuadrado MJ, Mujic F, Taub NA, Hunt BJ, Hughes GRV. The management of thrombosis in the antiphospholipid-antibody syndrome. N Engl J Med 1995;332:993–7.
57. Finazzi G. A prospective study of 360 patients with antiphospholipid antibodies (APA). Lupus 1994;3:360.
58. Carreras LO, Vermylen JG. 'Lupus' anticoagulant and thrombosis – possible role of inhibition of prostacyclin formation. Thromb Haemostasis 1982;48:38–40.
59. Rustin MHA. Bull HA, Machin SJ et al. Effects of the lupus anticoagulant in patients with systemic lupus erythematosis on endothelial cell prostacyclin release and procoagulant activity. J Invest Dermatol 1988;90:744–8.
60. Hasselaar P, Derksen RHWM, Blokzijl L, de Groot PG. Thrombosis associated with antiphospholipid antibodies cannot be explained by effects on endothelial and platelet prostanoid synthesis. Thrombo Haemostasis 1988;59:80–5.
61. Angles-Cano E, Sultan Y, Clauvel JP. Predisposing factors to thrombosis in systemic lupus erythematosus: Possible relation to endothelial cell damage. J Lab Clin Med 1979;94:312–23.
62. Malia RG, Kitchen S, Greaves M et al. Inhibition of activated protein C and its cofactor protein S by antiphospholipid antibodies. Br J Haematol 1990;76:101–7.
63. Cosgriff TM, Martin BA. Low functional and high antigenic antithrombin III level in a patient with the lupus anticoagulant and recurrent thrombosis. Arthritis and Rheumatism 1981;24:94–6.
64. Haemostasis and Thrombosis Task Force. The investigation and management of thrombophilia. In: Roberts B. (ed.). Standard haematology practice Oxford: Blackwell Scientific Publications: 1991.
65. Hirsh J, Hull RD, Raskob GE. Clinical features and diagnosis of venous thrombosis. J Am Coll Cardiol 1986;8:221–2.

66. Fotherby K. The progesterone only pill and thrombosis. Br J Family Planning 1989;15:83–5.
67. Conard J, Horellou MH, van Dreden P, Lecompte T, Samama M. Thrombosis and pregnancy in congenital deficiencies of AT III, protein C or protein S: Study of 78 women. Thromb Haemostasis 1990;63:319–20.
68. Rosendaal FR. Heijboer H, Briet E et al. Mortality in hereditary antithrombin III deficiency 1830–1989. Lancet 1991;337:260–2.
69. Menache D, O'Malley JP, Schorr JB, Wagner B, Williams C, the Cooperative Study Group. Evaluation of the safety, recovery, half-life, and clinical efficacy of antithrombin III (human) in patients with hereditary antithrombin III deficiency. Blood 1990;75:33–9.
70. Allaart CF, Poort SR, Rosendaal FR, Reitsma PH, Bertina RM, Briët E. Hereditary protein C deficiency: Carriers of the genetic defect have an increased risk of venous thrombotic events in symptomatic families. Lancet 1993;341:134–8.
71. Dreyfuss M, Magny JF, Bridey F et al. Treatment of homozygous protein C deficiency and neonatal purpura fulminans with purified protein C concentrate. N Engl J Med 1991;325:1565–8.
72. Peters C, Castella JF, Marlar RA, Montgomery RR, Zinkman WH. Homozygous protein C deficiency: Observations on the nature of the molecular abnormality and the effectiveness of warfarin therapy. Paediatrics 1988;81:272–6.
73. Dahlbäck B. Physiological anticoagulation. Resistance to activated protein C and venous thromboembolism. J Clin Invest 1994;94:923–7.
74. Lockshin MD. Answers to the antiphospholipid-antibody syndrome? N Engl J Med 1995;332:1025–7.
75. Rai R, Regan L, Dave M, Cohen H. Prospective randomized trial of aspirin versus aspirin plus heparin in pregnant women with the antiphospholipid syndrome. Br J Haematol 1996; 93 Suppl. 1:5.
76. Rai R, Clifford K, Cohen H, Regan L. High prospective fetal loss rate in untreated pregnancies of women with recurrent miscarriage and antiphospholipid antibodies. Hum Reprod 1995;10:3301–4.
77. Ginsberg JS, Hirsh J. Anticoagulants during pregnancy. Ann Rev Med 1989;40:79–86.
78. Iturbe-Alessio I, Fonseca MC, Mutchinik O, Santos MA, Zajarias A, Salazar E. Risks of anticoagulant therapy in pregnant women with artificial heart valves. N Engl J Med 1986;315:1390–3.

32. Pulmonary embolism and venous thromboembolism

DEREK BELL

Pulmonary embolism is the most serious complication associated with venous thrombosis. Venous thrombosis usually forms in the lower limb veins, but may also originate from thrombus in the pelvic veins, the inferior vena cava, the right side of the heart and also from indwelling venous catheters.

Diagnosis of pulmonary embolism is notoriously poor because the clinical manifestations are nonspecific and the investigative pathway to confirm or refute the diagnosis can be complex. Clinical assessment often fails these patients, therefore stratifying an individual's risk factors with appropriate prophylaxis for venous thrombosis assumes importance. A consistent approach to investigation and treatment of patients is essential to ensure optimal management.

Epidemiology

Reliable estimates of the incidence of fatal and nonfatal pulmonary embolism are difficult. Based on two large autopsy studies, each with over 2000 patients, the incidence of fatal pulmonary embolism in hospital patients is approximately 8–10% [1, 2]. In the study by Sandler and Martin [1], only 25–30% of those dying with pulmonary embolism had undergone recent surgery or suffered serious trauma, the majority being treated for nonsurgical conditions.

The recognition that pulmonary embolism is common in hospitalized patients and that it is not solely confined to postoperative patients has led to the identification of important risk factors for venous thrombosis (Table 32.1). The degree of thromboembolic risk may be stratified as low, moderate or high (Table 32.2) and the risk to benefit of prophylaxis estimated. Hospital patients in the low-risk categories probably do not warrant prophylaxis. Moderate-risk patients have a 10–40% risk of deep vein thrombosis (DVT) and a 1% risk of pulmonary embolism. In high-risk patients the incidence rises to 40–80% for DVT and 10% for pulmonary embolism. Routine prophylaxis is indicated in moderate and high-risk patients and is considered cost-effective [3].

Table 32.1. Risk factors for venous thromboembolism in hospitalized patients.

Patient features	Disease or procedure
Age	Trauma/surgery (especially pelvis, hip or lower limb)
Obesity (probably with age)	Malignancy
Previous deep vein thrombosis or pulmonary embolism	Heart failure
Pregnancy (particularly puerperium)	Recent myocardial infarction
High-dose estrogen therapy	Paralysis lower limb(s)
Immobility (> 4 days)	Inflammatory bowel disease
Thrombophilia	Polycythemia
	Paraproteinemia

Table 32.2. Patient risk groups for venous thrombosis with estimates of likelihood of developing deep vein thrombosis (DVT) or a fatal pulmonary embolism (PE).

Patient groups		DVT	Fatal PE
Low risk	Minor surgery (< 30 min), no risk factor other than age Major surgery (> 30 min) age < 40, no other risk factors	< 10%	0.01%
Moderate risk	Major surgery, age > 40 or other risk factors Major medical illness Major trauma or burns Minor surgery, illness or trauma in patients with previous DVT or PE Minor surgery, illness or trauma in patients with thrombophilia	10–40%	0.1–1%
High risk	Fracture/major orthopedic surgery to pelvis, hip or lower limb Major pelvic/abdominal surgery for malignancy Major surgery, illness or trauma in patients with previous DVT or PE Major surgery, illness or trauma in patients with thrombophilia Hemiplegic stroke, paraplegia Major lower limb amputation	40–80%	1–10%

Clinical features

The approach to the diagnosis of pulmonary embolism should be no different from standard clinical practice and requires a careful history and examination with appropriate clinical investigations to confirm or refute the diagnosis. Unfortunately,

Table 32.3. Presenting symptoms and signs associated with pulmonary embolism (PE).

Symptoms
Breathlessness – on exertion
– at rest
Pleuritic chest pain ⎫ suggest pulmonary infarction
Hemoptysis ⎭
Central chest pain (massive PE)
Syncope (massive PE)

Signs
Tachycardia
Tachypnea
Possible abnormal findings on chest examination
Local chest wall tenderness ⎫ suggest pulmonary infarction
Pleural rub ⎭

Central cyanosis ⎫ suggest massive PE
Hypotension ⎭

there is often overemphasis on the presence of pleuritic chest pain or hemoptysis rather than the most common presenting symptom of breathlessness. Similarly, the possibility of pulmonary embolism presenting as syncope is often overlooked, particularly if the patient survives the initial episode.

Physical examination is nonspecific, (Table 32.3) although in approximately 25% of patients with pulmonary embolism there may be symptoms or signs of venous thrombus [4]. Most commonly the patient will be tachypneic and tachycardic. The clinical findings on chest examination are nonspecific and include inspiratory crackles, expiratory wheeze, rarely a pleural rub or evidence of pleural effusion. Lower chest wall tenderness can occur and can mislead the clinician into making a diagnosis of musculoskeletal pain. When present this usually indicates the presence of pulmonary infarction. Patients with massive pulmonary embolism usually have evidence of low cardiac output with cyanosis and elevated jugular venous pressure. An unexplained low grade pyrexia may also be present in patients with pulmonary embolism.

Investigations

It is important when considering the diagnosis of pulmonary embolism, to distinguish between routine tests and those which contribute to a definitive diagnosis.

The routine tests performed include resting electrocardiogram, chest radiograph and arterial blood gases. No routine blood test exists which is helpful in the diagnosis although studies are being undertaken to establish the role of plasma D-dimer [5].

The ECG may be useful in excluding important differential diagnosis such as acute myocardial infarction, but most commonly reveals sinus tachycardia or other nonspecific abnormalities [6]. The findings, which all medical students associate with pulmonary embolism, of right-axis shift and S, Q3, T3 pattern, although suggestive of massive pulmonary embolism, are uncommon and nonspecific [6, 7].

Most patients with pulmonary embolism have a normal chest X-ray; the other recognized changes such as oligemia, atelectasis, infiltrates and effusion are unfortunately nonspecific and are common in other conditions. However, the chest X-ray is important as it excludes alternative serious conditions such as pneumothorax or lobar pneumonia and is essential for accurate interpretation of the perfusion lung scan.

The presence or absence of hypoxia on arterial blood gases does not exclude pulmonary embolism. In 10–15% of cases of pulmonary embolism proven by pulmonary angiography, a PO_2 of 80 mmHg (10.6 KPa) or greater will be found [6, 8].

Although the electrocardiogram, chest radiograph and arterial blood gases are not diagnostic and are nonspecific, they aid clinical decision making when taken into account with clinical history and examination [9].

A combination of radioisotope lung scans, objective tests for venous thrombosis and/or pulmonary angiography are required to establish or exclude the diagnosis of pulmonary embolism. There are two main diagnostic approaches. The more common approach starts with a lung perfusion scan, which if normal excludes the diagnosis [9, 10]. However, even when abnormal, it should, in most instances, be combined with additional objective tests to make a definitive decision. Less commonly, it is possible to proceed directly to pulmonary angiography but this usually reflects the severity of clinical presentation.

Ventilation and perfusion lung scans

Perfusion lung scanning is performed after intravenous injection of ^{99m}Tc-labeled macroaggregates of albumin. These macroaggregates lodge in the perfused pulmonary capillaries and the patient is scanned using a gamma camera. A normal multiple view perfusion scan performed soon after the acute event effectively excludes pulmonary embolism [9, 10].

An abnormal perfusion scan does not confirm pulmonary embolism as many other disorders will produce altered pulmonary blood flow, including pneumonia or effusions (chest X-ray usually abnormal) or clinically silent chronic obstructive pulmonary disease or asthma (chest X-ray may be normal). In patients with abnormal perfusion scans, most centers now perform a combined ventilation scan. Two large studies have shown that patients with large perfusion defects, segmental or greater, and a ventilation mismatch [9, 11] have a high probability (approximately 90%) of pulmonary embolism as determined by pulmonary angiography (Figure 32.1). However, even in patients with a ventilation perfusion match or small perfusion defects the frequency of pulmonary embolism is not sufficiently low to exclude embolism, particularly if the clinical suspicions are high or uncertain. Unfortunately, the majority of patients suspected of suffering from pulmonary embolism have indeterminate or low probability ventilation and per-

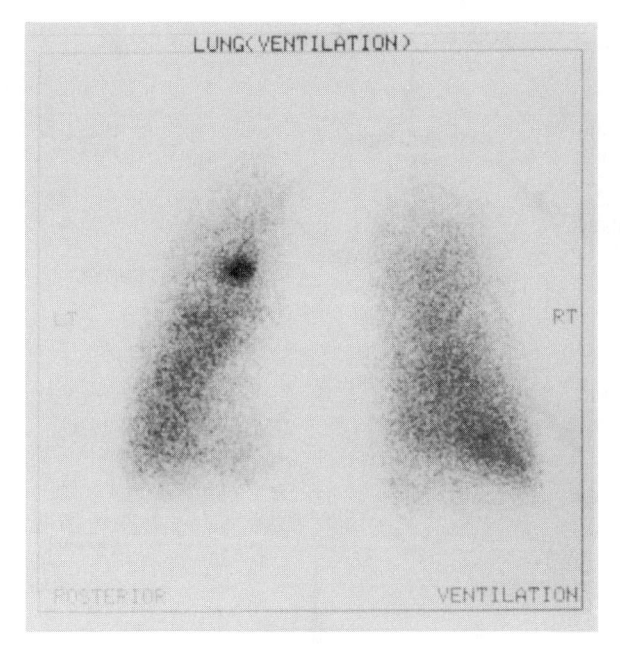

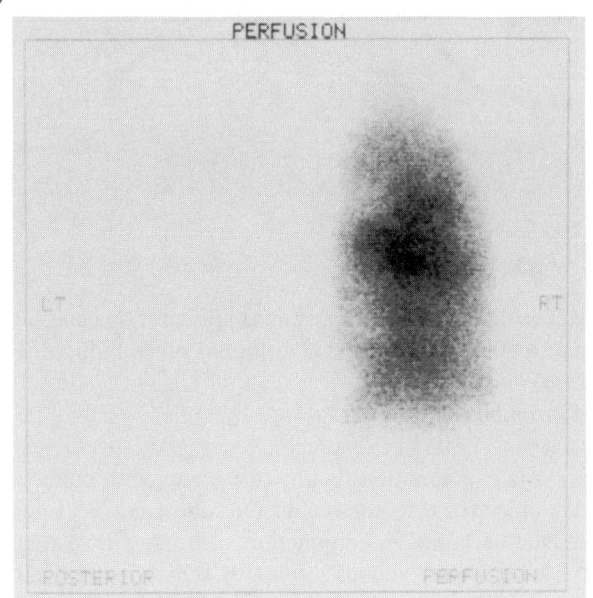

Figure 32.1. High probability ventilation (a) and perfusion scan (b) in the posterior view showing virtually absent perfusion in the left lung with well preserved ventilation.

```
                        PULMONARY EMBOLISM
                                │
                                ▼
                         CXR + V/Q SCAN
                        ╱       │       ╲
                       ╱        │        ╲
High Probability?     ╱         ▼         ╲    Normal?
                              INDETERMINATE
Treat as PE                                     Reconsider diagnosis
                                │
                                ▼
                         VENOGRAM/DOPPLER
                        ╱                ╲
                       ╱                  ╲
Positive?             ╱                    ╲
                                            Negative?
Treat as PE                       High clinical      Low clinical
                                  suspicion?        suspicion?

                                                    Reconsider diagnosis
                                       │
                                       ▼
                              PULMONARY ANGIOGRAPHY
                             ╱                    ╲
                            ╱                      ╲
                    Positive?                       Negative?

         Treat as PE: Thrombolysis?                 Reconsider diagnosis
```

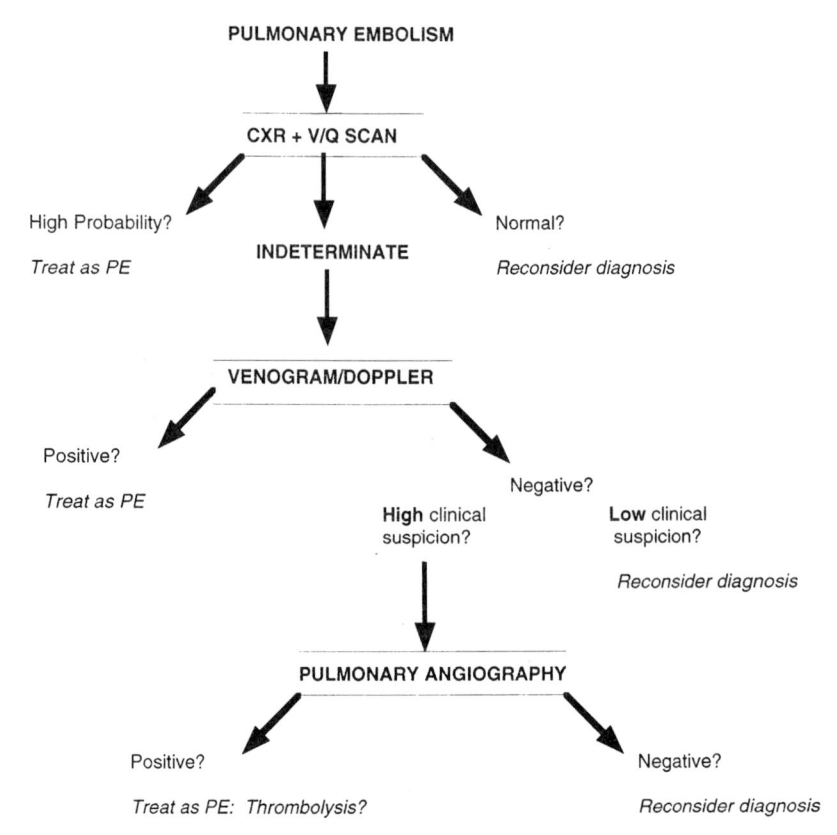

Figure 32.2. Suggested clinical algorithm to confirm or refute the diagnosis of pulmonary thromboembolism.

fusion scans and thus diagnostic strategies must allow for this and further objective tests are indicated. A suggested clinical algorithm is given in Figure 32.2.

Tests for venous thrombus

Deep vein thrombosis is a common finding in patients with pulmonary embolism [1, 12]. Therefore, objective tests for venous thrombosis are commonly used to increase the diagnostic certainty in conjunction with other investigations. Several methods can be used to detect venous thrombus. Which method is used will vary between institutions depending on availability and local expertise.

Venography remains the current standard reference test although other techniques are being evaluated [13]. The most reliable diagnostic criterion is the presence of an intraluminal filling defect which is consistent in all films and seen in at least two projections.

Although venography is the reference standard, disagreement between experienced radiologists has been reported in approximately 10% of venograms [14]. In addition, venography is invasive and associated with a potential risk of adverse reactions including hypersensitivity reaction, and potentially precipitating venous thrombus. It is contraindicated in patients with renal failure, known hypersensitivity or cellulitis of the affected limb. For these reasons venography is not usually used to screen for asymptomatic venous thrombus.

The two tests which appear most useful for screening, and when used in conjunction with ventilation and perfusion scanning help in the diagnosis of pulmonary embolism, are Doppler ultrasonography and impedance plethysmography. Both techniques are noninvasive and repeatable. Doppler ultrasound combines simultaneous real-time imaging with pulse-gated Doppler. In a large study compression ultrasonography has been shown to be highly specific and sensitive [15].

This method cannot yet reliably be used to detect venous thrombosis in the deep calf veins, although popliteal veins can be imaged with the patient in the prone position; proximal thrombosis is readily detected (Figure 32.3).

Impedance plethysmography is also sensitive and specific for proximal deep vein thrombosis provided a strict protocol is used [16]. More recent studies have cast doubt on the reliability of the technique [17] and for whatever reason it is not routinely used in most hospitals.

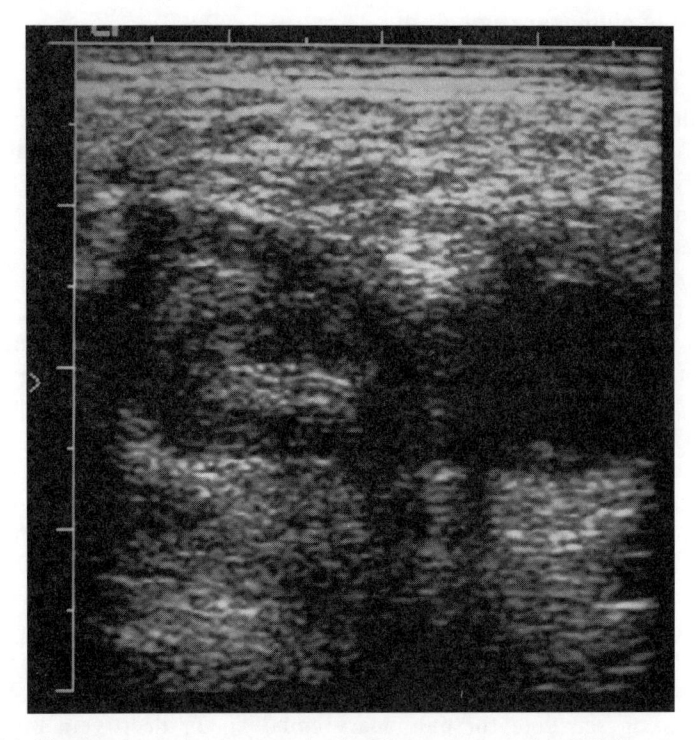

Figure 32.3. Ultrasound scan showing extensive thrombus in the femoral vein (left) and patent femoral artery.

Pulmonary angiography

Pulmonary angiography is the accepted reference standard for confirming or excluding pulmonary embolism. A negative pulmonary angiogram, in common with a normal perfusion scan, excludes the diagnosis of pulmonary embolism. Although nondiagnostic angiograms are uncommon, about 20–30% of patients will not be considered suitable for pulmonary angiography [18]. Pulmonary angiography has a mortality of approximately 0.5% with a major nonfatal complication rate of 1%. On the basis of the PIOPED study pulmonary angiography is said to be a sufficiently low-risk procedure to justify its use as a diagnostic tool in the appropriate clinical setting. Patients with pulmonary hypertension, right heart failure or respiratory failure are at greater risk of major complications, and the procedure should be undertaken carefully and after full assessment of the risk/benefit ratio. Elderly patients appear to be at greater risk of developing renal failure.

More recently a potential role for continuous volume computed tomography (helical or spiral CT) in the diagnosis of pulmonary embolism has been described. Although this technique looks promising many centers do not have sufficiently powerful scanners and the exact position in clinical algorithms has not yet been established [19].

Treatment of pulmonary embolism

Treating pulmonary embolism is essentially the same as the treatment of isolated venous thrombosis with anticoagulation being the mainstay of treatment. Thrombolytic therapy or interventional techniques are less commonly indicated.

An early study demonstrated the beneficial effect of anticoagulation [20]. At the present time, treatment for pulmonary embolism should be initiated with intravenous heparin, unless definite contraindications exist. More recent studies have demonstrated the efficacy of low molecular weight heparin in proximal venous thrombosis [21] and it is likely that this may become part of routine practice. Low molecular weight heparins are derivatives of heparin, which, because of predictable absorption, can be given as once daily subcutaneous injections without the need for monitoring [22]. This reduces medical and nursing time and offers the potential for outpatient based treatment.

Treatment with heparin should start at the time the clinical diagnosis is made, not when diagnosis is confirmed, because of the risk of further emboli. It is important to achieve adequate anticoagulation with heparin to prevent recurrence, and overlap heparin and warfarin therapy for at least 4–5 days. Overlap is considered necessary because it may take 7–10 days for the venous thrombus to become adherent, and the maximal effect of oral anticoagulation does not occur for up to 5 days, despite achieving a therapeutic prothrombin time or INR. This may be due to depression of protein C levels (a natural anticoagulant) by warfarin. Table 32.4 gives a suggested anticoagulation schedule for pulmonary embolism or deep vein thrombosis, including appropriate monitoring.

Table 32.4. Schedule for anticoagulating patients with pulmonary thromboembolism or deep vein thrombosis.

Heparin 5000 IU IV as a bolus loading dose
Heparin 1300–1400 IU/hour as a continuous infusion (calculations and adjustments simple if 50 000 IU heparin made up in 50 ml saline i.e. 1000 IU/ml)
Check APTT at 6 hours and adjust dose to maintain APTT 1.8–2.5 times control
Recheck APTT 6-hourly until therapeutic, then daily
Commence warfarin 10 mg at 24–72 hours – *check INR daily* (NB Starting warfarin early will reduce hospital length of stay)
Overlap heparin and warfarin for at least four days – check INR and APTT daily
Stop heparin after 5–7 days, provided INR is therapeutic (INR 2–3, unless recurrent disease, when 3–4.5)
Continue warfarin for at least 6 weeks in cases with a recognized cause, otherwise for at least 6 months

For most patients the daily warfarin requirement is 3–9 mg. The optimal duration of anticoagulation therapy remains uncertain, particularly as the relative risk of recurrence varies from patient to patient. A recent review has suggested that it is reasonable to anticoagulate patients for six weeks if they have identifiable reversible risk factors (such as recent surgery), but to continue for six months in patient with idiopathic venous thrombosis. A smaller group of patients require long-term anticoagulation. This includes patients with documented venous thrombosis or thromboembolism who have inherited thrombophilia, recurrent events, or have cancer and are undergoing active treatment [23].

The most common complication of anticoagulation with both heparin and warfarin is bleeding secondary to over-coagulation. As heparin has a short half-life it is usually sufficient to stop treatment. If bleeding is severe protamine sulfate can be given in a dose of 1 mg/100 IU heparin infused over the previous hour.

Patients on warfarin with minor bleeds can be given 1 mg vitamin K which will hasten normalization of the INR without making the patient resistant to warfarin. For life-threatening bleeds 5 mg vitamin K should be given intravenously with concentrates of factors II, IX and X. If concentrates are not available 1 L fresh frozen plasma can be given but this may be less effective [24]. Patients who develop bleeding complications of anticoagulants should be investigated for the source of the bleeding, and the bleeding not merely attributed to over-anticoagulation.

Heparin induced thrombocytopenia should be considered in patients developing a low platelet count following treatment. It is said to occur in 3–5% of cases and most commonly develops after 5–7 days, but may occur as early as 24–48 hours. The diagnosis should be confirmed by laboratory tests and an alternative source of heparin used if continued heparinization is necessary. Platelet counts should therefore be monitored daily while on heparin.

Although most clinicians are concerned about over-coagulation, there is compelling evidence that subtherapeutic anticoagulation is associated with an increased risk of recurrent venous thromboembolism [25]. Anticoagulation should therefore be monitored closely to ensure therapeutic treatment and avoid recurrent thrombosis or bleeding.

Thrombolytic therapy

The role of thrombolysis in the management of acute pulmonary embolism requires further research to identify the patients most likely to benefit. Thrombolysis leads to more rapid resolution of intrapulmonary thrombus (Figure 32.4) and the associated hemodynamic changes associated with pulmonary embolism, compared with heparin alone. These benefits are short-lived and by 5–7 days improvement in perfusion defects is similar in both groups of patients [26].

The Urokinase Pulmonary Embolism Trials (UPET) also showed no difference in mortality at 2 weeks between urokinase (6%) and heparin (7%). The number of bleeding complications in the urokinase group was higher but not statistically different [26].

There is no clear evidence from well performed randomized trials that thrombolysis improves clinical outcome, even in groups with hemodynamic compromise. However, the more rapid resolution of thrombus and hemodynamic parameters would suggest that critically ill patients are most likely to benefit. There appears to be no difference in clinical efficacy between streptokinase, urokinase or tissue-plasminogen activator, and all have been used to treat pulmonary embolism (Table 32.5). As with thrombolysis in myocardial infarction, a larger multicenter trial may be required to show the exact place of thrombolysis in the management of venous thromboembolism.

Invasive treatment of venous thromboembolism

Anticoagulation is the standard treatment for venous thromboembolic disease in both the acute and continuation phases of treatment. A proportion of patients will have contraindications to anticoagulation, usually a current source of bleeding or continued thromboembolic events which cannot be adequately treated despite therapeutic levels of anticoagulation. In these groups a number of options are available (Figure 32.5). The most commonly used is interruption of the inferior vena cava to prevent further thrombus dislodging from confirmed deep vein thrombosis. This is now currently performed under local anesthetic with insertion of a filter, usually via the femoral or jugular vein [27].

Table 32.5. Recommended thrombolytic regimens for pulmonary embolism.

Streptokinase	250 000 IU intravenously over 30 minutes Maintenance 100 000 IU/h for 24 hours
Urokinase	4400 IU/kg intravenously over 10 minutes Maintenance 4400 IU/kg/h for 24 hours
Tissue-plasminogen activator	100 mg intravenous infusion over 2 hours

All patients to be heparinized and anticoagulation monitored throughout treatment with APTT measurement

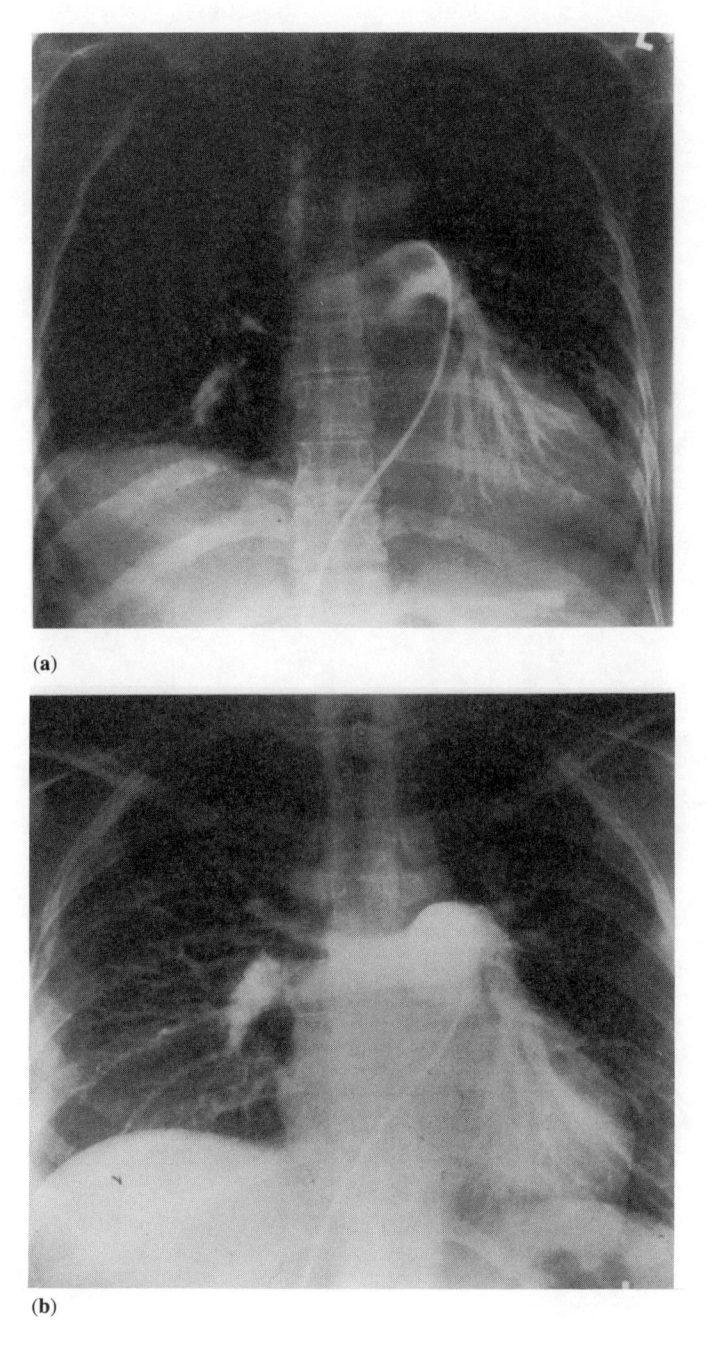

Figure 32.4. (a) Pulmonary angiogram showing extensive thrombus in the pulmonary artery trunk and right pulmonary artery; (b) pulmonary angiogram 24 hours after thrombolysis with streptokinase showing extensive revascularization.

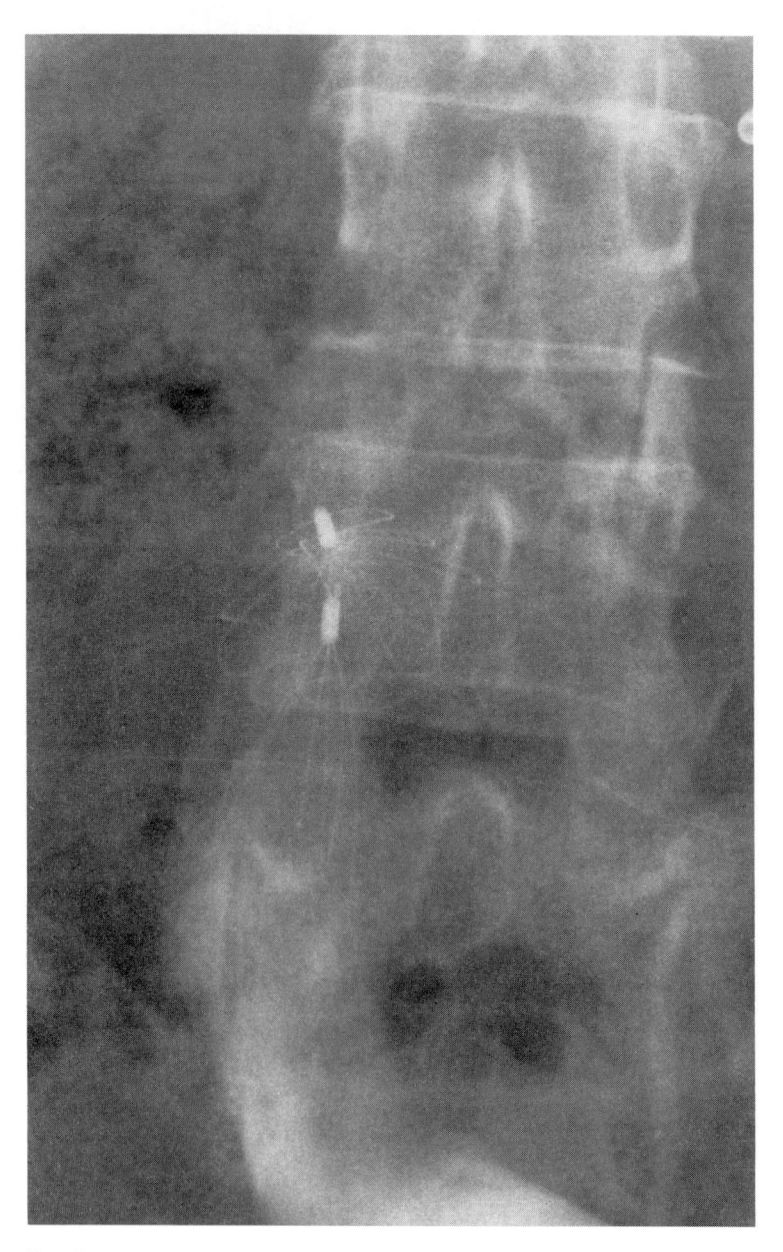

Figure 32.5. Venogram of inferior vena cava showing a caval filter *in situ*.

Summary

Currently our ability confidently to diagnosis thromboembolic disease, pulmonary embolism or deep vein thrombosis is poor. Ideally we require a simple blood test which is both specific and sensitive. At present we must rely on maintaining a high index of clinical suspicion and using objective tests to confirm or refute the diagnosis. The invasive tests remain the gold standards at present, but the use of duplex ultrasound for deep vein thrombosis appears to be a major step forward and the use of helical computed tomography or magnetic resonance imaging of pulmonary vessels may offer promise. Heparin remains the mainstay of acute therapy with warfarin in the maintenance phase. The exact role for low molecular weight heparin and thrombolytic therapy in the evidence based treatment of thromboembolic disease remains an area for major clinical research.

References

1. Sandler DA, Martin JF. Autopsy proven pulmonary embolism in hospital patients: Are we detecting enough deep vein thrombosis. J Roy Soc Med 1989;82:203–5.
2. Macintyre IMC, Ruckley CV. Pulmonary embolism: A clinical and autopsy study. Scot Med J 1974;19:20–4.
3. Bergquist D, Jenteg S, Lingren B, Matzsch T. The economics of general thrombolytic prophylaxis. World J Surg 1988;12:349–55.
4. Hull RD, Raskob GE, Coates G, Panju AA, Gill G. A new non-invasive management strategy for patients with suspected pulmonary embolism. Arch Intern Med 1989;149:2549–55.
5. Bounameaux H, de Moerlose P, Perrier A, Reber G. Plasma measurement of D-dimer as diagnostic aid in suspected venous thromboembolism: An overview. Thromb Haemostat 1994;71:1–6.
6. Stein PD, Dalen JE, McIntyre KM, Sasahara AA, Wenger NK, Willis PW. The electrocardiogram in acute pulmonary embolism. Prog Cardiovasc Dis 1975;17:247–57.
7. Szucs MM, Brooks HL, Grossman W et al. Diagnostic sensitivity of laboratory findings in acute pulmonary embolism. Ann Intern Med 1971;74:161–6.
8. Webber DM, Phillips JH Jr. A re-evaluation of electrocardiographic changes accompanying acute pulmonary embolism. Am J Med Sci 1966;251:381–91.
9. Bell WR, Simon TL, Demets DL. The clinical features of submassive and massive pulmonary embolism. Am J Med 1977;62:355–60.
10. The PIOPED Investigators. Value of the ventilation/perfusion scan in acute pulmonary embolism. Results of the prospective investigation of pulmonary embolism diagnosis. (PIOPED). J Am Med Assoc 1990;263:2753–59.
11. Hull RD, Raskob GE, Coates G, Panju AA. Clinical validity of a normal perfusion lung scan in patients with suspected pulmonary embolism. Chest 1990;97:23–6.
12. Hull RD, Hirsh J, Carter CJ, Raskob GE, Gill GJ, Jay RM. Diagnostic value of ventilation perfusion lung scanning in patients with suspected pulmonary embolism. Chest 1985;88:819–28.
13. Hull RD, Hirsh, J, Carter CJ. Pulmonary angiography ventilation lung scanning and venography for clinically suspected pulmonary embolism with abnormal perfusion scan. Ann Intern Med 1983;98:891–8.
14. Lensing AWA, Buler HR, Prandoni P et al. Contrast venography, the gold standard for the diagnosis of DVT: Improvement in observer agreement. Thromb Haemostat 1992;67:8–12.
15. Lensing AWA, Prandoni P, Brandje S et al. Detection of deep vein thrombosis by real time B-mode ultrasonography. N Engl J Med 1989;320:343–45.
16. Hull RD, Taylor DW, Hirsh J et al. Impedance plethysmography: The relationship between venous filling and sensitivity and specifically for proximal vein thrombosis. Circulation 1978;58:898–902.

17. Anderson SR, Lensing AWA, Wells PS, Levine MJ, Weitz JI, Hirsh J. Limitations of impedance of plethysmography in the diagnosis of clinically suspected deep vein thrombosis. Ann Intern Med 1993;118:25–30.
18. Stein PD, Athanasoulis C, Alvai A *et al.* Complications and validity of pulmonary angiography in acute pulmonary embolism. Circulation 1992;85:462–8.
19. Hansell DM, Padley SPG. Continuous volume computed tomography in pulmonary embolism: The answer or just another test. Thorax 1996;51:1–2.
20. Barritt DW, Jordan SC. Anticoagulant drugs in the treatment of PE: A controlled trial. Lancet 1960;i:1309–12.
21. Hull RD, Raskob GE, Pineo GF *et al.* Subcutaneous low-molecular weight heparin compared with continuous heparin in the treatment of proximal vein thrombosis. N Engl J Med 1992;326:975–82.
22. Hirsh J, Levine MN. Low molecular weight heparin. Blood 1992;79:1–17.
23. Hirsh J. The optimal duration of anticoagulant therapy for venous thrombosis. N Engl J Med 1995;332:1710–1.
24. British Society for Haematology. Guidelines on oral anticoagulation. J Chem Path 1990;43:177–83.
25. Hull RD, Raskob GI, Hirsh J *et al.* Continuous intravenous heparin compared with intermittent subcutaneous heparin in the initial treatment of proximal vein thrombosis. N Engl J Med 1986;315:1109–14.
26. The urokinase pulmonary embolism trial. A national cooperative study. Circulation 1973;47(Suppl.1):1–108.
27. Magnant JG, Walsh DB, Juravasky LI, Cronenwett JL. Current use of inferior vena cava filters. J Vasc Surg 1992;16:701–06.

33. Vascular restenosis

PHILIP CHAN

Restenosis is the process of recurrent stenosis of a vessel that may follow an intervention to bypass or mechanically widen the stenosis. It is recognized as probably the single most important complication of vascular procedures targeted at occlusive disease. Restenosis occurs in every vascular location, coronary, carotid, and limb arteries, and veins, after every procedure. There is no technique of vascular intervention, surgical or endovascular, that is immune to restenosis.

Restenosis in the clinical setting is usually obvious, with symptoms and physical findings suggesting recurrence of ischemic symptoms that preceded the intervention. However, many restenoses have progressed to occlusion by the time clinical events recur, and significant restenoses may be underway without major symptoms before occlusion [1]. For objectivity, an agreed definition of restenosis should involve quantification, and in most studies, this involves imaging of the intervention site.

The current gold standard for diagnosis of restenosis is angiography. This does show recurrent luminal compromise, but is subject to errors of underestimation from vascular remodeling, which tends to enlarge the vessel eccentrically to compensate for luminal narrowing [2], and from the uniplanar artefact of a three-dimensional stenosis being less evident when visualized in a flat two-dimensional plane. There are still problems with definition: any hemodynamically significant stenosis at the intervention site might be regarded as restenosis, and this definition is probably adequate for a procedure like vein grafting, where there was no major preexisting stenosis of this kind; but the definition is flawed by inclusions of less successful primary angioplasty procedures that did not fully restore the lumen.

Any change from an image after the primary procedure may be taken as restenosis, and defined as a measured change greater than two standard deviations from observer and repeat imaging error; this is flawed by the inclusion of very minimal restenosis, which may well be functionally unimportant after a major restoration of the lumen. In coronary angioplasty studies, 50% loss of initial luminal gain is often regarded as restenosis; again this measure is highly dependent upon whether that initial gain was large or small.

Application of different definitions of restenosis can result in important variations in the estimate of restenosis rates. Beatt *et al.* applied the the first two definitions (any hemodynamic stenosis and any change from post-procedure image) to a single set of pre- and post-coronary angioplasty images, and defined restenosis rates of 24% and 33% respectively; less than 50% of patients included in one definition were also included in the other definition [3].

For these reasons and also the practical problems associated with invasive study of asymptomatic patients, angiography is less established for the diagnosis of restenosis than previously. Ultrasound methods have the advantage of being less invasive (with the exception of intravascular ultrasound) and imaging the vessel wall as well as residual lumen. Duplex ultrasound criteria for restenosis in leg bypasses have been established, based on the increased velocity of blood flow through a stenosis [4].

Pathology

Restenosis is a mechanical obstruction to flow, recurrent after a vascular procedure. The structural basis of restenosis is characterized by a substantial thickening of the intimal layer of the vessel wall. The thickened intima is composed of fibrocellular connective tissue of variable cellularity, surrounded by extracellular matrix of collagen and ground substance. The cells are vascular smooth muscle, which proliferate in the intima and secrete matrix protein, probably after initial migration from the vessel media. In the early stages, the cellular component is prominent; in mature lesions, more extracellular matrix is observed. This process is seen after all vascular injury, whether it proceeds to restenosis or not, and represents a stereotypical process of vascular healing.

These structural changes have been recognized since the early days of vascular surgery [5]. It has been referred to as 'fibrosis' of the artery or graft, and been variously named as intimal, neointimal or fibrous hyperplasia, early or accelerated atherosclerosis [6, 7]. The term myointimal hyperplasia (MIH), reflects the smooth muscle origin of the cellular proliferation.

The proliferation of cells in MIH is not without limit, and in most models, the hyperplastic lesion stops increasing in size before critical hemodynamic effects are seen; there is also a phase of resolution, when the lesion becomes less cellular and may decrease in size. In some cases, thickening of the vessel wall by MIH may cause substantial narrowing of the lumen amounting to restenosis, and leading to occlusion by thrombosis. It is important to note that MIH represents a physiological process of vascular healing; restenosis is a pathological extension of this, and might involve different or additional mechanisms.

Ultrastructural studies of the lesions of MIH have clarified its cellular basis. The predominant cell type involved is the smooth muscle cell. Cells with appearances similar to fibroblasts are also seen, as are cells of intermediate appearance. However, in the uninjured artery there are no fibroblasts present in the intima and media; vascular smooth muscle cells make up the major component of the media, with occasional representation in the intima. There is believed to be a continuum of histologic appearances between smooth muscle cell and fibroblast; implying that these are not distinct cell types, but can differentiate from a common origin in both directions [8]. There is support for this view from cell culture studies, in which cells of vascular smooth muscle origin can be induced to differentiate into contractile (smooth muscle-like) and synthetic (fibroblast-like) phenotypes [9].

These cellular appearances account for the historical confusion between vascular 'fibrosis' and the cellular appearance of MIH. The proliferating smooth muscle cell (SMC) can adopt a phenotype similar to a fibroblast, and secrete collagen and ground substance, producing a copious extracellular matrix. Thus arterial and venous 'fibrosis' represents the mature lesion of MIH.

Is MIH and restenosis different in different parts of the circulation? Risk factors for restenosis are inconsistent from one series to another. The incidence of restenosis is remarkably similar (25–40%) after all procedures in all arterial beds. Histologic appearance of restenosis shows similar cell types and tissue architecture in all sites, ranging from coronary angioplasty to prosthetic surgical bypass, to venous reconstruction and arteriovenous fistula. We have reported data that a cellular trait in human vascular smooth muscle that is associated with restenosis is apparent in all parts of the circulation, arterial and venous, within a single individual [10]. There does not appear to be prima facie evidence to believe that restenosis varies from site to site.

The source of the proliferating SMC is probably from the medial layer underlying the lesion. Certainly, after grafting of uninjured vein into the arterial circulation, there are associated medial changes, with SMCs becoming hypertrophic, adopting the synthetic phenotype, and elaborating extracellular matrix and collagen. These medial SMCs probably migrate into the intima, where in some way they become free from the normal growth control mechanisms, and proliferate excessively [11].

The stimulus to MIH is vessel wall trauma. The mechanism that induces cellular proliferation is mediated by peptide growth factors. The course of events probably begins with endothelial denudation and the accumulation of platelets at that site. Platelet activation and degranulation release a number of factors that are stimulatory to medial SMCs, particularly the platelet-derived growth factor (PDGF), but also including TGFβ, serotonin and platelet factor 4, among others. Damaged vascular wall cells release basic fibroblast growth factor (bFGF). These factors are mitogenic for smooth muscle [12] and also chemotactic for SMCs [13] and will stimulate both proliferation and migration of medial SMC into the intima.

There may be a contribution from growth factors elaborated from proliferating SMCs themselves, allowing the process to continue after the resolution of the original platelet stimulation [14, 15]. The existence of such paracrine stimulation may be important in determining which lesions will progress and which remain self-limiting.

The relative importance of different growth factors in the etiology of MIH in humans is not known. PDGF transcripts have been found by *in situ* hybridization in atherosclerotic plaques [16] and a PDGF-like mitogen is secreted by cultured VSMCs derived from anastomotic hyperplastic lesions [17]. PDGF is expressed by cultured human venous endothelium [18] and by intimal cells in healing PTFE grafts [19]. TGFβ transcripts are expressed more in restenosis tissue than in atherosclerotic plaques from human coronary arteries [20].

Intimal hyperplasia may be important in the development of atherosclerosis. Ross and Glomset [21, 22] and Ross [23] theorize that the key initial event in atherogenesis is vessel wall injury, and VSMC proliferation. Subsequent development of the atherosclerotic lesion depends on 'progression factors', including VSMC proliferative capacity, lipid uptake, and inflammatory response. Vascular injury may be physical, with endothelial denudation and platelet activation as described above, or biochemical, perhaps associated with lipid peroxidation. The 'response to injury' hypothesis has become the dominant modern theory, and has given another dimension of interest to the VSMC and its growth characteristics.

Models of restenosis

Clowes et al. have studied in detail the cellular events following arterial injury with a balloon catheter in the rat carotid. Maximal SMC proliferation occurs just 2–4 days after arterial wall injury, as measured by labeled thymidine incorporation. Continued SMC proliferation appears to depend on endothelial coverage; in arterial segments covered by endothelium, the thymidine index returned to baseline values 4–8 weeks after injury, but remained high in arterial segments that were chronically denuded.

Luminal narrowing occurred early, around 2 weeks after injury; it was initially caused by SMC contraction. This vasoconstriction produced up to 75% luminal stenosis. Intimal thickening occurs measurably from the first week, becoming prominent at 4–12 weeks after injury. Between 2–12 weeks the number of intimal VSMCs appears to be roughly static; thickening of the arterial wall at this stage occurs mainly by synthesis and accumulation of connective tissue by these cells [24].

The rat carotid balloon injury model is the best studied model of vascular healing. Numerous other models exist, involving a bewildering array of models of vascular injury in all accessible vessels, in virtually all species of common laboratory animals. In addition, there is a variety of surgical approaches using autogenous and prosthetic bypasses in conditions of varying blood flow to study hemodynamic influences on MIH.

There is no confirmation that the proliferative process of MIH is the same in humans as in animals, particularly as restenosis is relatively common in humans and rare in animal models. Animal models have been used to validate therapies against MIH, and to study mechanical factors that may be involved in stimulating MIH. It is disturbing that considerable differences appear to exist between species in the response of vascular smooth muscle cells to growth factor stimulus and inhibition [25].

Mechanical factors and restenosis

Mechanical factors, in particular those related to blood flow, have been implicated in the etiology of MIH, particularly in animal models. Hemodynamic factors have been shown to correlate with the development of MIH. The normal laminar flow pattern in arteries produces a relatively slower-moving layer next to the artery wall called the boundary layer. In conditions of slow flow or turbulence, flow in the boundary layer may be static or even reversed, and this is known as boundary layer separation. It has been theorized that prolonged contact with platelets and other blood constituents in an area of boundary layer separation may contribute to arterial wall pathology. In the same conditions of low flow or turbulence, the normal laminar low pattern is disturbed, and a complex pattern ensues. Micro-areas of low flow in the complex pattern produce low tangential, or shear stress on the neighboring arterial wall.

Measurement of these areas in a dog femoro-femoral crossover bypass model produces a rather weak correlation between areas of low shear stress and of subsequent intimal hyperplasia [26]. In a plexiglass model of an end-to-side 45° anastomosis, a complex helicospiral flow pattern is produced at normal arterial pressure and pulsation: the areas of localized low shear stress roughly correspond with two of the sites of predilection for intimal hyperplasia; at the toe of the anastomosis and the floor of the recipient artery opposite the aperture [27, 28].

Confusingly, high shear stress has also been postulated as a factor in intimal hyperplasia. Placement of a vein graft into the arterial circulation results in a high wall shear stress, and the vein wall thickening that occurs returns the wall shear stress toward normal. Rigid external support of the vein graft reduces the high shear stress, and ends to reduce intimal hyperplasia [29]. There is support for this from human studies on femoropopliteal bypass and arteriovenous fistulas (constructed for dialysis access) using vessel wall Doppler tracking, in which high shear stress is associated with restenosis in both contexts [30].

Fillinger *et al.* have examined measures of turbulence, particularly the Reynolds number, in a canine arteriovenous femoral PTFE loop model, and found that turbulence correlates with the development of intimal hyperplasia [31, 32]. Graft compliance has been implicated in the development of intimal hyperplasia, more in hope apparently, than by direct experimentation. The hypothesis is that at an anastomosis, where the stiff artificial graft meets the compliant artery, there is a 'compliance mismatch', which is responsible for setting up deleterious patterns of blood flow, with areas of low/high shear stress, boundary layer separation, etc., which ultimately result in intimal hyperplasia. This is unlikely to be important in autogenous vein grafts, or in MIH occurring after angioplasty. Direct evidence is based on an experiment in just 14 dogs, in which paired glutaraldehyde-treated autografts which differed only in compliance, were placed in the femoral arteries, resulting in thrombosis of eight stiff and two compliant grafts within three months [33]. Hofstra *et al.*'s studies in human prosthetic grafts do not show any relation between compliance mismatch and restenosis [34].

In summary, using various animal models, and often on the basis of rather weak correlations, many mechanical factors including measures of turbulence, high flow, low flow, high shear stress, low shear stress, variation of shear stress with the cardiac cycle, the presence of a branch, boundary layer separation, and anastomotic compliance have been postulated as important determinants of intimal hyperplasia. Some of these factors are of course interrelated; they may all correlate with sites of excessive endothelial and intimal injury, setting into train the mechanism described above. It is not clear whether all these hemodynamic parameters can be practically addressed; there are limits to the hemodynamic results that can be achieved by anastomotic and angioplasty techniques. As MIH is essentially a cellular, proliferative process, it is clear that physical factors, even if influential, must act through the biological growth control mechanism.

Treatment for restenosis

Treatment of an established restenosis is not different in principle from that of the primary stenosis. There is apparently an individual predisposition to restenosis; the incidence of second restenosis is 50–60%, compared with 30–40% for first restenoses in coronary angioplasty. The incidence of second restenoses is higher even if the first restenosis occurred in a vessel remote from the second operative site [35, 36]. The most powerful risk factor identified for restenosis from the register of all early coronary angioplasties was that of having suffered a previous restenosis [37]. Correction of restenosis is worthwhile, as this influence is not 100% failure of correction; however, every practicing clinician in vascular medicine has individual patients who have restenosed multiple times, often failing multiple procedures in multiple sites.

The aim of most restenosis research is to define a strategy to prevent restenosis after intervention. There have been two main lines of research: to develop new procedures that might have lesser restenotic complication; and to discover drugs that reduce restenosis after standard procedures.

Development of new procedures is always attended by great hopes; in the vascular field, most of these hopes have centered upon reduction in restenosis. It is difficult to comment on new device results; the majority of these devices have not been subject to properly conducted trials and published results are usually more promising that subsequent experience in practice. It is clear however, that laser angioplasty has no advantage over, and may have more restenosis than conventional angioplasty [38]. Atherectomy in the coronary arteries or the femoropopliteal segment results in no reduction of restenosis compared to angioplasty [39, 40] and might result in more restenosis. Stenting of coronary arteries in two large multicenter trials showed a modest reduction in restenosis rates from around 35% to around 25% [41, 42]. Stenting of peripheral arteries is less well studied, and conclusions cannot be reached about their efficacy in reduction of restenosis.

Do improvements in existing techniques improve restenosis? In particular, does leaving a smoother intimal outline, or dilating an angioplasty site more widely, or handling a vein bypass more gently lead to less restenosis? Improvements in general technique will produce better results in most cases. Unfortunately, little of this improvement is attributable to effects on restenosis. Human data are sparse; depth of angioplasty as evidenced by medial fissuring exhibited by angiography has no effect on restenosis, nor does the recovery of deeper layers of the arterial wall by more substantial atherectomy [43, 44]. Experimental data indicate that change in anastomotic angle or in techniques of preparation of a vein bypass influenced the degree of MIH very little [45–48].

The range and number of candidate drugs in the prevention of restenosis is truly impressive. Over 50 agents have completed the course from promising *in vitro* and animal experiments through to randomized trials, usually in coronary angioplasty restenosis. No agent has however been acceptably shown to prevent human restenosis. It remains extremely puzzling why a large number of agents, indubitably shown to reduce MIH in animal vascular injury, have not inhibited restenosis in humans (Table 33.1).

What accounts for the disparity between animal and human results? It has been argued for some agents that the human trial was really a false negative: that the agent did in reality affect restenosis, but was administered in too low dosage (heparin [49]), in too high dosage (angiopeptin [50]), at incorrect frequency (cilazipril [51]), or that the methodology of quantitative angiography was too demanding a criterion. My view, while acknowledging some specific points about specific studies, is that credibility is strained to believe that all 40 plus studies have been incorrectly performed. The more likely explanation is that existing animal methods do not correctly model human restenosis, probably because those methods study physiological MIH rather than pathological restenosis. This view further

Table 33.1. Candidate drugs for the prevention of restenosis.

Class of agent	Agent	Trial acronym (if any)	Numbers in trial
Heparin	Unfractionated		419
	enoxaparin LMW	ERA	458
Antiplatelet agents	Aspirin/dipyridamole		203, 453, 79, 40, 249, 207,
	Ticlopidine		236, 179
	Ketanserin		43, 658
	Thromboxane A_2 synthase inhibitors	CARPORT, M-HEART, GRASP	707, 33, 755, 1089
	Prostacyclin		311, 286
Anticoagulant	Warfarin		110, *119*
	Coumadin		248
Fish oils	EPA preparations	FORT	82, 108, 204, 194, 108, 1 107, 204
ACE inhibitors/angiotensin II Antagonists	Cilazipril	MERCATOR, MARCATOR	595, 1436
	Enalapril		95
	Quinapril	QUIET	Ongoing
Calcium channel blockers	Diltiazem		94, 201
	Nifedipine		241
Steroids	Methylprednisolone	M-HEART	66, 722, 102,
Lipid-lowering agents	Lovastatin		157, 404
	LDL-apheresis	L-ART	66
Growth factor antagonist	Angiopeptin		553
	Trapidil	STARC	72, 254
Antiproliferative agents	Colchicine	CART	197, 253

implies that restenosis is not just 'too much MIH', but involves different or additional mechanisms.

Clearly the development of future strategies to reduce restenosis will involve research into processes of human restenosis. Of the shorter-term future, there is currently much interest in systems of local delivery and in gene therapy. Local delivery systems, for example through angiographic catheters, may be used to target drugs in high-dose formulations [52], or other agents, such as the seeding of intact endothelium [53], into the actual site of arterial injury after angioplasty. It is hoped that this approach will allow higher doses of drugs to be targeted more selectively at the site in question. Initial results show qualified promise.

Gene therapy relies on local delivery of nucleotide material into vascular wall at the site of injury. In metaphor, this approach takes the view of the restenosis process as a computer-controlled machine; drugs and devices target the moving parts and circuitry of the machine, but gene therapy aims at reprogramming the computer at its heart [54]. This approach is certainly exciting in principle. However, the nucleotide tools available at this time are crude, and target genes are known to be involved in cell proliferation of all kinds; the approach therefore offers little advantage at present over conventional cytostatic and cytotoxic agents. The hope of defining genetic sequences specific to vascular smooth muscle restenosis may prove optimistic.

Is restenosis important? It is true that some drugs used in coronary angioplasty trials have reported improvements in clinical events, such as the need for second procedures, and recurrent symptoms, even without improvements in restenosis [50, 55]. It is also true that limb bypasses can buy time for limb salvage through collateralization, and that even after restenosis and failure of the graft, the limb may remain viable. In some cases restenosis can undergo a degree of resolution [56], and established coronary restenosis, at least in the group < 70% stenosed, may remain static and not progress to vessel occlusion [57]. Nevertheless it is worth repeating that restenosis remains the single most common cause of failure of all surgical and endovascular procedures. It remains worthwhile to find a strategy to avoid this major complication; exceptional cases and certain defined groups might come to little harm from restenosis, but it is still the case that restenosis is undesirable, and will likely cause harm to the patient.

Conclusions

Work in the restenosis field is difficult. There is no universal definition, measurement is inconsistent, and risk factors are not readily identified. There are a huge number of randomized trials, but no treatment has been acceptably shown to reduce restenosis, except stenting in the coronary arteries; and even that is attended with an appreciable 25% incidence of restenosis. There is an urgent need to define models of human restenosis other than animal vascular injury and MIH. There is an urgent need to define pathophysiological processes in human restenosis that are distinct from those of normal vascular healing.

References

1. Taylor PR, Wolfe JH, Tyrrell MR, Mansfield AO, Nicolaides AN, Houston RE. Graft stenosis: Justification for one year surveillance Br J Surg 1990;77:1125–8.
2. Glagov S. Intimal hyperplasia, vascular modeling and the restenosis problem. Circulation 1994;84:2888–91.
3. Beatt KJ, Serruys PW, Luitjen HE et al. Restenosis after coronary angioplasty: The paradox of increased lumen diameter and restenosis. J Am Coll Cardiol 1992;19:258–66.
4. Grigg MJ, Nicolaides AN, Wolfe JHN. Detection and grading of femorodistal vein graft stenoses: Duplex velocity measurements compared with angiography. J Vasc Surg 1988;8:661–6.
5. Carrel A, Guthrie CC. Uniterminal and biterminal venous transplantation. Surg Gynecol Obstet 1906;2:266–86.
6. Imparato AM, Bracco A, Kim GE, Zeff R. Intimal and neointimal fibrous proliferation causing failure of arterial reconstructions. Surgery 1972;72:1007–17.
7. DeWeese JA, Rob CG. Autogenous vein grafts: Ten years later. Surgery 1977;82:775.
8. Sottiurai VS, Yao JST, Flinn WR, Batson RC. Intimal hyperplasia and neointima: An ultrastructural analysis of thrombosed grafts in humans. Surgery 1983;93:809–17.
9. Chamley-Campbell JH, Campbell GR, Ross R. The smooth muscle cell in culture. Physiol Rev 1979;59:1–61.
10. Munro E, Chan P, Patel M et al. Consistent responses of the human vascular smooth muscle cell in culture: Implications for restenosis. J Vasc Surg 1994;20:482–7.
11. Dilley RJ, McGeachie JK, Prendergast FJ. A review of the histologic changes in vein-to-artery grafts, with particular reference to intimal hyperplasia. Arch Surg 1988;123:691–6.
12. Ross R, Glomset JA. Atherosclerosis and the arterial smooth muscle cell. Science 1973;180:1332–9.
13. Bell L, Madri JA. Effect of platelet factors on migration of cultured bovine endothelial and smooth muscle cells. Circ Res 1989;65:1057–65.
14. Sjolund M, Hedin U, Sejersen T, Heldin CH, Thyberg J. Arterial smooth muscle cells express PDGF a chain mRNA, secrete a PDGF-like protein, and bind exogenous PDGF in a phenotype and growth state dependent manner. J Cell Biol 1988;106:403–13.
15. Golden MA, Au YPT, Kenagy RD, Clowes AW. Growth factor gene expression by intimal cells in healing PTFE grafts. J Vasc Surg 1990;11:580–5.
16. Wilcox JN, Smith KM, Williams LT, Schwartz SM, Gordon D. PDGF mRNA detection in human atherosclerotic plaques by in situ hybridisation. J Clin Invest 1988;82:1134–43.
17. Birinyi LK, Warner SJC, Salomon RN, Callow AD, Libby P. Observations on human SMCs from hyperplastic lesions of prosthetic bypass grafts: Production of a PDGF-like mitogen and expression of a gene for PDGF receptor – a preliminary study. J Vasc Surg 1989;10:157–65.
18. Limmani A, Fleming T, Molina R et al. Expression of genes for PDGF in adult human venous endothelium. J Vasc Surg 1988;7:10–9.
20. Nikol S, Isner JM, Pickering JG, Kearney M, Leclerc G, Weir L. Expression of transforming growth factor beta 1 is increased in human vascular restenotic lesions. J Clin Invest 1992;90:1582–92.
21. Ross R, Glomset JA. The pathogenesis of atherosclerosis Part 1. N Engl J Med 1976;295:369–77.
22. Ross R, Glomset JA. The pathogenesis of atherosclerosis Part 2. N Engl J Med 1976;295:420–5.
23. Ross R. The pathogenesis of atherosclerosis; a perspective for the 1990s. Nature 1993;362:801–9.
24. Clowes AW, Reidy MA, Clowes MM. Mechanisms of stenosis after arterial injury. Lab Invest 1983;49:208–15.
25. Castellot JJ, Pukac LA, Caleb BJ, Wright TC, Karnovsky MJ. Heparin selectively inhibits a protein kinase C dependent mechanism of cell cycle progression in calf aortic smooth muscle cells. J Cell Biol 1989;109:3147–55.
26. Rittgers SE, Karayiannicos PE, Guy JF. Velocity distribution and intimal proliferation in autogenous vein grafts in dogs. Circ Res 1978;42:792–801.
27. Bassiouny HS, White S, Glagov S, Choi E, Giddens DP, Zarins CK. Anastomotic intimal hyperplasia: Mechanical injury or flow induced. J Vasc Surg 1992;15:708–17.

28. Ojha M, Ethier CR, Johnston KW, Cobbold RS. Steady and pulasatile flow fields in an end-to-side anastomosis model. J Vasc Surg 1990;12:747–53.
29. Kohler TR, Kirkman T, Clowes AW. The effect of rigid external support on vein graft adaptation to the arterial circulation. J Vasc Surg 1989;9:277–85.
30. Hofstra L, Bergmans D, Leunissen K et al. Anastomotic intimal hyperplasia in prosthetic arteriovenous fistulas for hemodialysis is associated with initial high shear rate and not with mismatch in elastic properties. PhD Thesis, University of Limburg, Maastricht.
31. Fillinger MF, Reinitz ER, Schwartz RA, Resetarits DE, Paskanik AM, Bredenberg CE. Beneficial effect of banding on venous intimal-medial hyperplasia in arteriovenous loop grafts. Am J Surg 1989;158:87–94.
32. Fillinger MF, Reinitz ER, Schwartz RA et al. Graft geometry and venous intimal-medial hyperplasia in arteriovenous loop grafts. J Vasc Surg 1990;11:556–66.
33. Abbott WM, Megerman JM, Hasson JE, L'Italien G, Warnock D. Effect of compliance mismatch upon vascular graft patency. J Vasc Surg 1987;5:376–82.
34. Hofstra L, Hoeks A, Tordior J, Bergmans D, Daemen M, Kitslaar P. Mechanical factors predisposing to intimal hyperplasia in peripheral bypass grafts constructed with the use of autologous vein; a prospective analysis. PhD. Thesis, University of Limburg, Maastricht.
35. Bresee SJ, Jacobs AK, Garber GR et al. Prior restenosis predicts restenosis after coronary angioplasty of a new significant narrowing. Am J Cardiol 1991;68:1158–62.
36. Berger PB, Bell MR, Holmes DR, Hammes L, Kosanke JL, Bresee SJ. Effect of restenosis after an earlier angioplasty at another coronary site on the frequency of restenosis after a subsequent coronary angioplasty. Am J Cardiol 1992;69:1086–9.
37. Holmes DR, Vlietstra RE, Smith HC et al. Restenosis after percutaneous transluminal coronary angioplasty: A report from the PTCA registry of the National Heart, Lung and Blood Institute. Am J Cardiol 1984;53:77C–81C.
38. Lammer J, Pilger E, Ddecrinirs M, Quehenberger F, Klein GE, Stark G. Pulsed excimer laser versus continuous wave laser versus conventional angioplasty of peripheral arterial occlusions: Prospective controlled randomised trial. Lancet 1993;340:1183–8.
39. Vroegindeweij D, Tielbeek AV, Buth J, Schol F, Hop W, Landman G. Directional atherectomy versus balloon angioplasty in segmental femoropopliteal artery disease: Two year follow-up with color-flow duplex scanning. J Vasc Surg 1995;21:255–69.
40. Holmes DR, Topol EJ, Adelman AG, Cohen EA, Califf RM. Randomised trials of directional coronary atherectomy: Implications for clinical practice and future investigation. J Am Coll Cardiol 1994;24:431–9.
41. Serruys PW, deJaegere P, Kiememeij F et al. A comparison of balloon-expandable stent implantation with balloon angioplasty in patients with coronary artery disease. N Engl J Med 1994;331:489–95.
42. Fischman DL, Leon MB, Baim DS et al. and Stent Restenosis Study Investigators. A randomised comparison of coronary stent placement and balloon angioplasty in the treatment of coronary artery disease. N Engl J Med 1994;331:496–501.
43. Hermans W, Rensing B, Foley D et al. Therapeutic dissection after successful coronary balloon angioplasty; no influence on restenosis or clinical outcome in 693 patients. J Am Coll Cardiol 1992;20:767–80.
44. Kuntz RE, Hinohara T, Safian RD, Selmon MR, Simpson JB, Baim DS. Restenosis after directional coronary atherectomy; effect of luminal diameter and deep wall excision. Circulation 1992;86:1394–9.
45. Storm FK, Gierson ED, Sparks FC, Barker WF. Autogenous vein bypass grafts: Biological effects of mechanical dilatation and adventitial stripping in dogs. Surgery 1975;77:261–7.
46. Bond MG, Hostetler JR, Karayannacos PE, Geer JC, Vasko JS. Intimal changes in arteriovenous bypass grafts. J Thorac Cardiovasc Surg 1976;71:907–16.
47. Breyer RH, Spray TL, Kastl DG, Roberts WC. Histologic changes in saphenous vein aortocoronary bypass grafts. J Thorac Cardiovasc Surg 1976;72:916–24.
48. Quigley MR, Bailes JR, Kwaan HC, Cerullo LJ, Block S. Comparison of myointimal hyperplasia in laser-assisted and sutured anastomosed arteries, a preliminary study. J Vasc Surg 1986;4:217–9.

49. Ellis SG, Roubin GS, Wilentz J, Douglas JS, King SB. Effect of 18-to 24-hour heparin administration for prevention of restenosis after uncomplicated coronary angioplasty. Am Heart J 1989;117:777–82.
50. Emmanuelsson H, Beatt KJ, Bagger JP *et al.* Long term effects of angiopeptin in coronary angioplasty. Reduction in clinical events but not angiographic restenosis. Circulation 1995;91:1689–96.
51. Faxon DP and MARCATOR study group. Effect of high dose angiotensin converting enzyme inhibition on restenosis: Final results of the MARCATOR study, a double blind, placebo controlled trial of cilazipril. J Am Coll Cardiol 1995;2:362–9.
52. Lambert TL, Dev V, Rechavia E, Forrester JS, Litvack F, Eigler NL. Localised arterial wall drug delivery from a polymer coated removable metallic stent. Circulation 1994;90:1003–11.
53. Thompson MM, Budd JS, Eady SL, Underwood MJ, James RF, Bell PR. The effect of transluminal endothelial seeding on myointimal hyperplasia following angioplasty. Eur J Vasc Surg 1994;8:423–34.
54. Ohno T, Gordon D, San H *et al.* Gene therapy for vascular smooth muscle cell proliferation after arterial injury. Science 1994;265:781–4.
55. Topol EJ, Califf RM, Weisman HF *et al.* Randomised trial of coronary intervention with antibody against platelet IIb/IIIa integrin for reduction of clinical restenosis: Results at six months. EPIC investigators. Lancet 1994;343:881–6.
56. Morinaga K, Eguchi H, Miyazaki T, Okadome K, Sugimachi K. Development and regression of intimal thickening of arterially transplanted autogenous vein grafts in dogs. J Vasc Surg 1987;5:719–30.
57. Gordon PC, Friedrich SP, Piana RN *et al.* Is 40% to 70% diameter narrowing at the site of previous stenting or directional coronary atherectomy clinically significant? Am J Cardiol 1994;74:26–32.

34. Vascular emergencies

MAURO BARTOLO and ANNA RITA TODINI

The term 'vascular emergency' appears in modern literature [1]. This kind of emergency can or cannot be 'postponed': for example it can be postponed in cases of peripheral embolism, whereas it cannot be postponed in other conditions such as rupture of an aneurysm. The emergency entails not only the treatment of its cause but also of the shock, which is generally hypovolemic and not very frequent.

Acute ischemia of lower limbs

This is an asphyxial condition caused by acute obstruction of the main artery of a limb [2, 3]. The causes of this obstruction include embolism, thrombosis, and arterial injuries; each will be described separately. Diagnosis must be carried out as soon as possible as it takes only a few hours for an irreversible tissue ischemia to affect the patient.

The subjective symptoms affecting one or both limbs are characterized by sudden acute continuous pain which does not lessen spontaneously or with analgesics. This pain is accompanied by functional impotence because nervous ischemia is very precocious. The patient feels an unpleasant sensation of cold limbs. The following may be observed: disappearance of peripheral pulses; hypothermia of the ischemic limb, appearing pale at first and then cyanotic and streaky; veins are empty and seem flattened; and sensitivity tends to lessen or disappear – during palpation, the patient feels pain in his muscles and especially in the gastrocnemius muscle which, because of ischemic retraction, can lead to a club-foot like attitude. Neurologic damage is expressed by the paralysis of the external and/or internal sciatic–popliteal nerve.

Skin damage, such as blisters and necrosis, appears later when ischemia is irreversible and hypoxic damage affecting the microcirculation is accompanied by venular thrombosis. At this stage, called the 'devascularization syndrome' because of cellular lysis and release of toxic metabolites, worsening of the general state of the patient and humoral index is observed; acute renal insufficiency, acidosis, and hyperkalemia may develop.

There are different stages of arterial obstruction. The most serious case of acute ischemia is when there is an obstructing lesion of the aorta, both limbs are affected by ischemia and the abdominal wall is streaky; the more damaged is the general state of the patient, who can be affected by shock or heart failure, the more serious is the ischemia. Particular locations are: obstruction of the anterior tibial artery causing the anterior tibial compartment syndrome; and obstruction of the axillary and humeral arteries of the upper limb.

The etiology of embolic ischemia relates to:

1. valvular, ischemic, prosthetic, tumoral cardiopathy;
2. arteriopathy (atheromatous plaques at all levels, mainly at the level of the aortic arch, aneurysms); and
3. venous pathology caused by paradoxical embolus.

Atherosclerosis, thrombosis of an aneurysm, and thromboangitis obliterans are the causes of acute thrombotic ischemia, whereas acute thrombosis can be caused by blood alterations such as thrombocytosis, circulating antibodies, LAC, antiphospholipid antibodies and polyglobulism (Vaquez). Although the most important differential diagnosis is between embolism and acute thrombotic obstruction, the embolus may stop on stenotic plaques.

Embolism is the likely diagnosis when: atrial fibrillation appears; the patient presents symptoms indicating a previous arrhythmic paroxysm; transthoracic and transesophageal echocardiograms show either an intracardiac auricular or ventricular thrombus or a relevant aortic area; or symptoms appear suddenly and all other vascular districts are uninjured. In 50% of patients, the embolus stops in the femoral artery followed by: iliac arteries, saddle aorta, and popliteal arteries. Bifurcations are preferred sites. Acute thrombosis is the likely diagnosis when: common pulse locations show signs of vasosclerosis; the patient has a history of limping on one side; or pain is less acute. In this case pain is less acute because the collateral circulation starts working; in embolism this does not happen.

In these situations, angiography is compulsory and has the objectives of diagnosis and, if needed, treatment. The shape of the embolus is characteristic: when arterial profiles are normal, the interruption of flow is segmentary and sometimes the superior profile of the obstruction is slightly convex. The most obvious defect however is poor collateral circulation.

Therapy

Surgery with the Fogarty probe is generally preferred. It is advisable not to inject urokinase into arteries after surgery, because this fibrinolytic substance can further damage the endothelium, which has been affected by the probe. Instead of embolectomy with the Fogarty probe, small doses of urokinase can be locally injected into arteries (30 000–60 000 units per hour after a 200 000-unit bolus locally injected by means of the same catheter used during arteriography). The infusion should continue for 2 or 3 days, depending on the results obtained. Heparin is given during or following the local fibrinolytic treatment. If this treatment succeeds, the feet and all the limbs, previously cold, pale and with a thermal step 4 fingers lower than the location of the embolus, will become red and warm, emptied veins will fill up again and acute pains will disappear.

The postsurgery period is monitored by vascular echography. During infusion treatment, the local vascular situation is monitored with consecutive arteriographies by means of a catheter *in situ*. In some cases, acute obstruction could be caused by a thrombophilic condition due to a tumor which could still be clinically latent. In these patients, retrothrombosis will occur frequently.

If intimal lesions are not excessive, the Fogarty probe can also be used in acute thrombosis. An attempt can be made using the Fogarty probe to eliminate the obstruction in cases presenting with serious local damage. Afterwards, treatment continues with low molecular weight dextran and other hemorrheologic drugs. If cardiac dysrhythmia is confirmed anticoagulants will be required permanently.

False acute ischemia in diabetics should be mentioned. A phlegmon may hide a necrosis because in these cases perception of pulses is hindered by medial calcinosis of vessels. Warm feet and the detection of an infectious focus, which must be immediately treated, make the distinction possible and avoid amputation.

Revascularization syndrome

This syndrome is present in all forms of acute ischemia, when circulation recovers and limb ischemia lasts for a long period of time. Compartment post-ischemic edema is characteristic of this syndrome and is very painful. More serious are humoral changes related to tissue necrosis; they are comparable to the manifestations of this syndrome, and are characterized by hyperkalemia, myoglobinuria, increased creatine kinase LDH, and SGOT, with renal insufficiency [4].

The seriousness of the situation can lead, if not successfully treated, to amputation or dialysis and sometimes to death. Death can immediately follow arterial declamping. Fasciotomy can be performed locally. General treatment includes: metabolic rebalancing and treatment of possible sepsis.

Tibial compartment syndrome

Some vascular districts are particularly exposed to district pathologies [5] and some arteries are unaffected by injuries and hence rarely diseased, e.g. peroneal arteries used as emergency vessels in case of tibial obstruction. The anterior tibial artery can however thrombose at a very early stage of development and be easily compressed in its compartment.

If there is an obstruction, the whole anterior tibial compartment swells and hardens, while the foot dangles because the external popliteal sciatic nerve has been damaged [6]. It is a very painful condition which risks fasciotomy [7]. This is the only arterial syndrome accompanied by local edema.

In phlebothrombosis, the edema is generally harder and more widespread. Pressure measurements both of arterial and venous vessels, by means of a Doppler scan, permit differential diagnosis.

Blue toe syndrome

This is a peculiar and very painful condition where one or more fingers or one or both limbs appear cyanotic. The syndrome is caused by movement of the catheter inside the aorta and it occurs more often during coronography than during peripheral angiography. Microemboli of cholesterol crystals detach from plaques damaged by the point of the catheter. Aneurysms may represent another focus of emboli [8]. Pain is severe due to the lack of collateral circulation in vessels measuring a few microns. Necrosis sometimes affects one or more digital pulps and the sole and heel become streaky.

Cholesterol crystals have been found in peripheral and renal biopsies (as kidneys are almost always affected, it is believed that the upper part of the aorta tends to form emboli) and in the eyeground. If renal function is not damaged, low molecular weight dextran can be injected with care. Recidivations occur frequently because the aortic area often presents very friable ulcerous lesions. Anticoagulants, used over a long period of time, can worsen the situation; in fact the fibrin sheath, capable of limiting the tendency of plaque to form emboli, cannot deposit on the plaque itself.

Acute ischemia of the upper limbs

Compared to acute ischemia of the lower limbs, this occurs less frequently. The collateral circulation is richer and most of the time pain is limited to the fingers. Generally the cause of this syndrome differs from the cause of the lower limbs syndrome. Arteriosclerosis appears more frequently in lower limbs, while emboli stemming from the cardiac area, caused by subclavian aneurysms [9] or clinical emboli caused by accidental intraarterial injection of drugs or ergotamine occur more frequently in upper limbs.

These emboli, of medium size, can be successfully treated with the Fogarty probe or with located thrombolysis. Otherwise, chemical sympathicolysis or prostanoids can be used.

Ischemia and mesenteric infarct

Chronic forms of intestinal ischemia can lead, step by step, to intestinal necrosis. Acute forms of ischemia however, can rapidly lead to intestinal infarct, because the obstruction, mainly affecting the superior mesenteric artery, occurs in an environment where compensating collateral circulation is lacking [10, 11].

Acute intestinal ischemia is caused by:

1. Thrombosis (atherogenesis).
2. Embolism (cardiac embolism).
3. Functional intestinal ischemia (low output).
4. Venous thrombosis of the mesenteric vein.

The main symptom of embolic forms is widespread abdominal pain or partial and more acute pain, while pain is duller in phlebitis and low output ischemia.

Diagnosis must be carried out by means of arteriography; therapy for thrombosis is surgical: local thrombolysis or embolectomy in embolic forms and venous thrombectomy in venous thrombosis. Medical therapy plays a supporting role. If these forms preceding infarct are not detected and treated, they rapidly lead to intestinal infarct accompanied by the symptoms described above and a worsening of the general state: paralytic ileus, shock, and enterorrhagia in 50% of cases. The only accurate diagnosis is arteriography; surgery is the only therapy and it must be accompanied by supporting medical therapy including anticoagulants, antibiotics, plasma, and blood transfusions.

Arterial injuries

Arterial injuries can be caused by war or civil life: injury rate can vary from 20 per 1000 in the former, to 2–3 per 1000 in the latter. However, iatrogenic injuries, due to endovascular diagnosis or therapy, as well as mechanical–chemical arteritis in addicts are increasing.

The injuries of most interest are civil emergencies: car accidents or occupational injuries. According to Vollman's [12] classification, there are two kinds of injury:

- direct injuries (contusions, injuries); and
- indirect injuries (hematoma compression, fracture and sprain).

In direct injuries caused by firearms and other weapons, hemorrhage can be internal or external. In contusion injuries, there can be a lesion of the intima or intima and media accompanied by thrombosis, or a lesion of the whole artery followed by hemorrhage.

Arterial injuries are often not isolated, hence, diagnosis and treatment are very complex. Acute limb ischemia is the dominant syndrome in all kinds of injury. A precocious ultrasound diagnosis confirmed by arteriography to detect the location and number of lesions is essential. In serious and distal ischemia, surgery to restore the artery and surrounding tissue may be accompanied by fasciotomy of tibial compartments. Fasciotomy can sometimes disimpact un-thrombosed arteries. Supporting medical therapy includes anticoagulants with small doses of heparin to avoid thrombosis, hemorrheologics, and antibiotics.

Aneurysms

A significant vascular emergency is complications caused by aortic, inferior limb, and dissecting aneurysms [13]. Aneurysm complications cannot be avoided because the pathology is often asymptomatic and undetected; rupture may be the first symptom. Aneurysm complications are:

- compression of close organs (veins, ureter, sciatic nerve);
- thrombosis;
- embolism;
- rupture; and
- sepsis.

Only embolism, acute thrombosis of the aneurysmal sac, and rupture, the most serious complication, are vascular emergencies. Peripheral embolization of an aneurysm is caused by the detachment of an intraluminal thrombus fragment which can affect both or only one limb or cause the blue finger syndrome. Acute thrombosis of an aneurysm causes ischemia in the area where the aneurysm is located: in both limbs if it is aortic; in one limb if it is iliac or femoral; and in one leg if it is popliteal. Rupture of an aneurysm is the most serious complication because the patient's life is at risk.

In abdominal aortic aneurysm, rupture can be retroperitoneal or intraperitoneal with a high death rate varying from 60 to 80%. Most ruptures are in two phases. It is essential to make a diagnosis during the first phase, when the so-called 'cleavage syndrome' appears, a few hours or days before rupture. Clinical signs of cleavage are:

- acute abdominal pains, sudden and sore pains which can simulate any acute abdominal disease;
- temporary decrease of arterial pressure;
- presence of abdominal pulse mass; and
- biochemical modifications such as a decrease in red cells and hematocrit.

Diagnosis and surgery can avoid the phase of retropertioneal rupture where the above-mentioned symptoms can be accompanied by backache, oliguria, or anuria. Pulse mass is difficult to delimit, arterial pressure reduces, and the general state worsens rapidly.

Rupture of an aneurysm in the peritoneum causes a hematoperitoneum accompanied by the typical acute abdomen syndrome and shock. Any aneurysm of any size, including parietal blisters, can break; parietal blisters with a diameter larger than 5 cm have a higher rupture rate. Arterial hypertension is an aggravating factor. Rupture can also affect false aneurysms caused by intraluminal diagnosis and therapy or detachment of a vascular prosthesis. Rupture occurs less often at the femoral-popliteal level [14]. A thrombosed aneurysm is essentially detected by echography. TC and arteriography of the abdominal aorta before surgery are essential to understand the links with the celiac trunk, mesenteric artery, and renal arteries, of which often a double district exists. Peripheral arteries are also examined echography.

Therapy for broken abdominal-aortic aneurysms is surgery. Local fibrinolytic treatment can avoid limb amputation in popliteal thrombosed aneurysms.

Aortic dissection

Aortic dissection emergency has the highest death rate both in the acute phase and later [15]. Three percent of patients die when the first symptom, pain, appears; 38%

of patients die in the first 24 hours; 48% of patients die after 2 days; 70% after one week; and 80% after two weeks. The highest death rate (80%) is caused by aortic rupture, essentially intrapericardial rupture. One year later, prognosis is poor with respect to aortic or myocardic insufficiency, or hypertension.

The seriousness of the clinical situation depends on the location of the dissection [16]. Media degeneration by cleavage causes dissection. An intimal entry door connects the vascular lumen with the dissected media and enables blood under pressure to enter. Media detachment can begin from the ascending aorta and either affect the whole aorta (type I of De Bakey's classification) [17] or stop on the media artery (type II); otherwise it can detach from the descending aorta and reach the whole downstream area (type III). If collateral aortic branches are affected, they can become obstructed, causing cerebral, intestinal, medullary, or renal ischemia of superior or inferior limbs; an aortic dissection can therefore begin with a limb ischemia.

Thoracic pain, sometimes accompanied by shock, is typical of aortic dissection; it may be confused however with pulmonary infarct or embolism. Other symptoms apart from pain are: AI systolic murmur; myocardial infarct caused by coronary dissection and ischemia at different levels; hemiplegia and paraplegia with convulsions; acute abdomen; and anuria [18].

Diagnosis must be carried out by arteriography, although an initial screening can be carried out by transesophageal and peripheral echography; Doppler scans together with duplex scans can detect the typical flapping sound and visualize the double lumen.

Medical therapy is mainly aimed at reducing blood pressure. Surgical therapy is fundamental and is performed by heart surgeons.

Arterial hypertension

Hypertensive emergencies must be treated within a short period of time which varies from a few minutes to one hour [19]. The most commonly used drugs are sodium nitroprusside, nitroglycerin, nifedipine, verapamil, ACE-inhibitors, labetalol, and diuretics.

Hypertensive encephalopathy, accompanied by serious headache, nausea, vomiting, and visual deficit, can be treated with nitroprusside, labetalol, nifedipine, and verapamil. Eclampsia can be treated with labetalol and nifedipine. Nitroprusside and labetalol can be used for hemorrhagic stroke or cerebral infarct. In aortic dissection, arterial hypertension is treated with nitroprusside and beta-blockers without intrinsic sympathomimetic side-effects.

Phlebothrombosis of lower limbs

A pre-emergency situation is: echographic visualization of a thrombus (floating, pedunculated, moving back and forth) becoming an emergency for pulmonary embolism.

Leukophlegmasia, phlegmasia cerulea and venous gangrene are emergencies. Leukophlegmasia is caused by arteriospasm with secondary ischemia, while phlegmasia cerulea entails microcirculatory stasis at venular level. When blisters appear, the situation becomes very serious because a venous gangrene is beginning. Fasciotomy, especially in the anterolateral tibial compartment, which is generally hard and affected by stasis, is essential to avoid gangrene [20].

The most appropriate therapy is: urokinase infusion (200 mg/h) for a few days, with continuous monitoring of fibrinogenic levels which must not be lower than 80 mg%. Heparin can be given together with urokinase, especially at the beginning of the treatment.

Local venous treatment with urokinase has not been as successful as expected. In some cases, thrombectomy can be performed. If these measures are inadequate, especially in paraneoplastic forms where the tendency to form thrombi is very intense (cell-mediated thrombophlebitis according to Neri–Sarneri), it can be observed that necrosis appears under the sole, according to Lejart's venous sole drawing. Amputation is rare.

Pulmonary embolism

During the clinical course of phlebothrombosis, pulmonary embolism is still possible and symptoms such as tachycardia, hyperpnea, and clicking rales, can be suspicious. Echography and especially echocolor are reliable means by which a venous thrombosis can be monitored. By daily monitoring of the thrombus, it can be seen that at a certain moment its head starts floating then detaches, leaving *in situ* a remaining part with an oblique edge, like a flute. Venous vessels opening out obliquely and with a high flow into the thrombosed vein are responsible for the strength of the cut, the larger size of the thrombus and its consequent detachment (killer veins) [21].

Sometimes the venous wall detaches from the thrombus and not vice versa, enabling the thrombus to migrate; this can happen during a Valsalva maneuver unconsciously performed by the patient (sudden movements, cough, constipation, etc.) – patients must be told about the possible consequences of their behavior.

Despite treatment, some patients (the percentage can vary) are affected by pulmonary embolism [22] accompanied by serious symptoms such as dyspnea, cyanosis, tachycardia, and decubitus caused by the compulsory sitting position. Perfusional scintigraphy followed, if needed, by ventilatory scintigraphy, can be carried out in cases where symptoms are weak.

If symptoms are acute, an immediate pulmonary angiography enabling a more accurate and localized diagnosis, together with local infusion of urokinase (30 000–50 000 units/h) are preferred; although unnecessary, it is preferable to control the hematologic content of fibrinogen. Heparin therapy should continue. When blood gases are controlled, oxygen can be given by inhalation, but this is not always acceptable. The electrocardiogram and echocardiogram can show right cardiac strain. If pulmonary embolism is not accompanied by symptoms of phlebothrombosis, transesophageal echography will show the presence of thrombi in the right auricle.

If, despite phlebothrombosis control, the patient suffers pulmonary embolism and risks another embolism in the future, it is good practice to insert a filter in the inferior vena cava. Either a temporary filter, inserted by means of a catheter used to inject a fibrinolytic drug, or a definitive filter can be used. However, use of the first kind of filter is decreasing because of thrombotic stimulation caused by the catheter and filter. These methods have replaced the previously used caval clips. If pulmonary embolism begins with cardiac shock, emergency resuscitation is essential. If the condition is still serious, a possible embolectomy during extracorporeal circulation must be considered on the basis of the results of pulmonary angiography.

References

1. Pellis G, Offer G. Valutazione dei fattori di rischio in chirurgia vascolare d'urgenza. In: Pietri P. (ed.), Arteriopatié periferiche. Torino: Minerva Medica, 1982:17–24.
2. Cormier JM. Ischémie aigue des membres inferieures. In: Rouffy J, Natali J. (eds), Artériophaties atheromateuses des membres inferieurs. Paris: Masson, 1989:449–56.
3. Savage PEA. Problems in peripheral vascular disease. Lancaster: MPT Press, 1983:33–7.
4. Haimovici H. Vascular emergencies. New York: Appleton Century Grofts, 1984:267–89.
5. Mubarak SJ, Hargens AR. Acute compartment syndromes. Surg Clin N Am 1983;63:539–65.
6. Wilson EG. Diary of the Terra Nova Expedition to the Antartic, 1910–12. London: Blandford Press, 1972:238.
7. Patman RD, Thompson JE. Fasciotomy in peripheral vascular surgery. Arch Surg 1970;101:663–70.
8. Bartolo M, Todini AR, Antignani PL, Izzo AM. Les artériopathies ectasiantes: un chapitre oublié. J Mal Vasc 1990;15:109–13.
9. Kieffer E, Denis J, Benhamou JP et al. Complication artérielles du syndrome de la traversée thoracobrachiale. Traitment chirurgical de 38 cas. Chirurgie 1983;109:714–22.
10. Chiandussi L. L'ischemia mesenterica in Beretta Anguissola: Trattato delle malattie cardiovascolari. Torino: Utet, 1987:1297–300.
11. Masera N, Ferrara L, Namo M. Chirurgia geriatrica. Torino: Minerva Medica, 1990:225–32.
12. Vollman J. Surgical experience with 197 traumatic arterial lesion (1953–66). In: Hiertonn T, Rybeck B, (eds), Traumatic arterial lesion. Stockholm: Forvarets Forskningsanstalt, 1968.
13. Cormier JM, Gedeon A. Symposium sur la maladie anéurismale. J Mal Vasc Paris: Masson 1984:251–4.
14. Natali J. Anéurismes artériels des membres: Rev Prat 1966;16:599–614.
15. Blondeaau P. Dissection de l'aurte. In: Olivier C. Merlen JF (eds), Précis des maladies des vaisseaux. Paris: Masson, 1983:210–6.
16. Lellonche D, Benhaiem N, Sigaux EP. Dissection de l'aorte. Encycl-Méd chir. Paris (Coeur-Vaisseaux) 11311 A^{105}–1985:1–12.
17. De Bakey ME, Henly WS, Cooley DA, et al. Surgical management of dissecting aneurysms of aorta. J Thorac Cardiovasc Surg 1965;49:130–49.
18. Slater EE, De Sanctis RW. The clinical recognition of dissecting aortic aneurysm. Am J Med 1976;50:(5)625–33.
19. Ambrosioni E. Emergenze ipertensive. In enciclicl. Med. Ital. Aggiorn I. Firenze: Uses Ed. Scient, 1991:4001–12.

20. Brownse NL, Burnand KG, Thomas LM. Disease of the veins. London: Edward Arnold, 1988:476–8.
21. Todini AR, Ricci A, Paiella ML, Izzo AM, Bartolo M. Typologie de la thrombose veinouse profonde et embolie pulmonaire. Comunication: European Chapter International Union of Angiology XX Congrés Societé d'Angiologie de langue francaise. Beanne, 6–8 Octobre 1993.
22. Prandoni P, Vigo M. La diagnosi della trombosi venosa profonda e dell'embolia polmonare. Padova: Piccin, 1992:75–81.

35. Prevention of cardiovascular disease

MAHMOUD BARBIR, FAWZI LAZEM and CHARLES ILSLEY

Cardiovascular disease (CVD), including coronary heart disease (CHD), stroke, and occlusive peripheral arterial disease (PAD) remains the most common cause of mortality and morbidity despite the significant decline in the death rate during the last two decades both in Europe and the United States.

In industrialized countries, CHD is the leading cause of mortality in men over 45 years and in women over the age of 65 years [1–3]. Furthermore CVD is a major financial burden on both medical and social services in all countries. For example in the United States the estimated cost of treating heart disease is 56 billion dollars annually [4]; with increasing prevalence due to the ageing population, both primary and secondary prevention of CHD have been given a major public health importance. The majority of people today are more aware of health issues and disease and are demanding an emphasis on health promotion and disease prevention.

There is enthusiasm for understanding the pathogenesis of atherosclerosis and the development of high-tech diagnostic procedures together with an aggressive approach to the treatment of CHD. The same enthusiasm has not been given to measures to reduce or modify those risk factors that are known to be linked with the development of atherosclerosis and cardiovascular events.

Coronary risk factors are major determinants of subsequent cardiovascular events in those with established coronary artery disease as well as in healthy individuals. Moreover, the presence of known coronary artery disease dramatically increases the likelihood of an additional cardiac event [5]. In contrast to the lesser benefit in survival that can be achieved in healthy individuals with reductions in coronary risk factors, i.e. smoking, hypertension and high serum cholesterol (primary prevention) [6], considerable evidence supports a substantial effect of risk factor modification in those with established coronary artery disease (secondary prevention) [7]. Evidence from major clinical trials indicates that interventions to control risk factors, such as smoking cessation, avoidance of obesity, maintenance of a physically active lifestyle, lowering cholesterol level, treatment of hypertension, and maintenance of normal glucose tolerance, have contributed to the reduction of cardiovascular mortality and long-term disability [8].

Atherosclerosis and vascular biology

Atherosclerosis is a complex interaction of serum cholesterol with the cellular component of the arterial wall, and it is the fundamental underlying cause of occlusive cardiovascular disease, with subsequent development of clinical events. It is a chronic disease process that has its origin in childhood. Fatty streaks are found in children as young as 3 years of age [9], and intimal plaques have been found in adolescents [10–15] which gradually progress leading to an adverse clinical outcome in adulthood.

The endothelium of the blood vessels serves as a 'barrier' against circulating molecules and substances that may be detrimental to vascular integrity [16, 17]. Furthermore the normal endothelium also maintains a non-thrombogenic environment. Its cells are aligned in the direction of blood flow to create a flat surface, and it synthesizes and releases substances that retard the adhesion of platelets, monocytes, and other leukocytes [18–20].

A large number of vasoactive substances are secreted within the vessel wall. Within the endothelium, angiotensin II, endothelin and a variety of endothelium-derived constricting substances (e.g. thromboxane A_2) can cause contraction of smooth muscle cells [21], whereas other substances such as prostacyclin, nitric oxide (NO) and endothelium-derived hyperpolarizing factor cause relaxation of the blood vessel [22]. Therefore the vessel wall can promote both vasodilation and vasoconstriction. The pathological determinants of atherosclerosis in youth (PDAY) study, a multicenter study of the relation between CVD risk factors and post-mortem atherosclerosis in young people between 15–34 years of age, demonstrated a significant correlation between elevated levels of LDL, VLDL-cholesterol and low levels of HDL in post-mortem serum and the extent and severity of lesions in both the aorta and right coronary artery [10].

Cigarette smoking as assessed by post-mortem serum thiocyanate concentration was strongly associated with lesions in the aorta [10]. A high level of lipoprotein (a) (Lp(a)), a lipoprotein comprising a molecule of LDL covalently linked to apo(a) (apoprotein homologous to plasminogen), is a strong independent predictor of atheroma and an important risk factor for ischemic heart disease [23]. Children with high Lp(a) levels have been shown retrospectively to have an increased incidence of parental myocardial infarction at a young age [24]. Furthermore it is well established that coagulation factors, (fibrinogen, factor VII and factor X) and fibrinolytic factors (tissue plasminogen activator and plasminogen activator inhibitor) are strong predictors of cardiovascular disease. Various prospective epidemiological studies demonstrated that elevated fibrinogen level increases the risk and is an independent predictor of cardiovascular disease [25–33]. Fibrinogen level is higher in post-menopausal women [34]; in addition post-menopausal women on hormone replacement therapy have lower fibrinogen levels than those who do not receive such therapy [35]. Plasma fibrinogen level is also associated with physical activity; it increases with physical inactivity and decreases with regular physical exercises [36, 37].

Central to the pathogenesis of atherosclerosis is an abnormally functioning endothelium and a consequent loss of vascular integrity. Endothelial dysfunction may be caused by the biochemical or hemodynamic effect of established risk factors including high LDL-cholesterol, hypertension, diabetes mellitus and cigarette smoking. It has been reported that one of the markers of endothelial function is endothelial-dependent relaxation [38] which is closely related to nitrous oxide activity [39]. Current data suggest that in early atherosclerotic lesion nitrous oxide activity is reduced because of increased oxidative process [40].

Objectives of cardiovascular disease prevention

Coronary atherosclerosis used to be considered a gradually progressive disease for which there was little hope of an anatomic reversal after the pathological process had begun. Recently it has been demonstrated that regression of atherosclerosis is possible in humans. Autopsy studies performed in war-time Norway found severe calorie restriction to be associated with marked decrease in the severity and pathologic extent of vascular disease and in its associated mortality [41]. However convincing evidence in humans remains absent because sufficient means of altering the lipid profile or documenting changes in coronary vessels are not available. The results of clinical investigation of regression of atherosclerosis in humans will be reviewed later in the chapter.

The objective of cardiovascular disease prevention both in asymptomatic high-risk subjects (primary prevention) and in those with clinically established disease (secondary prevention) is to reduce their chance of developing cardiovascular disease and the risk of subsequent cardiovascular events, thereby reducing mortality and long-term disability.

Multiple risk factor intervention has been tested using clinical outcomes in multiple risk factor intervention trials [42] and using arteriographic endpoint in two multifactor, lifestyle risk reduction trials [43, 44]. Both studies demonstrated reduced rate of coronary artery narrowing and less disease progression in those who selected the risk reduction program versus those selecting the usual care. It has been shown that minimal reduction in multiple risk factors is likely to reduce risks more than aggressive reduction of a single risk factor while ignoring others [45].

The relationship between high serum cholesterol and CHD was first noted by Muller [46] and Thannhauser and Magendantz [47]. In the 1930s they demonstrated increased prevalence of CHD in patients with hereditary xanthomatosis. Since that time many epidemiological and observational studies confirmed that association [48–50].

In addition more than 30 randomized trials testing the effect of cholesterol-lowering therapy on CHD morbidity and mortality have been carried out; they have included both primary and secondary prevention trials [51–59]. The interventions have included diet and drugs to reduce cholesterol as well as other adjunctive therapy to reduce other risk factors, such as cessation of smoking and treatment of hypertension.

From these considerations the objective should be to reduce the total risk, which includes cessation of smoking, avoidance of obesity, encouragement of physical activity, and treatment of hypertension, diabetes mellitus, and of hyperlipidemia. Aggressive secondary prevention with all proven interventions, including cholesterol-lowering therapy, should be offered to CHD patients with hypercholesterolemia.

In asymptomatic individuals requiring primary prevention, treatment decisions concerning cholesterol reduction must be based on individual clinical assessment and the presence or absence of other CVD risk factors. The World Health Organisation expert committee on prevention of coronary heart disease [60] considered that comprehensive CHD prevention has to include three components:

1. Population strategy, for altering modifiable risk factors, e.g., lifestyle and socioeconomic factors, which are the underlying cause of mass occurrence of CHD in the entire population (primary prevention).
2. Identification of high-risk individuals and applying measures to reduce these risk factors.
3. Secondary prevention, to prevent the recurrence of CVD events and progression of the disease in patients with clinically established CVD.

The Task Force of the European Society of Cardiology, European Atherosclerosis Society and European Society of Hypertension [61] recommended priorities for CHD prevention in clinical practice in order to direct the preventive action most appropriately (see Table 35.1).

Table 35.1. Priorities of coronary heart disease prevention in clinical practice.

1.	Patients with established CHD or other atherosclerotic vascular disease.
2.	Asymptomatic subjects with particularly high risk (subjects with severe hypercholesterolemia or other forms of dyslipidemia, diabetes mellitus, hypertension and subjects with a cluster of several risk factors).
3.	Close relatives of patients with early onset CHD or other atherosclerotic vascular disease, asymptomatic subjects with particularly high risk.
4.	Other individuals met in connection with ordinary clinical practice.

Cardiovascular risk factor modification

Lifestyle

Lifestyle and related modifiable risk factors are known to be associated with risk of atherosclerotic vascular disease, however the underlying mechanism is not yet understood. The World Health Organisation committee report emphasized the concept that lifestyle associated with Western culture, such as tobacco smoking, diet rich in saturated fats and calories, and physical inactivity, has an important role in the development of CHD within populations [62].

Smoking

Smoking is a well-established risk factor for CHD [63–66] and other atherosclerotic diseases [67–69] in both sexes, of all ages and ethnic groups, and in subjects with and without declared CHD. In the United States 29% of CHD deaths are attributed to smoking [70]; in addition smokers sustain their CHD events at a much earlier age [71]. The relationship between smoking and CHD risk is modified, in particular, by plasma lipid levels. It has been demonstrated that in populations with low mean plasma cholesterol levels (such as the Japanese), the CHD disease incidence can remain low despite the high prevalence of smoking [72]. Smoking cessation is associated with significant reduction in CHD risk among all risk groups. Within one year CHD risk decreases by 50% and after several years, ex-smokers have similar CHD risk as non-smokers [70].

The risk of myocardial infarction is directly related to the number of cigarettes smoked; smoking low-tar cigarettes does not result in lower carbon monoxide or nicotine exposure [73] and is not associated with lower risk of myocardial infarction [70, 74]. Other additional randomized trials [75, 76] have shown that nicotine patch use is safe and results in higher short-term abstinence rates, although abstinence rates at 1 year were disappointing – 9.3% versus 5% in patch and placebo groups, respectively [77]. Smoking cessation is particularly important, not only because it reduces risk for cardiovascular disease, but also because it minimizes the incidence of lung cancer and other smoking-related diseases such as peptic ulceration.

Hypertension

Most studies have concentrated on elevated diastolic blood pressure; systolic pressure is however also a strong predictor of risk for cardiovascular disease [78]. The mortality increases progressively above a systolic blood pressure of 120 mmHg or more and the majority of CHD deaths occur among persons with systolic blood pressure of 130–139 mmHg or stage I hypertension (140–159 mmHg), despite higher relative risk among those whith more severe hypertension [79]. A randomized controlled trial of drug treatment for isolated elevation of systolic blood pressure has demonstrated benefit in terms of reduction in the incidence of cardiovascular complications including stroke, heart failure and CHD [80]. Based on the multiple risk factor intervention trial dataset, it has been estimated that the 11.6-year CHD death rate could be lowered by 35% by the primary prevention of hypertension in general practice.

The fifth report of the Joint National Committee on detection, evaluation and treatment of high blood pressure has emphasized the special importance of treating hypertension in those with evidence of target organ disease [81]. Therapy should be initiated with lifestyle modification, including minimizing sodium and alcohol intake, weight loss, and increased physical activity.

A meta-analysis of trials of blood pressure reduction looking at the mortality results in the control groups, demonstrated that the greatest benefit is seen in high-risk patients [82], and concluded that even a modest reduction in blood pressure in multiple risk factor patients and those with established vascular disease or severe hypertension can produce substantial benefits in terms of prevention of cardiovascular events or related deaths. Another meta-analysis trial showed that antihypertensive treatment resulted in 16% reduction in CHD events and CHD mortality; fatal stroke was reduced by 40% [83]. The choice of antihypertensive therapy in patients with preexisting CHD is based on individual clinical diagnosis. Beta-blockers are used in post-myocardial infarction patients; they reduce subsequent ischemic events and sudden death [84]. In patients with diabetes mellitus [85–87] and/or left ventricular dysfunction [88], ACE inhibitors are the drugs of choice.

Physical activity

Physical exercise improves functional work capacity and usually lowers heart rate and blood pressure, two major determinants of myocardial oxygen demand [89].

Pooled data from cardiac rehabilitation trials have shown significant reductions in long-term cardiovascular mortality in men and women of all ages [90]. In addition, exercise helps to reduce weight, lower serum triglyceride level, increase HDL-cholesterol level, decrease platelet adhesiveness, enhance fibrinolysis, and lessen the adrenergic response to stress [91, 92].

Sustained benefit for up to 10 years after myocardial infarction has recently been reported in the Swedish multifactorial cardiac rehabilitation trial [91]. Total mortality (42.2% versus 57.6%), cardiac mortality (35.7% versus 49.1%) and reinfarction rates (28.6% versus 39.9%) were significantly reduced in men and women in the intervention group, and return to work was higher (58% versus 22%). Only non-smokers and ex-smokers achieved a significant reduction in mortality. Exercise in patients with CHD can also alter the natural history of coronary disease progression. It has been demonstrated in a 1-year angiographic trial that exercise training significantly increases regression and reduces progression in the intervention group (28% versus 6% and 10% versus 45%, respectively). Exercise intensity and angiographic changes were related: 1400 kcal/week of leisure time activity was required to improve cardiovascular fitness, 1533 kcal/week to stabilize coronary lesions and 2200 kcal/week (5–6 hours of exercise per week) to induce regression [93].

A sedentary lifestyle should be considered an important modifiable risk factor for cardiovascular disease, therefore physicians' encouragement of regular exercise should represent a major goal in both primary and secondary prevention programs of cardiovascular disease.

Avoidance of obesity

Obesity has been established as a cause or has adverse influence on a number of other cardiovascular risk factors, including diabetes mellitus, hypertension, and lipid abnormalities [92, 94, 95].

In large-scale prospective studies by the American Cancer Society [96], and in the Framingham Heart Study [97], a strong positive association between relative weight and heart disease was demonstrated in both men and women. Obese individuals were doubly at risk compared to subjects at desirable weight [98]. More recently in an eight-year follow up of over 115 000 women, the relative risk of coronary disease was 3.3 (95 percent confidence interval, 2.3–4.5) in severely obese women (body-mass index, 29); in women who were mildly or moderately overweight (body-mass index, 25-28.9) there was an 80% increase in risk [99]. In this cohort study 40% of coronary events were attributable to being overweight; furthermore a weight gain of 10 kg between early and mid-adulthood was associated with an approximate doubling of the risk. The cardiovascular risk of obesity was amplified by other coronary risk factors [99].

Fat distribution, particularly fat deposition in the abdomen and upper body (andreoid type of obesity) may have an important effect on the risk of myocardial infarction [100-102].

The effect of weight reduction on the risk of coronary heart disease remains uncertain because of the small number of subjects with sustained weight loss in prospective studies. However, recent evidence suggests that weight loss induced by either dieting or increased exercise has favorable effects on several other coronary risk factors, such as glucose tolerance, blood pressure, HDL and triglyceride levels [94, 95, 103].

To achieve and maintain weight loss in obese patients is one of the most difficult problems facing the physician in clinical practice. The failure rate of treatment for obesity approached 60-90% for five years [104]; therefore an effective program of treatment must be multifaceted, including a hypocaloric diet, nutrition education, behavior modification counseling, emphasis on increased physical activity, and psychological and social support [105, 106].

Preventing obesity in childhood and adulthood is of paramount importance as are the detection and treatment of other diseases for which the obese patient is substantially at risk, such as hypertension, diabetes mellitus, and lipid abnormalities.

Plasma lipids

Epidemiological studies have consistently established a positive relation between serum cholesterol level and risk of CHD. Moreover the relationship has been shown as continuous over a wide range of baseline cholesterol levels and it appears that there is no evidence of a threshold serum cholesterol level below which there is no CHD risk [72, 107]. Recently the 25-year mortality follow-up of the cohorts of a seven-countries study (5 European countries, the United States, and Japan) has been completed and showed the relationship between serum total cholesterol level and 25-year mortality from CHD in different cultures [108]. It concluded that the relative increase in CHD risk with an increase in serum total cholesterol was comparable in different cultures [109]. However, the absolute increase was quite different from culture to culture since the absolute level of CHD risk differs substantially among cultures. Therefore, from a public health prospective, it is not enough to focus solely on serum cholesterol level to decrease the burden of CHD in populations. It appears that reduction in serum total cholesterol levels is not likely to bring cultures with a high CHD risk – such as the United States and Northern Europe – back to a CHD mortality level characteristic of the Mediterranean and Japanese cultures, unless other factors are also changed.

It is recommended that LDL-cholesterol be reduced to below 100 mg/dl (2.5 mmol/L) and HDL-cholesterol elevated to above 35 mg/dl (0.8 mmol/L) in patients with established disease [110]. HDL-cholesterol management should be most aggressive in patients with increased triglycerides, increased LDL-cholesterol, or both. This is in contrast to the less aggressive recommendations for primary prevention in those without multiple coronary risk factors. Around 60–70% of serum cholesterol is transported in the LDL-fraction, and there is a strong and direct relation between plasma and LDL-cholesterol and risk of subsequent CHD events [111–114]. This association is found in both men and women and also applies to patients with established CHD who run a higher risk of subsequent CHD events than asymptomatic individuals [115–117].

A series of randomized clinical trials testing the effect of cholesterol-lowering therapy on CHD morbidity and mortality demonstrated that reduction of LDL-cholesterol decreases the risk of subsequent development of heart disease. A recent overview of more than 20 trials of diets or drugs has shown an overall reduction in risk of 23% (95% CI, 18–28%, $P < 0.0001$), which was directly related to the amount and duration of blood cholesterol reduction [118]. The Scandinavian Simvastatin Survival Study [119], has removed any residual doubt about the benefits of cholesterol lowering in patients with hypercholesterolemia and established coronary heart disease. A total of 4444 patients (35–70 years of age, 81% men) with angina pectoris or previous myocardial infarction and serum cholesterol 5.5–8.0 mmol/L were randomly assigned to treatment with either simvastatin (3-hydroxy-3-methylglutaryl-coenzyme A reductase inhibitor) or placebo. Compared with placebo, treatment with simvastatin resulted in reduction of 25% and 35% in total and LDL-cholesterol levels, respectively, and an 8% increase in HDL-cholesterol levels; there were no essential changes in cholesterol levels in the placebo group. After a median follow-up period of 5.4 years, the simvastatin group had a 37% reduction in nonfatal myocardial infarction, a 37% decrease in the need for coronary revascularization, and a 42% reduction in deaths attributable to ischemic heart disease, compared with the placebo group.

HDL-cholesterol plasma levels, in contrast to those of total and LDL-cholesterol are inversely related to the risk of CHD [120–123]. In a multi-risk factor interventional trial and follow-up data from the lipid research clinic prevalence study, [43, 124, 125], the inverse relation between HDL-cholesterol and CHD remained significant even after control for age, LDL-cholesterol level, triglyceride level, body mass index, blood pressure, and smoking status [53, 126].

Plasma HDL-cholesterol has a physiological relation with the metabolism of triglycerides and very low density lipoproteins. Women usually have higher HDL-cholesterol levels than men and this difference persists after the menopause which might partially explain the low incidence of CHD among women compared to men. HDL-cholesterol is lowered by physical inactivity, smoking, and obesity, and modification of these risk factors may reverse these effects [127, 128].

The role of elevated triglycerides as an independent CHD risk factor remains unclear. In most case-control and prospective studies, the serum triglyceride level positively correlated with CHD rates by univariate analysis [129, 130], and in some multivariate analyses raised serum triglyceride was the best discriminant between patients with CHD and controls [131]. However, when total cholesterol and HDL-cholesterol are included in a multivariate analysis, triglycerides have been reported to lose their power to predict CHD in several studies [132–134].

Elevated triglyceride levels are often associated with reduced HDL-cholesterol levels [135–137], and to the extent that low HDL levels are atherogenic, elevated triglycerides likewise might be considered atherogenic [138]. There is however debate as to whether low HDL-cholesterol levels induced by high triglycerides are atherogenic.

Lipoprotein (a) (LP(a)) is an independent predictor of coronary artery disease [139]. The newborn baby has a very low Lp(a) concentration and the level slowly increases in the first weeks of life. It remains relatively constant during childhood, there is a small increase in men between 16 and 25 years of age, another increase between 36 and 45 years, and it eventually levels off. Post-menopausal women show a marked increase in average Lp(a) level [139]. Unlike LDL cholesterol, Lp(a) is resistant to modification.

Diabetes mellitus

Diabetes mellitus, whether insulin-dependent or non-insulin-dependent, accelerates atherosclerosis and increases the risk of cardiovascular disease, particularly in women [140–145]. Overall the increased risk of atherosclerosis among diabetics is considerable [146]. Patients with juvenile onset diabetes mellitus were followed for 20–40 years; 25% died of CHD compared to 9% of a comparable group without diabetes [147]. Adjusted mortality rates for coronary heart disease are 2–3 times higher among diabetic men and 3–7 times higher among diabetic women than among non-diabetics [144, 148–150].

Coronary risk factors such as hypertension, dyslipoproteinemia, and clinically manifest cardiovascular disease are present in excess at the time of diagnosis of non-insulin-dependent diabetes mellitus. Diabetes seems to accelerate the development of traditional coronary risk factors as well as independently increasing the risk of myocardial infarction [151–152]. Mechanisms postulated for its independent effect are an increased tendency to thrombosis, cardiac autonomic neuropathy and diabetic-cardiomyopathy [153–155]. Improved glucose control in the diabetic patient has to date not been proved experimentally to improve the risk of cardiovascular disease or outcomes for either primary or secondary prevention. However, achieving normoglycemia in the diabetic patient is extremely difficult with diet, oral hypoglycemic drugs or conventional subcutaneous insulin therapy, but it can be achieved in subgroups of patients with extensive insulin therapy [156].

Reduction of CHD risk in diabetic individuals depends more on control of other coexisting risk factors such as obesity, hypertension, smoking, physical inactivity, and blood lipid abnormalities [157].

Insulin resistant syndrome

This has been described recently as a metabolic syndrome characterized by elevated plasma triglycerides, low HDL-cholesterol, hypertension, impaired glucose tolerance, and central type of obesity. These individuals show decreased sensitivity of peripheral tissue, in particular skeletal muscle, to insulin [158–160]. It appears to be associated with an increased risk of CHD.

Clotting factors

The components of the coagulation system (fibrinogen, factors VII and X, and fibrinolytic factors (tissue plasminogen activator and plasminogen activator inhibitor) are strong predictors of cardiovascular disease [161–164]. Ernst and Resch [165] surveyed data from six prospective epidemiological studies on fibrinogen level, there was a two to threefold increase in risk and fibrinogen level is therefore an independent predictor of cardiovascular disease. It has been found that increased platelet aggregation is associated with increased risk of cardiovascular events [166, 167]. The currently available methods for the assessment of platelet aggregation are however not consistent and therefore cannot be used in risk stratification. Furthermore, there is a large body of evidence from randomized controlled trials demonstrating the beneficial effect of antiplatelet drugs (mainly aspirin) in the prevention of vascular events (nonfatal myocardial infarction, nonfatal stroke or vascular death) in patients with clinically established CHD or other atherosclerotic vascular disease [168]. Meta-analysis of these trials shows that low-dose aspirin (75–325 mg daily) reduces vascular events by 25%.

Post menopausal estrogen replacement therapy

Endogenous estrogen seems to have a protective role against CHD in premenopausal women because after menopause the risk begins to increase. The effect of exogenous estrogen replacement therapy on the risk of myocardial infarction has been reported in more than 32 published epidemiological studies; nearly half of these were prospective and half case-control or cross-sectional studies [169, 170]. Of the prospective studies only the Framingham Study reported an increased risk [171]. This was not statistically significant when angina pectoris was omitted.

An overview of 32 available observational studies estimates the reduction in the risk of coronary disease attributable to estrogen replacement therapy to be 44% [169]. The same results were obtained in a 10-year follow up from a nurses health study; a 44% reduction in the risk of coronary heart disease was also observed among current users of estrogen replacement.

The exact mechanisms of the apparent protective effect of estrogen are not fully understood; however it has a wide range of physiological effects on serum lipid profile, reducing total cholesterol and LDL levels and often increasing HDL-cholesterol [172–174], and improving endothelium-dependent vasoactivity [175]. Recent evidence suggests that estrogen as well as combined estrogen–progestin may favorably influence lipoprotein (a) level [35, 176]. Other postulated mechanisms include the inhibition of endothelial hyperplasia and atherosclerosis [177], inhibition of the vasoconstrictive effect of acetylcholine [178], and enhancement of the production of prostacyclin [179]. Combined estrogen–progesterone regimens have antioxidant properties [180], including inhibition of the modification and uptake of LDL-cholesterol in atherosclerotic leasions [181]. Estrogen has been associated with reduced blood pressure in some clinical trials [182]; this remains inconclusive. Despite the apparent cardiovascular benefits of postmenopausal estrogen therapy [183–185], they must be considered in the light of known risks [169, 186, 187]. Estrogen is a well-recognized cause of endometrial cancer, increases the incidence of gallbladder disease, and may increase the incidence of breast cancer. At present the evidence that estrogen replacement therapy prevents CHD is strong but not conclusive.

The conclusive evidence on the role of hormone replacement therapy (HRT) in the prevention of cardiovascular events may emerge only from comprehensive, randomized, controlled clinical trials among postmemopausal women. It will also be important to assess the effects of combination preparations that include estrogen and progestin which are currently used to avoid excess risk from endometrial cancer. Risk stratification analysis which takes into account women's baseline level of risk for various conditions, provides valuable information to aid the individual and her physician in making a decision whether to use HRT or not.

Alcohol

Alcohol abuse has been shown to increase the risks of myocardial infarction, stroke, and mortality from CHD. However, there is a substantial body of observational epidemiological evidence to suggest that moderate consumption of alcohol reduces the risk of heart disease [188].

Case control and large prospective cohort studies [189–192] have shown inverse association between moderate alcohol consumption and the risk of myocardial infarction. This reduction appears to be independent of the type of beverage consumed [193], suggesting that alcohol itself rather than components of the drinks is responsible for the observed effects. The possible mechanisms for the protective role include the alcohol-mediated increase in HDL-cholesterol subfractions HDL2 and HDL3 being inversely related to risk of myocardial infarction [194–196].

Other postulated mechanisms include the effects of alcohol on platelet aggregation [197] the release of plasminogen activator and fibrinogen [198]. Evidence of the effect of alcohol on coronary disease and cardiac events is based on data from observational prospective cohort studies comparing risk in individuals according to their level of consumption, [189–192]. No data from randomized trials are available. Therefore, when considering alcohol consumption as a modality for CHD prevention, potential adverse effects on health and behavior have to be carefully weighed against the potential benefits; general recommendations in favor of alcohol consumption do not appear justified.

Prophylactic low-dose aspirin

The role of prophylactic low-dose aspirin in reducing the risk of cardiovascular disease in apparently healthy individuals has been tested in two large randomized clinical trials of primary prevention in men [199, 200]. The US physician health study of 22 071 men aged 40–84 years, observed a statistically significant 44% reduction in the risk of first myocardial infarction ($P < 0.00001$) [198], where as the British Doctors trial of 5139 men aged 50–79 years showed no significant reduction

[200]. However a meta-analysis of both these trials demonstrated a significant 33% reduction in the risk of a first nonfatal myocardial infarction ($P \lesssim 0.0002$) [201]. In these two trials the data on the role of aspirin in the primary prevention of stroke and death from vascular causes are inconclusive [199, 200]. The favorable effects of aspirin in patients with coronary artery disease have been most clearly demonstrated in patients with acute myocardial infarction.

The second international study of infarct survival (ISIS-2), which enrolled 17 187 patients with suspected acute myocardial infarction, demonstrated that aspirin was approximately equivalent to thrombolytic therapy in reducing short-term mortality (23%) [202]. The incidence of reinfarction was reduced by 44% and stroke by 46%. Despite the apparent increase in the rate of minor bleeding (32%) the major bleeds requiring transfusion declined (–6%). A meta-analysis of long-term use of aspirin has shown that vascular mortality was reduced by 13% and subsequent cardiovascular events by 23% [203]. These data strongly support the routine short- and long-term use of aspirin in patients with suspected or demonstrated coronary artery disease without contraindications [204–206].

Angiotensin-converting enzyme (ACE) inhibitors

ACE inhibitors have been shown to be effective in reducing morbidity and mortality in patients with symptomatic and asymptomatic left ventricular dysfunction, both in chronic heart failure and after myocardial infarction. The results of several trials [206–212] suggest that patients with chronic left ventricular dysfunction (ejection fraction 35–40%), irrespective of the etiology or whether symptomatic or asymptomatic, can safely be treated with an ACE inhibitor unless otherwise contraindicated or not tolerated by the patient. A significant reduction of 14–28% in the incidence of myocardial infarction and other ischemic cardiac events has been demonstrated in these studies [207, 208, 213]. The effect of ACE inhibitors on the progression of coronary atherosclerosis remains unknown.

Beta-adrenergic blockers

Before the introduction of thrombolytic therapy, the use of beta-adrenergic blockers in acute Q-wave myocardial infarction was demonstrated to reduce one-year reinfarction and mortality by about 20% [204, 205]. In high-risk patients and in those with hyperadrenergic states, the immediate administration of beta-adrenergic blockers appears to be most effective. Beta-blockers decrease thrombosis and reduce the incidence of arrhythmia. However, they may actually increase vasoconstriction and the progression of atherosclerosis, because of their adverse effects on lipids. Currently there are few data available on the use of beta-adrenergic blockers with thrombolytic therapy. The thrombosis in myocardial infarction (TIMI IIB) study randomly assigned immediate and delayed use of beta-adrenergic blockers to patients receiving thrombolytic therapy, who were also assigned to invasive and conservative management strategies [214]. These data support the continued short-

and long-term use of beta-blockers in patients experiencing Q-wave myocardial infarction.

Antioxidants

In cardiovascular disease it has been hypothesized that antioxidant vitamins might inhibit the oxidation of LDL-cholesterol into a particularly atherogenic form and preserve endothelial function. Observational epidemiological data from both case control and cohort studies, have suggested that persons with a high intake of antioxidant vitamins through either their diet or vitamin supplements have somewhat lower than average risk of cardiovascular disease. However the relative impact of vitamin C, vitamin E, β-carotene, and flavonoids remains unclear.

The Nurses Health Study [215] and The Health Professionals follow-up study [216] showed a 34% and 36% reduction in CHD events, respectively, in the top quintiles of vitamin E consumption. In the European Community Multicenter Study on antioxidants, myocardial infarction and breast cancer (EURAMIC) trial [217], high β-carotene intake was protective only among smokers in the latter study; vitamin C intake showed no relationship with CHD.

At present definitive recommendations for antioxidant therapy are not justified.

Conclusion

In this brief chapter we have demonstrated that there is considerable and consistent evidence at the epidemiological, clinical, biochemical, cellular, and molecular levels, which suggests that CVD risk factors are present in childhood and adolescence. Therefore it is reasonable that such young persons who are likely to be at high risk for CVD should be identified and treated. Many of the risk factors are modifiable and early modification is associated with substantial reduction in mortality and morbidity. Furthermore it is easier to control a young child's health behavior than that of an older child or an adult and this can be undertaken in three settings as suggested by the American Heart Association Scientific Statement, a special report by Muller *et al.* on cardiovascular health and disease in children [218].

At home

Over the last two decades it has become normal for both parents to work and this has affected children's dietary habits with more consumption of fast food and prepacked foods. The number of hours spent by a young person on the computer and watching television has increased and correlates with the level of serum cholesterol and obesity. In addition parents can be influential role models and their behavior, particularly in regard to smoking, is important; therefore health education of children and a healthy lifestyle of parents will undoubtedly reflect positively in the children's lifestyle.

At school

Schools are another important site for development of health habits through classroom activity, school lunch program and physical education. The classroom is an ideal site for health education, and teachers, like parents, can be influential role models.

At the physician's office

Health care supervision, which includes preventive care, is the major role of the general physician. Traditionally the physician focused such care on areas of immediate concern such as accident prevention or immunization. Prevention of chronic diseases such as atherosclerosis has not been stressed, therefore this has to be reinforced in the physician's training program and given sufficient time.

References

1. Tuomilehto J, Kuulasmaa K, Torppa J. WHO; MONICA project: Geographic Variation in mortality from cardiovascular disease. World Health Stat Q 1987;40:171–84.
2. Uemura K. Pisa 2. Trends in cardiovascular disease mortality in industrialized countries since 1950. World Health Stat Q 1988;41:155–78.
3. Uemura K. International trends in cardiovascular disease in the elderly. Eur Heart J 1988;9(Suppl.D):1–8.
4. American Heart Association. Heart and stroke facts 1944. Statistical supplement. Dallas: American Heart Association, 1993.
5. Pekkanen J, Linn S, Heiss G et al. Ten year mortality from cardiovascular disease in relation to cholesterol level among men with and without preexisting cardiovascular disease. N Engl J Med 1990;322:1700–7.
6. Tsevat J, Weinstein MC, Williams LW, Tosteson ANA, Goldman L. Expected gains in life expectancy from various coronary heart disease risk modifications. Circulation 1991;83:1194–201.
7. Vogel RA. Comparative clinical consequences of aggressive lipid management, coronary angioplasty and bypass surgery in coronary heart disease. Am J Cardiol 1992;69:1229–33.
8. Haskell WL, Alderman EL, Fair JM et al. Effect of intensive multiple risk factor reduction on coronary atherosclerosis and clinical cardiac events in men and women with coronary artery disease. The Stanford Coronary Risk Intervention Project (SCRIP). Circulation 1994;89:975–90.
9. Holman RL, McGill HC Jr, Strong JP, Geer JC. The natural history of atherosclerosis: The early aortic lesion as seen in New Orleans in the middle of the 20th Century. Am J Pathol 1958;34:209–35.
10. PDAY Research Group. Relationship of atherosclerosis in young men to serum lipoprotein cholesterol concentration and smoking. A preliminary report from pathological determinants of atherosclerosis in youth (PDAY) research group. J Am Med Assoc 1990;264:3018–24.
11. Enos WF Jr, Beyer JC, Holmes RH. Pathogenesis of coronary disease in American soldiers killed in Korea. J Am Med Assoc 1955;158:912–4.
12. McNamara JJ, Molot MA, Stremple JF, Cutting RF. Coronary artery disease in combat casualties in Vietnam. J Am Med Assoc 1971;216:1185–7.
13. Newman WP III, Wattigney W, Berenson GS. Autopsy studies in United States. Children and adolescents: Relationship of risk factors to atherosclerotic lesions. Ann NY Acad Sci 1991;623:16–25.
14. Freedman DS, Newman WP III, Tracy RE et al. Black-white differences in aortic fatty streaks in adolescence and early adulthood. The Bogalusa Heart Study. Circulation 1988;77:856–64.

15. Strong JP. Landmark perspective coronary atherosclerosis in soldiers: A clue to the natural history of atherosclerosis in the young. J Am Med Assoc 1986;256:2863–6.
16. Dzan VJ, Gibbons GH, Cooke JP, Omugui N. Vascular biology and medicine in the 1990s. Scope concepts potention and perspective. Circulation 1993;87:705–19.
17. Gibbon GH, Dzan VJ. The emerging concept of vascular remodeling. N Engl J Med 1993;330:1431–8.
18. Ross R. The pathogenesis of atherosclerosis, a perspective for the 1990s. Nature 1993;362:801–9.
19. Levesque MJ, Nerem RM. The elongation and orientation of cultured endothelial cells in response to sheer stress. Biomech Eng 1985;107:341–7.
20. Luscher TF. Imbalance of endothelium-derived relaxing and contracting factors. A new concept in hypertension. Am J Hypertens 1990;3:317–30.
21. Van JR, Anggard EE, Boltingham R. Regulatory functions of the endothelium. N Engl J Med 1990;323:27–36.
22. Flabahan NA, Vanhoutte PM. Endothelium-derived hyperpolarizing factor. Blood Vessels 1990;27:238–45.
23. Rader DJ, Hoeg JM, Brewer HB Jr. Quantitation of plasma apolipoproteins in the primary and secondary prevention of coronary artery disease. Ann Intern Med 1994;120:1012–25.
24. Racial (black and white) differences in serum lipoprotein (a) distribution and its relation to parental myocardial infarction in children. Bogalusa Heart Study. Circulation 1991;84:160–7.
25. Ernst E, Resch KL. Fibrinogen as a cardiovascular risk factor. A meta-analysis and review of the literature. Ann Intern Med 1993;118:956–63.
26. Mead TW, Mellows S, Brozovic N et al. Haemostatic function and ischaemic heart disease. Principle result of Northwick Park heart study. Lancet 1986;533–7.
27. Wilhelmsen L, Svardsudd K, Korsan-Bengtsen K, Larsson B, Welin L, Tibblin J. Fibrinogen as a risk factor for stroke and myocardial infarction. N Engl J Med 1984;311:501–5.
28. Fuster V, Badimon L, Bardimon JJ, Chesebro JH. The pathogenesis of coronary artery disease and acute coronary syndromes. N Engl J Med 1992;326:242–50.
29. Kannel WB, Wolf PA, Castelli WP, D'Agustino RB. Fibrinogen and risk of cardiovascular disease. The fibrinogen study. J Am Med Assoc 1987;258:1183–6.
30. Yarnell JW, Baker IA, Sweetman et al. Fibrinogen viscosity and white blood cell count are major risk factors for ischaemic heart disease. Circulation 1991;83:836–44.
31. Thompson SG, Kienast J, Pyke SDM, Haverkate F, Van de loo JCW. Haemostatic factors and the risk of myocardial or sudden death in patients with angina pectoris. N Engl J Med 1995;332:635–41.
32. Balleisen L, Schulte H, Assmann G, Epping PH, Van De Loo J. Coagulation factors and progress of coronary heart disease. Lancet 1987;1:461.
33. Cremer P, Nagel D, Bottcher B, Seidel D. Fibrinogen ein koronarer risikofaktor. Diag Labor 1992;42:28–35.
34. Brunner EJ, Marmot MG, White IR et al. Gender and employment grade differences in blood cholesterol. Apolipoproteins and haemostatic factors in the Whitehall II study. Atherosclerosis 1993;102:195–207.
35. Nabulsi AA, Folsom AR, White A et al. For the atherosclerosis risk in communities study investigators. Association of hormone replacement therapy with various cardiovascular risk factors in post menopausal women. N Engl J Med 1993;328:1069–75.
36. Rankinen T, Rauraman R, Vaeisanen S et al. An inverse relationship between physical activity and plasma fibrinogen in post menopausal women. Atherosclerosis 1993;102:181–6.
37. Wood PC, Yarnell JWG, Pickering J, Fehily AM, O'Brien JR. Exercise, fibrinogen and other risk factors for ischaemic heart disease. Caerphilly prospective heart disease study. Br Heart J 1993;69:183–7.
38. Jaykody L, Kappagoda T, Senaratane MPJ, Thomson ABR. Impairment of endothelium dependent relaxation: An early marker of atherosclerosis in the rabbit. Br J Pharmacol 1988;94:335–46.
39. Luscher TF, Richard V, Tschudi M, Yang Z, Boulanger C. Endothelial control of vascular tone in large and small coronary arteries. J Am Coll Cardiol 1990;15:519–27.
40. Harrison DG, Freiman PC, Armstrong MI, Marcus ML, Heisted DD. Alteration of vascular reactivity in atherosclerosis. Circ Res 1987;61(Suppl.II):1174–80.

41. Strom A, Jensen RA. Mortality from circulatory disease in Norway 1940-1945. Lancet 1951;1:126-9.
42. Multiple risk factor intervention research group. Multiple risk factor intervention trial: Risk factor changes and mortality results. N Engl J Med 1982;248:1465-77.
43. Ornish D, Brown SE, Scherwitz LW et al. Can life style changes reverse coronary heart disease? Lancet 1990;336:129-33.
44. Schuler G, Hambrech R, Schlierf G et al. Regular physical exercise and low fat diet: Effects on progression of coronary artery disease. Circulation 1992;86:1-11.
45. Anderson KM, Wilson PWF, Odell PM, Kennel WB. An updated coronary risk profile: A statement for health professionals. Circulation 1991;83:356-62.
46. Muller C. Xanthomata, hypercholesterolaemia, angina pectoris. Acta Med Scand 1938;89:(Suppl.)75-84.
47. Thannhauser SJ, Magendantz H. The different clinical groups of xanthomatous disease: A clinical physiological study of 22 cases. Ann Intern Med 1938;11:1662-746.
48. Goldbourt U, Yaari S. Cholesterol and heart disease mortality. A 23 year follow up study of 9902 men in Israel. Atherosclerosis 1990;10:512-9.
49. Pekkanen J, Nussinen A, Punsar S, Karvonen MJ. Short and long term association of serum cholesterol with mortality: The 25 year follow-up of the Finnish cohorts of the seven countries study. Am J Epidemiol 1992;135:1251-8.
50. Isles CG, Hole DJ, Gillis CR, Hawthorne VM, Lever AF. Plasma cholesterol coronary heart disease and cancer in the Renfrew and Paisley survey. Br Med J 1989:298;920-4.
51. Leren P. The Oslo diet heart study. Eleven year report. Circulation 1970;42:935-42.
52. Coronary Drug Project Research Group. Clofibrate and niacin in coronary heart disease. J Am Med Assoc 1975;231:360-81.
53. Carlson LA, Danielson M, Ekberg I, Klintemar B, Rosenhamer G. Reduction of myocardial infarction by the combined treatment with clofibrate and nicotinic acid. Atherosclerosis 1977;28:81-6.
54. Committee of principle investigator. A co-operative trial in the primary prevention of ischemic heart disease using clofibrate. Br Heart J 1978;40:1069-118.
55. Lipid Research Clinics Program. The lipid research clinics coronary primary prevention trial results. J Am Med Assoc 1984;251:351-74.
56. Frick MH, ELO O, Happa K et al. Helsinki Heart Study: Primary prevention with gemfibrozil in middle-aged men with dyslipaemia. N Engl J Med 1987;317:1237-45.
57. Canner PL, Berge KG, Wenger NK et al. Fifteen year mortality in coronary drug project patients. Long term benefit with niacin. J Am Coll Cardiol 1986;8:1245-55.
58. Buchwald H, Varlo RL, Matt JP et al. Effect of partial ileal bypass surgery on mortality and morbidity from coronary heart disease in patients with hypercholesterolaemia. Report of the program on the surgical control of the hyperlipidemias (POSCH). N Engl J Med 1990;323:946-55.
59. Law MR, Wald NJ, Thompson SG. By how much and how quick does reduction in serum cholesterol concentration lower risk of ischaemic heart disease? Br Med J 1994;308:367-73.
60. Eleventh Bethesda Conference. Prevention of coronary heart disease. September 27-28, 1980. Bethesda, Maryland. Am J Cardiol 1981;47:713-76.
61. Pyorala K, Backer DE, Graham I, Pool Wilson P. Wood D. On behalf of the task force prevention of coronary heart disease in clinical practice. Eur Heart J 1994;15:1300-31.
62. Prevention of coronary heart disease, report of WHO expert committee. WHO technical report series 678. Geneva: World Health Organisation, 1982.
63. US Surgeon General. Cardiovascular disease, the health consequences of smoking. Washington, DC: US Department of Health and Human Services, Public Health Service, Office on Smoking and Health, 1983 (DHHS publication no. (PHS) 84-50204-384P).
64. US Surgeon General. Reducing the consequences of smoking: 25 years of progress. Bethesda, MD: US Department of Health and Human services, Public Health Services, Office on Smoking and Health, 1989 (DHSS publication no. (CDC) 89-8411. 703P).
65. Willett WC, Green A, Stampler MJ et al. Relative and absolute excess risks of coronary heart disease among women who smoke cigarettes. N Engl J Med 1987;317:1303-9.

66. Lacroix AZ, Lang J, Scherr P et al. Smoking and mortality among older men and women in three communities. N Engl J Med 1991;324:1614–25.
67. Wolf PA, D'Agostino RB, Kannel WB, Bonita R, Belanger AJ. Cigarette smoking as a risk factor for stroke. The Framingham Study. J Am Med Assoc 1988;259:1025–9.
68. Liedberg E, Person BM. Age, diabetes and smoking in lower limb amputations for arterial occlusive disease. Acta Orthop Scand 1983;54:383–8.
69. Strachan DP. Predictors of death from aortic aneurysm among middle aged men. The Whitehall Study. Br J Surg 1991;78:401–4.
70. Jonas MA, Oates JA, Ockene JK, Hennekens CH. AHA position statement. Statement on smoking and cardiovascular disease for health care professionals. Circulation 1992;86:1664–9.
71. Hensen EF, Andersen LT, Von Eyben FE. Cigarette smoking and age at first acute myocardial infarction and influence of gender and extent of smoking. Am J Cardiol 1993;71:1439–42.
72. Keys A, (ed.). Seven countries. A multivariate analysis of death and coronary heart disease. Cambridge, MA: Harvard University Press, 1980.
73. Coultas DB, Stidley CA, Samet JM. Cigarette yields of tar and nicotine and marker of exposure to tobacco smoke. Am Rev Respit Dis 1993;148:435–40.
74. Negri E, Franzosi MG, La Vecchia C, Santoro L, Nobili A, Tognoni G, on behalf of Gissi – E FRIM Investigators. Tar yield of cigarette and risk of acute myocardial infarction. Br Med J 1993;306:1567–70.
75. Fiore MC, Jorenby DE, Baker TB, Kenford SL. Tobacco dependence and the nicotine patch. Clinical guidelines for effective use. J Am Med Assoc 1992;268:2687–94.
76. Imperial cancer research fund general Research Group. Effectiveness of nicotine patch in helping people stop smoking. Results of a randomized trial in general practice. Br Med J 1993;306:1304–8.
77. Russell MAH, Stapleton JA, Teyerabend C et al. Targeting heavy smokers in general practice. Randomized control trial of transdermal nicotine patches. Br Med J 1993;306:1309–12.
78. Kannel WB, Dawber TR, McGee DL. Perspective on systolic hypertension. The Framingham Study. Circulation 1980;61:1179–82.
79. Stamler J, Stamler R, Neaton JD. Blood pressure, systolic and diastolic and cardiovascular risks. Arch Intern Med 1993;153:598–615.
80. SHEP Co-operative Research Group. Prevention of stroke by antihypertensive drug treatment in older persons with isolated systolic hypertension. Final results of the systolic hypertension in the elderly program (SHEP). J Am Med Assoc 1991;265:3255–64.
81. The Joint National Committee on detection, evaluation and treatment of high blood pressure. The fifth report of the Joint National Committee on detection, evaluation and treatment of high blood pressure. Bethesda National Institute of health. National heart lung and blood institute. NIH publication 93–1088, 1993.
82. Hoes AW, Grobbee DE, Lubsen J. Does drug treatment improve survival? Reconciling the trials in mild to moderate hypertension. Hoes AW. Non potassium sparing diuretics and sudden cardiac death in hypotensive patients, pharmacoepidemiological approach. Thesis, Erasmus University, Rotterdam, 1992.
83. Hebert PR, Moser M, Mayer J, Glynn RJ, Hennekens CH. Recent evidence on drug therapy of mild to moderate hypertension and decreased risk of coronary heart disease. Arch Intern Med 1993:578–81.
84. Lace J, Antmann EM, Silva JJ, Kupelnick B, Mosteller F, Chalmers JC. Cumulative meta-analysis of theraputic trials for myocardial infarction. N Engl J Med 1992;327:248–54.
85. Christleib AR. Treatment selection consideration for the hypertensive diabetic patient. Arch Intern Med 1990;150:1167–74.
86. Ravid M, Savin H, Jutrin I, Bental T, Katz B, Lishner M. Long term stabilizing effect of angiotensin converting enzyme inhibitors on plasma creatinine and proteinuria in normotensive type II diabetic patients. Ann Intern Med 1993;118:577–81.
87. Magenson CE. Angiotensin converting enzyme inhibitors and diabetic nephropathy. Br Med J 1992;304:327.

88. Groden DL. Vasodilator therapy for congestive heart failure, lessons from mortality trials. Arch Intern Med 1993;153:445–54.
89. Maskin CS. Aerobic exercise training in cardiopulmonary disease. In: Weber KT, Janicki JS (eds), Cardiopulmonary exercise testing. Physiological principles and clinical applications. Philadelphia: Saunders, 1986:317–32.
90. Bittner V, Oberman A. Efficacy studies in coronary rehabilitation. Cardiol Clin 1993;11:333–47.
91. Hedbaeck B, Perk J, Woldin P. Long term reduction of cardiac mortality after myocardial infarction. 10 year results of a comprehensive rehabilitation programme. Eur Heart J 1993;14:831–5.
92. Van Itallie TB. Obesity: Adverse effect on health and longevity. Am J Clin Nutl 1979;32(Suppl.):2723–33.
93. Hambrecht R, Niebauer J, Marburger C et al. Various intensities of leisure time physical activity in patients with coronary artery disease. Effect on cardiorespiratory fitness and progression of atherosclerotic leasions. J Am Coll Cardiol 1993;22:468–77.
94. Bierman EL, Hirsch J. Obesity. In: Williams RH (ed.), Textbook of endocrinology. 6th ed. Vol I. Philadelphia: Saunders, 1981:906–21.
95. Mann GV. The influence of obesity on health. N Engl J Med 1974;291:178–85,226–32.
96. Lew EA, Gardinkel L. Variations in mortality by weight among 750 000 men and women. J Chronic Dis 1979;32:563–76.
97. Hubert HB, Feinleib, McNamara PM, Castelli WP. Obesity as an independent risk factor for cardiovascular disease. A 26 year follow-up of participants in the Framingham heart study. Circulation 1983;67:968–77.
98. Simopolous AP, Van Itallie TB. Bodyweight health and longevity. Ann Intern Med 1984;100:285–95.
99. Manson JE, Celditz GA, Stampler MJ et al. A prospective study of obesity and risk of coronary heart disease in women. N Engl J Med 1990;322:882–9.
100. Kissebah AH, Vydelingum N, Murray R et al. Relation of body fat distribution to metabolic complications of obesity. J Clin Endocrinol Metab 1982;54:254–60.
101. Krotkiewski M, Bjorntorp P, Sjostrom L, Smith U. Impact of obesity on metabolism in men and women. Importance of regional adipose tissue distribution. J Clin Invest 1983;72:1150–62.
102. Bjorntrop P. Regional patterns of fat distribution. Ann Intern Med 1985;103:994–5.
103. Wood PD, Stefanick ML, Dreon DM et al. Change in plasma lipid and lipoproteins in overweight men during weight loss through dieting as compared with exercise. N Engl J Med 1988;319:1173–9.
104. Committee on diet and health. Diet and health implication for reducing chronic disease risk. Washington, DC: National Academy Press, 1989.
105. Dwyer JT. Treatment of obesity. In: Bjorntorp P, Porodoff BN (eds), Conventional programme and fat-diet in obesity. Philadelphia: JB Lippincott, 1992:662–76.
106. Bjorntorp P. Physical exercise in treatment of obesity. Philadelphia: JB Lippincott, 1992:708–11.
107. Chen Z, Peto R, Collins R, MacMahon S, Luj, LIW. Serum cholesterol and coronary heart disease in population with low cholesterol. Br Med J 1991;303:276–82.
108. Menotti A, Keys A, Krumhout D et al. Inter cohort differences in coronary heart disease mortality in the 25 year follow-up of the Seven Countries Study. Eur J Epidemiol 1993;9:527–36.
109. Verschuren WM, Jacobs DR, Bloemberg BP et al. Serum total cholesterol and long-term coronary heart disease mortality in different cultures. J Am Med Assoc 1995;274:131–6.
110. Summary of the second report of the National Cholesterol Education Program (NCEP): Expert panel on detection, evaluation and treatment of high blood cholesterol in adults (adult treatment panel II). J Am Med Assoc 1993;269:3015–23.
111. Ragland DR, Brand RJ. Coronary heart disease mortality in western collaborative group study follow-up experience of 22 years. Am J Epidemiol 1988;127:462–75.
112. Neaton JD, Blackburn H, Jacobs D et al. Serum cholesterol level and mortality findings for men screened in the multiple risk factor intervention trial. Arch Intern Med 1992;152:1490–500.
113. Davey-Smith G, Shipley MJ, Marmot MG, Rose G. Plasma cholesterol and mortality. The Whitehall Study. J Am Med Assoc 1992;267:70–6.

114. Chenz, Peto R, Collins R, MacMahon S, Luj, LIW. Serum cholesterol concentration and coronary heart disease in a population with low serum cholesterol concentration. Br Med J 1991;303:276–82.
115. Ulvenstram G, Bergstrand R, Johansson S et al. Prognostic importance of cholesterol levels after myocardial infarction. Prev Med 1984;13:355–66.
116. Pekkanen J, Linn S, Heiss J et al. 10 years mortality from cardiovascular disease in relation to cholesterol level among men with and without preexisting cardiovascular disease. N Engl J Med 1990;322:1700–7.
117. Wong ND, Wilson PWF, Kannel WB. Serum cholesterol as a prognostic factor after myocardial infarction. The Framingham Study. Ann Intern Med 1991;115:687–93.
118. Yusuf S, Wittes J, Friedman L. Overview of results of randomised clinical trials in heart disease II. Unstable angina, heart failure, primary prevention with aspirin and risk factor modification. J Am Med Assoc 1988;260:2259–63.
119. Scandinavian Simvastatin Survival Study Group. Randomised trial of cholesterol lowering in 4444 patients with coronary heart disease. The Scandinavian Simvastatin Survival Study (4S). Lancet 1944;344:1383–9.
120. Miller GJ, Miller NE. Plasma high density lipoprotein concentration and development of ischaemic heart disease. Lancet 1975;1:16–9.
121. Miller NE, Forde OH, Thelle DS, MJQS OD. The Tromso heart study of high density lipoprotein and coronary heart disease – prospective case control study. Lancet 1977;1:965–8.
122. Gordon T, Castelli WP, Hjortland MC, Kannel WB, Dawber TR. High density lipoprotein as a protective factor against coronary heart disease. Am J Med 1977;62:707–14.
123. Castelli WP, Garrison RJ, Wilson PWF, Abbott RD, Kalousdian S, Kannel WB. Incidence of coronary heart disease and lipoprotein cholesterol levels. The Framingham Study. J Am Med Assoc 1986;256:2835–8.
124. Sherwin RW, Wentworth DN, Cutler JA, Hulley SB, Kuller LH, Stamler J. Serum cholesterol levels and cancer mortality in 301, 662 men screened for the multiple risk factor intervention trial. J Am Med Assoc 1987;257:943–8.
125. Jacobs DR Jr, Mebane IL, Bangdiwala SI, Criqui MH, Tyroler HA. High density lipoprotein cholesterol as a predictor of cardiovascular disease mortality in men and women. The follow-up study of the lipid research clinic prevalence study. Am J Epidemiol 1990;131:32–47.
126. Manninen V, Elo MO, Frick H et al. Lipid alterations and decline in the incidence of coronary heart disease in the Helsinki Heart Study. J Am Med Assoc 1988;260:641–51.
127. Robinson D, Fern JA, Bevan EA, Stock J, Williams PT, Galton DJ. High density lipoprotein subfractions and coronary risk factors in normal men. Arteriosclerosis 1987;7:341–6.
128. Haffner SM, Applebaum-Bowden D, Wahl PW et al. Epidemiological correlates of high density lipoprotein subfraction apolipoproteins, A-I, A-II and D, and lecithin cholesterol acetyl transferase E: Effect of smoking, alcohol and adiposity. Anteriosclerosis 1985;5:169–77.
129. Criqui MH, Heiss G, Cohn K et al. Plasma triglyceride level and mortality from coronary heart disease. New Engl J Med 1993;328:1220–5.
130. Austin MA. Plasma triglycerides as a risk factor for coronary heart disease: The epidemiologic evidence and beyond. Am J Epidemiol 1989;129:249–57.
131. Barbir M, Wile D, Tayner I, Aber VR, Thompson GR. High prevelance of hypertriglyceridaemia and apolipoprotein abnormalities in coronary artery disease. Br Heart J 1988;60:397–403.
132. Pocock SJ, Shaper AG, Philips AN. Concentration of high density lipoprotein cholesterol, triglycerides and total cholesterol in ischaemic heart disease. Br Med J 1989;298:998–1002.
133. Assmann G, Schulte H. Triclycerides and atherosclerosis: Results from the prospective cardiovascular munster study. In: Gotto AM Jr, Paoletti R (eds), Atherosclerosis reviews Vol. 22. New York: Raven Press, 1991:51–7.
134. Wilson PWF, Anderson KM, Castelli WP. The impact of triglycerides on coronary heart disease: The Framingham Study. In: Gotto AM Jr, Paoletti R (eds), Atherosclerosis reviews Vol. 22. New York: Raven Press, 1991:59–63.
135. Rhoads GG, Gulbrandsen CL, Kagan A. Serum lipoproteins and coronary heart disease in a population study of Hawaii Japanese men. N Engl J Med 1976;294(6):293–8.

136. Davis CE, Gordon D, LaRosa J, Wood PD, Halperin M. Correlations of plasma high density lipoprotein cholesterol level with other plasma lipids and lipoprotein concentrations: The lipid research clinics programme prevalence study. Circulation 1980;62(4pt2):24–30.
137. Albrink MJ, Krauss RM, Lindgren FT, Vonder Groeben J, Pan S, Wood PD. Inter correlations among high density lipoprotein, obesity and triglycerides in a normal population. Lipids 1980;15:668–78.
138. Grundy SM, Vega GL. Two different views of the relationship of hypertriglyceridemia to coronary heart disease. Arch Intern Med 1992;152:28–34.
139. Heinrich J, Sankamp M, Kokott R, Schulte H, Assmann G. Relationship of lipoprotein (a) to variables of coagulation and fibrinolysis in a healthy population. Clin Chem 1991;37:1950–4.
140. West KM. Epidemiology of diabetes and its vascular lesions. New York: Elsevier, 1978.
141. Butler WJ, Ostrander LD Jr, Carman WJ, Lamphiear DE. Mortality from coronary heart disease in the Tecumseh study: Long term effect of diabetes mellitus, glucose tolerance and other risk factors. Am J Epidemiol 1985;121:541–7.
142. Kannel WB, McGee DL. Diabetes and glucose tolerance as risk factor for cardiovascular disease. The Framingham Study. Diabetes Care 1979;2:120–6.
143. Heyden S, Heiss G, Bartel AG, Hames CG. Sex differences in coronary mortality among diabetics in Evans County, Georgia. J Chronic Dis 1980;33:265–73.
144. Barrett-Connor E, Wingard DL. Sex differential in ischaemic heart disease mortality in diabetics. A prospective population based study. Am J Epidemiol 1983;118:489–96.
145. Morrish NJ, Stevens LK, Head J, Fuller JH, Jarrett RJ, Keen H. A prospective study of mortality among middle-aged diabetic patients (the London cohort of the WHO multi-national study of vascular disease in diabetics). II Associated risk factors. Diabetologia 1990;33:542–8.
146. Krolewski AS, Warram JH, Rand LI et al. Epidemiologic approach to the etiology of type I diabetes mellitus and its complications. N Engl J Med 1987;317:1390–8.
147. Krolewski AS, Kosinski EJ, Warram JH et al. Magnitude and determinants of coronary artery disease in juvenile onset, insulin dependent diabetes mellitus. Am J Cardiol 1987;59:750–5.
148. Manson JE Colditz GA, Stampler MJ et al. A prospective study of maturity onset diabetes mellitus and risk of coronary heart disease and stroke in women. Arch Intern Med 1991;151:1141–7.
149. Pan WH, Cedres LB, Liu K et al. Relationship of clinical diabetes and asymptomatic hyperglycaemia to risk of coronary heart disease mortality in men and women. Am J Epidemiol 1986;123:504–16.
150. Kannel WB, McGee DL. Diabetes and cardiovascular disease. The Framingham Study. J Am Med Assoc 1979;241:2035–8.
151. Jarrett RJ. The epidemiology of coronary heart disease and related factors in the context of diabetes mellitus and impaired glucose tolerance. In: Jarrett RJ (ed.), Diabetes and heart disease. Amsterdam: Elsevier, 1984:1–23.
152. Renderman NB, Handenschild C. Diabetes as an atherogenic factor. Prog Cardiovasc Dis 1984;26:373–412.
153. Fleischer N, Fein FS, Sonnenblick EH. The heart and endocrine disease. In: Hurst JW (ed.), The heart arteries and veins. 7th ed. New York: McGraw-Hill, 1990:1497–513.
154. Chakratti R, Meade TW. WHO multination group, clotting factors, platelet function and fibrinolytic activity in diabetics and in a comparison group. Diabetologia 1976;12:383 (Abstract).
155. Mayne EE, Bridges JM, Weaver JA. Platelet adhesiveness, plasma fibrinogen and factor 8 levels in diabetes mellitus. Diabetologia 1970;6:436–40.
156. DCCT Research Group. Diabetes control and complication trial (DCCT) results of feasibility study. Diabetes Care 1987;10:1–19.
157. Kannel WB. Lipids, diabetes and coronary heart disease. Insights from the Framingham Study. Am Heart J 1985;110:1100.
158. Rosengren A, Wellin L, Tsipogianni A, Wilhelmsen L. Impact of cardiovascular risk factors on coronary heart disease and mortality among middle aged diabetic men. A general population study. Br Med J 1989;299:127–31.
159. Manson JE, Golditz GA, Stampfer MJ et al. A prospective study of maturity-onset diabetes mellitus and risk of coronary heart disease and stroke in women. Arch Intern Med 1991;151:1141–7.

160. Stamler J, Vaccaro O, Neaton J, Wentworth D for the multiple risk factor intervention trial research group. Diabetes, other risk factors and 12 years cardiovascular mortality for men screened for the multiple risk factor intervention trial. Diabetes Care 1993;16:434–49.
161. Wilhelmsen L, Svardsudd K, Korsan-Bengtsen K, Larson B, Welin L, Tibblin J. Fibrinogen as a risk factor for stroke and myocardial infarction. N Engl J Med 1984;311:501–5.
162. Mead TW, Mellow S, Brozovic M et al. Haemostatic function and ischaemic heart disease: Principal results of the Northwick Park hospital study. Lancet 1986;ii:533–7.
163. Kannel WB, Wolf PA, Castelli WP, D'Agostino RB. Fibrinogen and risk of cardiovascular disease. J Am Med Assoc 1987;258:1183–6.
164. Meade TW. Fibrinogen and other clotting factors in cardiovascular disease. In: Francis RB Jr (ed.), Atherosclerotic vascular disease, haemostatis and endothelial function. New York: Marcel Dekker, 1992:1–34.
165. Ernst E, Resch KL. Fibrinogen as a cardiovascular risk factor. A meta-analysis and review of the literature. Ann Intern Med 1993;118:956–63.
166. Thaullow E, Erikssen J, Sandvik K-L et al. Blood platelets count and function related to total and cardiovascular health in apparently healthy men. Circulation 1991;84:613–7.
167. Elwood PC, Renaud S, Sharp DS, Beswick AD, O'Brien Jr, Yarnell JW. Ischaemic heart disease and platelets aggregation. The Caerphilly collaborative heart disease study. Circulation 1991;83:38–44.
168. Antiplatelets Trialist Collaboration. Collaborative overview of randomized trials of antiplatets therapy – I: Prevention of death, myocardial infarction and stroke by prolonged antiplatelets therapy in various categories of patients. Br Med J 1994;308:81–106.
169. Stampfer MJ, Colditz GA. Estrogen replacement therapy and coronary heart disease: A quantitative assessment of the epidemiologic evidence. Prev Med 1991;20:47–63.
170. Stampfer MJ, Colditz GA, Willett WC et al. Postmenopausal estrogen therapy and cardiovascular disease: Ten-year follow up from the nurses health study. N Engl J Med 1991;325:756–62.
171. Wilson PWF, Garrison RJ, Castelli WP. Post menopausal estrogen use, cigarette smoking and cardiovascular morbidity in women over 50: The Framingham Study. N Engl J Med 1985;313:1038–43.
172. Henderson BE, Ross RK, Paganini-Hill A, Mack TM. Estrogen use and cardiovascular disease. Am J Obstet Gynecol 1986;154:1181–6.
173. Bush TL, Miller VT. Effects of pharmacologic agents used during menopause. Impact on lipids and lipoproteins. In: Mishell DR JR (ed.), Menopause: Physiology and pharmacology. Chicago: Year Book Medical Publishers, 1987:187–208.
174. Lobo RA. Estrogen and cardiovascular disease. Ann NY Acad Sci 1990;592:286–94.
175. Belchetz PE. Hormonal treatment of postmenopausal women. N Engl J Med 1994;330:1062–71.
176. Soma M, Fumangalli R, Paoleti R et al. Plasma Lp (a) concentration after estrogen and progestragen in post menopausal women. Lancet 1991;337:612.
176. Hegele RA. Lipoprotein (a): An emerging risk factor for atherosclerosis. Can J Cardiol 1989;5:263–5.
177. Fischer GM, Cherian K, Swain ML. Increased synthesis of aortic collagen and elastin in experimental atherosclerosis. Inhibition by contraceptive steroid. Atherosclerosis 1981;39:463–7.
178. La Rosa JC. Estrogen: Risk versus benefit for the prevention of coronary artery disease. Coronary Artery Dis 1993;4:588–94.
179. Chang WC, Nakao J, Orimo H, Murota S-I. Stimulation of prostaglandin cyclo-oxygenase and synthetase activities by estradiol in rat aortic smooth muscle cells.
180. Sack MN, Rader DJ, Cannon RO. Oestrogen and inhibition of oxidation of low-density lipoproteins in post-menopausal women. Lancet 1994;243:269–70.
181. Haarbo J, Leth-Espensen P, Stender S, Christiansen C. Estrogen monotherapy and combined estrogen–progestogen replacement therapy attenuates aortic accumulation of cholesterol in ovariectomized cholesterol fed rabbits. J Clin Invest 1991;87:1274–9.
182. Coronary Drug Project Research Group. Influence of adherence to treatment and response of cholesterol on mortality in the coronary drug project. N Engl J Med 1980;303:1038–41.
183. Rosenberg L, Armstrong B, Jick H. Myocardial infarction and estrogen therapy in post menopausal women. N Engl J Med 1976;294:1256–9.

184. Rosenberg L, Slone D, Shapiro S, Kaufmann D, Strolley PD, Miettinen. Non contraceptive estrogens and myocardial infarction in young women. J Am Med Assoc 1980;244:339–42.
185. Jick H, Dinah B, Rothman KJ. Non contraceptive estrogens and non fatal myocardial infarction. J Am Med Assoc 1978;239:1407–8.
186. Barrett-Connor E, Bush TL. Estrogen and coronary heart disease in women. J Am Med Assoc 1991;265:1861–7.
187. Ernster VL, Bush TL, Huggins GR, Hulka BS, Kelsey JL, Schottenfeld D. Benefits and risks of menopausal estrogen and/or progestin hormone use. Prev Med 1988;17:201–23.
188. Hennekens CH. Alcohol. In: Kaplan N, Stamler J (eds), Prevention of coronary heart disease, practical management of the risk factors. Philadelphia: Saunders, 1983:130–8.
189. Kannel WB, Gordon T. Some characteristics of the incidence of cardiovascular disease and health. Framingham Study: 16 year follow-up. Section 26 of the Framingham Study. Washington, DC: Government Printing Office, 1970.
190. Yano K, Rhoads GG, Kagan A. Coffee, alcohol and risk of coronary heart disease among Japanese men living in Hawaii. N Engl J Med 1977;297:405–9.
191. Stampfer MJ, Colditz GA, Willett EC, Speizer FE, Hennekens CH. A prospective study of moderate alcohol consumption and the risk of coronary disease and stroke in women. N Engl J Med 1988;319:267–73.
192. Rimm EB, Giovannucci EL, Willett WC et al. A prospective study of alcohol consumption and risk of coronary disease in men. Lancet 1991;338:464–8.
193. Hennekens CH, Willett W, Rosner B, Cole DS, Mayrent SL. Effects of beer, wine, liquor on coronary deaths. J Am Med Assoc 1979;242:1973–4.
194. Thornton J, Symes C, Heaton K. Moderate alcohol intake reduces bile cholesterol saturation and raises HDL cholesterol. Lancet 1983;2:819–22.
195. Stampfer MJ, Sacks FM, Salvini S, Willett WC, Hennekens CH. A prospective study of cholesterol apolipoproteins and the risk of myocardial infarction. N Engl J Med 1991;325:373–81.
196. Buring JE, O Connor GT, Goldhaber SZ et al. Decreased HDL2 and HDL3 cholesterol Apo A-I and Apo A-II and increased risk of myocardial infarction. Circulation 1992;95:22–9.
197. Toivanen J, Ylikorkalo O, Vinikkal. Ethanol inhibits platelets' thromboxane A2 production but has no effect on lung prostacyclin synthesis in humans. Thromb Res 1984;33:1–8.
198. Laing WE. Ethyl alcohol enhances plasminogen activation secretion by endothelial cells. J Am Med Assoc 1983;250:772–6.
199. Steering Committee of the Physicians Health Study research group. Final report on the aspirin component of the ongoing Physicians Health Study. N Engl J Med 1989;321:129–35.
200. Peto R, Gray R. Collins R et al. Randomised trial of prophylactic daily aspirin in British male doctors. Br Med J 1988;296:313–6.
201. Hennekens CH, Peto R, Hutchinson GB, Doll R. An overview of the the British and American aspirin studies. N Engl J Med 1988;318:923–4.
202. ISIS-2 Collaborative Group. Randomised trial of IV streptokinase, oral aspirin, both or neither among 17187 cases of suspected acute myocardial infarction. Lancet 1988;ii:349–60.
203. Antiplatelets Trialists's collaboration. Secondary prevention of vascular disease by prolonged antiplatelets treatment. Br Med J 1988;269:320–31.
204. Yousuf S, Sleight P, Held P, McMahon S. Routine medical management of acute myocardial infarction: Lessons from overviews of recent randomised controlled trials. Circulation 1990;82(Suppl.II):117–34.
205. Yusuf S, Witters J, Friedman L. Overview of results of randomised clinical trials in heart disease. I. Treatments following myocardial infarction. J Am Med Assoc 1988;260:2088–93.
206. The Consensus Trial Study Group. Effect of enalapril on mortality in severe congestive heart failure. N Engl J Med 1987;316:1429–35.
207. The SOLVD Investigations. Effect of enalapril on survival in patients with reduced left ventricular ejections and congestive heart failure. N Engl J Med 1991;325:293–302.
208. The SOLVD Investigations. Effect of enalapril on mortality and the development of heart failure in asymptomatic patients with reduced left ventricular ejection fractions. N Engl J Med 1992;327:685–91.

209. ISIS IV. Collaborative group. ISIS-4 (Fourth international study of infarct survival): Randomised study of oral captopril in over 50 000 patients with suspected acute myocardial infarction. Circulation 1993;88:1394 (Abstract).
210. Swedberg K, Held P, Kjekshus J, Rasmussen K, Ryden L, Wedel H on behalf of the Consensus II Study Group. Effects of the early administration of enalapril on mortality in patients with acute myocardial infarction. Results of the North Scandinavian Enalapril Survival Study (Consensus II). N Engl J Med 1992;327:678–84.
211. The acute infarction ramipril efficacy (AIRE) study investigators. Effect of ramipril on mortality and morbidity of survivors of acute myocardial infarction with clinical evidence of heart failure. Lancet 1993;342:821–8.
212. Yusuf S, Pepine CJ, Garces C et al. Effect of enalapril on myocardial infarction and unstable angina pectoris in patients with low ejection fractions. Lancet 1922;340:1173–8.
213. Pfeffer MA, Poranunwald E, Moye LA et al. on behalf of SAVE Investigations. Effect of captopril on mortality and morbidity in patients with left ventricular dysfunction after acute myocardial infarction: Results of survival and ventricular enlargement trial. N Engl J Med 1992;327:669–77.
214. Yusuf S, Peto J, Lewis J, Collins R, Sleight P. Beta blockade during and after myocardial infarction: An overview of the randomised trials. Prog Cardiovas Dis 1985;27:335–71.
215. Stampfer MJ, Hennekens CH, Manson JAE, Goldlitz GA, Rosner B, Willett WC. Vitamin E consumption and the risk of coronary disease in women. N Engl J Med 1993;328:1444–9.
216. Rimm EB, Stampfer MJ, Ascherio A, Giuvahnucci E, Coldlitz GA, Willett WC. Vitamin E consumption and risk of coronary disease in men. N Engl J Med 1993;328:1450–6.
217. Kardinaal AFM, Kok FJ, Kinstad J et al. Antioxidants in adipose tissue and risk of myocardial infarction: The Euramic Study. Lancet 1993;342:1379–84.
218. Moller JH, Taubert KA, Allen HD et al. Cardiovascular health and disease in children. Current status. Circulation 1984;89:923–30.

Index

A-2318 117
abaximab 39
acetylcholine 434
activated coagulation factor X(Xa) 33–4
activated protein C resistance (APCR) 405
Addison's disease 437
adenosine 114–15, 132
　syndrome X 183
adenosine diphosphate/triphosphate 55
adhesion molecules 26, 54
albumin 55
alcohol 505
　consumption, stroke risk 78–9
　lower limb arterial disease 281–2
α_2-antiplasmin 35
α-adrenergic receptors 433
α-blocker(s) 114
　α_1 367(table)
aminophylline 195–6
aneurysm(s), complications 489–90
angina
　chronic, stable 167–9, 173
　epidemiology 188–9
　fixed threshold 117–18
　functional classification 168(table)
　lifestyle associated 191
　natural history 189–90
　pectoris 123, 153
　primary 118
　relative cost/benefits of treatment 197(table)
　risk factors 191–3
　secondary 117
　stable 27
　treatment 190–1
　unstable 27, 169
　variant of Prinzmetal 118
angiography
　cerebral see cerebral angiography, extracranial vascular disease
　coronary 175–6
　coronary artery disease 129–30
　pulmonary 466, 469(fig.)
　renal 335
　restenosis, diagnosis 473
angioplasty
　balloon 103
　patch 102–3
　restenosis 478
angiotensin-converting-enzyme (ACE) inhibitors 196, 367(table), 369, 506
　gene 155
　　polymorphism 156
　　microalbuminuria 421
anticoagulant drugs 38

naturally occurring, acquired deficiencies 448–9
　oral 411–12, 414
　pregnancy 454–5
antihypertensive drugs 367(table)
antioxidants 278–9, 507
antiphospholipid antibodies, management 454
antiplatelet drugs 38–9, 313
antithrombin III 405
antithrombins (thrombin antagonists) 38
　deficiency
　　clinical manifestations 446–7
　　management 452
　hemostasis, normal 443–4
aortic aneurysm 209–17
　abdominal 299–300, 364
　atherosclerosis associated 211
　clinical presentation 213
　connective tissue degradation associated 211–12
　environmental factors 212
　epidemiology 210
　etiology 211
　genetic predisposition 212
　infra-renal 209
　management 214–17
　　abdominal 215–16
　　asymptomatic 215
　　outcome after surgery 216–17
　　ruptured aneurysm 214
　　symptomatic 214–15
　　thoracic 216
　　thoraco-abdominal 216
　mycotic aneurysm 212–13
　natural history 210–11
　non-ruptured 213–14
　ruptured 213
　thoracic 209–10
　thoraco-abdominal 210
aortic dissection 217–18, 364, 490–1
aortic valve, dicrotic notch 14
apolipoprotein(s) 278
　B (apo B) 278
　　gene 154
　E (apoE), gene 154
argobatran 38
arterial injuries 489
arterial wall, structure 67, 68(fig.)
arteriogram, instructions for patients 302–3
arteriography, policies 297(figs.)
arterioles 1
arterioral nephrosclerosis 365
Arvin 248
aspirin 38, 193, 196, 313, 411
　microalbuminuria 421
　prophylactic low-dose 505–6

A.-M. Salmasi and A. Strano (eds), Angiology in Practice, 519–526.
© *1996 Kluwer Academic Publishers. Printed in Great Britain.*

atheronecrosis 124
atherosclerosis 21–8
  atherogenetic cellular mechanisms 25–7
    lymphocytes 27
    monocytes 25–6
    smooth muscle cells 26–7
  carotid, investigation 88–91
  epidemiology 21
  fatty streak 23
  plaque 23–5, 27–8
    pathological–radiological correlation 27
    regression 28
    rupture 28
  risk factors 21–2
    age 21
    cigarette smoking 22
    diabetes mellitus 22
    hyperlipidemia 22
    hypertension 22
    race 22
    sex 21
  vascular biology 495–7
atrial fibrillation 80
atropine 434
autonomic dysfunction 431–40
autonomic neuropathy 423

basic fibroblast growth factor (bFGF) 475
Bayliss reflex 114
β-adrenergic receptors 432–3
β-agonists 110, 114
β-blockers 110, 114, 194, 196, 367(table), 506–7
  asthma 369
  diabetes mellitus 368
  obstructive airway disease 369
bioflavonoids 394
blood, non-Newtonian liquid 44–5
blood coagulation 34–5
  activation 406
blood flow 1–17, 18(fig.)
  disturbed/turbulent 7–8
  flow resistance 4
  geometry effects on profile 8–13
    bifurcations 11
    constrictions 11–13
    curved tubes 9–11
    inlet effect 8–9
  in vivo studies 51
  laminar flow 2(fig.), 3(fig.)
  large vessel 50
  microvascular 50–1
  pressure flow relationship 2–4
  pulsatile in elastic tubes 14–17
    compliance 14–15
    reflection of transient pulse 15–16
    velocity profiles 16–17
  resistance in single/multiple tubes 43
  steady flow in rigid tubes 2
  streamlined 43–4
  turbulent 43–4
  velocity 4–6, 12(fig.)
  viscosity 6–7
  volume flow 4–6
blood pressure 355–6
  measurement 355–6
  monitoring 345, 356
blood viscosity 41–3
  factors affecting 46–50

hematocrit 49
plasma viscosity 48
red cell deformability 48
rouleaux formation 46–8
shear rate 46
temperature 50
hyperviscosity 406
blue toe syndrome 488
Bradbury–Eggleston syndrome 436
brain 63–71
  aneurysm 63
  atherosclerotic plaque development 67–71
    calcification 68
    hemorrhage 70
    stenosis 71
    thrombus 70
    ulceration 69–70
  blood supply 63–6
    collateral circulation 65–6
  hemodynamics, atherogenic effect 66–7
  hemorrhagic stroke 63
  infarction 63
  transient ischemic attack (TIA) 63, 70
Buerger's disease 300
buflomedil 312

calcium antagonists 110, 194–5, 367(table), 369
calcium-heparin 314
cancer procoagulant 404
captopril 436
cardiac catheterization 175–6
cardiac glycosides 110
cardiovascular disease
  clotting factors 504–7
  prevention 497–8
  risk factor modification 498–503
carotid artery stenosis
  asymptomatic 81, 98
  management 97–105
  mild/moderate 98
  severe 97–8
  symptomatic 97
carotid body tumors 93
carotid disease, extracranial
  interventional techniques 99–103
    anesthesia 99–100
    balloon angioplasty 103
    eversion endarterectomy 102
    patch angioplasty 102–3
    shunting 103
    standard endarterectomy 100–2
    stenting 103
  investigations 87–94
  management 97–105
  operative measurements 104–6
    cerebral monitoring 104–5
    quality control 106
carotid murmurs 81
carotid sinus hypersensitivity syndrome 438
Casson's law 384
caval filters 416
celiac band syndrome 329–30
celiac occlusive disease 327–9
centella asiatica 394
cerebral angiography
  extracranial vascular disease 91–3
    complications 91–2
    embolic cerebrovascular disease 92–3

cerebral monitoring   104
chest pain, differential diagnosis   168(table), 173
CHIVA (cure conservatrice et chémodynamique de l'insufisance veineuse en ambulatoire)   391–2
cholesterol   148, 277
chronic venous insufficiency (CVI)   380–7
    classification   380
    development   380–2
    functional capillar density   386
    leukocytes activation   385–6
    lymphatic vessel permeability   386–7
    pressure variation   386–7
    recent acquisitions   382–3
    vasomotion/flow motion   384–5
cicaprost   39
cigarette smoking   22, 275, 362, 496, 498
    stroke risk   77
claudications   80
    β-blockers   369
    intermittent   258
        painfree walking distance measurement   258–60
    intermittent blood viscosity   280
    intermittent prevalence in men by age   273(fig.)
    mortality   274
    management   295(fig.)
clonidine   361–2, 436
clopidogrel   39
clotting factors   504–7
coaxial catheter system   103
complement system C_{4a}/C_{5a} 256
connective tissue remodeling   156
contraceptive pill   81–2
    deep vein thrombosis   405
    estrogen containing   362
    thrombophilia   451
coronary arteries
    atherectomy   478
    autonomic nervous system effects   113
    endothelium dependent relaxations   56
    endothelium factors   115–17
    epicardial, stenosis   117–18
    flow
        hemodynamics   109–18
            regulation   111–12
        metabolic control   114–15
        myogenic factors   114
    plaques   27
    relative coronary reserve   113
    resistance regulations   113
    risk factors   57–60
    spasm   59, 118
    stenting   478
    vasomotor tone regulation   113(fig.)
coronary artery bypass graft (CABG)   190
    asymptomatic carotid stenosis   99
    surgery   199–203
        risk   203–4
coronary artery disease   121–33, 139–56, 167–76
    angiography   129–30
    atherosclerotic   121–4
        longitudinal distribution   125–7
    atherosclerotic plaque   124–5, 136(fig.)
        disruption   127–9
    case definition   139–41
    case frequencies   144
    clinical manifestations   139–40, 167–9
    clinically overt   145–7
    coronary steal   123

covert preclinical disease   144–5
disease frequency   141–3
disease markers   144
echocardiography   173–4
    stress   175
ecological fallacy   143–4
electrocardiography   170–2
epidemiology   139
etiology   147
holter monitoring   172–3
ischemic consequences   123
ischemic impact reduction   127
ischemic preconditioning   132
management see coronary artery disease management
physical examination   169–70
postmortem examination   140–1
premature   154
radionuclide imaging   175
risk factors   147–56
    blood rheology   152–4
    coagulation   152–4
    essential fatty acids   152
    fetal/neonatal origins   151–2
    genetic polymorphism   154–6
    hyperlipidemia   148–9
study design   143–4
vasomotion   122–3
vasospasm   122–3
coronary artery disease management   187–205
    ACE inhibitors   196
    aminophylline   195–6
    aspirin   193, 196
    β-blockers   194
    calcium antagonists   194–5
    dihydropiridine   194–5
    diltiazem   195–6
    nitrates   193–4, 196
    ranolizine   196
    transcutaneous spinal stimulation   196
    trimetazine   196
    verapamil   195
    warfarin   193, 196
coronary heart disease, prevention/priorities   498(table)
coronary steal   123
coronary vasomotion   53–5
coumarin
    pregnancy   454–5
    skin necrosis   447
critical leg ischemia   307
    treatment   314–15
critical limb ischemia   262–3
Cushing's syndrome   352, 357
cyclooxygenase inhibitors   116
cystic adventitial arterial disease   301

D1/2 dopaminergic receptors   433
deep vein thrombosis   403–16
    definition   403
    diagnosis   407–11
    etiology   404–6
    history   403–4
    idiopathic   404
    pathogenesis   406–7
    prevalence   403–4
    prophylaxis   411–13
    risk factors   404–6
    therapy   413–16
defibrotide   314

dehydroergotamine 394
dextran 248, 411–12
diabetes mellitus 22, 503
   cardiovascular manifestations/complications 419–26
      epidemiology 419–20
      pathology 420–1
      presentation 424–6
      risk factors 421–4
   diabetic microangiopathy 258
   effect on peripheral arterial disease 308(table), 309
   glycemic control 422–3
   lower limb arterial disease 280
   stroke risk 80
dihydropyridine 194–5
   calcium antagonists 196
diltiazem 195–6
diosmin 394
diuretics
   loop 367(table)
   potassium-sparing 367(table)
dobutamine, stress 175
dopamine-beta-hydroxylase deficiency 436–7
dysfibrinogenemia, congenital 447
dyslipidemias, peripheral arterial disease associated 309

E-secreting tumors 437
echocardiography 173–4
   stress 174–5
electrocardiography 170–2
enalapril 436
endothelin 56–7, 59, 117, 255
   constrictor mechanisms 57
endothelium 32–3
endothelium-derived relaxing factor (EDRF) 54–5, 115, 116(fig.)
endarterectomy
   eversion 102
   standard 100–2
epinephrine 117
estrogen 362
   postmenopausal replacement therapy 504–5
   replacement, deep vein thrombosis 405
European Carotid Surgery Trial (ECST) 88–95

factor V 54
factor VII 36
   gene 155
factor Xa antagonists 38
Fahraeus–Lindqvist effect 255–6
familial dysautonomia 435–6, 437
fatty acids, essential 152, 278–9
fatty streaks 124
   children 496
female sex hormones 21
Fenn effect 110
fibrinogen 36, 79, 279
   defects 447
      management 454
fibrinolysis 407
   hemostasis, normal 443–4
fibrinolytic system 35, 36–7
fibromuscular dysplasia 301
fibronectin 33
flowmotion 384
functional capillary density (FCD) 386

gangrene
   dry 261, 262(fig.)

humid 261
genetic polymorphism 154–6
glomerulonephritis 22
glucose tolerance, impairment 79
GMP-140 256
guanabenz 436
guanethidine 248
Guillain–Barre syndrome 436

Hagen–Poiseuille law 253
haloperidol 436
hematocrit 49, 256
   polycythemia vera 406
   raised 79
hemodilution 311–12
hemorheology 41–51
hemostasis, normal 443–4
heparin 32, 38, 411–12, 413–15
   cofactor-2 255
   low molecular weight 411–12, 413
      induced thrombocytopenia 467
      pulmonary embolism treatment 466, 467(table)
   pregnancy 455
high-density lipoprotein 21–2, 148–9
hirudin 38
hirugen 38
hirulog 38
holter monitoring 172–3
Homan's sign 407
hyperaldosteronism, primary 348
hyperfibrinogenemia 406
hyperglycemia, asymptomatic 422
hyperinsulinemia 281, 423
hyperlipidemia 22, 148–9
   heriditary 22
   stroke risk 77–8
hypertension 22, 343–52, 355–69, 499
   age prevalence 350(table)
   blood tests 358–9
   chest X-ray 359
   children 346, 347(table)
   classification 343–5
   clinical examination 357–8
   clinical manifestations 351–2
   complications 363–5
   crises/emergencies 345–6
   elderly patient 346–7
   electrocardiography 359
   emergencies 491
   epidemiology 349–50
   history 357
   investigations 352
      specialised 359–62
   lower limb arterial disease associated 279
   management, therapeutic 365–9
   mineralocorticoid 361
   peripheral arterial disease associated 309
   pregnant patient 347, 348(table)
   renovascular see renovascular hypertension 324–5
   risk factors 350–1, 362–3
   screening 356–9
   secondary forms 347–9
   secondary, guidelines 360(table)
   stroke risk 76–7
   urine tests 358
hypertension see also blood pressure
hypertriglyceridemia 155
hyperviscosity syndrome 51

Index 523

hypotension 431–40
  postural, causes 435–6

iloprost 39
imipramine 184, 436
indobufen 313
innominate artery stenosis 226–8
innominate steal syndrome 222–3, 231–6
innominate syndrome 222, 230(fig.)
insulin resistance 281
insulin resistant syndrome 503–4
γ-interferon 27
integrins 256
interleukins 256
intestinal ischemia
  acute 328–9
  chronic 329
ischemic heart disease, mortality 187(fig.)

Javid shunt 103

ketanserin 247, 312–13

left bundle branch block, syndrome X 182
left ventricular function assessment 176
left ventricular hypertrophy 80
leukotrienes 118, 256
levonorgestrel 82
linoleic acid 152
lipoprotein(s) 278
  a[Lp(a)] 36–7, 149
lisinopril 436
long QT syndrome 440
low density lipoprotein 22, 25, 58–9, 124
  receptor genes 154
low-density lipoprotein 148–9
lower limb arterial disease 271–83, 289–303
  acute thromboembolism, assessment 298–9
  aneurysm assessment 299–300
  assessment of atherosclerotic, stenotic, occlusive disease 293–8
  clinical assessment 289–303
    color-Doppler ultrasound scanning 291–2
    continuous-wave Doppler ultrasound 290
    intraarterial digital subtraction angiography 292
    pressure indices 290
  critical ischemia management 295(fig.)
  epidemiology 271–4
    asymptomatic disease 273
    morbidity 273–4
    mortality 274
    natural history 273
  factors worsening macrocirculation 307(table), 308(table)
  femopopliteal disease 298
  peripheral obstructive disease 307–17
    diabetes mellitus effect 308(table)
    fatal/non-fatal endpoints 315
    hygienic-dietetic measures 310–11
    interventional therapy 315–17
    pharmacological therapy 311–15
    risk factor correction 308–9
  risk factors 274–82
    alcohol 281–2
    antioxidants 278–9
    apolipoproteins 278
    cholesterol 277
    diabetes mellitus 280

    essential fatty acids 278–9
    glucose intolerance 280–1
    hemostatic factors 279–80
    hyperinsulinemia 281
    hypertension 279
    insulin resistance 281
    lipids 275
    lipoproteins 278
    personality 281
    physical activity 282
    smoking 275
    triglycerides 276
  stenosis degree evaluation 291(table)
lower limb arteries 251–68
  big toe
    cyanosis 261(fig.)
    laser-Doppler output signal 266(fig.)
  blood flow 253
  blood pressure 252–3
  blood velocity 251, 252(fig.)
  clinical features 258–63
  critical limb ischemia 261–3
  Doppler continuous wave 264(fig.)
  instrumental examination 263–8
  laser Doppler output signal 254(fig.)
  microcirculation 253–8
    geometry of microvessels 255–6
    leukocytes 256–8
    microhemodynamics 253–5
    platelets 256
    red cells 256
  pathophysiology 258–63
  peripheral arterial disease measurement 267–8
  peripheral obstructive disease 307–17
  strain gauge plethysmography 265(fig.)
lower limb venous system
  anatomy 373–9
  physiology 373–9
lower limb(s)
  acute ischemia 485–7
    therapy 486–7
  phlebothrombosis 491–2
lung scans
  radioisotope 462
  ventilation/perfusion 462–4
lupus-like anticoagulant 405
lymphocytes 27

magnesium ions 118
magnetic resonance angiography (MRA) 93–4
Magnus effect 386
mastocytes 118
mesenteric artery
  infarct 488–9
  ischemia 488–9
mesenteric ischemia 338–9
mesenteric occlusive disease 327–9
methyl-dopa 247
Mialhe stentor 299–300
microalbuminuria 421
microcirculatory unit, schematic representation 381(fig.)
microvascular defense system (MDS) 256–7
microvascular flow regulating system (MFRS) 255
mimetics, non-peptide 39
Moens–Korteweg equation 14
monocytes 25–6
multiple system atrophy 436

myocardial infarction 80, 131–2, 169
  complications 174
  subendocardial 131
myocardial ischemia
  detection 173–4
  syndrome X 182–3
myocardial oxygen consumption 109–11
myocardial oxygen delivery 122
myointimal hyperplasia 474–6
myxedema 22

naftidrofuryl 313
nailfold capillaroscopy 247
Newtonian fluid 3, 7, 14
  equation 42–3
nitrates 193–4, 196
nitric oxide 32, 54–5, 255
  syntase 54–5
North American Symptomatic Carotid Endarterectomy Trial (NASCET) 88–91, 95

obesity 78
occlusive digital hypothermic challenge test 244–6
oculovagal reflex syndrome 440
Ohm's law 4, 43

Palmaz stent 103
papillary muscle dysfunction 174
paraproteinemias 51
parasympathetic nervous system, anatomical/chemical organization 433–40
pentasaccharide (synthetic) 38
pentolinium 436
pentoxifylline 248, 312
peptides (synthetic) 39
percutaneous transluminal angioplasty (PTA) 333, 336–8
percutaneous transluminal coronary angioplasty (PTCA) 190, 197–9
pericapillary fibrin cuff phenomenon 382
peripheral plasma renin activity (PRA) 334
peripheral vascular disease 80–1
  diabetes mellitus 420
Perthes' test 390
phenothiazine 436
phenoxybenzamine 436
phentolamine 436
pheochromocytoma 348, 349(tables), 352, 357, 361–2
  postural hypotension 437
phlebectomy (Muller's technique) 391–2
phorbol-ester 117
phosphodiesterase inhibitors 110
placental ratio 75
plasma renin determination 333–4
plasma skimming 255–6
plasma viscosity 44, 48
plasmapheresis 51
plasminogen activator inhibitor-1 (PAI-1) 35–6, 54, 153
platelet activating factor (PAF) 256
platelet-derived growth factor (PDGF) 124, 256
  restenosis 475
platelets 33–4, 37
  adhesion 33
  aggregation 33
  release reaction 33
  shape change 33
plethysmography, impedance 465

Poiseuille law 3
  flow 17, 42(fig.), 44–5
polycystic renal disease 352, 357, 361
popliteal entrapment syndrome 301
post-micturition syncope 439
postphlebitic syndrome 380, 383(fig.)
prazosin 247, 436
primary thrombophilic conditions 405
procainamide 110–11
propionyl-L-carnitine (PLC) 312
prostacyclin 32, 54–6, 255
prostaglandin E1 248
protein C 405
  activated resistance 446
  antithrombin deficiency 446–7
  deficiency 446
    management 452–3
  hemostasis, normal 443–4
  resistance activated management 454
protein S 255, 405
  deficiency 446
    management 453
  hemostasis, normal 443–4
proteoglycans 32
Pruitt–Inahara shunt 103
pulmonary embolism 403–4, 459–71
  clinical features 460–1
  epidemiology 459–60
  investigations 461–6
  prophylaxis 459
  symptoms/signs associated 461(table)
  treatment 466–71
  vascular emergency 492–3
purinergic reception 433
purpura fulminans
  management 453
  neonatorus 447

radionuclide imaging 175
ranolozine 196
Raynaud's phenomenon 50
Raynaud's syndrome 241–8
  associated conditions 246(table)
  clinical presentation 241–2
  diagnosis 244–7
  epidemiology 244
  pathophysiology 242–4
  screening investigations 247(table)
  treatment 247–8
red cells
  deformity 48
  rouleaux formations 46–8, 50
renal vein renin ratio (RVRR) 334
renal vein renin/systemic renin index (RSRI) 334
renin–angiotensin system 156
renography/scintigraphy, radionucleotide 334–5
renovascular disease 360–1
  treatment 335–8
    percutaneous transluminal angioplasty 337–8
    pharmacological therapy 336
    surgery, results 337
    surgical therapy 336–7
renovascular hypertension 324–5
  clinical clues 348(table)
  evaluation 333–5
    intravenous urogram 334
    plasma renin determination 333–4
    radionucleotide renography/scintigraphy 334–5

renal angiography   335
renal sonography   335
renovascular insufficiency   326–7, 333
renovascular occlusive disease   323–7
  clinical manifestations   324
  incidence   323–4
reperfusion syndrome   258
reserpine   247
restenosis, vascular   473–80
  mechanical factors   476–8
  models   476
  pathology   474–6
  prevention, candidate drugs   479(table)
  treatment   478–80
retinopathy   365
retrograde femoral puncture   296
revascularization syndrome   487
Reynolds numbers   8, 11, 13, 253
Riley–Day syndrome   435–7
rutin   394

saphenous vein
  great, stripping   391
  small, stripping   392
Schwartz's test   390
serotonin   118, 256
shear stress   67
shunting   103
Shy–Drager syndrome   435–6
silent ischemia   168
single photon emission computed tomography (SPECT)   175
single-gene syndrome   154
sleep clonidin test   361–2
smoking, peripheral arterial disease associated   309
smooth muscle cell   26–7
sonography
  duplex   87
  renal   335
spiral CT angiography   94
ST-segment   171
  depression, non-coronary causes   172(table)
steal syndrome   175
  homolateral   225–6
  intermittent   225
  latent   225
steal syndrome *see also* innominate steal syndrome; subclavian steal syndrome
stenting   103
streptokinase   415, 468
stroke   73–82
  acute   99
    endarterectomy   99
  CT scan   74(table)
  epidemiology   73
  ischemic, causes of   75(table)
  mortality   74
  risk factors   76–82
    acute myocardial infarction   80
    age   79–80
    alcohol consumption   78–9
    asymptomatic carotid stenosis   81
    atrial fibrillation   80
    cigarette smoking   77
    contraceptive pill   81
    diabetes mellitus   80
    fibrinogen, raised   79
    hematocrit, raised   79

hyperlipidemia   77–8
hypertension   76–7
impaired glycose tolerance   79
left ventricular hypertrophy   80
peripheral vascular disease   80
physical activity   79
sex   80
transient ischemic attacks   81
truncal obesity   78
variations   74–5
stroke volume   1, 110
stromelysin   156
subclavian artery
  obstruction   236
  stenosis   226–8
  therapy   236–9
subclavian steal syndrome   219–20, 223–5, 228–31
  diseases leading to   220(table), 221(fig.)
  physiopathology   219–21
  therapy   236–9
subendocardial ischemia   112
sudden death   132–3
  diabetes mellitus, autonomic neuropathy   424
sulfinpyrazone   38–9
sulodexide   38
swallow syncope   439
sympathetic nervous system, anatomic/chemical organization   431–3
syndrome X   179–84
  alternative syndrome   180
  clinical presentation   180–1
  definition   179–80
  differential diagnosis   180
  pathogenesis   181
    adenosine release   183
    increased pain reception   184
    ischemic cardiomyopathy   183–4
    myocardial ischemia   182
  prognosis   184
  treatment   184
systemic circulatory system   1

Takayasu's disease   300–1, 364
tension time index   110
thiazide   367(table)
thrombin   55, 117–18
thrombin antagonists (antithrombins)   38
thrombin receptor antagonist peptides   38
thrombin–antithrombin complex (TAT)   153
thromboembolism   31–9
  pulmonary
    algorithm to confirm/refuse diagnosis   464
    anticoagulation protocol   467(table)
  venous
    invasive treatment   468–70
    risk factors in hospitalized patients   460(table)
thrombolysis   415
thrombolytic therapy, pulmonary embolism   468
thrombomodulin   32
thrombophilia
  acquired   448–9
  hemostatic defects predisposing   445–8
  laboratory investigations   450–1
  management   451–5
  suspected, approach to the patient   449–50
thrombosis   31–9
  atherosclerosis associated   36–7
    factor VII   36

526   Index

thrombosis   (cont'd.)
  fibrinogen   36
  fibrinolytic system   36–7
    platelet   37
    vessel wall   37
  coagulation system   34–5
  endothelium   32–3
  fibrinolytic system   35
  pathogenetic factors   31–5
  platelets   33–4
  therapy   37–9
    anticoagulant drugs   38
    antiplatelet drugs   38–9
thromboxane A2   33, 118, 256
thromboxane receptor antagonists   39
thromboxane synthase inhibitors   39
thymoxamine   248
tibial compartment syndrome   487
tick anticoagulant peptide   38
ticlopidine   39, 313–14
tissue plasminogen activator   35, 255, 416, 468
transcranial Doppler   104–5
transcutaneous spinal stimulation   196
transforming growth factor β   124
transient ischemic attacks, stroke risk   81
Trendelenburg test   390
triglycerides   276
trimetazine   196
Troxerutin   394
tumor necrosis factor α   256

ultrasound   87–8, 91
upper limb arteries disease   219–39
  diagnosis   226–36
  physiopathology   219–26
  therapy   236–9
upper limbs, acute ischemia   488
urogram, intravenous   334
urokinase   416, 468

Valsalva maneuver   423
varicose veins/ulcers   371–99
  clinical examination   387
  definition   371–2

  epidemiology   372–3
  instrumental testing   394–9
    Doppler ultrasonography   394–5
    dynamic capillaroscopy   398–9
    laser Doppler   397
    microlymphography   399
    real-time echotomography   395–6
    reflected light rheography   396–7
    transcutaneous oxymetry   398
  medical therapy   393–4
  patient history   388
    objective   389–90
  primitive
    etiopathogenetic hypothesis   379–80
    risk factors   379–80
  surgical treatment   390–3
vascular emergencies   485–93
vascular endothelium   53–60
  coronary vasomotion   53–5
  dysfunction, coronary risk factors   57–60
  vasoconstriction, endothelium derived   56
  vasorelaxation, endothelium derived   55–6
vasodepressor syncope   437
vasomotion   384
vasospasm   243
vasovagal syncope   437
venogram   470(fig.)
venography   464–5
venous disease see also chronic venous insufficiency
venous thromboembolism see also thrombophilia
ventricular septal rupture   174
verapamil   195
vertebral subclavian steal syndrome   225–6, 227(fig.), 232–4(figs)
vessel bifurcations   1
vessel wall   37
vitamin K   467

warfarin   38, 193, 196
  pregnancy   455
  pulmonary embolism   467
  skin necrosis, management   453
whortleberry anticyanocides   394
Willebrand factor   33, 153

Developments in Cardiovascular Medicine

96. I. Cikes (ed.): *Echocardiography in Cardiac Interventions.* 1989
    ISBN 0-7923-0088-2
97. E. Rapaport (ed.): *Early Interventions in Acute Myocardial Infarction.* 1989
    ISBN 0-7923-0175-7
98. M.E. Safar and F. Fouad-Tarazi (eds.): *The Heart in Hypertension.* A Tribute to Robert C. Tarazi (1925-1986). 1989 ISBN 0-7923-0197-8
99. S. Meerbaum and R. Meltzer (eds.): *Myocardial Contrast Two-dimensional Echocardiography.* 1989 ISBN 0-7923-0205-2
100. J. Morganroth and E.N. Moore (eds.): *Risk/Benefit Analysis for the Use and Approval of Thrombolytic, Antiarrhythmic, and Hypolipidemic Agents.* Proceedings of the 9th Annual Symposium on New Drugs and Devices (1988). 1989 ISBN 0-7923-0294-X
101. P.W. Serruys, R. Simon and K.J. Beatt (eds.): *PTCA - An Investigational Tool and a Non-operative Treatment of Acute Ischemia.* 1990 ISBN 0-7923-0346-6
102. I.S. Anand, P.I. Wahi and N.S. Dhalla (eds.): *Pathophysiology and Pharmacology of Heart Disease.* 1989 ISBN 0-7923-0367-9
103. G.S. Abela (ed.): *Lasers in Cardiovascular Medicine and Surgery.* Fundamentals and Technique. 1990 ISBN 0-7923-0440-3
104. H.M. Piper (ed.): *Pathophysiology of Severe Ischemic Myocardial Injury.* 1990
    ISBN 0-7923-0459-4
105. S.M. Teague (ed.): *Stress Doppler Echocardiography.* 1990 ISBN 0-7923-0499-3
106. P.R. Saxena, D.I. Wallis, W. Wouters and P. Bevan (eds.): *Cardiovascular Pharmacology of 5-Hydroxytryptamine.* Prospective Therapeutic Applications. 1990
    ISBN 0-7923-0502-7
107. A.P. Shepherd and P.A. Öberg (eds.): *Laser-Doppler Blood Flowmetry.* 1990
    ISBN 0-7923-0508-6
108. J. Soler-Soler, G. Permanyer-Miralda and J. Sagristà-Sauleda (eds.): *Pericardial Disease.* New Insights and Old Dilemmas. 1990 ISBN 0-7923-0510-8
109. J.P.M. Hamer: *Practical Echocardiography in the Adult.* With Doppler and Color-Doppler Flow Imaging. 1990 ISBN 0-7923-0670-8
110. A. Bayés de Luna, P. Brugada, J. Cosin Aguilar and F. Navarro Lopez (eds.): *Sudden Cardiac Death.* 1991 ISBN 0-7923-0716-X
111. E. Andries and R. Stroobandt (eds.): *Hemodynamics in Daily Practice.* 1991
    ISBN 0-7923-0725-9
112. J. Morganroth and E.N. Moore (eds.): *Use and Approval of Antihypertensive Agents and Surrogate Endpoints for the Approval of Drugs affecting Antiarrhythmic Heart Failure and Hypolipidemia.* Proceedings of the 10th Annual Symposium on New Drugs and Devices (1989). 1990 ISBN 0-7923-0756-9
113. S. Iliceto, P. Rizzon and J.R.T.C. Roelandt (eds.): *Ultrasound in Coronary Artery Disease.* Present Role and Future Perspectives. 1990 ISBN 0-7923-0784-4
114. J.V. Chapman and G.R. Sutherland (eds.): *The Noninvasive Evaluation of Hemodynamics in Congenital Heart Disease.* Doppler Ultrasound Applications in the Adult and Pediatric Patient with Congenital Heart Disease. 1990
    ISBN 0-7923-0836-0
115. G.T. Meester and F. Pinciroli (eds.): *Databases for Cardiology.* 1991
    ISBN 0-7923-0886-7
116. B. Korecky and N.S. Dhalla (eds.): *Subcellular Basis of Contractile Failure.* 1990
    ISBN 0-7923-0890-5
117. J.H.C. Reiber and P.W. Serruys (eds.): *Quantitative Coronary Arteriography.* 1991
    ISBN 0-7923-0913-8
118. E. van der Wall and A. de Roos (eds.): *Magnetic Resonance Imaging in Coronary Artery Disease.* 1991 ISBN 0-7923-0940-5
119. V. Hombach, M. Kochs and A.J. Camm (eds.): *Interventional Techniques in Cardiovascular Medicine.* 1991 ISBN 0-7923-0956-1
120. R. Vos: *Drugs Looking for Diseases.* Innovative Drug Research and the Development of the Beta Blockers and the Calcium Antagonists. 1991 ISBN 0-7923-0968-5

Developments in Cardiovascular Medicine

121. S. Sideman, R. Beyar and A.G. Kleber (eds.): *Cardiac Electrophysiology, Circulation, and Transport.* Proceedings of the 7th Henry Goldberg Workshop (Berne, Switzerland, 1990). 1991 ISBN 0-7923-1145-0
122. D.M. Bers: *Excitation-Contraction Coupling and Cardiac Contractile Force.* 1991
 ISBN 0-7923-1186-8
123. A.-M. Salmasi and A.N. Nicolaides (eds.): *Occult Atherosclerotic Disease.* Diagnosis, Assessment and Management. 1991 ISBN 0-7923-1188-4
124. J.A.E. Spaan: *Coronary Blood Flow.* Mechanics, Distribution, and Control. 1991
 ISBN 0-7923-1210-4
125. R.W. Stout (ed.): *Diabetes and Atherosclerosis.* 1991 ISBN 0-7923-1310-0
126. A.G. Herman (ed.): *Antithrombotics.* Pathophysiological Rationale for Pharmacological Interventions. 1991 ISBN 0-7923-1413-1
127. N.H.J. Pijls: *Maximal Myocardial Perfusion as a Measure of the Functional Significance of Coronary Arteriogram.* From a Pathoanatomic to a Pathophysiologic Interpretation of the Coronary Arteriogram. 1991 ISBN 0-7923-1430-1
128. J.H.C. Reiber and E.E. v.d. Wall (eds.): *Cardiovascular Nuclear Medicine and MRI.* Quantitation and Clinical Applications. 1992 ISBN 0-7923-1467-0
129. E. Andries, P. Brugada and R. Stroobrandt (eds.): *How to Face 'the Faces' of Cardiac Pacing.* 1992 ISBN 0-7923-1528-6
130. M. Nagano, S. Mochizuki and N.S. Dhalla (eds.): *Cardiovascular Disease in Diabetes.* 1992 ISBN 0-7923-1554-5
131. P.W. Serruys, B.H. Strauss and S.B. King III (eds.): *Restenosis after Intervention with New Mechanical Devices.* 1992 ISBN 0-7923-1555-3
132. P.J. Walter (ed.): *Quality of Life after Open Heart Surgery.* 1992
 ISBN 0-7923-1580-4
133. E.E. van der Wall, H. Sochor, A. Righetti and M.G. Niemeyer (eds.): *What's new in Cardiac Imaging?* SPECT, PET and MRI. 1992 ISBN 0-7923-1615-0
134. P. Hanrath, R. Uebis and W. Krebs (eds.): *Cardiovascular Imaging by Ultrasound.* 1992 ISBN 0-7923-1755-6
135. F.H. Messerli (ed.): *Cardiovascular Disease in the Elderly.* 3rd ed. 1992
 ISBN 0-7923-1859-5
136. J. Hess and G.R. Sutherland (eds.): *Congenital Heart Disease in Adolescents and Adults.* 1992 ISBN 0-7923-1862-5
137. J.H.C. Reiber and P.W. Serruys (eds.): *Advances in Quantitative Coronary Arteriography.* 1993 ISBN 0-7923-1863-3
138. A.-M. Salmasi and A.S. Iskandrian (eds.): *Cardiac Output and Regional Flow in Health and Disease.* 1993 ISBN 0-7923-1911-7
139. J.H. Kingma, N.M. van Hemel and K.I. Lie (eds.): *Atrial Fibrillation, a Treatable Disease?* 1992 ISBN 0-7923-2008-5
140. B. Ostadel and N.S. Dhalla (eds.): *Heart Function in Health and Disease.* Proceedings of the Cardiovascular Program (Prague, Czechoslovakia, 1991). 1992
 ISBN 0-7923-2052-2
141. D. Noble and Y.E. Earm (eds.): *Ionic Channels and Effect of Taurine on the Heart.* Proceedings of an International Symposium (Seoul, Korea , 1992). 1993
 ISBN 0-7923-2199-5
142. H.M. Piper and C.J. Preusse (eds.): *Ischemia-reperfusion in Cardiac Surgery.* 1993
 ISBN 0-7923-2241-X
143. J. Roelandt, E.J. Gussenhoven and N. Bom (eds.): *Intravascular Ultrasound.* 1993
 ISBN 0-7923-2301-7
144. M.E. Safar and M.F. O'Rourke (eds.): *The Arterial System in Hypertension.* 1993
 ISBN 0-7923-2343-2
145. P.W. Serruys, D.P. Foley and P.J. de Feyter (eds.): *Quantitative Coronary Angiography in Clinical Practice.* With a Foreword by Spencer B. King III. 1994
 ISBN 0-7923-2368-8

Developments in Cardiovascular Medicine

146. J. Candell-Riera and D. Ortega-Alcalde (eds.): *Nuclear Cardiology in Everyday Practice.* 1994 ISBN 0-7923-2374-2
147. P. Cummins (ed.): *Growth Factors and the Cardiovascular System.* 1993
ISBN 0-7923-2401-3
148. K. Przyklenk, R.A. Kloner and D.M. Yellon (eds.): *Ischemic Preconditioning: The Concept of Endogenous Cardioprotection.* 1993 ISBN 0-7923-2410-2
149. T.H. Marwick: *Stress Echocardiography.* Its Role in the Diagnosis and Evaluation of Coronary Artery Disease. 1994 ISBN 0-7923-2579-6
150. W.H. van Gilst and K.I. Lie (eds.): *Neurohumoral Regulation of Coronary Flow.* Role of the Endothelium. 1993 ISBN 0-7923-2588-5
151. N. Sperelakis (ed.): *Physiology and Pathophysiology of the Heart.* 3rd rev. ed. 1994
ISBN 0-7923-2612-1
152. J.C. Kaski (ed.): *Angina Pectoris with Normal Coronary Arteries: Syndrome X.* 1994
ISBN 0-7923-2651-2
153. D.R. Gross: *Animal Models in Cardiovascular Research.* 2nd rev. ed. 1994
ISBN 0-7923-2712-8
154. A.S. Iskandrian and E.E. van der Wall (eds.): *Myocardial Viability.* Detection and Clinical Relevance. 1994 ISBN 0-7923-2813-2
155. J.H.C. Reiber and P.W. Serruys (eds.): *Progress in Quantitative Coronary Arteriography.* 1994 ISBN 0-7923-2814-0
156. U. Goldbourt, U. de Faire and K. Berg (eds.): *Genetic Factors in Coronary Heart Disease.* 1994 ISBN 0-7923-2752-7
157. G. Leonetti and C. Cuspidi (eds.): *Hypertension in the Elderly.* 1994
ISBN 0-7923-2852-3
158. D. Ardissino, S. Savonitto and L.H. Opie (eds.): *Drug Evaluation in Angina Pectoris.* 1994 ISBN 0-7923-2897-3
159. G. Bkaily (ed.): *Membrane Physiopathology.* 1994 ISBN 0-7923-3062-5
160. R.C. Becker (ed.): *The Modern Era of Coronary Thrombolysis.* 1994
ISBN 0-7923-3063-3
161. P.J. Walter (ed.): *Coronary Bypass Surgery in the Elderly.* Ethical, Economical and Quality of Life Aspects. With a foreword by N.K. Wenger. 1995 ISBN 0-7923-3188-5
162. J.W. de Jong and R. Ferrari (eds.), *The Carnitine System.* A New Therapeutical Approach to Cardiovascular Diseases. 1995 ISBN 0-7923-3318-7
163. C.A. Neill and E.B. Clark: *The Developing Heart: A 'History' of Pediatric Cardiology.* 1995 ISBN 0-7923-3375-6
164. N. Sperelakis: *Electrogenesis of Biopotentials in the Cardiovascular System.* 1995
ISBN 0-7923-3398-5
165. M. Schwaiger (ed.): *Cardiac Positron Emission Tomography.* 1995
ISBN 0-7923-3417-5
166. E.E. van der Wall, P.K. Blanksma, M.G. Niemeyer and A.M.J. Paans (eds.): *Cardiac Positron Emission Tomography.* Viability, Perfusion, Receptors and Cardiomyopathy. 1995 ISBN 0-7923-3472-8
167. P.K. Singal, I.M.C. Dixon, R.E. Beamish and N.S. Dhalla (eds.): *Mechanism of Heart Failure.* 1995 ISBN 0-7923-3490-6
168. N.S. Dhalla, P.K. Singal, N. Takeda and R.E. Beamish (eds.): *Pathophysiology of Heart Failure.* 1995 ISBN 0-7923-3571-6
169. N.S. Dhalla, G.N. Pierce, V. Panagia and R.E. Beamish (eds.): *Heart Hypertrophy and Failure.* 1995 ISBN 0-7923-3572-4
170. S.N. Willich and J.E. Muller (eds.): *Triggering of Acute Coronary Syndromes.* Implications for Prevention. 1995 ISBN 0-7923-3605-4
171. E.E. van der Wall, T.H. Marwick and J.H.C. Reiber (eds.): *Advances in Imaging Techniques in Ischemic Heart Disease.* 1995 ISBN 0-7923-3620-8
172. B. Swynghedauw: *Molecular Cardiology for the Cardiologist.* 1995
ISBN 0-7923-3622-4

Developments in Cardiovascular Medicine

173. C.A. Nienaber and U. Sechtem (eds.): *Imaging and Intervention in Cardiology.* 1996
     ISBN 0-7923-3649-6
174. G. Assmann (ed.): *HDL Deficiency and Atherosclerosis.* 1995   ISBN 0-7923-8888-7
175. N.M. van Hemel, F.H.M. Wittkampf and H. Ector (eds.): *The Pacemaker Clinic of the 90's. Essentials in Brady-Pacing.* 1995   ISBN 0-7923-3688-7
176. N. Wilke (ed.): *Advanced Cardiovascular MRI of the Heart and Great Vessels.* 1996
     ISBN 0-7923-3720-4
177. M. LeWinter, H. Suga and M.W. Watkins (eds.): *Cardiac Energetics: From Emax to Pressure-volume Area.* 1995   ISBN 0-7923-3721-2
178. R.J. Siegel (ed.): *Ultrasound Angioplasty.* 1995   ISBN 0-7923-3722-0
179. D.M. Yellon and G.J. Gross (eds.): *Myocardial Protection and the K_{ATP} Channel.* 1995   ISBN 0-7923-3791-3
180. A.V.G. Bruschke, J.H.C. Reiber, K.I. Lie and H.J.J. Wellens (eds.): *Lipid Lowering Therapy and Progression of Coronary Atherosclerosis.* 1996   ISBN 0-7923-3807-3
181. A.-S.A. Abd-Eyattah and A.S. Wechsler (eds.): *Purines and Myocardial Protection.* 1995   ISBN 0-7923-3831-6
182. M. Morad, S. Ebashi, W. Trautwein and Y. Kurachi (eds.): *Molecular Physiology and Pharmacology of Cardiac Ion Channels and Transporters.* 1996 ISBN 0-7923-3913-4
183. A.M. Oto (ed.): *Practice and Progress in Cardiac Pacing and Electrophysiology.* 1996   ISBN 0-7923-3950-9
184. W.H. Birkenhäger (ed.): *Practical Management of Hypertension.* Second Edition. 1996   ISBN 0-7923-3952-5
185. J.C. Chatham, J.R. Forder and J.H. McNeill (eds.): *The Heart in Diabetes.* 1996
     ISBN 0-7923-4052-3
186. J.H.C. Reiber and E.E. van der Wall (eds.): *Cardiovascular Imaging.* 1996
     ISBN 0-7923-4109-0
187. A-M. Salmasi and A. Strano (eds.): *Angiology in Practice.* 1996 ISBN 0-7923-4143-0

Previous volumes are still available

KLUWER ACADEMIC PUBLISHERS – DORDRECHT / BOSTON / LONDON